BIOPSY INTERPRETATION SERIES

BIOPSY INTERPRETATION OF THE CENTRAL NERVOUS SYSTEM

Second Edition

Matthew J. Schniederjan, MD
Neuropathologist
Children's Healthcare of Atlanta
Assistant Professor
Department of Pathology and Laboratory Medicine
Emory University School of Medicine
Atlanta, Georgia

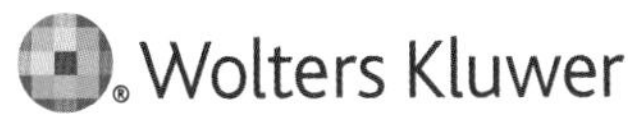
Wolters Kluwer

Philadelphia • Baltimore • New York • London
Buenos Aires • Hong Kong • Sydney • Tokyo

Acquisitions Editor: Ryan Shaw
Editorial Coordinator: Alexis Pozonsky
Marketing Manager: Dan Dressler
Design Coordinator: Stephen Druding
Production Product Manager: Bridgett Dougherty
Manufacturing Coordinator: Beth Welsh
Prepress Vendor: Aptara, Inc.

2nd edition

9 8 7 6 5 4 3 2 1

Printed in China

Library of Congress Cataloging-in-Publication Data

Names: Schniederjan, Matthew J., author.
Title: Biopsy interpretation of the central nervous system / Matthew J. Schniederjan.
Other titles: Biopsy interpretation series.
Description: Second edition. | Philadelphia : Wolters Kluwer, [2018] |
Series: Biopsy interpretation series | Includes bibliographical references and index.
Identifiers: LCCN 2017039563 | ISBN 9781496382634
Subjects: | MESH: Central Nervous System Diseases—diagnosis | Central
Nervous System Diseases—pathology | Central Nervous System—pathology | Biopsy—methods
Classification: LCC RC386.6.B55 | NLM WL 141 | DDC 616.8/04758—dc23
LC record available at https://lccn.loc.gov/2017039563

LWW.com

RRS1709

DEDICATION

To my wife, Stephanie, whose patience and kind support made this work possible.

PREFACE TO THE FIRST EDITION

This new book carries on a strong tradition of diagnostically oriented texts established by the Biopsy Interpretation Series, in the present case focused on lesions of the central nervous system. Our purpose is to provide a practical guide and concise reference that can be a companion text for general surgical pathologists, trainees in pathology and neuropathology, and clinicians who treat patients with neurologic diseases that require surgical sampling. Given the heavy orientation of the Biopsy Interpretation Series to the busy and serious-minded diagnostician, we have taken this opportunity to create something new and, we think, useful. While there are certainly several excellent books on neuropathology and surgical neuropathology, the majority are reference texts that are comprehensive and encyclopedic, making them less than optimal on a daily basis to assist with interpretation. Because the central concern here is with establishing the correct diagnosis, the content is aimed at anticipating difficult diagnostic decisions and providing a direct and reliable guide to their resolution.

The text contains relatively little discussion of historical background, disease mechanisms, or basic research findings unless they are clinically relevant. Rather, the emphasis is on highlighting the distinguishing histologic features and helpful ancillary testing necessary to make a confident and competent diagnosis, as well as to place each lesion in the setting of its clinical significance. For the discussion of neoplastic diseases, we have relied on the most current *World Health Organization Classification of the Central Nervous System*, 4th edition, as our guide for classification and grading.

Current practice of surgical neuropathology, perhaps more than most pathologic subspecialties, requires knowledge of the clinical and neuroimaging features of a lesion to generate a differential diagnosis. The differential diagnosis of a sellar/suprasellar lesion in a teenaged girl is completely distinct from that of a frontal lobe lesion in a middle-aged man. While slapping the H&E-stained slide on the stage in the absence of clinical and imaging context may occasionally suffice for a correct diagnosis (craniopharyngioma comes to mind), in the long run this practice will almost certainly generate anxiety, uncertainty, and less than adequate diagnoses. To emphasize this necessity in practice, we have started the discussion of each individual entity with a section on Clinical Context, setting the stage for discussion of histopathologic features, ancillary studies, and differential diagnosis, maximizing the efficiency and utility of the book as both a reference and a tool for education.

Matthew J. Schniederjan, MD
Daniel J. Brat, MD, PhD

PREFACE TO THE SECOND EDITION

In the years since the publication of the first edition of this book, as a result of large-scale efforts to understand the genetics of brain tumors, surgical neuropathology has shifted further toward a multifaceted approach to tumor categorization, similar to the field of hematopathology. This is evident in the updated 4th edition of the *World Health Organization Classification of Tumours of the Central Nervous System*, in which genetic features are now defining elements for several major categories of CNS tumors. This edition reflects those changes and, in an attempt to increase its longevity in the face of a rapidly advancing literature, seeks to anticipate some of the changes in classification that may be ahead.

New to this edition is a brief chapter on intraoperative consultation as pertains to CNS specimens, a topic not usually covered in neuropathology texts, yet of significant interest to many pathologists. I hope that this new section will provide a succinct and basic foundation for pathologists who find themselves performing neuropathology intraoperative consultations with limited prior experience.

Also different in this edition is the departure of my outstanding mentor, colleague, and coauthor from the previous edition, Dan Brat, to whom I owe an enormous debt of gratitude for his wise guidance and excellent training. I am honored to be given the opportunity to produce this edition as a solo effort.

The purpose of this book continues to be, as with the other volumes in the Biopsy Interpretation Series, to serve as a compact, practically oriented resource for the surgical pathologist and pathology trainee. To that end, this edition retains a strong focus on diagnosis that places histopathology in the context of important clinical, neuroimaging, and genetic findings, relatively free of discussion of mechanisms and other aspects that are less directly related to diagnostic practice. I hope that you find it useful.

Matthew J. Schniederjan, MD

CONTENTS

BIOPSY INTERPRETATION SERIES

BIOPSY INTERPRETATION OF THE CENTRAL NERVOUS SYSTEM

1

BENIGN CYSTS AND SELECTED DEVELOPMENTAL ANOMALIES

BENIGN ENDODERMAL CYSTS (RATHKE CLEFT, COLLOID, ENTEROGENOUS, NEURENTERIC, AND NEUROEPITHELIAL CYSTS)

General

Endodermal cysts are benign developmental lesions that contain epithelia resembling those derived from the endodermal germ layer, specifically respiratory and gastrointestinal. They occur outside of the central nervous system (CNS) paraspinally as bronchogenic and enteric cysts, respectively. In the CNS, those with respiratory epithelium may go by different names depending on the site; in the sellar and suprasellar spaces, they are Rathke cleft cysts; those in the third ventricle are colloid cysts. Those with gastrointestinal epithelium are often referred to as enterogenous or neurenteric cysts. In any location, any of the above may be more generically termed endodermal or neurenteric cysts.

Clinical Context

Endodermal cysts are common surgical neuropathology specimens, most often presenting as Rathke cleft or colloid cysts. They rarely present congenitally, although most are resected in early and middle adulthood. The signs and symptoms with which endodermal cysts present depend on location: Rathke cleft cyst with hypopituitarism and/or visual problems; colloid cyst with headache and hydrocephalus (and occasionally sudden death (1)); and spinal cord lesions with weakness. Rathke cleft cysts have also been described to present with "Rathke cleft cyst apoplexy," in which sudden hemorrhage into the cyst cavity produces acute enlargement and rapid onset of severe headache, visual disturbance, and pituitary insufficiency (2). Colloid cysts have been noted in familial clusters, typically in females, but it is not clear whether this represents a specific genetic defect or coincidence (3,4).

Neuroimaging of endodermal cysts shows a sharply circumscribed round to ovoid mass that is usually intradural and extra-axial, or, for colloid cysts, intraventricular. Less commonly, some examples are intraparenchymal (5). Again, endodermal cysts occur throughout the length of the neuraxis, yet are most common around the base of the brain and in the posterior fossa. Although variable, the cyst contents are most often hyperintense on T1-weighted magnetic resonance sequences and hyperintense on T2-FLAIR, sometimes with a partial rim of contrast enhancement, reflecting reactive changes in surrounding tissue (6). Computed tomography (CT) images infrequently show calcification of the cyst wall.

Grossly, the cyst lining is an inconspicuous membrane that holds variable contents from thin, clear, or cloudy liquid to inspissated, translucent, thyroid-like colloid.

Simple surgical excision is the preferred treatment for endodermal cysts, resulting in generally favorable outcomes. The overwhelming majority of endodermal cysts are benign, yet several cases with malignant progression and/or dissemination have been described (7–9).

Histopathology

The linings of endodermal cysts reflect the variety of endodermally derived surface epithelia seen in the digestive and respiratory tracts, in most cases (Figure 1-1). Cells range from cuboidal to tall columnar and may be pseudostratified. Cilia often project from the apical surface. Mucin-bearing goblet cells may be interspersed between columnar cells and less commonly can form the vast majority, creating a gastric foveolar-type surface. Squamous metaplasia is uncommon but can be extensive and overwhelm the other elements (Figure 1-2). By metaplastic production and accumulation of keratinaceous debris, what originated as an endodermal cyst can metamorphose into a lesion similar to an epidermoid cyst over time.

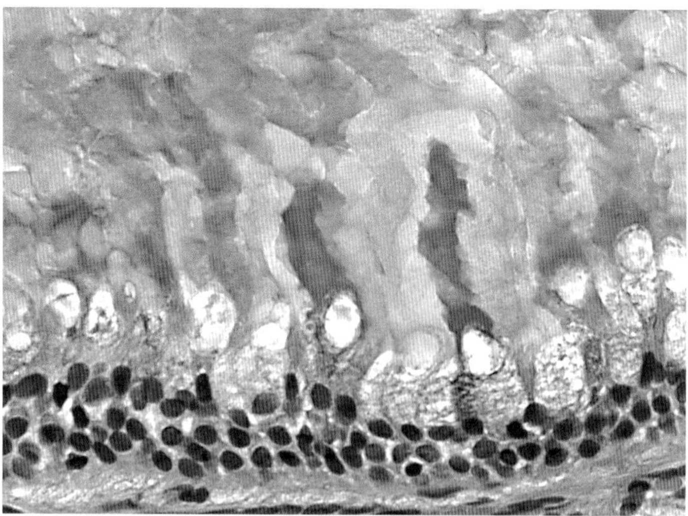

FIGURE 1-1 The epithelial lining of endodermal cysts is frequently composed of ciliated columnar cells and interspersed goblet cells.

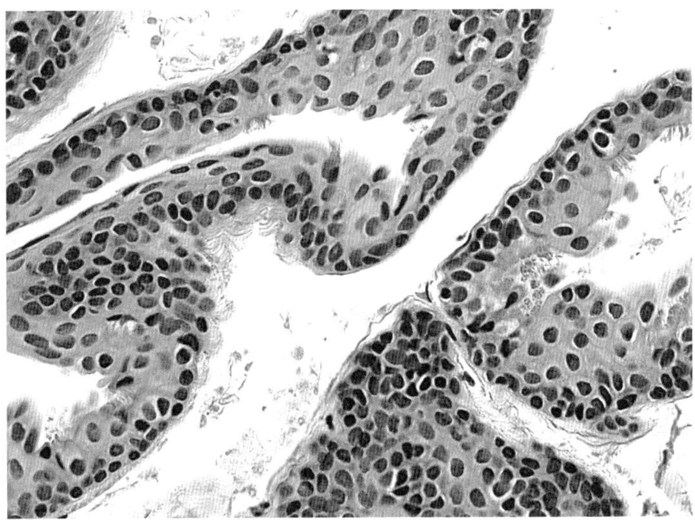

FIGURE 1-2 Only scattered ciliated columnar cells remain among metaplastic squamous cells in this endodermal cyst. Note the absence of a granular layer and the presence of intracystic keratin flakes.

Rathke cleft cysts occasionally contain such squamous metaplasia, and this feature can be misleading in the sellar–suprasellar area because craniopharyngiomas may also sometimes incorporate ciliated respiratory epithelium. Metaplasia in Rathke cleft cysts should therefore be interpreted with caution and invoked only when clear maturation to dry keratin flakes is observed. This topic is discussed further in Chapter 8 with craniopharyngiomas.

Another source of confusion regarding Rathke cleft cysts is that long-term degeneration of hemorrhage into the cavity can produce contents similar to those of adamantinomatous craniopharyngiomas: “machine oil” fluid containing xanthogranulomatous debris and cholesterol crystals. In such cases, this material may mislead the radiologist, neurosurgeon and, potentially, the pathologist. Such cyst contents are more common in craniopharyngiomas, but cannot necessarily be taken as evidence for that diagnosis.

Nondescript, loose fibrous tissue typically underlies the epithelium of endodermal cysts; smooth muscle, or possibly other mucosa-associated tissues, may be present (10).

EPIDERMOID AND DERMOID CYSTS

Clinical Context

These common CNS lesions occur in patients of all ages with no clear predominance in either sex. The anatomic distribution for epidermoid cysts is diffuse, with examples from every location along the neuraxis. They are most frequent in the posterior fossa, especially near the cerebellopontine angles (11). Patients often present with headache and/or cranial nerve dysfunction (12). In contrast, dermoid cysts tend to occur as midline lesions in younger patients. These cysts may have a sinus tract to the skin surface that allows for cyst infection (13). Either may occur as cystic, intraosseous skull lesions.

Magnetic resonance imaging (MRI) of most epidermoids and dermoids shows a T1-hypointense, T2-hyperintense mass that does not enhance with contrast material (11,12). Like abscesses, the contents of epidermoid cysts impede the free motion of water molecules, causing "restricted diffusion" on diffusion-weighted MR sequences and providing an important diagnostic cue for radiologists (14). The cyst contents are hypodense on CT scan.

Because the surrounding tissues may be densely adherent to the cyst wall, total resection may be difficult. Nevertheless, even with subtotal resection, the outcome after surgery is generally favorable, with little difference in recurrence rates from totally resected cases in one review of the literature (12). Rarely, epidermoid or dermoid cysts undergo malignant transformation (15–17). Rupture of cyst contents into the cerebrospinal fluid (CSF) precipitates chemical meningitis.

Histopathology

The epidermoid/dermoid cyst lining, by definition, consists of keratinizing squamous epithelium, with dermal adnexa in the case of dermoid. The squamous cells mature normally toward the center and accumulate as sheets of anucleate keratin, which constitute the majority of the tumor mass. In contrast to craniopharyngioma and metaplastic endodermal cysts, the other squamous primary lesions of the CNS, epidermoid, and dermoid cysts have a granular layer (Figure 1-3).

Differential Diagnosis

Papillary craniopharyngiomas are also squamous lesions, but they are readily distinguished from dermoid/epidermoid cysts because they lack the keratohyalin granular layer and accumulation of mature flakes of "dry" keratin seen in the latter. The calcified and inflamed cellular debris of adamantinomatous craniopharyngiomas is also not a feature of epidermoid cysts.

Mature teratomas histologically and clinically overlap with dermoid cysts, but contain additional tissues derived from other germ layers, whereas dermoid cysts only contain ectodermally derived tissue.

A keratin-filled cyst can arise from metaplasia in an endodermal lesion but cannot be diagnosed as such, unless corresponding epithelium is identified. Lack of a granular layer in a keratinaceous cyst epithelium suggests a metaplastic process.

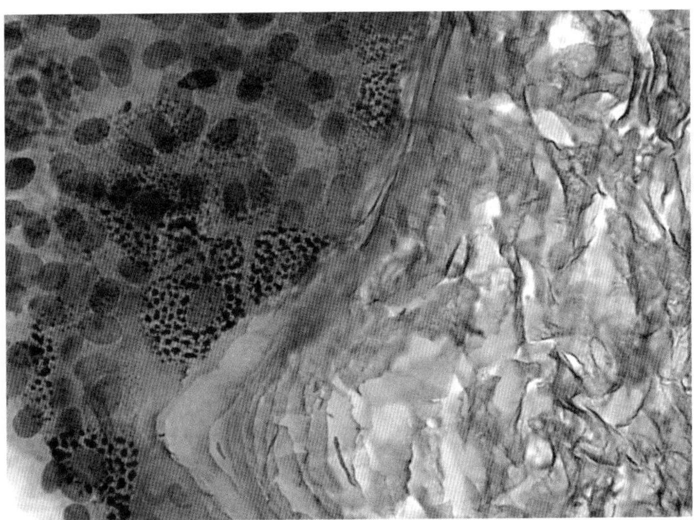

FIGURE 1-3 This oblique section through the lining of an epidermoid cyst accentuates the maturation sequence though the granular layer into "dry" keratin flakes.

NEUROGLIAL HETEROTOPIAS

Developmental anomalies occasionally sequester brain tissue in extra-CNS locales, sometimes as glial heterotopias in midline nasopharyngeal areas, referred to variably as glial heterotopia, glial choristoma, glial hamartoma, or, inappropriately, "nasal glioma." Other similar lesions include parasellar (18) and intradural spinal cerebellar tissue (19). Microscopic examination reveals a mixture of fibrillar glial cells and collagen, perhaps with mature neurons. The lesion may become fibrotic or sclerotic, obscuring the glia, but glial fibrillary acidic protein (GFAP), S100, and CD56 antibodies all highlight the heterotopic cells.

ARACHNOID CYST

Clinical Context

Arachnoid cysts are usually encountered in pediatric patients who present with headache, nausea, vomiting, and/or other signs of increased intracranial pressure. Radiologically, they are thin-walled, unilocular cysts containing CSF. They can occur anywhere throughout the neuraxis, but they are most commonly situated superficially in the temporal fossa (20,21). Chronic subdural hematomas can form adjacent to arachnoid cysts after even minor trauma (22). The term arachnoid cyst is also sometimes dubiously applied to superficial cyst-like lesions that remain after resorption of subdural hematomas.

Arachnoid cysts can be associated with autosomal dominant polycystic kidney disease, in which case they are typically asymptomatic and do not require treatment (23). Germline abnormalities at 16q and 11p15 have also been described in cases of familial arachnoid cysts (24,25).

Endoscopic or open fenestration or cystoperitoneal shunting are the main treatments for arachnoid cysts, with generally favorable long-term outcome (26).

Histopathology

The cyst wall is a thin, collagenous leptomeningeal membrane with scattered meningothelial cells. Because these lesions may be simply fenestrated and not resected, tissue may not always be submitted for pathologic review.

CHOROID PLEXUS CYST

Clinical Context

These developmental anomalies are frequently detected in utero within the lateral ventricles by ultrasonography. Among these fetuses, the probability of trisomy 18 (Edward syndrome) is greater than for the general population, leading many to be karyotyped (27–29). Those choroid plexus cysts occurring outside of Edward syndrome have no discernible effect (30). Only a handful of cases have been reported to cause symptoms, some of which are in adults (31–34).

Histopathology

The cyst contains thin, CSF-like fluid and is lined by a scalloped profile of choroid plexus cells that may be normal or flattened by chronic pressure.

MENINGEAL CYST

These CSF-filled cavities form along the spine due to defects in the dural sac that convey CSF between the extradural cyst and the subarachnoid space. Symptomatic cases, which generally present with back or leg pain, may represent cysts that have lost their communication and pressurize from buildup of fluid (35). Histologic examination shows a thick, fibrous capsule that may not have any arachnoid lining (36).

LIPOMA

Clinical Context

In the CNS, lipomas are nonneoplastic, developmental defects and are most associated with occult spinal dysraphism in spinal cord cases and agenesis or hypoplasia of the corpus callosum in intracranial cases (37,38). Spinal cord lipomas are typically located in the conus medullaris and filum terminale and are more often associated with symptoms, usually due to tethering of the cord. Such symptoms may include back

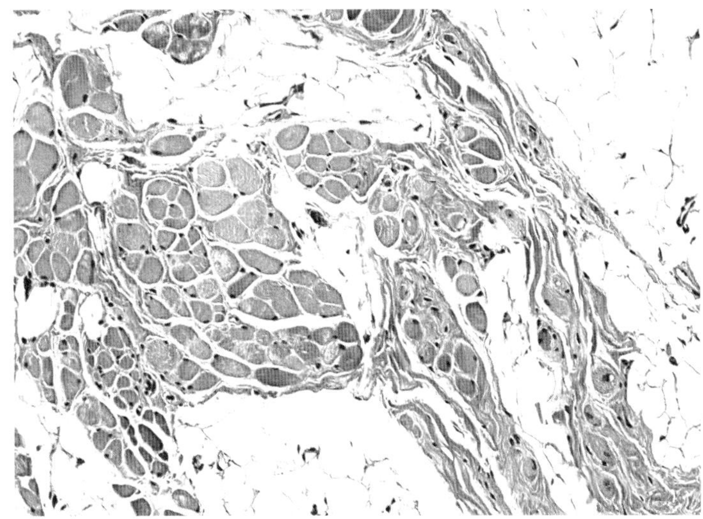

FIGURE 1-4 Other mesenchymal elements may be present in filum lipomas, such as skeletal muscle, seen here.

pain, leg weakness, or bowel and bladder dysfunction. Spinal cord lipomas are only removed when symptomatic.

Most intracranial lipomas are found in the midline at the anterior corpus callosum, in the quadrigeminal cistern, and in the sellar region. These lesions are usually asymptomatic and stable, so are generally not removed unless symptoms develop.

Radiologically, lipomas appear as discreet masses that are markedly hyperintense in T1-weighted MR images due to their high lipid content.

Surgeons resect spinal lipomas with generally favorable results, yet a subset have patterns of macroscopic growth that are difficult to resect entirely, sometimes leading to a recurrence or progression of symptoms (39).

Histopathology

Sections in spinal cord lipomas show mature adipose tissue, usually with adjacent dense fibrous tissue, peripheral nerve, and prominent blood vessels when arising in the filum. Neuroglial and ependymal tissue may also be present in filum lipomas. Other mesenchymal tissues, such as skeletal muscle, are occasionally seen (Figure 1-4).

ECCHORDOSIS PHYSALIPHORA

Clinical

Remnants of the embryonic notochord may lie stranded along the midline intradurally and are known as ecchordosis physaliphora. These lesions are usually pea-sized and located anterior to the ventral pons along the basilar artery. Occasional osseous ecchordoses may be difficult to distinguish

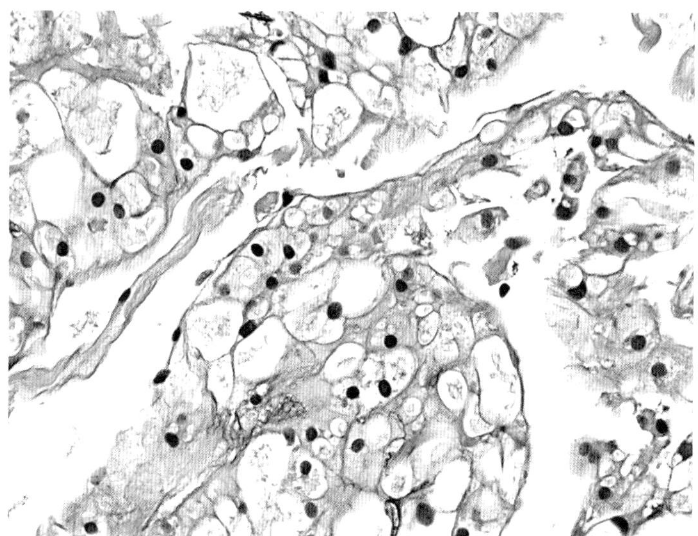

FIGURE 1-5 The large, irregularly vacuolated cells and small hyperchromatic nuclei of ecchordosis physaliphora closely match the physaliphorous component of chordoma.

from chordomas (40). The vast majority are asymptomatic, but a few cases have hemorrhaged (41,42) or caused CSF leakage (43,44).

On MRI, ecchordoses are T1 hypointense, T2 hyperintense, and lack contrast enhancement (45).

Histopathology

Ecchordoses are characterized by "physaliphorous" (*Greek: bubble-bearing*) cells with numerous large, clear, cytoplasmic vacuoles in a scant background of basophilic ground substance (Figure 1-5). Scattered epithelioid cells with pink cytoplasm can be seen, but are not generally in the chains and clusters of chordoma. The nuclei are monotonous and small, with no mitosis and no visible nucleoli.

The immunohistochemical profile of ecchordosis physaliphora is essentially identical to that of chordoma (46,47), except that markers of proliferation should show minimal, if any, staining. The differential diagnosis of chordoma and ecchordosis is discussed in the section on chordoma in Chapter 17.

Pineal cysts are discussed in Chapter 12 with pineal region tumors and hypothalamic hamartomas are included among sellar/suprasellar lesions in Chapter 8.

REFERENCES

1. Demirci S, Dogan KH, Erkol Z, et al. Sudden death due to a colloid cyst of the third ventricle: report of three cases with a special sign at autopsy. *Forensic Sci Int.* 2009;189(1–3):e33–e36.
2. Chaiban JT, Abdelmannan D, Cohen M, et al. Rathke cleft cyst apoplexy: a newly characterized distinct clinical entity. *J Neurosurg.* 2011;114(2):318–324.

3. Nader-Sepahi A, Hamlyn PJ. Familial colloid cysts of the third ventricle: case report. *Neurosurgery.* 2000;46(3):751–753.
4. Socin HV, Born J, Wallemacq C, et al. Familial colloid cyst of the third ventricle: neuroendocrinological follow-up and review of the literature. *Clin Neurol Neurosurg.* 2002;104(4):367–370.
5. Kachur E, Ang LC, Megyesi JF. Intraparenchymal supratentorial neurenteric cyst. *Can J Neurol Sci.* 2004;31(3):412–416.
6. Preece MT, Osborn AG, Chin SS, et al. Intracranial neurenteric cysts: imaging and pathology spectrum. *Am J Neuroradiol.* 2006;27(6):1211–1216.
7. Dunham CP, Curry B, Hamilton M. Malignant transformation of an intraaxial-supratentorial neurenteric cyst—case report and review of the literature. *Clin Neuropathol.* 2009;28(6):460–466.
8. Perry A, Scheithauer BW, Zaias BW, et al. Aggressive enterogenous cyst with extensive craniospinal spread: case report. *Neurosurgery.* 1999;44(2):401–404; discussion 404–405.
9. Sahara Y, Nagasaka T, Takayasu M, et al. Recurrence of a neurenteric cyst with malignant transformation in the foramen magnum after total resection. Case report. *J Neurosurg.* 2001;95(2):341–345.
10. Sampath S, Yasha TC, Shetty S, et al. Parasellar neurenteric cyst: unusual site and histology: case report. *Neurosurgery.* 1999;44(6):1335–1337; discussion 1337–1338.
11. Talacchi A, Sala F, Alessandrini F, et al. Assessment and surgical management of posterior fossa epidermoid tumors: report of 28 cases. *Neurosurgery.* 1998;42(2):242–251; discussion 251–242.
12. Schiefer TK, Link MJ. Epidermoids of the cerebellopontine angle: a 20-year experience. *Surg Neurol.* 2008;70(6):584–590; discussion 590.
13. Caldarelli M, Massimi L, Kondageski C, et al. Intracranial midline dermoid and epidermoid cysts in children. *J Neurosurg.* 2004;100(5 Suppl Pediatrics):473–480.
14. Hu XY, Hu CH, Fang XM, et al. Intraparenchymal epidermoid cysts in the brain: diagnostic value of MR diffusion-weighted imaging. *Clin Radiol.* 2008;63(7):813–818.
15. Ge P, Luo Y, Fu S, et al. Recurrent epidermoid cyst with malignant transformation into squamous cell carcinoma. *Neurol Med Chir (Tokyo).* 2009;49(9):442–444.
16. Lewis AJ, Cooper PW, Kassel EE, et al. Squamous cell carcinoma arising in a suprasellar epidermoid cyst. Case report. *J Neurosurg.* 1983;59(3):538–541.
17. Sawan B, Vital A, Loiseau H, et al. Squamous cell carcinoma developing in an intracranial prepontine epidermoid cyst. *Ann Pathol.* 2000;20(3):258–260.
18. Chang AH, Kaufmann WE, Brat DJ. Ectopic cerebellum presenting as a suprasellar mass in infancy: implications for cerebellar development. *Pediatr Dev Pathol.* 2001;4(1):89–93.
19. Chung CJ, Castillo M, Fordham L, et al. Spinal intradural cerebellar ectopia. *Am J Neuroradiol.* 1998;19(5):897–899.
20. Helland CA, Lund-Johansen M, Wester K. Location, sidedness, and sex distribution of intracranial arachnoid cysts in a population-based sample. *J Neurosurg.* 2010;113(5):934–939.
21. Wester K. Peculiarities of intracranial arachnoid cysts: location, sidedness, and sex distribution in 126 consecutive patients. *Neurosurgery.* 1999;45(4):775–779.
22. Domenicucci M, Russo N, Giugni E, et al. Relationship between supratentorial arachnoid cyst and chronic subdural hematoma: neuroradiological evidence and surgical treatment. *J Neurosurg.* 2009;110(6):1250–1255.
23. Schievink WI, Huston J, 3rd, Torres VE, et al. Intracranial cysts in autosomal dominant polycystic kidney disease. *J Neurosurg.* 1995;83(6):1004–1007.
24. Arriola G, de Castro P, Verdú A. Familial arachnoid cysts. *Pediatr Neurol.* 2005;33(2):146–148.
25. Bilguvar K, Ozturk AK, Bayrakli F, et al. The syndrome of pachygyria, mental retardation, and arachnoid cysts maps to 11p15. *Am J Med Genet.* 2009;149A(11):2569–2572.

26. Shim KW, Lee YH, Park EK, et al. Treatment option for arachnoid cysts. *Child's Nerv Syst.* 2009;25(11):1459–1466.
27. Gabrielli S, Reece EA, Pilu G, et al. The clinical significance of prenatally diagnosed choroid plexus cysts. *Am J Obstet Gynecol.* 1989;160(5 Pt 1):1207–1210.
28. Nava S, Godmilow L, Reeser S, et al. Significance of sonographically detected second-trimester choroid plexus cysts: a series of 211 cases and a review of the literature. *Ultrasound Obstet Gynecol.* 1994;4(6):448–451.
29. Platt LD, Carlson DE, Medearis AL, et al. Fetal choroid plexus cysts in the second trimester of pregnancy: a cause for concern. *Am J Obstet Gynecol.* 1991;164(6 Pt 1):1652–1655; discussion 1655–1656.
30. DiPietro JA, Costigan KA, Cristofalo EA, et al. Choroid plexus cysts do not affect fetal neurodevelopment.*J Perinatol.* 2006;26(10):622–627.
31. Dempsey RJ, Chandler WF. Choroid plexus cyst in the lateral ventricle causing obstructive symptoms in an adult. *Surg Neurol.* 1981;15(2):116–119.
32. Hatashita S, Takagi S, Sakakibara T. Choroid plexus cyst of the lateral ventricle in an elderly man. Case report. *J Neurosurg.* 1984;60(2):435–437.
33. Kariyattil R, Panikar D. Choroid plexus cyst of the third ventricle presenting as acute triventriculomegaly. *Childs Nerv Syst.* 2008;24(7):875–877.
34. Jeon JH, Lee SW, Ko JK, et al. Neuroendoscopic removal of large choroid plexus cyst: a case report. *J Korean Med Sci.* 2005;20(2):335–339.
35. Davis SW, Levy LM, LeBihan DJ, et al. Sacral meningeal cysts: evaluation with MR imaging. *Radiology.* 1993;187(2):445–448.
36. Sato K, Nagata K, Sugita Y. Spinal extradural meningeal cyst: correct radiological and histopathological diagnosis. *Neurosurg Focus.* 2002;13(4):ecp1.
37. Yilmaz N, Unal O, Kiymaz N, et al. Intracranial lipomas–a clinical study. *Clin Neurol Neurosurg.* 2006;108(4):363–368.
38. Niwa T, de Vries LS, Manten GT, et al. Interhemispheric lipoma, callosal anomaly, and malformations of cortical development: a case series. *Neuropediatrics.* 2016;47(2):115–118.
39. Pang D, Zovickian J, Oviedo A. Long-term outcome of total and near-total resection of spinal cord lipomas and radical reconstruction of the neural placode, part II: outcome analysis and preoperative profiling. *Neurosurgery.* 2010;66(2):253–272; discussion 272–253.
40. Rengachary SS, Grotte DA, Swanson PE. Extradural ecchordosis physaliphora of the thoracic spine: case report. *Neurosurgery.* 1997;41(5):1198–1201; discussion 1201–1192.
41. Alkan O, Yildirim T, Kizilkiliç O, et al. A case of ecchordosis physaliphora presenting with an intratumoral hemorrhage. *Turkish Neurosurg.* 2009;19(3):293–296.
42. Fracasso T, Brinkmann B, Paulus W. Sudden death due to subarachnoid bleeding from ecchordosis physaliphora. *Int J Legal Med.* 2008;122(3):225–227.
43. Alli A, Clark M, Mansell NJ. Cerebrospinal fluid rhinorrhea secondary to ecchordosis physaliphora. *Skull Base.* 2008;18(6):395–399.
44. Macdonald RL, Cusimano MD, Deck JH, et al. Cerebrospinal fluid fistula secondary to ecchordosis physaliphora. *Neurosurgery.* 1990;26(3):515–518; discussion 518–519.
45. Mehnert F, Beschorner R, Kuker W, et al. Retroclival ecchordosis physaliphora: MR imaging and review of the literature. *Am J Neuroradiol.* 2004;25(10):1851–1855.
46. Macdonald RL, Deck JH. Immunohistochemistry of ecchordosis physaliphora and chordoma. *Can J Neurol Sci.* 1990;17(4):420–423.
47. Lagman C, Varshneya K, Sarmiento JM, et al. Proposed diagnostic criteria, classification schema, and review of literature of notochord-derived ecchordosis physaliphora. *Cureus.* 2016;8(3):e547.

2

INFLAMMATORY AND INFECTIOUS LESIONS

DEMYELINATING LESIONS

Clinical Context

The etiologies and patient characteristics associated with demyelinating lesions vary considerably. Most frequently encountered is the enigmatic autoimmune process of *multiple sclerosis,* in which multiple lesions occur over a discontinuous time course. Because solitary, monophasic lesions with identical histology also occur and have different clinical implications, multiple sclerosis as a diagnosis should generally be avoided by the pathologist in favor of a more generic and appropriate diagnosis of "demyelinating lesion." Other autoimmune central nervous system (CNS) demyelination syndromes include acute disseminated encephalomyelitis (ADEM), acute hemorrhagic leukoencephalopathy (AHL), and neuromyelitis optica.

Most plaques of demyelination are recognized as such by the clinical team either by the history of the illness or by the characteristic radiographic features of demyelination. All ages are affected, and those in the third and fourth decades are the most common, with a female predominance.

On neuroimaging, demyelinating lesions are typically hyperintense on T2/FLAIR MR images and show areas of contrast enhancement, likely due to increased vascular permeability. Mass effect is generally absent but can be seen in cases of "tumefactive" demyelination. By definition, demyelinating lesions are limited to the white matter and should not overtly extend into gray matter structures. Solitary and progressive demyelinating lesions are sometimes biopsied with the expectation of a diagnosis of glioblastoma because a pattern of contrast enhancement forms peripherally around the lesion. However, unlike the unbroken ring enhancement in glioblastoma, demyelinating lesions usually have an "open ring" or telltale gap on one side, typically the more superficial side (1). This finding, although relatively specific to demyelination, is not a sensitive indicator and is occasionally present in other types of lesions (2). When multiple similar lesions are present on neuroimaging, the preoperative suspicion is usually metastatic disease.

Some patients with biopsy-proven demyelinating disease go on to develop high-grade lymphomas at the site of their plaque. Whether these two processes are pathogenetically linked, or are merely unfortunate coincidences, remains to be demonstrated. At least some cases represent lymphomas treated with steroids that altered the histology to appear as a demyelinating lesion (3). The initial insult is often referred to as a *sentinel lesion* and may be chronologically distant from the subsequent lymphoma (4).

Treatment of multiple sclerosis and other demyelinating diseases is based on immunosuppressive agents, with highly variable outcomes. Severity of disease ranges from a single monophasic demyelinating lesion that recedes without recurrence to debilitating widespread disease that culminates in death.

ADEM is a demyelinating illness that typically occurs in children and young adults, in most cases closely following a viral infection or immunization. A single monophasic course is typical, although relapsing–remitting cases may occur and are termed multiphasic diffuse encephalomyelitis. As the name indicates, ADEM is diffuse in the brain and spinal cord white matter. MRI of ADEM typically reveals diffusion restriction in the acute phase, with resolution over time, as well as decreasing *N*-acetyl aspartate/choline ratios on spectroscopy (5). Most cases are diagnosed based on clinical and imaging findings alone and are not biopsied, yet unusual cases may require tissue diagnosis. Acute hemorrhagic leukoencephalitis is a severe form of ADEM with vascular involvement, hemorrhage, and necrosis.

Histopathology

Demyelinating lesions display a set of consistent histologic features, although their overall appearance and the prominence of different components vary somewhat with the age of the lesion.

Macrophages are always a part of the cellular milieu and can be so dense as to give a strong impression of neoplasm, especially in new onset lesions in which macrophages have less abundant cytoplasm (Figure 2-1). Occasional mitotic macrophages add to the illusion of neoplasia. Lymphoplasmacytic infiltrates are also usually present in a perivascular pattern (Figure 2-2), suggesting inflammatory nature of the macrophage infiltrate rather than a reaction to necrosis, that is, infarct (Table 2-1). Immunohistochemical reactivity for CD68 or HAM56 can support the identity of macrophages, although caution is warranted because CD68, a lysosomal marker, is also expressed in granular cell astrocytomas, which are also rich in lysosomes. HAM56 is a marker for macrophages that should not be positive in granular cell astrocytoma, but this hypothesis has not been systematically tested. CD163 is probably the most specific marker for macrophages in this setting (6).

Reactive astrocytes are present in all but the most nascent lesions, extending prominent cytoplasmic processes from enlarged and eosinophilic cell bodies. The astrocytes take up evenly spaced positions within

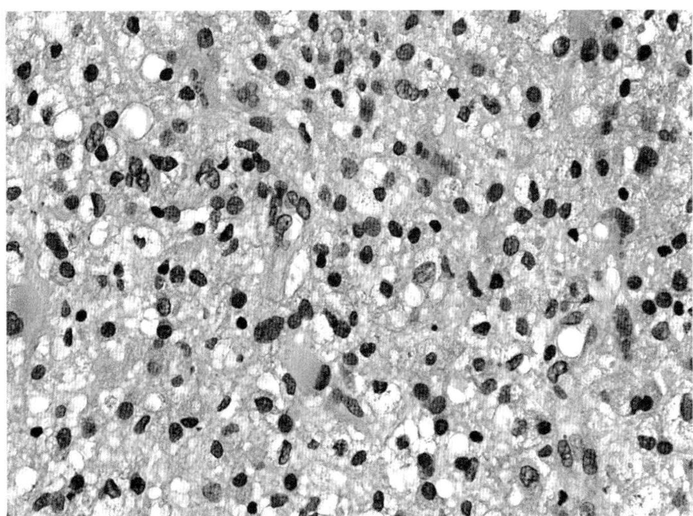

FIGURE 2-1 Hyperacute demyelinating lesions may be densely populated by macrophages, with small amounts of cytoplasm without obvious reactive astrocytes, mimicking the appearance of an infiltrating glioma.

the lesion and form a loose glial scar-like matrix in which the other cells are suspended (Figure 2-3). Occasional astrocytes display a starburst array of apparent chromosomes in place of the nucleus. These eye-catching *granular mitotic figures* (Figure 2-4) are often seen in reactive lesions, but cannot be considered by themselves as evidence of such because they also appear in neoplastic processes, including glioblastoma, albeit much less

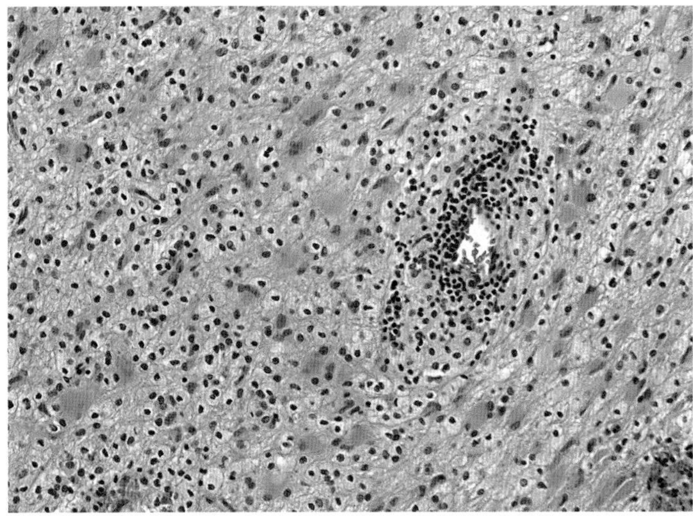

FIGURE 2-2 In demyelinating lesions, lymphocytes congregate around vessels, and reactive astrocytes are spread evenly with abundant space between each other.

TABLE 2-1 Diagnostic Considerations: Macrophage-Rich and Macrophage-Like Lesions

Diagnosis	Distinguishing Feature(s)
Demyelinating lesion	Lymphoplasmacytic inflammation, preserved axons
Infarct	Minimal lymphocytes or plasma cells, axon destruction
Progressive multifocal leukoencephalopathy	Inclusions in oligodendrocytes, atypical astrocyte nuclei, preserved axons, SV40 positive, inflammation with superimposed IRIS
Rosai–Dorfman Disease	Plasma cells, Russell bodies, large pale nuclei and prominent nucleoli, S100 reactivity, emperipolesis
Amebic meningoencephalitis	Perivascular, macrophage-like cells with too small nuclei and too big nucleoli, basophilic cysts (*Acanthamoeba*—wrinkled, *Balamuthia*—double layer), meningeal involvement
Granular cell astrocytoma	Highly proliferative, GFAP-positive, preserved myelinated axons, "targetoid" cytoplasm, sometimes necrosis
Erdheim–Chester Disease	Also bone lesions, spindle-shaped tumor cells in parenchyma, *BRAF* V600E mutant (~50–60%)

frequently. The *Creutzfeldt astrocyte* is conceptually a granular mitotic figure in which the dense chromatin fragments have inflated to pale micronuclei (Figure 2-3). These generally occur in proximity with granular mitotic figures.

Demyelinating lesions are generally exclusive to the white matter and do not extend significantly into areas of gray matter, although special staining can reveal loss of sparse intracortical myelin in some cases. When examining macrophage-rich lesions, lack of overt gray matter involvement is one of the most helpful clues in distinguishing between demyelination and infarct. The presence of ischemic, "red" neurons indicates gray matter and strongly favors infarct.

When one is lucky enough to have it included in the biopsy, the transition from demyelinating plaque to adjacent brain is sharp and well delineated. This feature is accentuated and often visible to the naked eye following myelin staining with Luxol fast blue (Figure 2-5).

The resident axons of the white matter are left more or less intact in demyelinating lesions, the damage being most severe to the myelinating

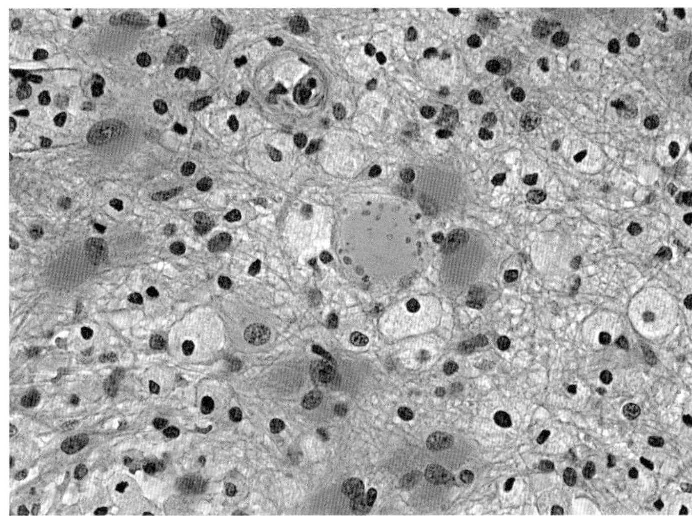

FIGURE 2-3 In demyelinating lesions, macrophages are suspended in a scaffold of reactive astrocytes with open chromatin and prominent nucleoli. In the center, a *Creutzfeldt astrocyte* contains numerous pale nuclear fragments.

oligodendrocytes. This is one of the cardinal features of demyelinating lesions, although it is difficult to appreciate on hematoxylin and eosin (H&E)-stained sections and usually requires application of immunostaining for neurofilament (Figure 2-6) or of Bielschowsky silver stain. Variable, but generally modest, degrees of axonal fragmentation and swelling can be

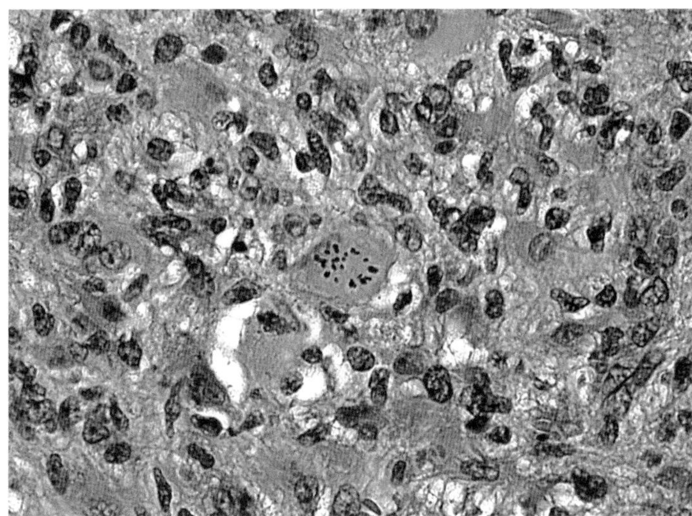

FIGURE 2-4 Granular mitotic figures, seen here in a glioblastoma, contain dark chromatin fragments that frequently arrange themselves in a starburst pattern.

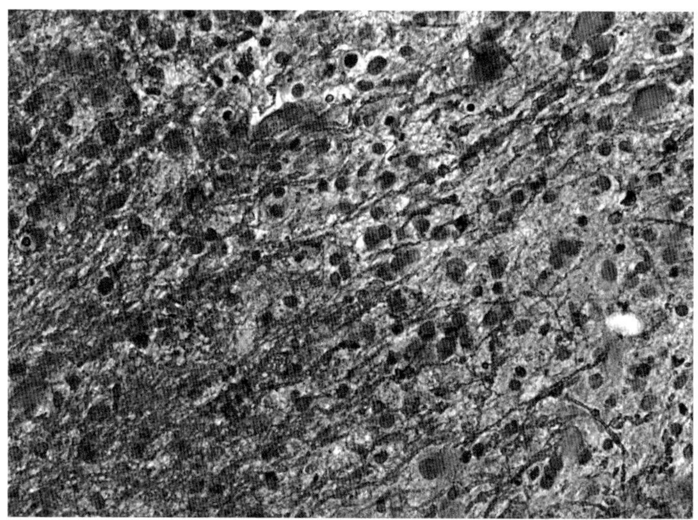

FIGURE 2-5 Luxol fast blue staining shows loss of blue staining in demyelinated areas (upper right), which can be well circumscribed.

noted in florid lesions, whereas infarcts show widespread and marked disruption of axons.

ADEM is also typically a macrophage-rich demyelinating process, yet it has a perivenular distribution of smaller lesions that distinguishes it from multiple sclerosis-type lesions. AHL has a similar pattern to ADEM with the additional features of necrosis and hemorrhage.

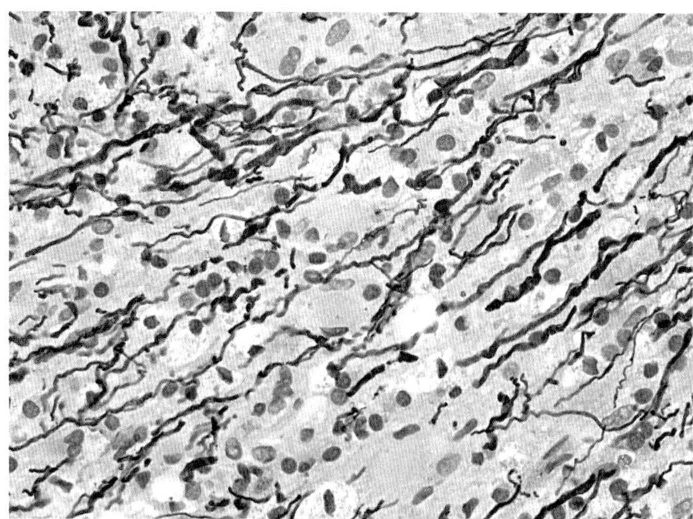

FIGURE 2-6 Immunohistochemistry for neurofilament shows preservation of axons within demyelinating plaques, a feature not seen in macrophage-rich infarcts.

Differential Diagnosis

Because the diagnosis of multiple sclerosis depends on identifying anatomically and temporally distinct lesions, it is fundamentally a clinical endeavor and cannot be issued on the basis of biopsy alone. Although many demyelinating lesions occur in the context of multiple sclerosis, the biopsy diagnosis should in most cases be limited to what is histologically demonstrable. The diagnosis "demyelinating lesion" fulfills this criterion and provides the clinician with sufficient information for proper management.

Increased sophistication and diagnostic accuracy of imaging techniques prevent all but a rare infarct from biopsy. When biopsy is performed, though, the infarct will often contain dense macrophage infiltrates comparable with those of demyelinating lesions. However, there are several key features that separate the two histologically. Unlike demyelinating lesions, infarcts affect the gray matter, destroy axons, and usually lack lymphocytes and plasma cells. Infarcts also induce endothelial hypertrophy in nearby vessels, and cause them to stand out against the parenchymal background.

Although technically a demyelinating disease itself, progressive multifocal leukoencephalopathy (PML) is pathophysiologically distinct, in that it results from unchecked replication of the JC virus in oligodendroglia due to severe immunosuppression. Most of the histologic features of PML are similar to those of other demyelinating diseases, with two exceptions. First, the presence of viral cytopathic effects, such as ground glass nuclear inclusions in oligodendrocytes and atypical nuclear features in astrocytes, is restricted to PML and not seen in autoimmune lesions. Also, perivascular lymphoplasmacytic inflammation is usually absent in PML. However, PML patients with immune reconstitution inflammatory syndrome (IRIS) may have brisk superimposed T and B cell infiltrates due to rapid recovery of immune function and response to the virus (7). Although macrophage infiltrates can be dense in PML, they are typically less than in multiple sclerosis.

The cellularity and nuclear uniformity of early demyelinating lesions can recreate the features of an oligodendroglioma or even diffuse astrocytoma. This misapprehension can be convincing in frozen sections that distort the cellular features, necessitating examination of smear preparations, which greatly facilitate the identification of macrophages (Figure 2-7). Perivascular lymphocytes and sharp circumscription are not features typically associated with infiltrating gliomas, yet are common in demyelinating disease.

Lymphomas that are treated with corticosteroids can have an appearance very similar to demyelinating lesions, but may show some necrosis and scattered apoptotic debris, both of which are unusual in the latter.

Granular cell astrocytomas are rare and aggressive infiltrating gliomas that have perivascular lymphocytic infiltrates and contain cells with ample cytoplasm and numerous lysosomes that react with antibodies to CD68, leading to a pathologic appearance that closely resembles demyelinating

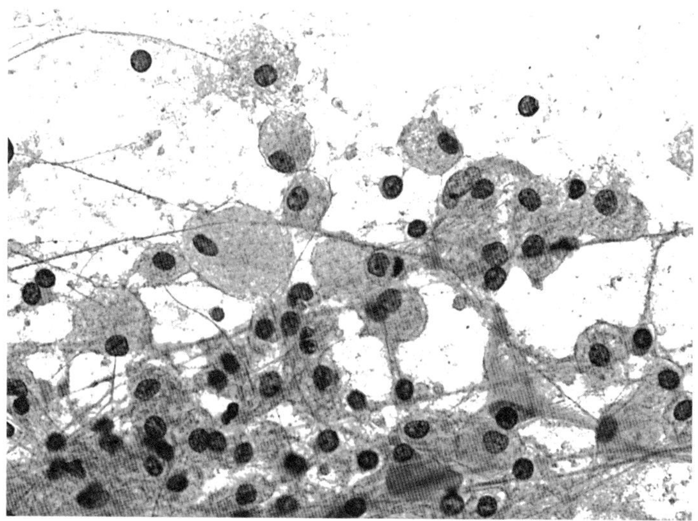

FIGURE 2-7 Smear preparations preserve the nuclear regularity and foamy cytoplasm of histiocytes during intraoperative consultation, facilitating their recognition.

disease. Comparison of the features of demyelinating lesions and granular cell astrocytoma is discussed in the section on anaplastic astrocytomas in Chapter 3.

SARCOIDOSIS

Clinical Context

This systemic inflammatory disease can affect any organ, but it has a proclivity for the lungs and hilar lymph nodes. CNS involvement occurs in approximately 5% to 20% of sarcoidosis patients and typically manifests as a cranial neuropathy, more often involving the optic nerves (8,9). Sarcoidosis maintains a worldwide distribution, including all races, although incidence is three to four times higher among people of African descent than among Caucasians (10).

The radiologic features of neurosarcoidosis are highly variable, famously mimicking several other disease processes, but can be distilled to several neuroimaging patterns that encompass most cases. The most common findings are of cranial nerve enlargement with contrast enhancement, correlating with cranial nerve deficits, or discontinuous dural thickening and enhancement that sometimes appears similar to a meningioma on MRI (9,11,12). The other major pattern is leptomeningeal enhancement, usually around the skull base and occasionally extending into the brain along perivascular spaces (12). Multiple enhancing and nonenhancing parenchymal lesions are less common but not unusual. Single intraparenchymal mass lesions are rare but may simulate neoplasia and require biopsy (13–16).

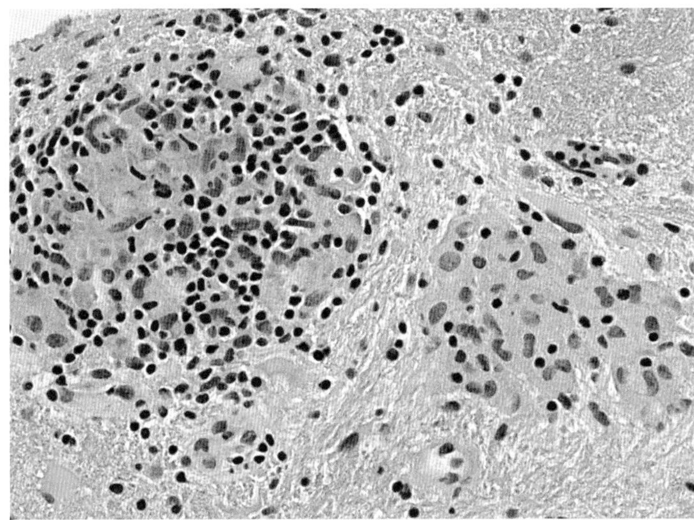

FIGURE 2-8 Small epithelioid granulomas are seen in most cases of neurosarcoidosis.

Histopathology

Noncaseating, epithelioid granulomas are the footprints of sarcoidosis, although several other processes may leave similar tracks. In general, the granulomas are small and formed of epithelioid histiocytes (Figure 2-8), although multinucleated giant cells are also seen. *Asteroid bodies,* cytoplasmic inclusions with a sea urchin shape, are occasionally seen in multinucleated giant cells but are not specific to sarcoidosis (17). A corona of lymphocytes rings many granulomas. Because other processes can also cause noncaseous granulomas, a diagnosis of "nonnecrotizing granulomatous inflammation" is generally appropriate because differentiating features are not histologically apparent.

Although necrosis is generally thought to exclude sarcoid granulomas, necrotizing granulomas have been demonstrated in the setting of sarcoid, although very rarely in the brain (18). The diagnosis of necrotizing sarcoid granulomatosis is difficult to establish with certainty and is essentially one of exclusion. Extensive necrosis is more often seen in infectious granulomas.

The differential diagnosis for sarcoid granulomas includes fungal or mycobacterial infection, germinoma, or another autoimmune illness. Application of stains for microorganisms decreases the likelihood of missing an infectious granuloma. In the case of granulomas from the pineal gland, posterior third ventricle, suprasellar region, or other midline locations, the thought of germinoma should be considered. Because germinoma can be greatly masked by inflammation, OCT4 or placenta-like alkaline phosphatase (PLAP) immunostaining can be useful to highlight tumor cells. The features of other autoimmune diseases are discussed later in this chapter.

OTHER SYSTEMIC AUTOIMMUNE DISEASES

Autoimmune connective tissue diseases can affect the CNS, but they are seldom the presenting symptom and are therefore rarely biopsied. The typical epidemiologic and clinical characteristics vary with each individual entity. Their imaging and histologic appearances are briefly mentioned here.

Behçet disease is a rare syndrome of oral ulcers, genital ulcers, and uveitides and has a high rate of CNS involvement. Neuro-Behçet disease usually occurs late in the course and is diagnosed clinically, yet a small number of cases present with CNS complaints. MRI shows T2 hyperintensities in the brainstem in most cases, with involvement of the cerebral white matter and basal ganglia also being common (19,20). Histologically, neuro-Behçet disease displays necrotizing perivascular neutrophilic infiltrates (21,22).

Rheumatoid arthritis most commonly causes a meningitis with contrast enhancement on MRI and lymphocytic infiltrate, vasculitis, and scattered necrobiotic rheumatoid nodules on histology (23).

Granulomatosis with polyangiitis (formerly Wegener granulomatosis) may attack the CNS through direct extension from sinonasal inflammation, as individual granulomas or as a CNS vasculitis (24). Mass lesions are rare (25,26).

Systemic lupus erythematosus commonly affects the CNS, usually as a multifocal cortical process on MRI (27). The histopathology of such lesions is not well documented in the literature.

Sjögren syndrome in the CNS appears similar to multiple sclerosis radiologically, with multiple white matter lesions (28). One postmortem series found meningitis with mixed inflammatory infiltrates, as well as vasculitis and hemorrhage (29). An inflammatory pseudotumor is reported in the choroid plexus (30).

GOSSYPIBOMA (TEXTILOMA)

Occasionally, a patient with a prior history of resected tumor will develop a subsequent mass lesion in the tumor bed which, instead of being recurrent neoplasm, is merely an inflammatory reaction to retained foreign material, which is usually gelatin sponge (Gelfoam) (Figure 2-9), oxidized cellulose (Surgicel) (31–33), or cotton (Figure 2-10) in the CNS. These lesions contain the offending foreign material admixed with fibrosis and granulomatous inflammation, although the material may be entirely degraded by the time of resection (31). Microfibrillar collagen (Avitene), another hemostatic agent, may induce a brisk eosinophilic infiltrate in addition to other reactive changes (34).

RADIATION NECROSIS

Clinical Context

Death of normal brain tissue is a late complication of radiation therapy and usually develops between 6 months and 2 years following exposure,

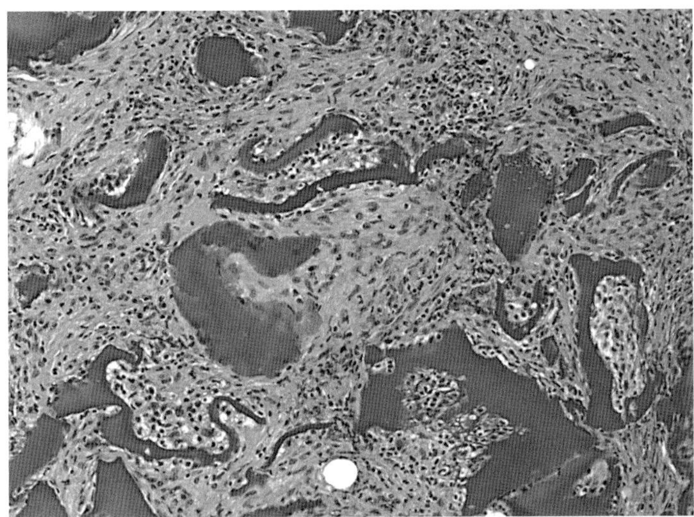

FIGURE 2-9 Foreign body reaction to Gelfoam that mimicked recurrent lymphoma.

mostly at doses of 50 Gy and above (35). Infiltrating gliomas frequently undergo such radiotherapy, which, while an effective measure to slow down the advance of disease, creates a diagnostic dilemma for the treating clinician, who must then attempt to distinguish between changes due to tumor recurrence and those due to radionecrosis on subsequent surveillance imaging. If imaging studies are inconclusive or the patient is symptomatic, the lesion may be biopsied or resected.

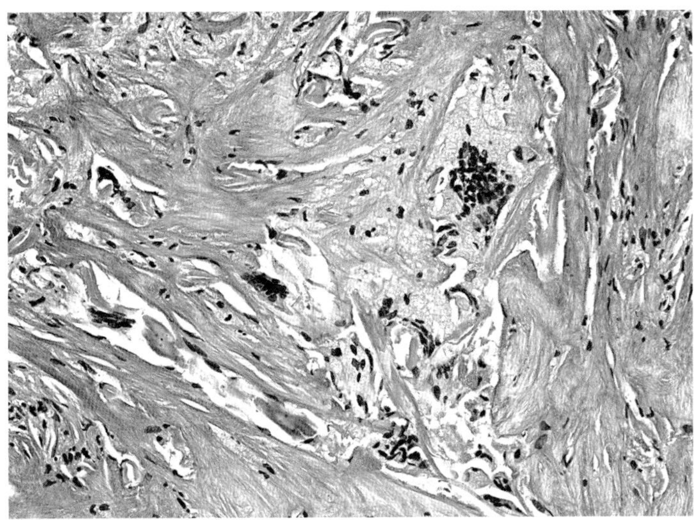

FIGURE 2-10 These cotton fibers and giant cells clinically simulated recurrent sinonasal carcinoma.

The MRI appearance of radiation necrosis consists of a contrast-enhancing lesion that generally lacks mass effect, but generates an impressive corona of edema, imbuing a similarity to the appearance of high-grade glioma or lymphoma. Several radiologic techniques have been used to interrogate possible radionecrosis, including diffusion-weighted imaging (36), thallium uptake (37), positron-emission tomography (38), and spectroscopy (39), with mixed results.

Treatment for radiation necrosis may consist of surgical resection, corticosteroids or bevacizumab, an angiogenesis inhibitor (40).

Histopathology

Coagulative necrosis, with pale outlines of once-living structures, heterogeneously involves white matter and contains a sparse population of residual glial cells (Figure 2-11). Inflammatory cells are generally minimal, with only a sparse contingent of foamy macrophages, if any. The blood vessels react to the insult with fibrinoid necrosis, thickening and hyalinization of the media, and breakdown of the endothelial layer, which presumably causes the thrombi seen in many of the damaged vessels. Alternatively, some blood vessels may be proliferating, even floridly, under hypoxic conditions. The endothelial cells are generally atrophic but may be enlarged with radiation atypia. Deposits of hemosiderin, proteinaceous debris, and calcium occur as the lesion ages.

The differential diagnosis of radiation necrosis almost invariably includes recurrent tumor, and the course of the patient's ongoing treatment often depends on which diagnoses are returned. If the interpretation is recurrent/progressive tumor, then the treatment regimen will most

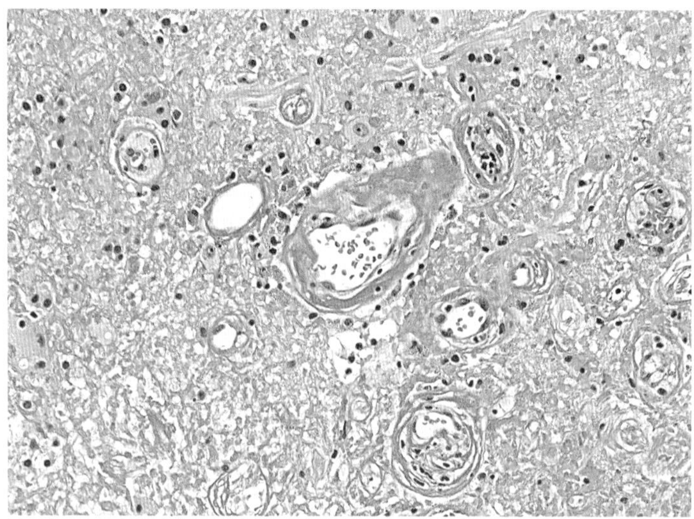

FIGURE 2-11 Radiation necrosis with thickened hyalinized vessels, reactive astrocytosis, and necrosis.

likely be changed to another antineoplastic therapy, but a diagnosis of radiation necrosis will shift treatment focus to alleviate its effects. In the strictest sense, some residual tumor is always present in cases of infiltrating glioma, but the interpretation should reflect the overall theme of the biopsy tissue. Scant atypical cells do not justify a diagnosis of recurrence in the context of large amounts of radiation necrosis. Mentioning both recurrent tumor and radiation necrosis in the diagnosis, and including a comment estimating the relative amounts of each may be helpful to avoid confusion.

In an infiltrating astrocytoma, radiation-induced necrosis should not be taken as a sign of progression to glioblastoma, although proving whether necrosis is due to treatment or tumor biology is difficult. Progression to glioblastoma should be considered when increased cellularity and/or pseudopalisading necrosis develop(s). Microvascular proliferation can also be seen following radiation, and therefore should be used with caution as a criterion for glioblastoma following radiation.

ABSCESS

Clinical Context

Suppurative bacterial infections arrive in the CNS hematogenously by direct extension from neighboring structures and from direct inoculation by a penetrating injury. In the subarachnoid and subdural spaces, this results in suppurative meningitis and subdural empyema, respectively, where the infection spreads along the tissue plane in a sheet-like fashion. Infections of the brain parenchyma progress rapidly from a focus of tissue destruction and neutrophilic inflammation (acute cerebritis) to a pocket of necroinflammatory debris sealed within a tough collagenous capsule, forming an abscess, usually after approximately 2 weeks.

In abscesses, the culpable bacterial genera are most commonly *Staphylococcus*, *Streptococcus*, or other gram-positive cocci, yet a large minority of cultured abscesses fail to grow organisms. Anaerobic and polymicrobial infections make up only small fractions of the total. Common sources of infection include pneumonia, dental abscess, sinusitis, otitis, and mastoiditis, each of which is associated with different bacterial species. People of all ages are affected with no strong predilection for any decade, but there is a consistent male predominance, by ratios of around 2:1 overall (41–45).

Abscesses proceed to surgery less and less often, most likely because imaging techniques have become accurate enough to diagnose most cases and antibiotic therapies are effective. Most abscesses have a characteristic appearance on MRI, with thin uniform rims of contrast enhancement around a nonenhancing core. The purulent contents consistently show *restricted diffusion* on diffusion-weighted imaging, meaning that the lesion's water molecules have limited random movement relative to adjacent tissue.

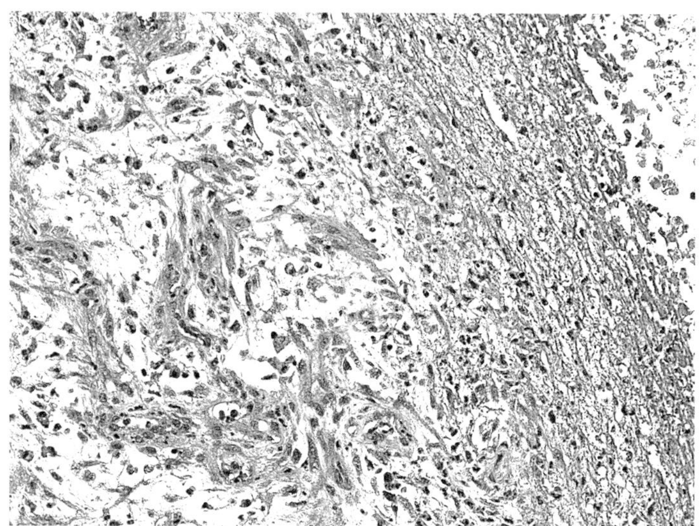

FIGURE 2-12 The proliferating fibroblasts of an abscess wall can create a neoplastic appearance but contain acute inflammatory cells.

This finding is closely associated with abscesses, but necrosis in other ring-enhancing lesions occasionally produces this phenomenon.

Histopathology

Acute cerebritis is characterized by tissue destruction, hemorrhage, and massive neutrophilic infiltration. The affected area liquefies and, over the course of several weeks, is sequestered within a multilayered abscess wall, surrounded by (from center to edge) granulation tissue and chronic inflammation, collagenous capsule, and reactive gliosis with mild vascular proliferation. The activated fibroblasts and proliferating blood vessels (Figure 2-12) can be worrisome on frozen section, especially if one's thoughts are primed by suspicions of glioblastoma. Recognition of prominent acute inflammatory infiltrates and collagen deposition will guide away from a neoplastic diagnosis.

MYCOBACTERIAL INFECTIONS

In the developing world, tuberculosis is a regular intruder in the CNS, but is uncommon in North America. CNS tuberculosis generally presents in one of three patterns: a chronic meningitis, one or more mass lesions (tuberculoma), or an abscess. In the United States, these are seen most often in immigrants and the immunosuppressed. Although CNS involvement is thought to be the most severe form of tuberculosis, each of these types of infection is amenable to treatment with antibiotics. Surgery may be indicated in large mass lesions, or if CSF flow is compromised (46).

The meningitis consists of a gelatinous, translucent suspension of lymphocytes, monocytes, and small caseous granulomas that extends slowly throughout the basal meninges, although any location is susceptible. Over time, fibrosis firms the affected area. Because CSF can be tested for *Mycobacterium tuberculosis* DNA, biopsy plays little role in diagnosing this meningitis.

Tuberculomas are irregularly contoured, solid masses of granulomatous inflammation and fibrosis, often around a central caseous, necrotic core.

True acute tuberculous abscesses are rare, but should be kept in mind when examining an otherwise quotidian pyogenic abscess in an immunosuppressed patient, where such lesions are preferentially found and exhibit neutrophilic inflammation (47). The histologic picture is essentially identical to a pyogenic abscess: pus, acute and chronic inflammation, and a collagenous capsule.

Ziehl–Neelsen acid-fast stain colors *M. tuberculosis* bacilli bright red, but the organisms also appear on other histochemical stains. Gomori methenamine silver (GMS) preparations accentuate the organisms in black, and Gram staining produces lightly gram-positive purple rods. The bacilli vary from short homogeneously staining rods to filamentous chains with a discontinuous, "beaded" staining pattern in all three stains.

Other acid-fast bacilli, especially *Mycobacterium avium intracellulare,* are occasionally seen in the CNS as mass lesions, generally in the immunocompromised (48).

WHIPPLE DISEASE

Cerebral infection by *Tropheryma whipplei* is rare in the absence of significant gastrointestinal infection. When it occurs, it can easily go unrecognized on brain biopsy. Affected patients are generally male and between the ages of 40 and 65. Presentations range from stroke-like symptoms (49) to progressive dementia (50), even Klüver–Bucy syndrome (51). T2/FLAIR-weighted MRI shows single or multiple lesions throughout the brain with variable contrast enhancement (52).

The histology of cerebral Whipple disease is that of a macrophage-rich lesion with variable amounts of lymphocytes and plasma cells. The macrophages contain irregular, polymorphous, sometimes sickle-shaped, fragments of PAS-positive, diastase-resistant material in otherwise foamy cytoplasm. A perivascular distribution of the macrophages is often apparent. Gram and GMS stains also label this organism.

TOXOPLASMOSIS

Infection with this protozoan parasite is widespread among mammals. Humans frequently encounter *toxoplasma* through exposure to oocysts in domestic cat feces. Most often, exposure results in only a mild flu-like

TABLE 2-2 Diagnostic Considerations: Acute Necrotizing Encephalitis

Diagnosis	Distinguishing Feature(s)
Angioinvasive fungus	Fungal hyphae or pseudohyphae, best seen on GMS staining
Toxoplasmosis	Round tissue cysts containing bradyzoites, possibly individual curved tachyzoites
Amebic meningoencephalitis	Perivascular, macrophage-like cells with too small nuclei and too big nucleoli, wrinkled basophilic cysts (*Acanthamoeba, Balamuthia*)
Acute viral encephalitis	Nuclear inclusions and atypia

illness. However, the organism is devastating to fetuses and the immunosuppressed, causing a potentially fatal necrotizing encephalitis. *Toxoplasma* appears as multiple irregular periventricular lesions that enhance with contrast, making them radiologically similar to primary CNS lymphomas, which also occur in the immunosuppressed (53). If *toxoplasma* is suspected clinically, the patient will be treated with pyrimethamine–sulfadiazine, reserving biopsy for cases that fail to respond.

Histologically, the overall picture is that of a necrotizing encephalitis (Table 2-2) with lymphocytes and plasma cells, although the inflammatory infiltrates can be virtually absent in severe immunosuppression (Figure 2-13). Within necrotic debris, especially around the edges of a lesion, two forms of

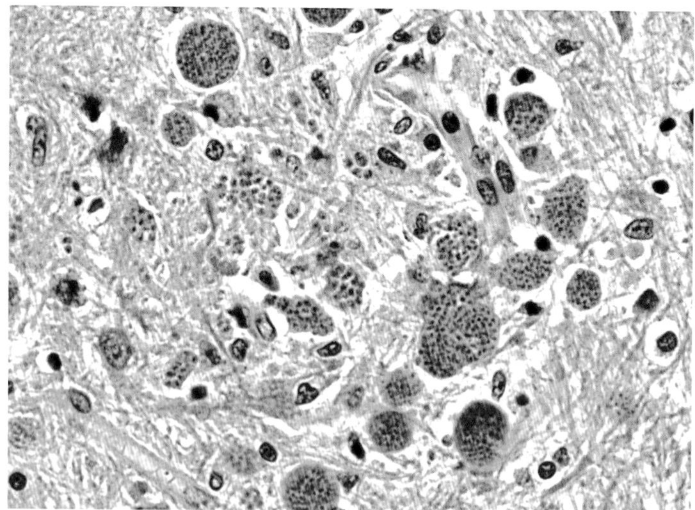

FIGURE 2-13 *Toxoplasma gondii* colonizes cells and produces pseudocysts containing numerous bradyzoites, provoking little inflammation in immunocompromised hosts, as seen here.

the *toxoplasma* organism can be seen on H&E staining. In one form, colonized cells swell with organisms in the bradyzoite stage, which are visible as multiple 1- to 2-μm amphophilic dots within the cytoplasm, the cell membrane forming a *pseudocyst* around them. When the bradyzoites mature to tachyzoites, the pseudocyst ruptures and releases organisms to colonize other cells. These 2-μm, vaguely banana-shaped tachyzoites are difficult to see on H&E staining, but are readily apparent on immunohistochemistry. Wright–Giemsa staining also accentuates the organisms and is useful in touch imprints of infected tissue.

FUNGI

Cryptococcus can cause disease anywhere in the body but has a tendency for neurotropism. Most CNS *Cryptococcus* infections are associated with immune deficiency and involve the species *Cryptococcus neoformans* (54). The species *Cryptococcus gattii* is less common and affects immunocompetent hosts in a majority of cases (55,56). This organism typically causes a disseminated and slowly progressive meningoencephalitis that can extend deeply into the brain along perivascular spaces. Cases that present with signs and symptoms of meningitis rarely receive biopsies, though occasional examples form solid masses of reactive fibrosis, granulomatous inflammation, and organisms, recreating the appearance of an aggressive neoplastic lesion on imaging (57). This organism is a yeast form that is variable in diameter with a thick polysaccharide capsule that lends a mucoid appearance to colonies grossly. In H&E-stained sections, the organism is a glassy, light blue orb with a clear halo of invisible mucoid material (Figure 2-14). The capsule, being a mucinous polysaccharide,

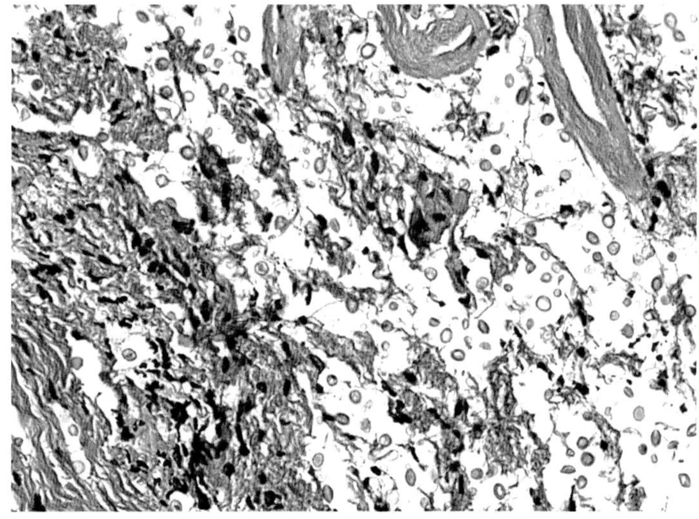

FIGURE 2-14 *Cryptococci* are dented glass-like orbs with peripheral clearing on H&E staining and sometimes form a mass lesion, or "cryptococcoma."

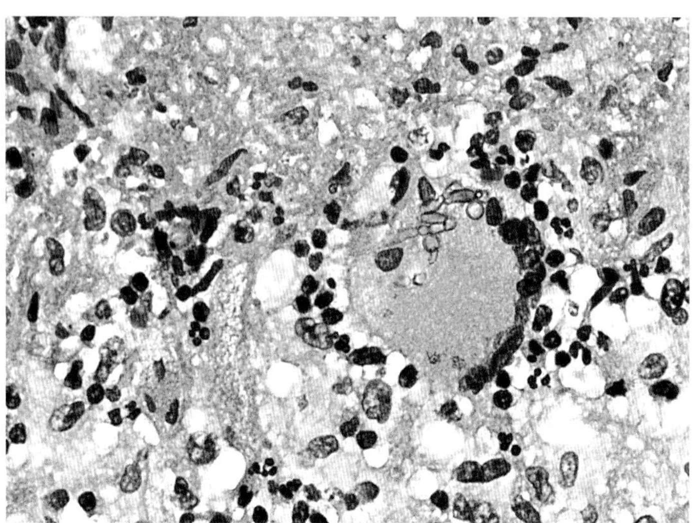

FIGURE 2-15 *C. bantiana* typically grows in brain tissue as pigmented, elliptical conidia in a background of granulomatous inflammation.

shows affinity for PAS, mucicarmine, and Alcian blue, while the cell wall is positive on Fontana-Masson and GMS stains (58).

Coccidioides immitis is endemic in the southwest United States and primarily causes self-limited pulmonary infections. It spreads to the CNS in a small fraction of cases where it causes a chronic progressive meningitis that is lethal over months to years without treatment, but is relatively curable with long-term fluconazole therapy (59). *C. immitis* causes abscess only in the rarest of patients (60). In tissue, the organisms form spherules measuring 10 to 100 μm that usually contain multiple 2- to 5-μm endospores, both of which are visible in routine H&E-stained sections (61).

Cladophialophora bantiana is a dematiaceous fungus that is highly neurotropic and more frequently affects immunocompetent patients, that is, it is likely to show up unexpectedly. The CNS is typically the only organ overtly involved in immunocompetent patients. The fungus forms a granulomatous mycetoma that may not have a single central cavity and is frequently presumed to be a neoplasm on neuroimaging. Histologically, a background of fibrosis and other inflammation contains granulomas with sparse, pigmented, elliptical, vaguely lemon-shaped conidia (Figure 2-15). Septate hyphae may be seen rarely.

Angioinvasive fungi that grow in tissue as hyphae, such as *Aspergillus*, *Rhizopus*, and *Mucor*, most often affect patients with immune insufficiency, but not those whose deficit results from human immunodeficiency virus (HIV) infection, rather favoring allograft recipients, cancer patients, and diabetic patients instead. *Aspergillus* is thought to spread to the CNS hematogenously from pulmonary sites. Although many details vary, the common theme among these organisms is an angioinvasive pattern of

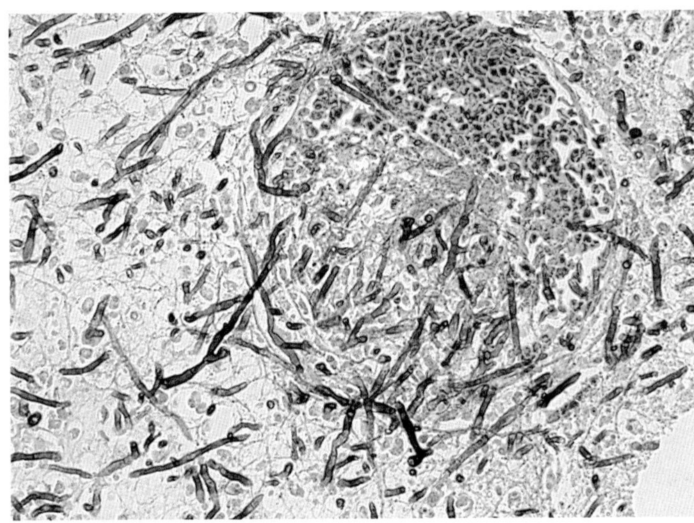

FIGURE 2-16 The septate hyphae of *Aspergillus* penetrate vessel walls and invade the surrounding tissue (Gomori methenamine).

growth in which blood vessels are destroyed, causing infarction of adjacent tissue. The inflammatory response depends on the immune status of the patient, but it is generally neutrophilic acutely and somewhat muted in extent. Aspergillus species grow as segmented, or septate, hyphae of uniform thickness that branch at acute angles (Figure 2-16), whereas *Rhizopus* and *Mucor* have variable thickness hyphae without septation that branch at right angles. Despite aggressive treatment with antifungal agents, many patients with cerebral angioinvasive fungi succumb to their disease.

CYSTICERCOSIS

Of tapeworms that infect humans, *Taenia solium* has the unique ability to disseminate throughout the host's tissues, but only when contracted by ingestion of ova from fecal matter. After hatching from the ova, *T. solium* larvae travel the bloodstream and implant in a variety of tissues, including the brain. Each larva then encysts, forming a cysticercus, and remains in an infective state. Patients with neurocysticercosis generally present with seizures when the lesions are intraparenchymal, and signs of CSF obstruction when the cysts are intraventricular, although many patients have cysts in both (62). In the United States, these patients mostly come from Mexico and elsewhere in Latin America (63). In active lesions, the imaging appearance is that of a 0.5- to 1.5-cm fluid-filled cyst with contents isointense to CSF on T1- and T2-weighted sequences, but after the organism dies, it becomes more T1 intense. Edema and calcification accompany many of the lesions (64). Large, multiloculated examples are less common and are termed *racemose* lesions, referring to their grape-cluster appearance (65).

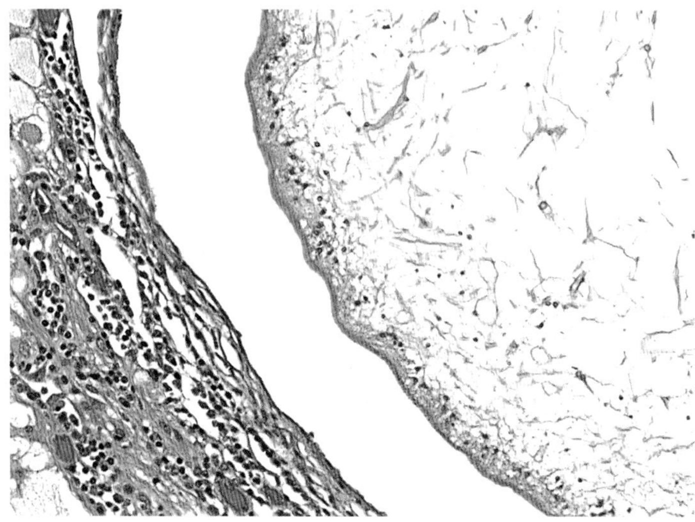

FIGURE 2-17 On the right is the surface of an intracerebral *T. solium* cyst with a cellular superficial layer and underlying reticular layer with scattered canaliculi.

Tissue sections of the cyst wall show a three-layered rind comprising a dense outer cuticle overlying a cellular band of small pinpoint nuclei and a loose inner reticulum with branching tubular canaliculi (Figure 2-17) (65). The head, or *scolex,* is a nodular protrusion into the cyst and microscopically displays internal organs and sharp chitinous hooklets that surround the organism's mouth. Necrotic and degenerating cysticerci may lack many of the aforementioned features and provoke a brisk acute and granulomatous inflammation.

Several other parasitic worms may breach the cerebral defenses at various phases of their life cycles, including *Equinococcus granulosus, Trichinella spiralis, Baylisascaris procyonis, Schistosoma japonicum,* and others.

AMEBIASIS

Three genera of amebas account for the vast majority of amebic CNS infections: *Acanthamoeba, Balamuthia,* and *Naegleria. Acanthamoeba* and *Balamuthia* typically infect immunocompromised hosts and establish a subacute or chronic meningoencephalitis that produces granulomatous inflammation (granulomatous amebic encephalitis [GAE]), although *Balamuthia* can also cause mixed or acute infiltrates (66). *Naegleria,* in contrast, infects healthy hosts and causes an acute purulent exudate (primary amebic meningoencephalitis [PAM]). The neuroimaging findings are nonspecific, generally showing single or multiple discreet lesions in GAE and more ill-defined lesions and infarcts in PAM (67). Rarely, the intestinal

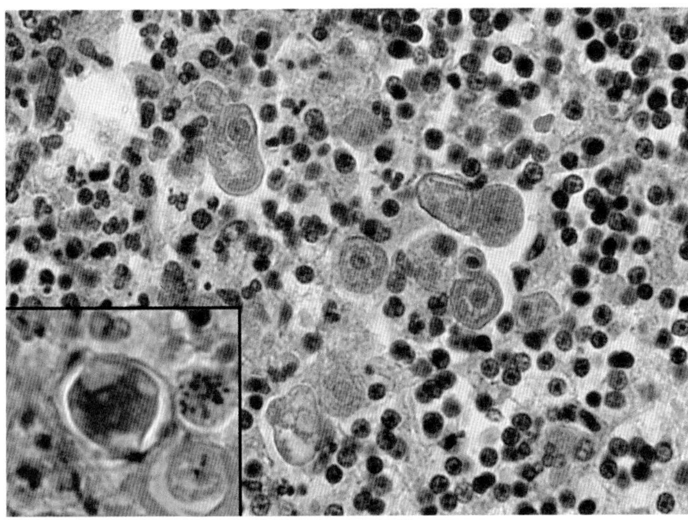

FIGURE 2-18 Amebas in the trophozoite stage appear similar to macrophages, with vacuolated cytoplasm and round nuclei. *Acanthamoeba* and *Balamuthia* may show cyst forms with wrinkled double membranes (inset).

parasite *Entamoeba histolytica* can spread to the CNS and cause meningoencephalitis.

In addition to acute and/or granulomatous inflammation, amebic CNS infections produce a necrotizing encephalitis with destruction and thrombotic occlusion of blood vessels. The organisms are most concentrated in the perivascular space (Figure 2-18) and are present as cysts and trophozoites in GAM, but only trophozoites are seen in PAM. *Acanthamoeba* and *Balamuthia* cysts have wrinkled "double-membrane" cyst walls, a round to stellate endocyst and measure 12 to 30 μm in diameter (68). GMS staining blackens the outer membrane of the cyst. Trophozoites from all three genera look like macrophages, with abundant vacuolated cytoplasm, but the nuclei are slightly smaller, more round, and have prominent nucleoli. Lack of staining for CD68 may help to differentiate the two. Definitive diagnosis in tissue sections may require assistance from the Centers for Disease Control and Prevention, where multiple genus-specific antibodies exist (66).

PROGRESSIVE MULTIFOCAL LEUKOENCEPHALOPATHY

Clinical Context

The JC virus is a member of the *Polyomaviridae* family and closely related to the BK virus and simian virus 40 (SV40). It infects the vast majority of humankind and causes disease only when the host's immune system fails to keep virus growth in check. The viral genome lies inactive in astrocytes and oligodendrocytes until a lapse in cell-mediated immunity allows replication, ultimately destroying the infected cells and leaving axons stripped of their myelin and unable to propagate signals. PML is most common among HIV-infected patients and is not frequently seen in other types of immunosuppression. However, some immunomodulatory agents, such as natalizumab (69) and rituximab (70), have a stronger association with PML than with other similar drugs.

On MRI, PML generally appears as multiple discreet white matter lesions that are T2/FLAIR hyperintense and do not affect the cortex but may involve the thalamus and basal ganglia (71). Enhancement after contrast administration is rare, setting the appearance of PML apart from lymphoma and toxoplasmosis, where enhancement is the rule (72,73). However, cases in which the patient has received antiretroviral therapy or has discontinued immunosuppressant therapy, contrast enhancement can be seen on MRI as a result of IRIS (74).

Treatment for PML is generally focused on reversing immunosuppression with highly active antiretroviral therapy in AIDS patients, leading to improved survival in recent years. In one nationwide cohort study, the overall median survival of patients with PML was only 90 days (75). The presence of JC virus–specific T cells in the circulation has been associated with longer survival in patients with PML, as have higher $CD4^+$ cell counts (75,76).

Histopathology

The histologic picture of PML, in broad strokes, is that of an unenthusiastic demyelinating lesion. The overall cellularity is lower in PML than in typical multiple sclerosis plaques, partially because lymphoplasmacytic infiltrates are absent or minimal, and also because of a lower turnout of macrophages. In contrast, lymphocytic infiltrates can be striking in cases of PML-IRIS where the patient's immune system is in the process of responding to the virus. Like multiple sclerosis plaques, a loose latticework of reactive and enlarged astrocytes forms in the background, but in PML, some of those cells display nuclear atypia due to viral cytopathy (Figure 2-19). The amount and severity of this nuclear atypia, along with apparent mitotic figures, can lure one toward a diagnosis of infiltrating glioma, yet the presence of macrophages should discourage such suspicions. Discreet Cowdry type A viral inclusions are not seen in PML. Subtle glassy-smooth nuclear inclusions are more common.

PML lesions resist Luxol fast blue staining because of myelin destruction, and contain well-preserved axons with neurofilament immunostaining or Bielschowsky silver staining. Because JC virus shares a highly conserved protein, the T antigen, with other polyoma viruses, immunostaining for SV40 can be used to detect JC virus in PML lesions. The staining is nuclear in distribution and may only be in scattered individual cells unless the tissue near the lesion edge is included (77).

The differential diagnosis in PML includes autoimmune demyelination and neoplasm. The former can be eliminated if there is evidence of

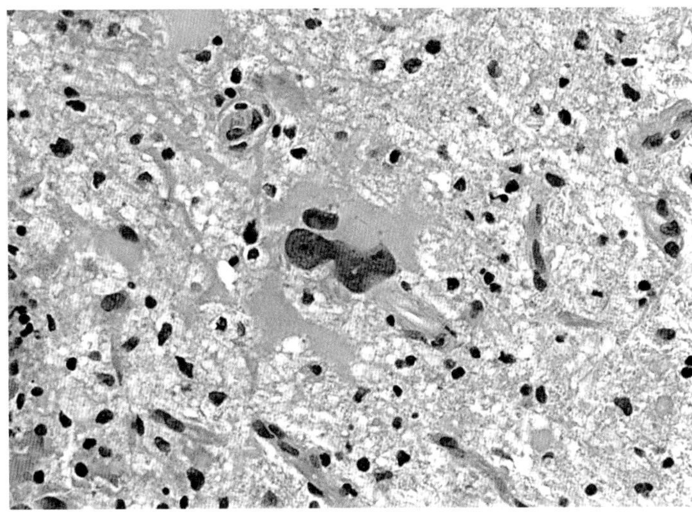

FIGURE 2-19 Progressive multifocal leukoencephalopathy can cause marked nuclear atypia in glia that should not be confused with neoplastic anaplasia.

viral infection, either by cytopathic effects or immunohistochemical staining.

VIRAL ENCEPHALITIDES

Because molecular diagnostic methods for most viruses can be performed on CSF without violating the cranial vault, brain biopsies for viral disease are rare.

Besides a few findings that identify specific virus types, the morphologic clues that suggest viral encephalitis are generic to the entire category and can even be seen in a few other conditions. Viral infection elicits a mild perivascular lymphocytic infiltrate and increases in the numbers of "rod cells," or microglia. Scattered loose congregations of microglia form *microglial nodules,* some of which have a neuron in the center (Figure 2-20). The neuron is said to be undergoing *neuronophagia.* Large, pill-shaped nuclear inclusions with narrow clear haloes (Cowdry type A inclusions) are often associated with cytomegalovirus (CMV) but may also be seen with other viruses, including herpes simplex virus (HSV), varicella zoster virus (VZV), measles, and others. Limited additional disease-specific findings are mentioned here.

HSV classically causes an acute necrotizing encephalitis that is centered in the temporal lobes, but asymmetrical in severity. Inflammation and infected cells can be seen diffusely (78).

CMV encephalitis is well known in the immunocompromised and in utero. It can also cause disease in patients with apparently intact immunity

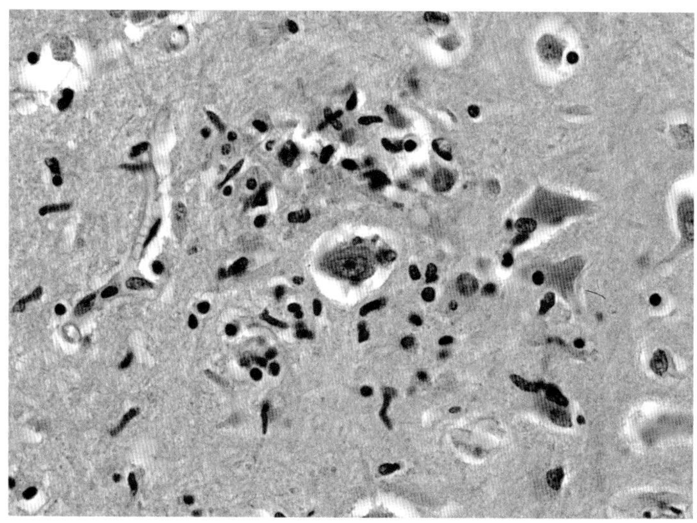

FIGURE 2-20 Elongate microglia form a microglial nodule that is characteristic of viral encephalitides, here involving a neuron (neuronophagia).

(79). A necrotizing encephalitis of the periventricular areas is typical, often with calcifications.

VZV infects and destroys oligodendrocytes (among others) and causes a concomitant vasculopathy of large or small arteries, resulting in a histologic pattern with varying amounts of both infarction and demyelination (80). Viral cytopathic effects are more likely to be seen in the small-vessel pattern (80).

HIV causes chronic or subacute diffuse encephalitis with the characteristic finding of multinucleated giant cells formed by the merger of microglia/histiocytes (Figure 2-21). Comorbid infections are common (81).

Rabies induces diffuse encephalitis with only scant inflammation, but with characteristic neuronal cytoplasmic inclusions (*Negri bodies*) (Figure 2-22), which are eosinophilic and typically oblong, ranging in size from 1 to 5 μm.

Subacute sclerosing panencephalitis and acute measles encephalitis are rare ever since the institution of measles vaccination programs in North America. Large nuclear and cytoplasmic inclusions in oligodendroglia, neurons, and astrocytes are typical. Neurons may contain globose neurofibrillary tangles.

Other cerebrotropic viruses, of which there are many, are even less likely to be explored with biopsy.

CREUTZFELDT–JAKOB DISEASE

Clinical Context

Of the several prion diseases that afflict humans, Creutzfeldt–Jakob disease (CJD) requires mention here because it is, by far, the most common prion

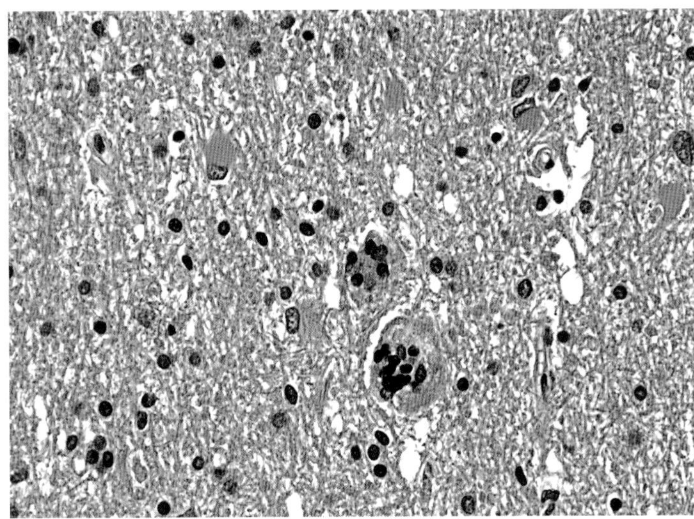

FIGURE 2-21 HIV encephalitis is characterized by multinucleated giant cells in a background of microgliosis.

disease, therefore the most likely to be biopsied. Most cases are sporadic (~90%), with familial and variant (transmitted) forms accounting for the rest. The sporadic disease preferentially affects the elderly (median age 68 years) and shows no significant skew toward either sex (82). The typical history is that of rapidly progressing dementia, generally over the course of less than 6 months, often with myoclonus, ataxia, and/or loss of vision (83). Patients with variant CJD have a longer course, usually over a year or more.

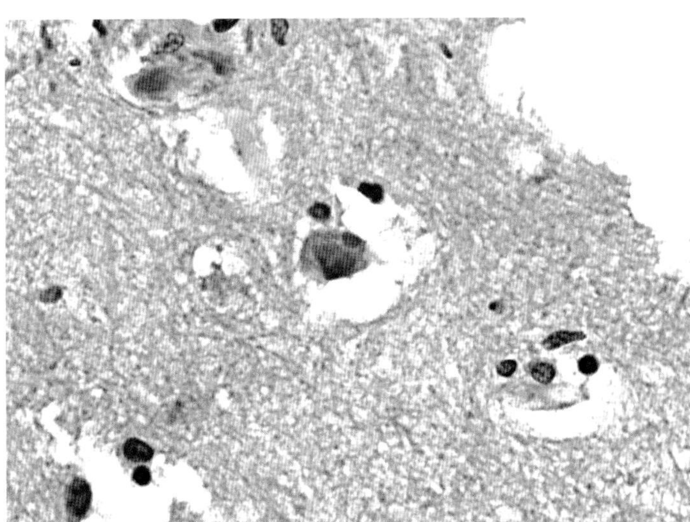

FIGURE 2-22 *Negri bodies* are eosinophilic cytoplasmic neuronal inclusions characteristic of rabies encephalitis.

Clinical diagnosis rests on history, electroencephalography (EEG), and CSF examination. EEG shows characteristic of "periodic sharp wave potentials" that are present in most sporadic cases. Analysis for the 14-3-3 protein, named for its elution and electrophoretic migration properties, reveals elevated CSF levels in CJD, although this finding only indicates active neuronal destruction. Neither EEG nor protein 14-3-3 studies are specific to CJD but are in combination, reliable indicators of disease when performed in the context of a suspicious clinical history (84). MRI patterns are variable but generally show T2/FLAIR hyperintensities in the cortex, putamen, and caudate nucleus in sporadic cases (85). Variant CJD, which results from ingestion of contaminated meat, shows characteristic bilateral pulvinar T2 changes on MRI (86).

In the event of biopsy for suspected CJD, the tissue should be handled in a way that minimizes potential contamination within the laboratory. Deferral of frozen sections is important, both because of contamination and destruction of histologic detail by the freezing process. However, a small amount of tissue, for example, one needle core, should be frozen for possible biochemical studies (see later). Biopsy tissue for histology should be fixed in 10% formalin for 24 hours before submersion in 90% formic acid for 1 hour, after which the tissue is processed normally (87). Contaminated disposable instruments should be incinerated, but reusable instruments can be decontaminated with undiluted sodium hypochlorite bleach or a 2*N* sodium hydroxide solution.

Histopathology

The histologic diagnosis of CJD requires the presence of gray matter, where the degenerative changes occur. The neuropil contains vacuoles of varying sizes throughout, with a mild reactive gliosis and loss of neurons, but no significant inflammatory infiltrate (Figure 2-23). As the disease

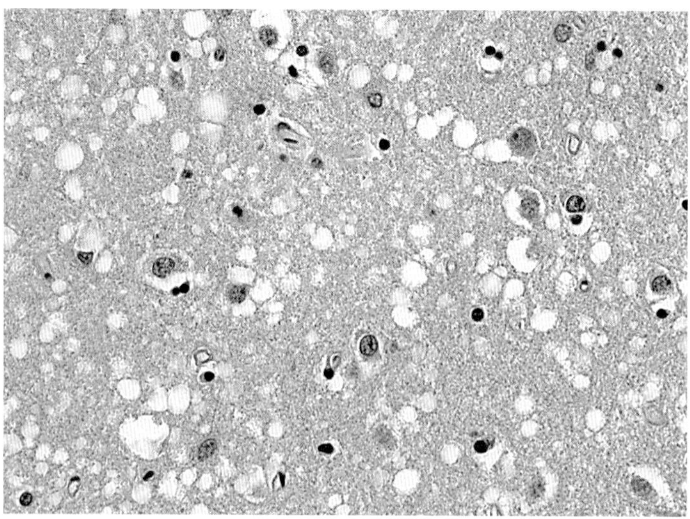

FIGURE 2-23 Spongiform encephalopathy of Creutzfeldt–Jakob disease is prominent vacuolation of cortex with relative sparing of the white matter (white matter not shown).

progresses, the vacuolations coalesce and impart a ragged appearance to the neuropil. If both white and gray matter is present, the vacuolation should be limited to the latter, or else the suspicion of CJD should be reevaluated. Other common causes for vacuolation of brain parenchyma include edema and a combination of Alzheimer disease and dementia with Lewy bodies (88).

If a biopsy shows changes consistent with CJD, the diagnosis should be confirmed by more specific methods. To that end, frozen biopsy tissue in the United States can be sent to the National Prion Disease Pathology Surveillance Center at Case Western Reserve University for Western blotting and other diagnostic testing at no charge.

ROSAI–DORFMAN DISEASE

Clinical Context

CNS cases of extranodal sinus histiocytosis are rare, with only a few dozen in the literature, mostly as case reports. In contrast to Langerhans cell histiocytosis, which is clonal and neoplastic, Rosai–Dorfman disease is an idiopathic, polyclonal inflammatory process (89). In the CNS, it is more reported in adults as an extra-axial mass, although intraparenchymal location has been reported (90), as have pediatric cases (91,92). The presentation parallels that of meningiomas, being a dural mass that enhances after gadolinium administration. Most patients with Rosai–Dorfman disease are cured after surgical resection, although some cases may behave aggressively (93,94). Radiation and corticosteroids are also sometimes used.

Histopathology

CNS lesions in Rosai–Dorfman disease contain similar mixed inflammatory cell infiltrates as peripherally located lesions, but are generally more fibrotic. The low-magnification appearance may be vaguely nodular or just with regionally variable cellularity. The histiocytes that characterize this lesion may be densely distributed or in scattered clusters, camouflaged by infiltrates of lymphocytes and plasma cells with a dusting of neutrophils. The histiocytes themselves have ample cytoplasm and large round to oval nuclei with obvious eccentric nucleoli and pale vesicular chromatin (Figure 2-24). Recognizing these nuclear features is key in distinguishing histiocytes of Rosai–Dorfman disease from other types. A contingent of the plasma cells are binucleate or contain spherical hyaline aggregates of eosinophilic immunoglobulin (Russell bodies), which, when there are multiple within the same plasma cell, constitute a *Mott cell.* The phenomenon of smaller inflammatory cells passing through the cytoplasm of lesional histiocytes, or emperipolesis, is a histologic hallmark of Rosai–Dorfman disease (Figure 2-24). However, it was seen only in 7 of 11 cases in one series and is therefore not an entirely sensitive criterion for its diagnosis (93).

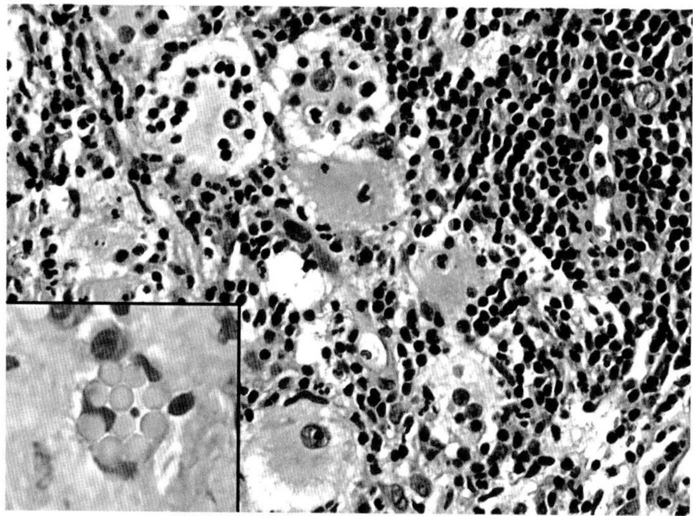

FIGURE 2-24 Extranodal Rosai–Dorfman disease is characterized by histiocytes with round central nuclei with prominent nucleoli, sometimes containing intracytoplasmic inflammatory cells. Mott cells with intracytoplasmic immunoglobulin droplets are common (inset).

Immunohistochemistry for S100 protein will show strong cytoplasmic reactivity in the histiocytes of Rosai–Dorfman disease, differentiating them from most other histiocytic infiltrates and often creating punched-out spaces at points of emperipolesis (Figure 2-25). Although the histiocytes of Langerhans cell histiocytosis are morphologically distinct from those in

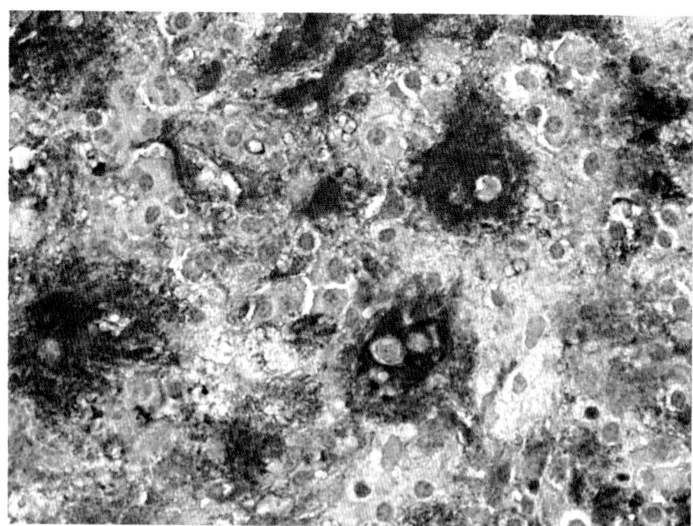

FIGURE 2-25 Immunohistochemistry for S100 protein stains the histiocytes of Rosai–Dorfman disease and accentuates emperipolesis.

Rosai–Dorfman, a lack of staining for CD1a assists in ruling out their presence.

PLASMA CELL GRANULOMA

This rare and somewhat vaguely defined inflammatory pseudoneoplasm usually arises on the dura. The exact nature of plasma cell granuloma is unknown, but it overlaps with Rosai–Dorfman disease in age, anatomic distribution, and in several histologic aspects (93,95). It is characterized by a plasmacytic infiltrate that contains binucleate forms and intracytoplasmic Russell bodies overlaid on a background of histiocytes, lymphocytes, neutrophils, and fibrosis. Histiocytes with emperipolesis have also been described in plasma cell granuloma (96). Many cases reported in the literature have escaped S100 immunohistochemistry, so it is difficult to rule out Rosai–Dorfman disease. Even in the absence of S100-protein–positive histiocytes, a terminal, "spent" phase of Rosai–Dorfman disease cannot be excluded. Nevertheless, should histiocytes within a CNS lesion with the above characteristics fail to express S100 protein, plasma cell granuloma may be a viable diagnosis. IgG_4-related inflammatory lesions may also fit the histologic description of plasma cell granuloma, so that diagnosis should also be considered.

CASTLEMAN DISEASE

Rarely, this idiopathic inflammatory lesion forms a dura-based mass that resembles a meningioma on neuroimaging. Castleman disease usually affects the lymph nodes, expanding them with numerous enlarged germinal centers with concentrically arranged lymphocytes and penetrating capillaries in the *hyaline vascular* variant, and follicular hyperplasia with intervening plasma cells in the *plasma cell* variant. Prognosis is very good for unicentric disease following resection. Immunoglobulin production should be polyclonal.

REFERENCES

1. Masdeu JC, Moreira J, Trasi S, et al. The open ring. A new imaging sign in demyelinating disease. *J Neuroimaging.* 1996;6(2):104–107.
2. Masdeu JC, Quinto C, Olivera C, et al. Open-ring imaging sign: highly specific for atypical brain demyelination. *Neurology.* 2000;54(7):1427–1433.
3. Alderson L, Fetell MR, Sisti M, et al. Sentinel lesions of primary CNS lymphoma. *J Neurol.* 1996;60(1):102–105.
4. Ng S, Butzkueven H, Kalnins R, et al. Prolonged interval between sentinel pseudotumoral demyelination and development of primary CNS lymphoma. *J Clin Neurosci.* 2007;14(11):1126–1129.
5. Balasubramanya KS, Kovoor JM, Jayakumar PN, et al. Diffusion-weighted imaging and proton MR spectroscopy in the characterization of acute disseminated encephalomyelitis. *Neuroradiology.* 2007;49(2):177–183.

6. Lau SK, Chu PG, Weiss LM. CD163: a specific marker of macrophages in paraffin-embedded tissue samples. *Am J Clin Pathol.* 2004;122(5):794–801.
7. Bauer J, Gold R, Adams O, et al. Progressive multifocal leukoencephalopathy and immune reconstitution inflammatory syndrome (IRIS). *Acta Neuropathol.* 2015;130(6): 751–764.
8. Joseph FG, Scolding NJ. Neurosarcoidosis: a study of 30 new cases. *J Neurol Neurosurg Psychiatry.* 2009;80(3):297–304.
9. Pawate S, Moses H, Sriram S. Presentations and outcomes of neurosarcoidosis: a study of 54 cases. *QJM.* 2009;102(7):449–460.
10. Rybicki BA, Maliarik MJ, Major M, et al. Epidemiology, demographics, and genetics of sarcoidosis. *Semin Respir Infect.* 1998;13(3):166–173.
11. Seltzer S, Mark AS, Atlas SW. CNS sarcoidosis: evaluation with contrast-enhanced MR imaging. *AJNR Am J Neuroradiol.* 1991;12(6):1227–1233.
12. Shah R, Roberson GH, Curé JK. Correlation of MR imaging findings and clinical manifestations in neurosarcoidosis. *AJNR Am J Neuroradiol.* 2009;30(5):953–961.
13. Grand S, Hoffmann D, Bost F, et al. Case report: pseudotumoral brain lesion as the presenting feature of sarcoidosis. *Br J Radiol.* 1996;69(819):272–275.
14. Kimball MM, Wind JJ, Codispoti KE, et al. Neurosarcoidosis presenting as an isolated intrasellar mass: case report and review of the literature. *Clin Neuropathol.* 2010;29(3): 156–162.
15. Uruha A, Koide R, Taniguchi M. Unusual presentation of sarcoidosis: solitary intracranial mass lesion mimicking a glioma. *J Neuroimaging.* 2011;21(2):e180–e182.
16. Veres L, Utz JP, Houser OW. Sarcoidosis presenting as a central nervous system mass lesion. *Chest.* 1997;111(2):518–521.
17. Cunningham JA. Characteristics of stellate inclusions in giant cells and the associated tissue reactions. *Am J Pathol.* 1951;27(5):761–781.
18. Markert JM, Powell K, Tubbs RS, et al. Necrotizing neurosarcoid: three cases with varying presentations. *Clin Neuropathol.* 2007;26(2):59–67.
19. Tali ET, Atilla S, Keskin T, et al. MRI in neuro-Behçet's disease. *Neuroradiology.* 1997; 39(1):2–6.
20. Lee SH, Yoon PH, Park SJ, et al. MRI findings in neuro-Behçet's disease. *Clin Radiol.* 2001;56(6):485–494.
21. Arai Y, Kohno S, Takahashi Y, et al. Autopsy case of neuro-Behçet's disease with multifocal neutrophilic perivascular inflammation. *Neuropathol.* 2006;26(6):579–585.
22. Shintaku M, Kaneda D. Binucleated neurons in the pontine nuclei in neuro-Behçet's disease: a study of 3 autopsy cases. *Clin Neuropathol.* 2012;31(5):379–385.
23. Matsushima M, Yaguchi H, Niino M, et al. MRI and pathological findings of rheumatoid meningitis. *J Clin Neurosci.* 2010;17(1):129–132.
24. Seror R, Mahr A, Ramanoelina J, et al. Central nervous system involvement in Wegener granulomatosis. *Medicine (Baltimore).* 2006;85(1):54–65.
25. Azuma N, Katada Y, Nishimura N, et al. A case of granuloma in the occipital lobe of a patient with Wegener's granulomatosis. *Mod Rheumatol.* 2008;18(4):411–415.
26. Berlis A, Petschner F, Bötefür IC, et al. Wegener granuloma in the fourth ventricle. *AJNR Am J Neuroradiol.* 2003;24(3):523–525.
27. Jennings JE, Sundgren PC, Attwood J, et al. Value of MRI of the brain in patients with systemic lupus erythematosus and neurologic disturbance. *Neuroradiology.* 2004;46(1): 15–21.
28. Delalande S, de Seze J, Fauchais AL, et al. Neurologic manifestations in primary Sjögren syndrome: a study of 82 patients. *Medicine.* 2004;83(5):280–291.

29. de la Monte SM, Hutchins GM, Gupta PK. Polymorphous meningitis with atypical mononuclear cells in Sjögren's syndrome. *Ann Neurol.* 1983;14(4):455–461.
30. Chang Y, Horoupian DS, Lane B, et al. Inflammatory pseudotumor of the choroid plexus in Sjögren's disease. *Neurosurgery.* 1991;29(2):287–290.
31. Kothbauer KF, Jallo GI, Siffert J, et al. Foreign body reaction to hemostatic materials mimicking recurrent brain tumor. Report of three cases. *J Neurosurg.* 2001;95(3):503–506.
32. Ito H, Onishi H, Shoin K, et al. Granuloma caused by oxidized cellulose following craniotomy. *Acta Neurochir (Wien).* 1989;100(1–2):70–73.
33. Sandhu GS, Elexpuru-Camiruaga JA, Buckley S. Oxidized cellulose (Surgicel) granulomata mimicking tumour recurrence. *Br J Neurosurg.* 1996;10(6):617–619.
34. Ribalta T, McCutcheon IE, Neto AG, et al. Textiloma (gossypiboma) mimicking recurrent intracranial tumor. *Arch Pathol Lab Med.* 2004;128(7):749–758.
35. Ruben JD, Dally M, Bailey M, et al. Cerebral radiation necrosis: incidence, outcomes, and risk factors with emphasis on radiation parameters and chemotherapy. *Int J Radiat Oncol Biol Phys.* 2006;65(2):499–508.
36. Asao C, Korogi Y, Kitajima M, et al. Diffusion-weighted imaging of radiation-induced brain injury for differentiation from tumor recurrence. *AJNR Am J Neuroradiol.* 2005; 26(6):1455–1460.
37. Tie J, Gunawardana DH, Rosenthal MA. Differentiation of tumor recurrence from radiation necrosis in high-grade gliomas using 201Tl-SPECT. *J Clin Neurosci.* 2008;15(12): 1327–1334.
38. Thompson TP, Lunsford LD, Kondziolka D. Distinguishing recurrent tumor and radiation necrosis with positron emission tomography versus stereotactic biopsy. *Stereotact Funct Neurosurg.* 1999;73(1–4):9–14.
39. Chernov M, Hayashi M, Izawa M, et al. Differentiation of the radiation-induced necrosis and tumor recurrence after gamma knife radiosurgery for brain metastases: importance of multi-voxel proton MRS. *Minim Invasive Neurosurg.* 2005;48(4):228–234.
40. Torcuator R, Zuniga R, Mohan YS, et al. Initial experience with bevacizumab treatment for biopsy confirmed cerebral radiation necrosis. *J Neurooncol.* 2009;94(1):63–68.
41. Carpenter J, Stapleton S, Holliman R. Retrospective analysis of 49 cases of brain abscess and review of the literature. *Eur J Clin Microbiol Infect Dis.* 2007;26(1):1–11.
42. Kao PT, Tseng HK, Liu CP, et al. Brain abscess: clinical analysis of 53 cases. *J Microbiol Immunol Infect.* 2003;36(2):129–136.
43. Nielsen H, Gyldensted C, Harmsen A. Cerebral abscess. Aetiology and pathogenesis, symptoms, diagnosis and treatment. A review of 200 cases from 1935–1976. *Acta Neurol Scand.* 1982;65(6):609–622.
44. Lu CH, Chang WN, Lin YC, et al. Bacterial brain abscess: microbiological features, epidemiological trends and therapeutic outcomes. *QJM.* 2002;95(8):501–509.
45. Roche M, Humphreys H, Smyth E, et al. A twelve-year review of central nervous system bacterial abscesses; presentation and aetiology. *Clin Microbiol Infect.* 2003;9(8):803–809.
46. Gropper MR, Schulder M, Sharan AD, et al. Central nervous system tuberculosis: medical management and surgical indications. *Surg Neurol.* 1995;44(4):378–384; discussion 384–375.
47. Vidal JE, Penalva de Oliveira AC, Bonasser Filho F, et al. Tuberculous brain abscess in AIDS patients: report of three cases and literature review. *Int J Infect Dis.* 2005;9(4): 201–207.
48. Sadek M, Yue FY, Lee EY, et al. Clinical and immunologic features of an atypical intracranial mycobacterium avium complex (MAC) infection compared with those of pulmonary MAC infections. *Clin Vaccine Immunol.* 2008;15(10):1580–1589.

49. Peters G, du Plessis DG, Humphrey PR. Cerebral Whipple's disease with a stroke-like presentation and cerebrovascular pathology. *J Neurol Neurosurg Psychiatry.* 2002;73(3):336–339.
50. Rossi T, Haghighipour R, Haghighi M, et al. Cerebral Whipple's disease as a cause of reversible dementia. *Clin Neurol Neurosurg.* 2005;107(3):258–261.
51. Leesch W, Fischer I, Staudinger R, et al. Primary cerebral Whipple disease presenting as Klüver-Bucy syndrome. *Arch Neurol.* 2009;66(1):130–131.
52. Gerard A, Sarrot-Reynauld F, Liozon E, et al. Neurologic presentation of Whipple disease: report of 12 cases and review of the literature. *Medicine.* 2002;81(6):443–457.
53. Schroeder PC, Post MJ, Oschatz E, et al. Analysis of the utility of diffusion-weighted MRI and apparent diffusion coefficient values in distinguishing central nervous system toxoplasmosis from lymphoma. *Neuroradiology.* 2006;48(10):715–720.
54. Cryptococcus neoformans Infection. 2015; https://www.cdc.gov/fungal/diseases/cryptococcosis-neoformans/index.html. Accessed May 8, 2016.
55. Li Q, You C, Liu Q, et al. Central nervous system cryptococcoma in immunocompetent patients: a short review illustrated by a new case. *Acta Neurochir (Wien).* 2010;152(1):129–136.
56. Cryptococcus gattii Infection. 2015; https://www.cdc.gov/fungal/diseases/cryptococcosis-gattii/index.html. Accessed May 8, 2016.
57. Cunliffe CH, Fischer I, Monoky D, et al. Intracranial lesions mimicking neoplasms. *Arch Pathol Lab Med.* 2009;133(1):101–123.
58. Lazcano O, Speights VO, Jr., Strickler JG, et al. Combined histochemical stains in the differential diagnosis of Cryptococcus neoformans. *Mod Pathol.* 1993;6(1):80–84.
59. Drake KW, Adam RD. Coccidioidal meningitis and brain abscesses: analysis of 71 cases at a referral center. *Neurology.* 2009;73(21):1780–1786.
60. Bañuelos AF, Williams PL, Johnson RH, et al. Central nervous system abscesses due to Coccidioides species. *Clin Infect Dis.* 1996;22(2):240–250.
61. Saubolle MA. Laboratory aspects in the diagnosis of coccidioidomycosis. *Ann N Y Acad Sci.* 2007;1111:301–314.
62. Teitelbaum GP, Otto RJ, Lin M, et al. MR imaging of neurocysticercosis. *AJR Am J Roentgenol.* 1989;153(4):857–866.
63. Winn W. Koneman's Color Atlas of Diagnostic Microbiology. Baltimore, MD: Lippincott Williams and Wilkins; 2006:1281–1284.
64. Martinez HR, Rangel-Guerra R, Elizondo G, et al. MR imaging in neurocysticercosis: a study of 56 cases. *AJNR Am J Neuroradiol.* 1989;10(5):1011–1019.
65. Pittella JE. Neurocysticercosis. *Brain Pathol.* 1997;7(1):681–693.
66. Guarner J, Bartlett J, Shieh WJ, et al. Histopathologic spectrum and immunohistochemical diagnosis of amebic meningoencephalitis. *Mod Pathol.* 2007;20(12):1230–1237.
67. Singh P, Kochhar R, Vashishta RK, et al. Amebic meningoencephalitis: spectrum of imaging findings. *AJNR Am J Neuroradiol.* 2006;27(6):1217–1221.
68. Martinez AJ, Visvesvara GS. Free-living, amphizoic and opportunistic amebas. *Brain Pathol.* 1997;7(1):583–598.
69. Clifford DB, De Luca A, Simpson DM, et al. Natalizumab-associated progressive multifocal leukoencephalopathy in patients with multiple sclerosis: lessons from 28 cases. *Lancet Neurol.* 2010;9(4):438–446.
70. Carson KR, Evens AM, Richey EA, et al. Progressive multifocal leukoencephalopathy after rituximab therapy in HIV-negative patients: a report of 57 cases from the Research on Adverse Drug Events and Reports project. *Blood.* 2009;113(20):4834–4840.
71. Post MJ, Yiannoutsos C, Simpson D, et al. Progressive multifocal leukoencephalopathy in AIDS: are there any MR findings useful to patient management and predictive of

patient survival? AIDS Clinical Trials Group, 243 Team. *AJNR Am J Neuroradiol.* 1999; 20(10):1896–1906.

72. Thurnher MM, Thurnher SA, Muhlbauer B, et al. Progressive multifocal leukoencephalopathy in AIDS: initial and follow-up CT and MRI. *Neuroradiology.* 1997;39(9):611–618.
73. Whiteman ML, Post MJ, Berger JR, et al. Progressive multifocal leukoencephalopathy in 47 HIV-seropositive patients: neuroimaging with clinical and pathologic correlation. *Radiology.* 1993;187(1):233–240.
74. Yousry TA, Pelletier D, Cadavid D, et al. Magnetic resonance imaging pattern in natalizumab-associated progressive multifocal leukoencephalopathy. *Ann Neurol.* 2012;72(5): 779–787.
75. Khanna N, Elzi L, Mueller NJ, et al. Incidence and outcome of progressive multifocal leukoencephalopathy over 20 years of the Swiss HIV Cohort Study. *Clin Infect Dis.* 2009;48(10):1459–1466.
76. Marzocchetti A, Tompkins T, Clifford DB, et al. Determinants of survival in progressive multifocal leukoencephalopathy. *Neurology.* 2009;73(19):1551–1558.
77. Greenlee JE, Keeney PM. Immunoenzymatic labelling of JC papovavirus T antigen in brains of patients with progressive multifocal leukoencephalopathy. *Acta Neuropathol.* 1986;71(1–2):150–153.
78. Kennedy PG, Adams JH, Graham DI, et al. A clinico-pathological study of herpes simplex encephalitis. *Neuropathol Appl Neurobiol.* 1988;14(5):395–415.
79. Studahl M, Ricksten A, Sandberg T, et al. Cytomegalovirus encephalitis in four immunocompetent patients. *Lancet.* 1992;340(8826):1045–1046.
80. Kleinschmidt-DeMasters BK, Amlie-Lefond C, Gilden DH. The patterns of varicella zoster virus encephalitis. *Hum Pathol.* 1996;27(9):927–938.
81. Lantos PL, McLaughlin JE, Schoitz CL, et al. Neuropathology of the brain in HIV infection. *Lancet.* 1989;1(8633):309–311.
82. Holman RC, Khan AS, Belay ED, et al. Creutzfeldt-Jakob disease in the United States, 1979–1994: using national mortality data to assess the possible occurrence of variant cases. *Emerg Infect Dis.* 1996;2(4):333–337.
83. Knight R. Creutzfeldt-Jakob disease: a rare cause of dementia in elderly persons. *Clin Infect Dis.* 2006;43(3):340–346.
84. Zerr I, Pocchiari M, Collins S, et al. Analysis of EEG and CSF 14-3-3 proteins as aids to the diagnosis of Creutzfeldt-Jakob disease. *Neurology.* 2000;55(6):811–815.
85. Meissner B, Kallenberg K, Sanchez-Juan P, et al. MRI lesion profiles in sporadic Creutzfeldt-Jakob disease. *Neurology.* 2009;72(23):1994–2001.
86. Collie DA, Summers DM, Sellar RJ, et al. Diagnosing variant Creutzfeldt-Jakob disease with the pulvinar sign: MR imaging findings in 86 neuropathologically confirmed cases. *AJNR Am J Neuroradiol.* 2003;24(8):1560–1569.
87. Brown P, Wolff A, Gajdusek DC. A simple and effective method for inactivating virus infectivity in formalin-fixed tissue samples from patients with Creutzfeldt-Jakob disease. *Neurology.* 1990;40(6):887–890.
88. Tschampa HJ, Neumann M, Zerr I, et al. Patients with Alzheimer's disease and dementia with Lewy bodies mistaken for Creutzfeldt-Jakob disease. *J Neurol Neurosurg Psychiatry.* 2001;71(1):33–39.
89. Paulli M, Bergamaschi G, Tonon L, et al. Evidence for a polyclonal nature of the cell infiltrate in sinus histiocytosis with massive lymphadenopathy (Rosai-Dorfman disease). *Br J Haematol.* 1995;91(2):415–418.
90. Juri G, Jaki -Razumovi J, Rotim K, et al. Extranodal sinus histiocytosis (Rosai-Dorfman disease) of the brain parenchyma. *Acta Neurochir (Wien).* 2003;145(2):145–149; discussion 149.

91. Di Rocco F, Garnett MR, Puget S, et al. Cerebral localization of Rosai-Dorfman disease in a child. Case report. *J Neurosurg.* 2007;107(2 Suppl):147–151.
92. Tian Y, Wang J, Ge Jz, et al. Intracranial Rosai-Dorfman disease mimicking multiple meningiomas in a child: a case report and review of the literature. *Childs Nerv Syst.* 2015;31(2):317–323.
93. Andriko JA, Morrison A, Colegial CH, et al. Rosai-Dorfman disease isolated to the central nervous system: a report of 11 cases. *Mod Pathol.* 2001;14(3):172–178.
94. Tian Y, Wang J, Li M, et al. Rosai-Dorfman disease involving the central nervous system: seven cases from one institute. *Acta Neurochir (Wien).* 2015;157(9):1565–1571.
95. Mirra SS, Tindall SC, Check IJ, et al. Inflammatory meningeal masses of unexplained origin. An ultrastructural and immunological study. *J Neuropathol Exp Neurol.* 1983;42(4):453–468.
96. Brandsma D, Jansen GH, Spliet W, et al. The diagnostic difficulties of meningeal and intracerebral plasma cell granulomas–presentation of three cases. *J Neurol.* 2003;250(11):1302–1306.

3

DIFFUSE GLIOMAS

The WHO classification of brain tumors has undergone great change in the 2016 update to the 4th edition with regard to the diffuse, or infiltrating, gliomas (1). The unifying feature of the entities in this group is their pattern of infiltrative growth, which prevents them from being completely excised and contributes to their inexorably progressive nature. Now, in addition to the classic histomorphologic, phenotypic diagnoses along lines of cell type, there is a further refinement and subcategorization into molecular genetic categories, primarily based on the presence of isocitrate dehydrogenase (IDH) mutations and whether chromosome arms 1p and 19q are deleted, creating a "layered" or integrated genetic and morphologic diagnosis. This approach has improved the correlation between pathologic diagnosis and clinical outcome and has provided a more consistently objective set of variables by which these entities are defined. Furthermore, it has brought closer the once separate categories of diffuse astrocytoma and oligodendroglioma based on their shared genetic characteristics. At the same time, the approach has provided a means to reliably and reproducibly sort the once ambiguous and oftentimes problematic category of mixed oligoastrocytomas discretely into either oligodendrogliomas or astrocytomas, drawing a more sharp and unambiguous border between the two.

Ultimately, the most important large-scale categorization of infiltrating gliomas is whether or not they exhibit *IDH1* or *IDH2* mutations. Broadly speaking, two tumors with identical histologic findings will have significantly different outcomes and responses to treatment if one is IDH mutant and the other is IDH wild type. IDH-mutant infiltrating gliomas do so much better than their wild-type counterparts that IDH-mutant cases of the highest histologic grade often have a better clinical course than the lowest histologic grade of IDH-wild–type cases. Caveat lector: there are rare cases of low-grade diffuse gliomas in children that have their own unique set of genetic findings and are exceptions to this generalization.

If one then separates the infiltrating gliomas into IDH mutant and IDH wild type and then arranges them in order of 1p/19q status and histologic grade, the entities form a rough spectrum of clinical outcomes, with IDH-mutant, 1p/19q codeleted, and histologically low-grade tumors at one end with the best outcomes, and IDH-wild–type, 1p/19q intact, histologically high-grade tumors at the other (Table 3-1). That is the approach taken here in presenting the diffuse gliomas that previously occupied entirely separate

TABLE 3-1 Diffuse Gliomas as Categorized by WHO 2016 Update to 4th Ed. Classification of Tumours of the Central nervous System

IDH Status	1p/19q Status	Histology	Diagnosis	Other Features
IDH mutant	Codeleted	<6 mit/10 hpf, no necrosis or MVP	Oligodendroglioma, IDH mutant, 1p/19q codeleted (WHO grade II)	*TERT* promoter mut.
		≥6 mit/10 hpf, necrosis or microvascular proliferation	Anaplastic oligodendroglioma, IDH mutant, 1p/19q codeleted (WHO grade III)	TERT promoter mut., deletion 9p, MGMTp meth.
		No/rare mitosis	Diffuse astrocytoma, IDH mutant (WHO grade II)	*TP53* mut., *ATRX* mut. MGMTp meth.
	1p/19q intact	Mitosis	Anaplastic astrocytoma, IDH mutant (WHO grade III)	*TP53* mut., *ATRX* mut., gain of 7, LOH 10q, MGMTp meth.
		Necrosis, microvascular proliferation	Glioblastoma, IDH mutant (WHO grade IV)	*TP53* mut., *ATRX* mut., gain of 7, LOH 10q, LOH 19q, MGMTp meth.
		No/rare mitosis	Diffuse astrocytoma, IDH wild-type (WHO grade II [rare])	Uncertain (provisional diagnosis)
IDH wildtype	1p/19q intact	Mitosis	Anaplastic astrocytoma, IDH wildtype (WHO grade III)	Similar to IDH-wildtype glioblastoma
		Necrosis, microvascular proliferation	Glioblastoma, IDH wildtype (WHO grade IV)	LOH 10q, EGFR amp., deletion 9p (p16), *TP53* mut., MGMTp unmeth.
		H3 K27M mutation, any histologic grade	Diffuse midline glioma, H3 K27M mutant (WHO grade IV)	Pons/thalamus/spinal cord, young age *TP53* mut., *PDGFRA* amp., *ACVR1* mut.

MGMTp, MGMT promoter; LOH, loss of heterozygosity.

chapters. In some cases, there are histologic patterns that are associated with one IDH status, but not consistently. To avoid redundancy, those patterns are discussed once under the heading that more typically characterizes them.

IDH-MUTANT INFILTRATING GLIOMAS

Isocitrate Dehydrogenase

IDH is a metabolic enzyme associated with the Krebs or citric acid cycle that converts isocitrate to α-ketoglutarate by removing a carboxylic group. There are at least three isoforms in humans: IDH3 being more in the mitochondria and directly involved in the citric acid cycle, whereas IDH1 and IDH2 are cytoplasmic and not involved directly in the citric acid cycle (2).

In 2008, Parsons et al. published findings of DNA sequencing in glioblastomas, including a recurring point mutation, R132H, in the gene *IDH1* that was associated with younger patient age and improved survival (3). That discovery led to finding *IDH1* and *IDH2* mutations in a large number of infiltrating gliomas, including most lower-grade lesions (4). Greater than 80% of IDH mutations are IDH1 R132H, the rest are other substitutions at codon 132 in *IDH1* or are in codon 172 of *IDH2.* We now understand that IDH mutations are an early, inciting event in gliomagenesis and that those tumors constitute a genetically and clinically distinct group.

The mechanism by which IDH mutations lead to gliomas is through a toxic gain of function in which the mutant protein produces D-2-hydroxyglutarate, an "oncometabolite" that promotes proliferation and induces a globally hypermethylated genome (5,6) In the context of IDH mutation, additional upregulation of telomere lengthening allows the tumor cells to divide indefinitely. Oligodendrogliomas do that through activating mutations in the promoter for the gene *TERT* and astrocytomas through inactivation of *ATRX,* which is an inhibitor of telomere lengthening through the alternative pathway (7,8).

Oligodendroglioma, IDH Mutant, 1p19q Codeleted (WHO Grade II), Anaplastic Oligodendroglioma, IDH Mutant, and 1p19q Codeleted (WHO Grade III)

Oligodendrogliomas constituted approximately 8% of all gliomas in a recent large tumor registry with an annual incidence of about 0.5 per 100,000 person-years, and a 2:1 ratio of grade II to grade III tumors (9). The vast majority of oligodendrogliomas occur in adults during the fourth through sixth decades of life with median ages of around 41 years for grade II tumors and 49 years for grade III (9). As with infiltrating astrocytomas, males have a somewhat higher incidence by a ratio of about 3:2 (10,11). No familial tumor predispositions are specifically linked to oligodendrogliomas. Oligodendrogliomas are rare in children, and only show IDH mutations and 1p19q codeletions occasionally, and then mostly in older children and adolescents, supporting the idea that the vast majority of pediatric "oligodendrogliomas" are in fact a distinct tumor type (12).

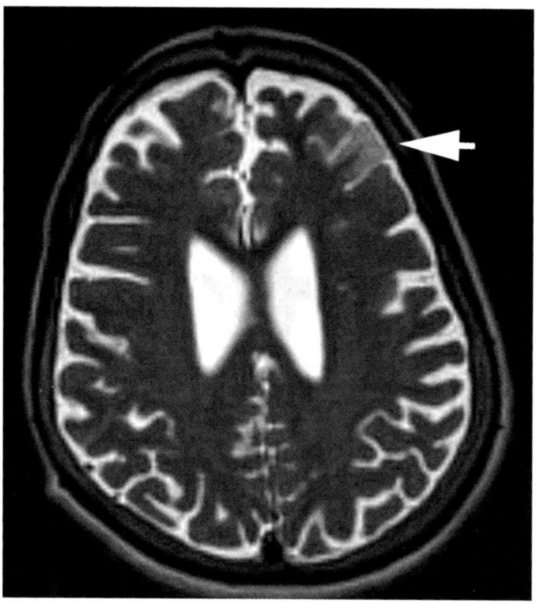

FIGURE 3-1 T2-weighted magnetic resonance imaging (MRI) showing a grade II oligodendroglioma, IDH mutant, 1p/19q codeleted, following the cortical contour, a feature commonly seen in such lesions.

Nearly all oligodendrogliomas arise within the cerebral hemispheres, and most of the rare cases affecting the brainstem, cerebellum, and spinal cord are of unknown IDH status, therefore unconfirmed. Within the hemispheres, the mass typically infiltrates along the cortex, causing expansion and loss of the gray–white matter junction. This corticotropism may explain the high rate of seizures as presenting complaints in oligodendroglioma. Other nonspecific signs and symptoms of mass lesions, such as headache, nausea/vomiting, and focal neurologic deficits, are also common (13,14).

RADIOLOGY. Magnetic resonance imaging (MRI) shows a variably infiltrative intra-axial lesion in the cerebral hemispheres that often is centered in or follows the contours of the cortex. Grade II oligodendrogliomas are generally poorly circumscribed, homogeneously T2/FLAIR hyperintense and T1 hypointense, and without contrast enhancement, whereas grade III cases enhance and tend toward more circumscribed outlines (15). Calcifications are common and are more readily identified on CT imaging. The expanding cortical ribbon seen in MRI of oligodendrogliomas is similar to that of dysembryoplastic neuroepithelial tumor (DNT) (Figure 3-1), even sometimes showing nodularity and satellite lesions.

TREATMENT AND PROGNOSIS. According to CBTRUS registry data, the 5-year survival rate for patients with grade II oligodendrogliomas is about 80%, significantly higher than the 50% for grade II astrocytomas, although these are not all genetically defined cases (9). Data from other series that include IDH status and codeletion also consistently show better survival for oligodendroglioma, albeit by varying margins (16,17). Anaplastic oligodendrogliomas, WHO grade III, have a 5-year survival rate of 55% to 60% (9). There is considerable individual variability in time to progression and overall survival. In the past, age was a powerful predictor of prognosis, with survival being inversely related to age at diagnosis. However, it's unclear whether this difference remains after excluding genetically defined astrocytomas.

Radiation and chemotherapy are effective against oligodendrogliomas, yet the effects are temporary, and even cases with a complete response tend to recur over time and progress to death from disease. Combination chemotherapy is a common and well-established initial treatment for oligodendrogliomas of either grade, consisting of procarbazine, lomustine (CCNU) and vincristine, known by abbreviation as "PCV," although grade II lesions may not be treated at all until recurrence after resection. Temozolomide, the typical chemotherapeutic agent for glioblastomas, is frequently used as a second-line agent for recurrent cases, and is now increasingly being used as a first-line agent, particularly with anaplastic oligodendrogliomas (18). Radiotherapy is additionally used in many cases when there is subtotal resection, anaplasia, or recurrence (19). The exact role of radiation relative to chemotherapy remains undecided in oligodendrogliomas.

HISTOPATHOLOGY. In their classical form, oligodendrogliomas are one of the iconic lesions of neuropathology, such that medical students with modest pathology instruction may recognize them; however, as a morphologic diagnosis, oligodendroglioma has shown great interobserver variability, especially with regard to mixed oligoastrocytic tumors (20). As a result of large collaborative studies of glioma genetics, it is now known that what was previously a "spectrum" diagnosis ranging from pure oligodendroglioma to pure astrocytoma, spanned by a poorly reproducible and ambiguous mixed category, is actually a sharply demarcated, binary distribution with regard to cell type. Oligodendrogliomas are now defined more by their genetic features, specifically IDH mutations and 1p/19q codeletion, than they are by histopathologic ones. Although the vast majority of oligodendrogliomas will have classical features, some will have histologic features that are more astrocytic. Regardless of how astrocytic the morphology appears, an infiltrating glioma with whole-arm 1p/19q codeletion and an IDH mutation is an oligodendroglioma. Below are the typical histologic features of oligodendrogliomas, none of which is present in all cases.

Nuclear features are consistent in oligodendrogliomas and are the most important histologic clue that an infiltrating glioma is oligodendroglial (14,21). Low-magnification views facilitate recognition of the uniformity of tumor nuclei, which is not usually seen in infiltrating astrocytomas. At higher magnification, the nuclei are round with regular contours and

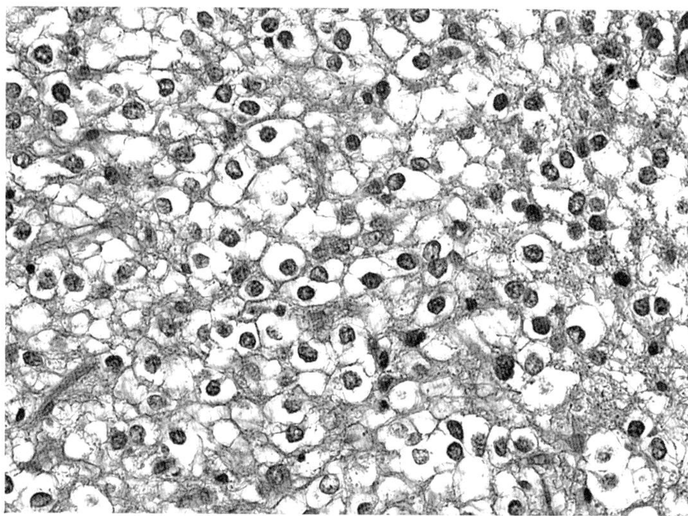

FIGURE 3-2 The typical histologic appearance of oligodendroglioma cells with uniform, round, regular nuclei containing pale chromatin and a single small nucleolus and surrounded by a small "halo."

robustly defined nuclear envelopes. Chromatin density is variable, but usually somewhat pale with a small, visible nucleolus (Figure 3-2). Although the nuclei in the preponderance of oligodendrogliomas exemplify this description, some grade III lesions can have marked atypia, especially following treatment (Figure 3-3).

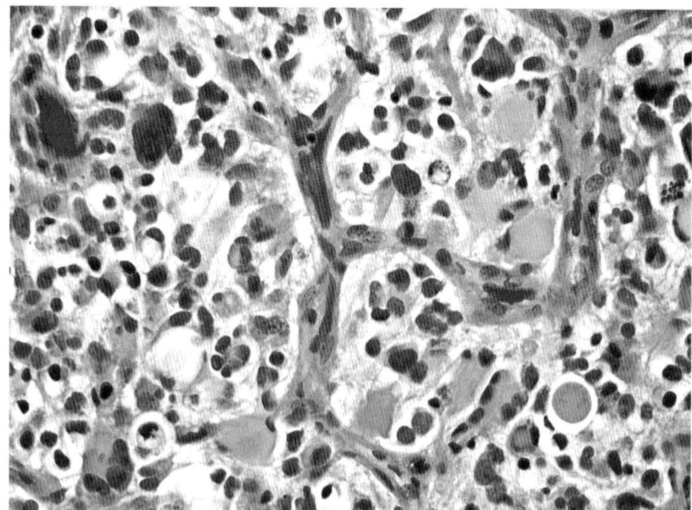

FIGURE 3-3 The uniformity of nuclear features of oligodendrogliomas deteriorates in some anaplastic oligodendrogliomas, but this finding is usually focal.

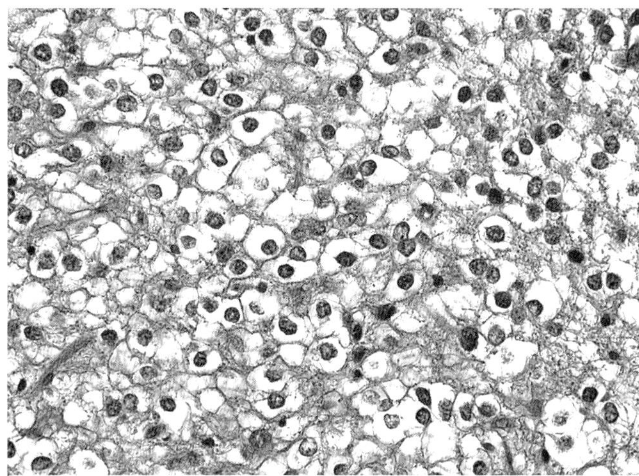

FIGURE 3-4 Cytoplasmic clearing results from delayed fixation and gives the impression of plant-like cell walls when prominent.

The cytoplasm of oligodendroglial cells is classically clear, forming a halo and giving the widely known "fried egg" appearance (Figure 3-4). However, this effect is the result of an autolytic process that is halted when the tissue is either frozen or rapidly fixed, limiting its diagnostic utility. This clearing can also appear in other tumor types, including astrocytomas, ependymomas, neurocytomas, and DNT. Few processes, as the roots *oligo* and *dendro* suggest, extend from the cytoplasm, a trait best seen on crush preparations (Figure 3-5). In some cells, eccentric orbs of eosinophilic

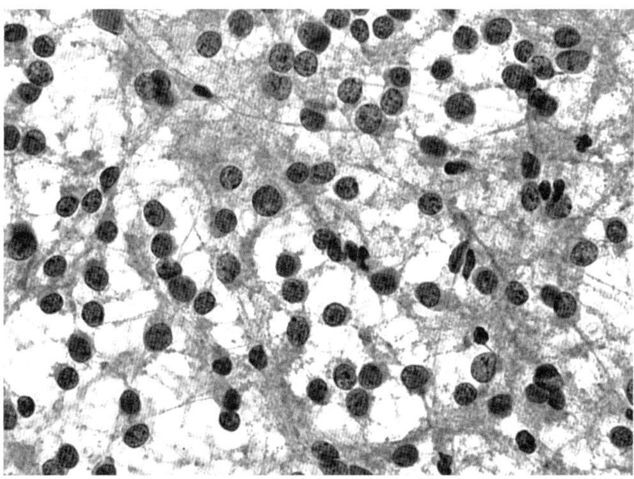

FIGURE 3-5 Smear preparations are necessary to demonstrate the nuclear features of oligodendroglioma at intraoperative consultation. Note the thin rims of cytoplasm and overall lack of cytoplasmic processes.

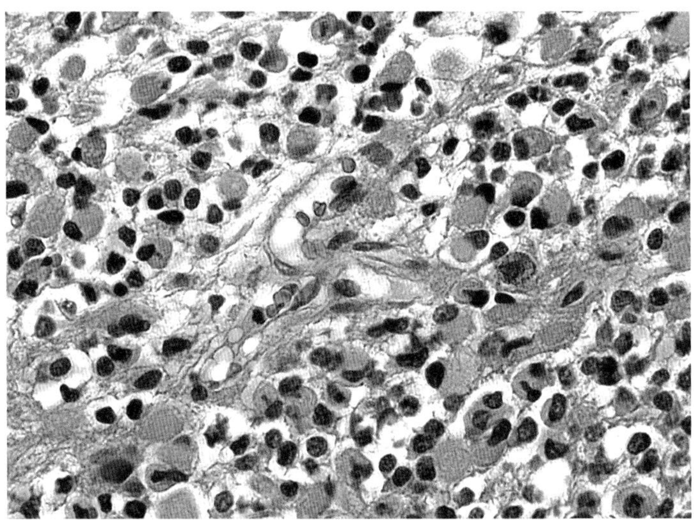

FIGURE 3-6 Minigemistocytes are characterized by process-poor smooth globose eosinophilic cytoplasm that indents the nucleus.

cytoplasm create *mini-* or *microgemistocytes* that resemble gemistocytic astrocytes, except smaller with more monotonous and regular nuclei and scant cytoplasmic processes (Figures 3-6 and 3-7). Occasional cells may contain refractile, GFAP-positive, eosinophilic granules that should not be confused with the eosinophilic granular bodies (EGBs) of pilocytic astrocytoma and ganglioglioma (Figure 3-8) (22).

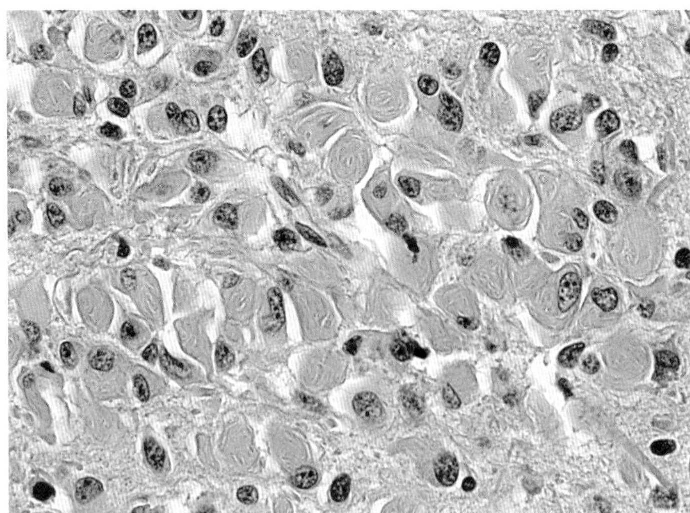

FIGURE 3-7 Some oligodendroglioma cells contain internally coarsely fibrillar cytoplasm but still extend few processes and are sometimes called "gliofibrillary oligodendrocytes."

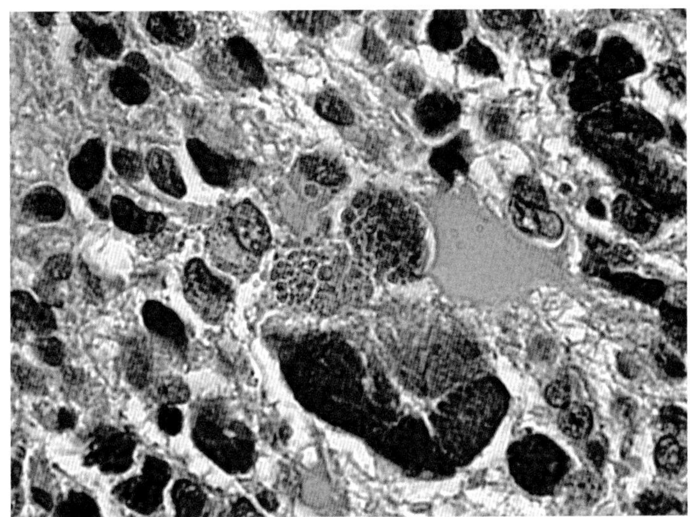

FIGURE 3-8 Scattered cells with eosinophilic granules appear in some anaplastic oligodendrogliomas and should not be confused with the eosinophilic granular bodies of lower-grade lesions.

Several other histologic findings are typical for oligodendrogliomas but are neither necessary nor sufficient for the diagnosis. Calcifications are common and can form among tumor cells (Figure 3-9) or precipitate within tumoral blood vessels. The vasculature comprises anastomosing delicate capillaries that resemble chicken wire or honeycomb (see Figure 3-9). Tumor cells collect along obstructions in their paths of invasion, making *secondary*

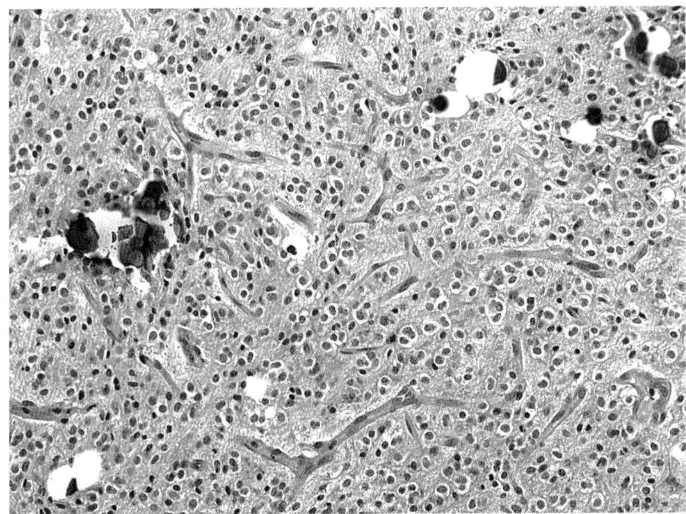

FIGURE 3-9 Many oligodendrogliomas also have a rich capillary vasculature and scattered calcifications.

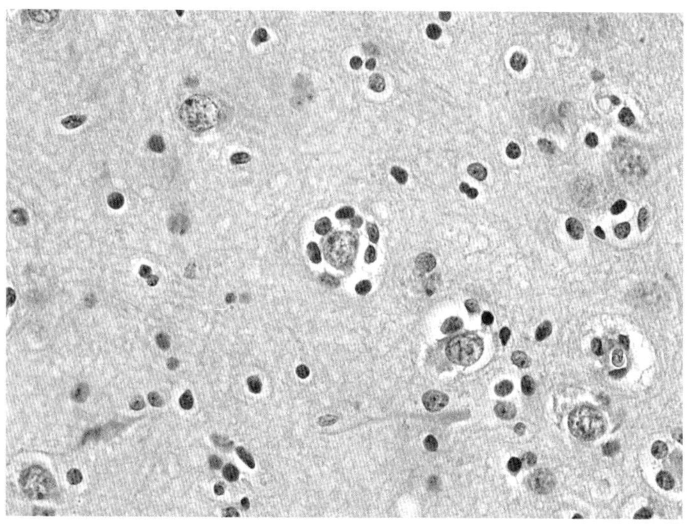

FIGURE 3-10 Perineuronal satellitosis is more characteristic of oligodendrogliomas, but it can also be seen in some infiltrating astrocytomas.

structures, seen as perivascular and subpial aggregates and perineuronal satellitosis (Figure 3-10). An abundant myxoid background is present in some oligodendrogliomas and may pool into microcystic spaces (Figure 3-11).

Occasional oligodendrogliomas show morphologic evidence of neurocytic differentiation, including nucleus-free zones of neuropil and fibrillar rosettes (23).

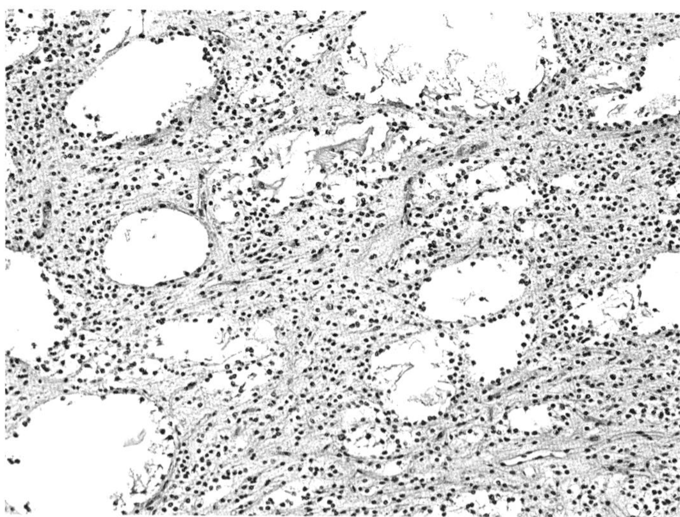

FIGURE 3-11 The mucoid ground substance produced by some oligodendrogliomas pools into microcystic spaces, resembling pilocytic astrocytoma and dysembryoplastic neuroepithelial tumor.

Grade III anaplastic oligodendrogliomas have features similar to their grade II counterparts but have microvascular proliferation or endothelial hypertrophy, necrosis, and/or high mitotic rates. These features are discussed further in the section Grading.

IMMUNOHISTOCHEMISTRY. The three most important immunostains for determining whether an infiltrating glioma is an oligodendroglioma are IDH1 R132H, ATRX, and p53. Greater than 90% of oligodendrogliomas will demonstrate cytoplasmic reactivity for the antibody to the mutant IDH1 protein, the remaining negative cases having alternate, nonimmunoreactive mutations of IDH1 or IDH2. Retained ATRX expression and a wild-type pattern of p53 staining further support the diagnosis of oligodendroglioma, although the latter can rarely be strong and diffuse (mutant pattern).

GFAP is positive in many oligodendrogliomas (~70%) but often only in a subset of cells, including the mini/microgemistocytes and "gliofibrillary oligodendrocytes" which contain a narrow perinuclear rim of staining and scant processes (24,25). The tumor cells also show variable amounts of staining for synaptophysin, ranging from none to strong and diffuse, depending on the specific antibody used. This immunohistochemical evidence of neuronal differentiation in oligodendrogliomas is supported by frequent ultrastructural observation of neurosecretory granules and synapses (26). Other markers of more mature neuronal phenotype, neuronal nuclear antigen (NeuN) and phosphorylated neurofilament, are not seen, although a surprising number react with antibodies against nonphosphorylated neurofilament (27). Neurofilament staining is most useful to demonstrate invasion of native neurons by infiltrating tumor cells. MIB-1 indices are variable, commensurate with the grade of the individual tumor. Nuclear reactivity for p53, a surrogate for *TP53* mutation, is uncommon in oligodendrogliomas and more typical of IDH-mutant astrocytomas (28).

GENETICS. The diagnosis of oligodendroglioma in adults requires the presence of an IDH1 or IDH2 mutation, unless the IDH status is unable to be assessed (see oligodendroglioma, NOS). IDH-wild–type cases diagnosed as oligodendroglioma in pediatric patients are discussed under oligodendroglioma, NOS.

Originally an indicator of prognosis and response to therapy, codeletion of chromosome arms 1p and 19q is now definitional in combination with IDH mutations for the diagnosis of oligodendroglioma (29–31). The codeletion almost always results from a translocation of nearly the entire 1p and 19q arms, t(1;19)(q10;p10), leading to loss of the derivative chromosome, thus deletion of those arms (32). For many years, fluorescence in situ hybridization (FISH) directed at 1p36 and 19q13 was the standard method of identifying 1p/19q codeletion. However, this method also detects small deletions of those loci without loss of the remaining arm. Because of this, FISH detects "codeletion" in other gliomas, such as IDH-wild–type glioblastoma, in approximately 5% of cases. Therefore, such false positives by FISH can result in a small number of IDH-mutant astrocytomas being misdiagnosed as oligodendrogliomas. Although FISH remains an acceptable method for detecting codeletion, other approaches that assess for whole-arm deletion may reduce the incidence of false positives due to focal deletions. Among these are loss of heterozygosity (LOH) by polymerase chain reaction (PCR), comparative genomic hybridization (CGH), or single nucleotide polymorphism (SNP) microarray.

Another genetic feature that is present in almost all cases of oligodendroglioma is activating mutations of the *TERT* promoter, although this finding is not specific (33). *TERT* is the gene for telomere reverse transcriptase, which is a component of the telomerase complex that functions to lengthen the repeat sequences at the ends of chromosomes; the telomeres, thereby increasing the number of times cells can divide. *TERT* promoter mutations in oligodendrogliomas result in higher expression of *TERT.* In the setting of an IDH-mutant infiltrating glioma, the presence of a *TERT* promoter mutation is strongly suggestive of a 1p/19q codeletion. However, *TERT* promoter mutations are also common in IDH-wild–type infiltrating astrocytomas, so diagnostic conclusions based on *TERT* promoter status should only follow thorough assessment of IDH1 and IDH2 mutation status. Even then, *TERT* mutations are also occasionally present in IDH-mutant astrocytomas (16,34).

Other common genetic findings in oligodendrogliomas include inactivating mutations of *CIC, FUBP1,* and *NOTCH1,* which may be present singly or in combination, and at least one of which is present in most cases of genetically defined oligodendroglioma. *FUBP1* and *CIC* are within deleted segments of 1p and 19q, respectively, and mutations in them are extremely rare in other gliomas. *NOTCH1* mutations may be seen in other infiltrating gliomas and are associated with progression in oligodendrogliomas.

TP53 mutations are uncommon in oligodendrogliomas with 1p/19q codeletion and IDH mutations, observed in only a few percent (28,35). Similar to astrocytomas, *CDKN2A* deletions are also common alterations associated with microvascular proliferation and contrast enhancement on MRI (36).

GRADING. Because IDH status was not available for incorporation into older series, looking at histologic grading of oligodendrogliomas, it's unclear to what degree any potential contamination with IDH-wild–type gliomas may have contributed to the conclusions of those studies. Nevertheless, there does appear to be a difference in survival among oligodendroglioma patients based on histologic grade (16,37).

The specific criteria for what constitutes anaplasia in oligodendrogliomas are not rigidly defined in the 2016 WHO update (1). Grade II oligodendrogliomas can show occasional mitotic figures, cytologic atypia, and dense hypercellularity. The minimum 2016 WHO criteria for grade III anaplastic oligodendroglioma are "brisk mitotic activity" and "conspicuous

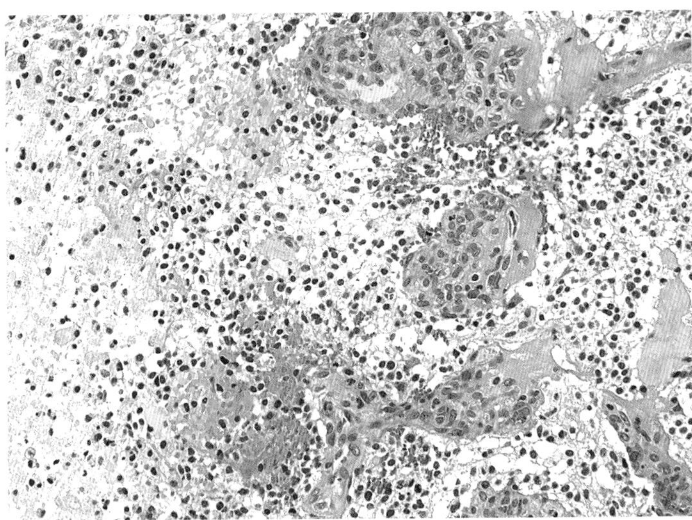

FIGURE 3-12 Vascular proliferation, necrosis, and frequent mitoses are all indications of anaplasia in oligodendrogliomas.

microvascular proliferation," without further definition. Mentioned, but not recommended, is the definition of brisk mitotic activity from a large series supporting the importance of that feature: 6 or more mitotic figures in 10 high-magnification (400×) fields (37). Necrosis, palisading or not, is another criterion for anaplasia that is widely accepted (Figure 3-12). As a soft sign, high-grade examples also commonly develop cytologic features that are more epithelioid, with increased cytoplasm, crisp cytoplasmic borders, and prominent nucleoli. A small number of grade III cases, especially those following treatment, also exhibit marked nuclear pleomorphism and/or coarsely granular tumor cells that resemble EGBs (Figure 3-13). Such nuclear pleomorphism may raise concern for glioblastoma, but oligodendroglial lesions will retain their paucity of fibrillar processes. Palisading of tumor cells around necrosis is uncommon but may occasionally be seen and should not be misconstrued as evidence of glioblastoma in an IDH-mutant, 1p/19q-codeleted tumor.

DIFFERENTIAL DIAGNOSIS. Although rounded nuclei with haloes are typical for oligodendrogliomas, they appear in myriad other CNS neoplasms; therefore, they are by no means specific. The adoption of IDH mutations and 1p/19q codeletion as definitional features in adult oligodendrogliomas has, however, made that diagnosis more objective and simplified the exclusion of morphologic mimics. After one has ruled out IDH mutations and 1p/19q codeletion in an oligodendroglial-appearing tumor, these other entities should be considered.

In children, pilocytic astrocytoma, DNT, and infiltrating astrocytoma are usually in the differential diagnosis with oligodendroglioma; however,

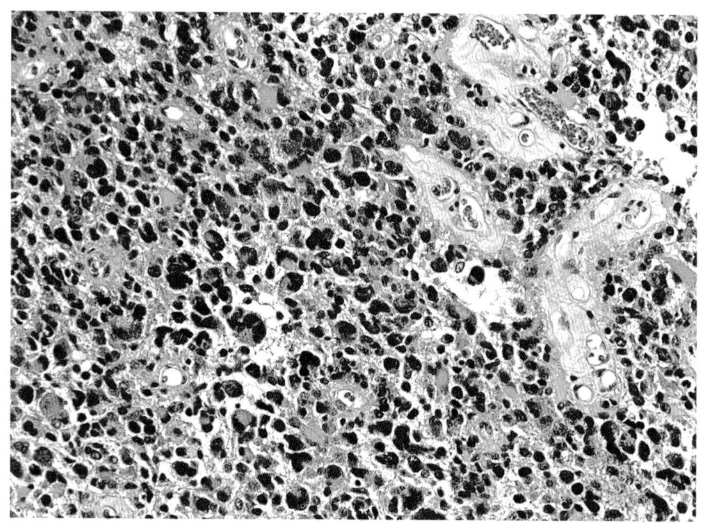

FIGURE 3-13 Striking nuclear pleomorphism in a treated oligodendroglioma. This tumor arose from a WHO grade II, IDH-mutant, 1p/19q codeleted oligodendroglioma years after initial treatment, with long-term survival.

the first two are much more likely in pediatric patients. The haloed round nuclei of DNT can intermingle in an infiltrative pattern with native brain, creating an appearance identical to oligodendroglioma, especially in small samples where more typical areas of DNT are lacking. Even when typical areas are present, myxoid and microcystic backgrounds may be seen in both and can significantly overlap. Nevertheless, several morphologic features can usually distinguish the two: compared with DNT, oligodendrogliomas have more open chromatin and prominent nucleoli, higher proliferation indices, and lack "floating neurons." Evidence of IDH mutation or whole-arm 1p/19q codeletion effectively rules out a diagnosis of DNT, although sample size and cellularity can occasionally make such testing difficult. Mutations or other alterations of FGFR1 and, to a lesser degree BRAF, have been described in DNTs and can support that diagnosis (38,39).

Typical cases with biphasic growth, EGBs, and Rosenthal fibers aside, pilocytic astrocytoma can appear almost identical to oligodendroglioma. These oligo-like cases are more common in the posterior fossa/cerebellum and are usually poorly infiltrative, containing few native axons. Any diagnosis of oligodendroglioma in the posterior fossa of a child that is both low grade and contrast enhancing is dubious, even with a diffuse growth pattern. Identification of a *KIAA1549-BRAF* gene fusion, which is present in most posterior fossa pilocytic astrocytomas, may be helpful in confirming that diagnosis and ruling out oligodendroglioma (40). In both pilocytic astrocytoma and DNT, curable grade I lesions, the distinction from oligodendroglioma is critical.

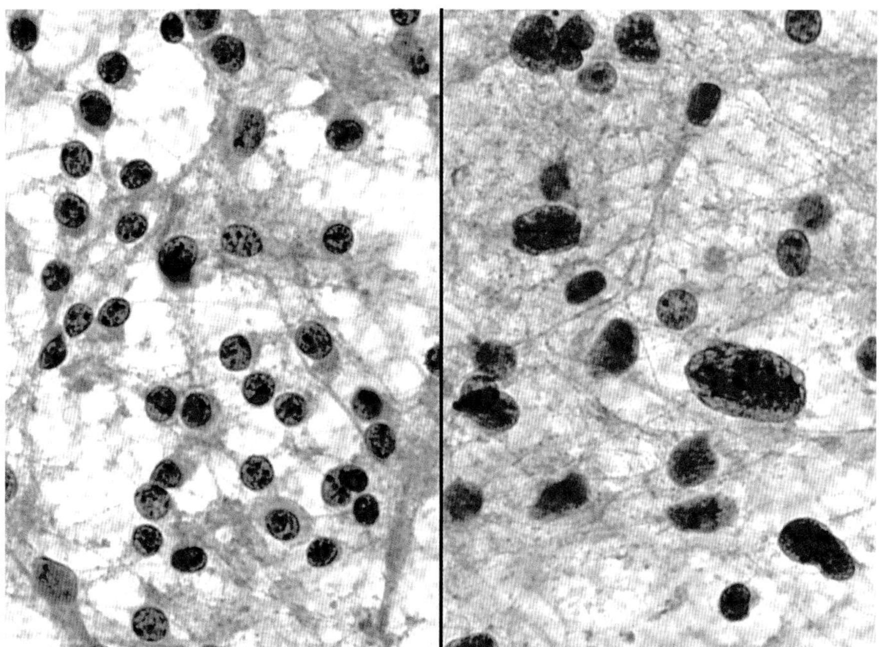

FIGURE 3-14 The classic nuclei of oligodendrogliomas (left) are round, regular, and uniform, whereas those of infiltrating astrocytomas (right) are elongate, irregular, and pleomorphic, seen here in smear preparation.

The distinction of oligodendroglioma from diffuse astrocytoma is now based on genetic characteristics. All infiltrating gliomas, regardless of morphology, should be tested for IDH mutations and 1p/19q codeletion. Morphologically, oligodendrogliomas have monomorphic, round, regular nuclei with open, fine chromatin, and small nucleoli. The nuclei of astrocytomas are more pleomorphic and elongate with irregular contours and denser chromatin. By analogy, the nuclei of oligodendrogliomas are like Florida oranges, and those of diffuse astrocytomas are like Idaho potatoes (Figure 3-14). Small-cell astrocytomas/glioblastomas are an exception and share many histologic features with oligodendroglioma, including monomorphic nuclei, haloes, capillary-rich vasculature, and microcalcifications. Immunostaining can usually strongly suggest oligodendroglioma in the context of the appropriate morphology. IDH1 R132H reactivity with retention of ATRX nuclear staining and lack of strong p53 expression make IDH-mutant astrocytoma highly unlikely.

Patients with long-standing epilepsy may accumulate an excess of nonneoplastic oligodendrocytes, resulting in hypercellular white matter with prominent perivascular accumulations that resemble secondary structures in oligodendroglioma (Figure 3-15). These hyperplastic cells are

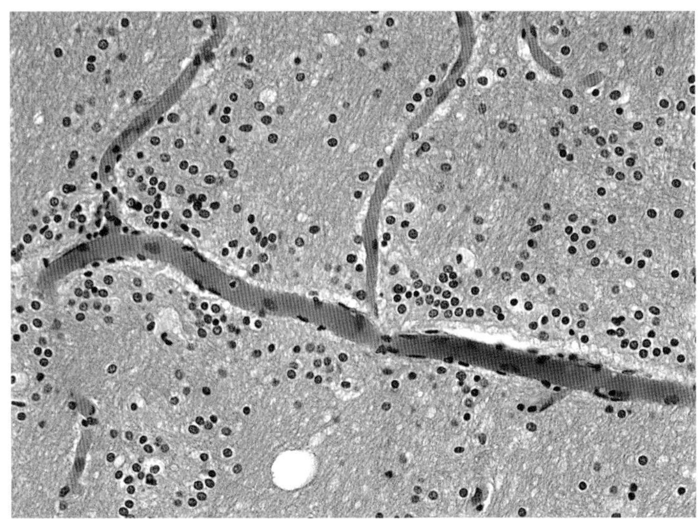

FIGURE 3-15 Nonneoplastic oligodendroglia accumulate in the white matter of patients with long-standing epilepsy, even forming false secondary structures around blood vessels.

indistinguishable from other native oligodendroglia, unlike neoplastic oligodendroglia that usually have slightly larger nuclei. Mitotic figures may even be encountered rarely. MRI showing T2-FLAIR hyperintensity favors a neoplastic lesion. Demonstration of 1p or 19q deletion or mutant IDH1 essentially rules out a reactive process.

Central and extraventricular neurocytomas are similar to oligodendrogliomas in monomorphism and capillary vasculature and are subject to the same perinuclear haloes with delayed fixation. Oligodendrogliomas can occasionally show significant immunoreactivity for synaptophysin, but generally lack anucleate zones of neuropil and fibrillar rosettes, with rare exceptions. Widespread immunoreactivity for NeuN is present in most neurocytomas and only rarely in oligodendrogliomas (41). Neurocytomas with 1p/19q codeletion have been reported, although their IDH status was unknown, so it is unclear whether they could have been oligodendrogliomas with neurocytic differentiation (42).

Diffuse leptomeningeal glioneuronal tumor (DLGT), a rare tumor that is usually low grade and occurs in children, has an oligodendroglial histology, similar immunohistochemical profile, and frequent deletions of 1p and/or 19q by FISH. However, there are no reported cases of this entity with IDH1 mutations and only a minority is 1p/19q codeleted (43,44). Furthermore, most DLGTs show *KIAA1549-BRAF* fusions similar to pilocytic astrocytomas (45).

The clear cell pattern of ependymoma also resembles oligodendroglioma in places, but it is noninfiltrating, has diastase-sensitive cytoplasmic

PAS positivity, and occurs most often in and around the ventricles of children. Most examples will also have areas of more typical ependymoma pattern.

Oligodendroglioma, NOS (WHO Grade II) and Anaplastic Oligodendroglioma, NOS (WHO Grade III)

In some cases with classic oligodendroglioma histology, assessment of IDH and/or 1p/19q status may not be feasible for whatever reason. In such cases, a diagnosis of "oligodendroglioma, NOS" may be issued with the understanding that it is "provisional." Even when immunohistochemistry strongly supports a diagnosis of oligodendroglioma (positive IDH1 R132H and ATRX and wild-type pattern p53), it is not a substitute for 1p/19q status, and the modifier NOS applies (1).

In most pediatric cases diagnosed as oligodendroglioma (WHO grade II), there is neither an IDH mutation nor whole arm 1p/19q codeletion. Although the 2016 WHO tacitly recognizes IDH-wild–type oligodendrogliomas, it is, in my opinion, a diagnosis to be strenuously avoided in children. Available data from sequencing arrays show that IDH-wild–type, grade II oligodendrogliomas in children have a similar set of genetic abnormalities as grade I tumors such as DNT, angiocentric glioma, and rosette-forming glioneuronal tumor (38,46,47). Such grade I lesions may recur over time but are indolent, rarely progress to malignancy and are potentially curable by surgery. A diagnosis of grade II oligodendroglioma, NOS may encourage less aggressive surgery, because such tumors are typically not resectable, increasing the likelihood of eventual recurrence and persistence of seizures, if present. That diagnosis may also result in unnecessary chemotherapy, or even radiation in some cases, both of which carry risk of harm to the patient. Anaplastic IDH-wild–type cases are rare and less controversial as regards treatment, yet there is little evidence beyond subjective morphologic impression that such cases are indeed oligodendrogliomas.

Oligoastrocytoma, NOS (WHO Grade II) and Anaplastic Oligoastrocytoma, NOS (WHO Grade III)

The 2016 WHO discourages use of the term oligoastrocytoma except in rare cases that are morphologically ambiguous and cannot be adequately tested for molecular markers of oligodendroglioma or astrocytoma, such as 1p/19q codeletion, TERT mutation, IDH mutation, ATRX loss, or p53 mutation. As with oligodendroglioma, NOS, it should be understood to be a provisional diagnosis. There are exceptionally rare "dual-genotype" cases in which there are two separate populations that show the genetic findings of oligodendroglioma and astrocytoma (48,49). Such cases could reasonably be called oligoastrocytomas after thorough workup, even though the "dual-genotype" cases explicitly do not constitute an official category in the WHO 2016 update (1).

Diffuse Astrocytoma, IDH Mutant (WHO Grade II) and Anaplastic Astrocytoma, IDH Mutant (WHO Grade III)

CLINICAL CONTEXT. Grade II and III astrocytomas are less common than glioblastomas, making up only about 8% of adult neuroepithelial tumors. Of those, around three-quarters contain a point mutation in the IDH1 or, less commonly, IDH2 gene (50). The incidence of IDH-mutant astrocytomas peaks in the third and fourth decades of life, with no significant differences between grades II and III (51). IDH mutations are rare in the pediatric population and primarily occur in adolescents. There is a modest male predominance for both grades (10,16). The signs and symptoms at presentation vary widely, ranging from acute onset of seizures to subtle and slowly progressive deficits in speech, mentation, movement, etc., sometimes over the course of months. Seizures are the most common presenting sign. IDH-mutant astrocytomas overwhelmingly occur in the cerebral hemispheres, showing a mild predilection for the frontal and temporal lobes, and are rare in the cerebellum, brain stem, and spinal cord. A larger proportion of grade II astrocytomas have IDH mutations than grade III, the latter having a higher frequency of IDH-wild–type cases.

Neuroimaging by magnetic resonance (MR) shows a poorly defined lesion with mild T1 hypointensity and T2 hyperintensity that often advances along white matter tracts (Figure 3-16). Increased T2 signal is thought to mark the presence of edema in areas infiltrated by tumor.

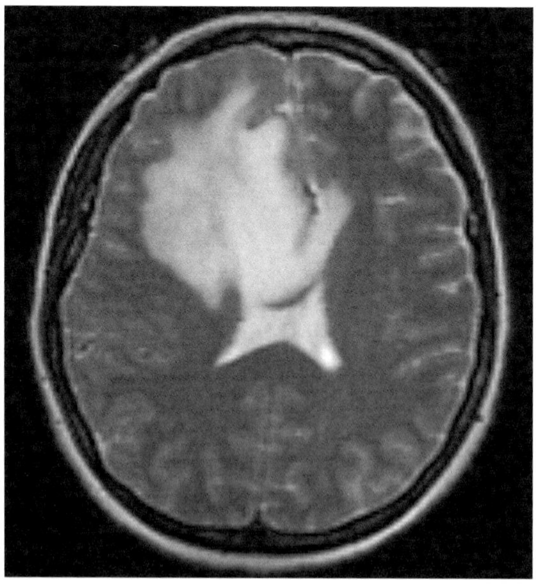

FIGURE 3-16 T2-weighted magnetic resonance imaging (MRI) shows increased signal in areas with higher water content (edema) and demonstrates the extension of grade II astrocytomas through white matter, here reaching to the contralateral hemisphere.

Gadolinium contrast material has no effect in grade II astrocytomas, whereas it causes enhancement in a subset of grade III cases, providing the radiologist a clue to higher grade (52). A lack of contrast enhancement, however, does not rule out the possibility of an anaplastic lesion. The tumor's epicenter usually lies within the white matter. Areas of brain permeated by neoplastic cells are often expanded, causing subtle mass effects on surrounding structures. Spread from one hemisphere to the other along the corpus callosum or a commissure is typical for infiltrating astrocytomas. Circumscription, cyst formation with or without a mural nodule, and contrast enhancement each argue strongly against a grade II astrocytoma. The differential diagnosis on imaging broadens for grade III lesions, but these cases typically present less of a challenge histologically because of their higher cellularity and nuclear pleomorphism.

Therapy protocols for grade II astrocytomas generally include radiation only when symptomatic or when surveillance imaging shows progression. Grade III astrocytomas receive radiotherapy upon diagnosis, sometimes accompanied by temozolomide chemotherapy. The behavior of diffuse astrocytomas is variable, yet virtually all progress in extent and grade over time and are resistant to therapy. Although many patients receive a gross total resection, due to the infiltrative nature of the tumor cells, microscopic residual disease is essentially always present.

In the past, there was a significant difference in survival between grade II and grade III diffuse astrocytomas (28,53–55). However, when segregated by IDH mutation status, the difference in survival among IDH-mutant cases based on WHO histologic grade decreases, around 11 years median overall survival for grade II and 9 years for grade III (51,56). Older series had also indicated a survival advantage in grade II and III astrocytomas for younger patients, although this was likely also due to greater numbers of IDH-wild–type tumors with shorter survival and higher age at diagnosis. There is little correlation with age and survival among IDH-mutant astrocytomas, grades II and III (51).

HISTOPATHOLOGY. The separate sections below are intended only to represent histologic patterns that may be seen in IDH-mutant astrocytomas, in order to facilitate their recognition. The following morphologic patterns are not suggestions for diagnostic terminology and should be taken to represent the variety of histologic appearances among grades II and III IDH-mutant astrocytomas. Diagnoses should be limited to the either **diffuse astrocytoma, IDH mutant (WHO grade II),** or **anaplastic astrocytoma, IDH mutant (WHO grade III).**

FIBRILLARY. The most common histologic pattern of both IDH-mutant and IDH-wild–type astrocytoma is the "fibrillary," which is composed of tumor cell nuclei distributed singly throughout brain parenchyma, imparting varying degrees of hypercellularity. The neoplastic cells most often appear as "naked nuclei" that have little or no discernible fibrillar cytoplasm on routine sections and are generally larger and have more folds and irregular

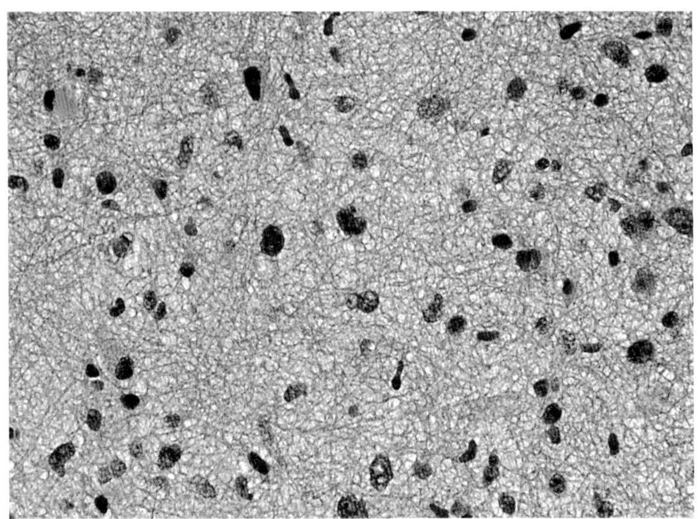

FIGURE 3-17 Grade II infiltrating astrocytomas are usually modestly cellular and contain large and hyperchromatic nuclei with irregular nuclear contours.

contours of the nuclear membrane than their nonneoplastic counterparts (Figure 3-17). The chromatin pattern ranges from the more common hyperchromatic and coarse to the occasional open and smooth. Nucleoli are usually subtle in infiltrating astrocytomas. Sometimes the nuclei lack hyperchromasia, enlargement and irregularity, making their morphologic recognition difficult without complementary methods. Perinuclear clearing, or "haloes," is a typical feature of oligodendrogliomas that can also appear in the cells of astrocytomas. In such cases, nuclear pleomorphism and irregularity favor astrocytic differentiation. By definition, necrosis and endothelial proliferation are absent. The WHO discourages diagnostic use of the term "fibrillary," and it is presented here more for historical context.

Although histologic grading appears not to have as much prognostic value in IDH-mutant astrocytomas, current WHO grading guidelines for them remain in effect (31). According to those guidelines, a single mitotic figure is not sufficient to raise the grade of an infiltrating astrocytoma to grade III. A single instance of mitosis must be considered in the context of the total area of the tissue section; a small needle or endoscopic biopsy may only need one to achieve grade III status, whereas one matters less in a large open biopsy. The rate of Ki-67/MIB1 staining is a useful adjunct to mitotic count in these situations. Correlation with radiology and clinical history may also be helpful. Other "soft" features that indicate grade III astrocytoma include greater degrees of hypercellularity and nuclear pleomorphism than grade II lesions (Figure 3-18).

GEMISTOCYTIC. Astrocytomas frequently produce cells with eccentric pink cytoplasm similar to that of reactive, nonneoplastic astrocytes, or

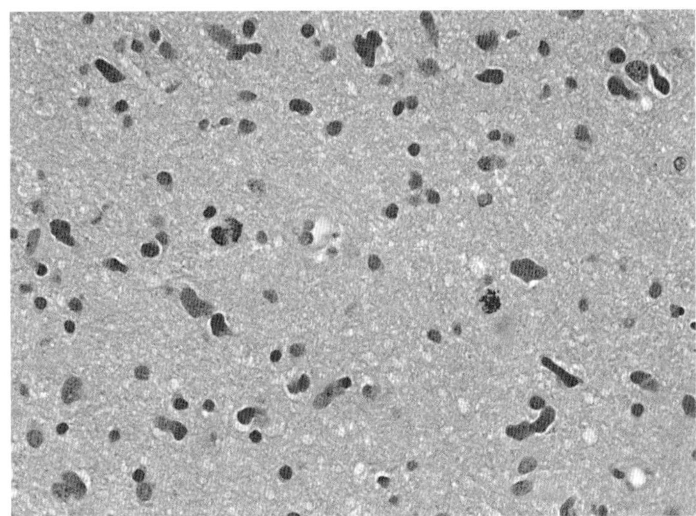

FIGURE 3-18 Mitotic figures are the only histologic feature that separates grade III anaplastic astrocytomas from grade II, although the difference in prognosis is small in IDH-mutant examples.

"gemistocytes." This change appears focally in many infiltrating astrocytomas, but only when an arbitrary threshold of 20% of tumor cells does the term "gemistocytic" apply. Gemistocytic astrocytoma, IDH mutant, is an official variant of IDH-mutant diffuse astrocytoma. Some cases are almost entirely gemistocytic. Analysis of *TP53* mutations has shown the gemistocytes to be neoplastic, but they have a low rate of proliferation and are probably terminally differentiated (57). A second component of smaller neoplastic cells with scant cytoplasm and higher nuclear pleomorphism is thought to drive the progression of this tumor (Figure 3-19). Additional distinguishing features are the presence of perivascular T lymphocytes (~60% of cases) and a higher frequency of *TP53* mutations than other patterns of diffuse astrocytomas (~85% to 90%) (54,58).

Lesions in this category are classically thought to be more aggressive than fibrillary pattern astrocytomas (28,59,60), but that assertion has been challenged (61,62). Although listed among the grade II IDH-mutant diffuse astrocytomas in the 2016 WHO system, gemistocytic astrocytomas may meet criteria for grade III or may lack IDH mutations in around a quarter of cases (63).

In contrast to the fibrillary pattern, gemistocytic lesions have a greater male predominance and occur exclusively in the supratentorial compartment (64). An early report noted a higher frequency of family cancer history in patients with gemistocytic astrocytoma than in those with other astrocytomas (60).

The differential diagnosis of gemistocytic astrocytomas includes reactive gemistocytic lesions and subependymal giant cell astrocytoma (SEGA).

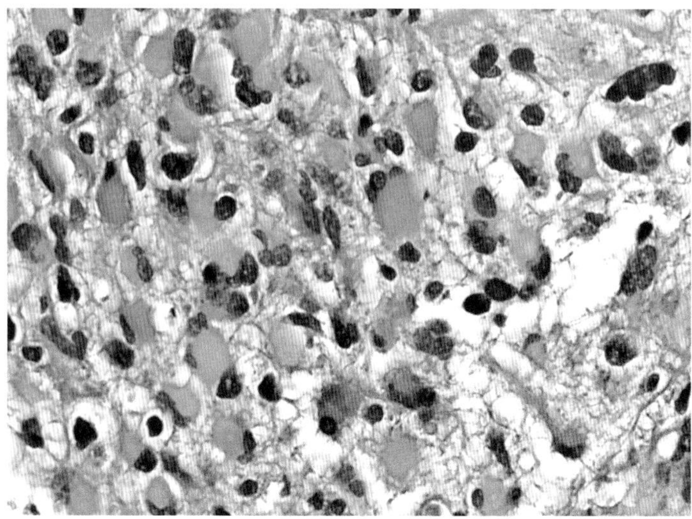

FIGURE 3-19 Gemistocytic astrocytomas have large cells with eccentric, smooth, pink cytoplasm-like reactive astrocytes but with greater nuclear atypia and interspersed anaplastic nuclei with scant cytoplasm.

Reactive gemistocytes tend to have more open chromatin and more prominent nucleoli than neoplastic gemistocytes and are spread more evenly throughout the lesion with long delicate cytoplasmic processes in smear preparations (Figures 3-20 and 3-21). Reactive cells should not show

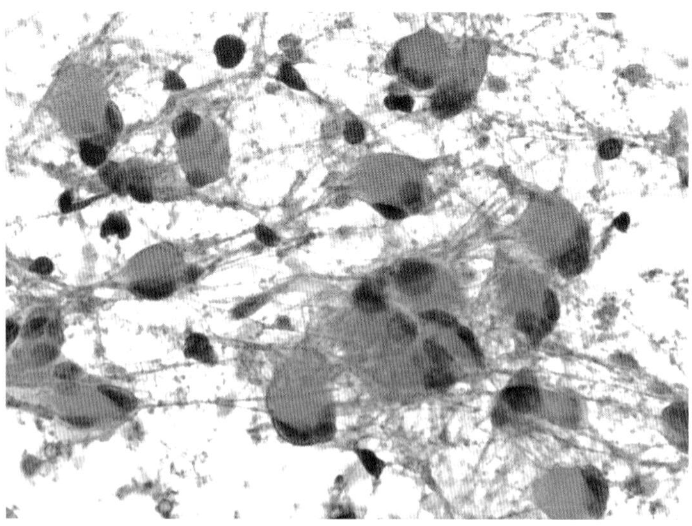

FIGURE 3-20 Neoplastic gemistocytes have fibrillar processes that are fewer, shorter, and less evenly distributed than reactive gemistocytes, causing them to spread more easily on smear preparations.

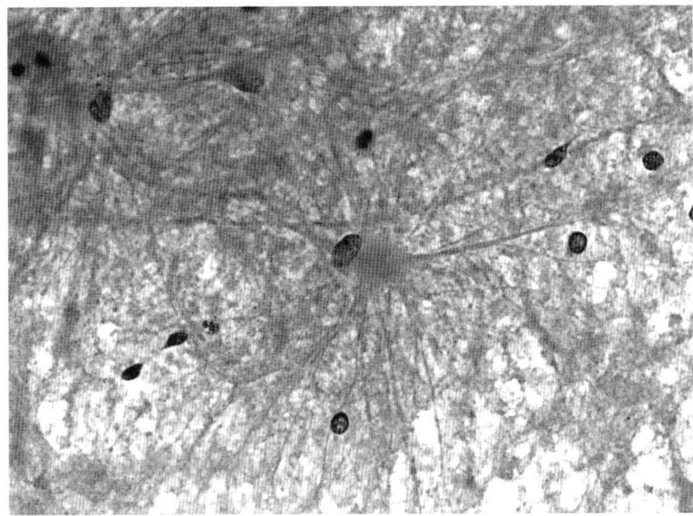

FIGURE 3-21 Reactive astrocytes have long and delicate cytoplasmic extensions that are evenly distributed around the cell, as seen here in smear preparation.

strong positivity for p53, or any expression of IDH1 R132H. Although SEGA may appear histologically similar to gemistocytic astrocytoma, its exophytic, circumscribed, intraventricular growth pattern is not seen in the latter. SEGA also tends to have more ganglioid nuclei with open chromatin and large nucleoli. Reactivity for p53 or IDH R132H also strongly favors gemistocytic astrocytoma over SEGA.

PROTOPLASMIC. This pattern is an uncommon part of the normal histologic variability of diffuse astrocytomas. Although no specific review of IDH mutations in protoplasmic astrocytomas has been published, the presence of p53 staining in some cases suggests the presence of IDH mutation. The low-power pattern of microcysts with a mucinous background is similar to that of DNT, as well as some oligodendrogliomas and pilocytic astrocytomas (Figure 3-22). The nuclei retain the pleomorphism, irregularity, and hyperchromasia typical of other infiltrating astrocytomas. The tumor is so named because its cells resemble the small "protoplasmic" astrocytes of the cortex, with smaller nuclei and scant cytoplasm with fewer processes. Only a few examples are documented, most showing low MIB1 proliferation indices (<5%). A minority are positive for p53 (65). Survival has been favorable in the few reported cases, and no grade III examples have been described (66).

NEUROPIL-LIKE ISLANDS. A small number of infiltrating astrocytomas contain round to oval areas of cortical fibrillarity surrounded by, or containing, monotonous small round cells (Figure 3-23). These areas and cells are positive for synaptophysin and negative for GFAP by immunohistochemistry. The remaining infiltrating glial component is morphologically similar

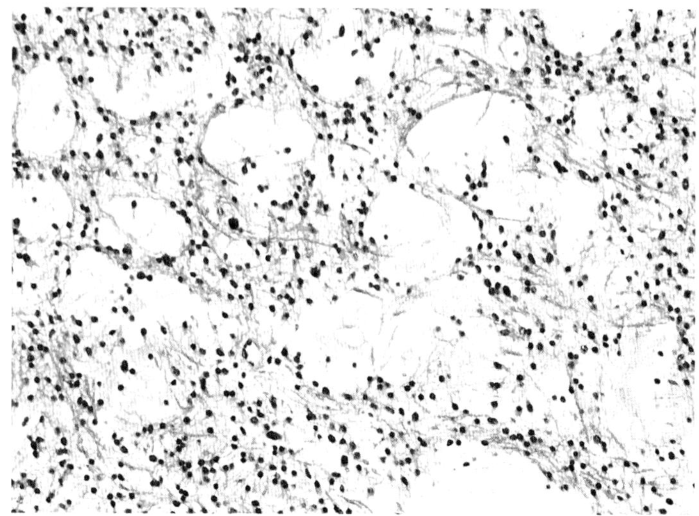

FIGURE 3-22 Some IDH-mutant astrocytomas have a myxoid appearance with microcysts, a pattern classically referred to as "protoplasmic" after the small, protoplasmic astrocytes of the cortex.

to infiltrating astrocytoma and expresses GFAP. Formerly considered a specific named pattern of infiltrating astrocytoma, "glioneuronal tumor with neuropil-like islands," it has been demonstrated that such lesions generally have evidence of IDH, TP53, and ATRX mutations, thus are a part of the histologic variety seen in IDH-mutant astrocytomas (67). One may also rarely see this pattern in IDH-wild–type astrocytomas.

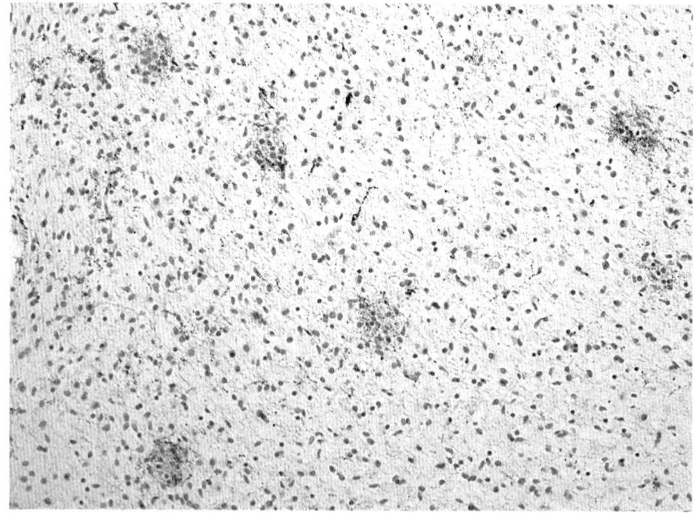

FIGURE 3-23 Synaptophysin immunostaining highlights foci of neuronal differentiation in some diffuse gliomas.

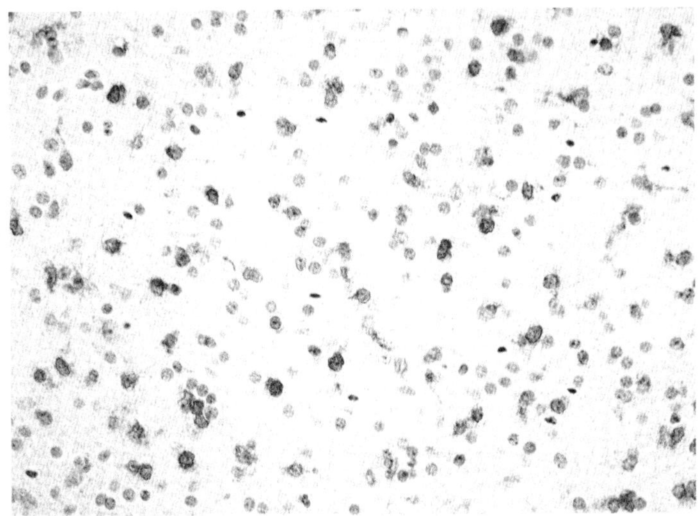

FIGURE 3-24 Monoclonal antibodies to IDH1 R132H reliably show cytoplasmic reactivity in IDH1-mutant tumors with the R132H allele.

IMMUNOHISTOCHEMISTRY AND ANCILLARY TESTING. Immunostains are essential to quickly and accurately categorize infiltrating gliomas. By definition, all IDH-mutant astrocytomas must harbor a mutation in either the *IDH1* or *IDH2* genes. The vast majority, around 90%, of these will be the *IDH1* R132H allele, the protein product of which has two reliable, commercially available antibodies (68). These antibodies (clones H09 and HMab-1) are standard for initial assessment of IDH status in infiltrating gliomas and are specific enough that positive staining is sufficient by itself as evidence of the mutation (Figure 3-24). However, because the prognosis of IDH-mutant astrocytomas is so much better than IDH-wild type–ones, grade II or III astrocytomas that are negative for the IDH1 R132H immunostain should be worked up further by DNA-based methods to rule out the presence of other IDH1 or IDH2 mutations.

The vast majority (~85% to 90%) of IDH-mutant astrocytomas will also have mutations or deletions of the *ATRX* gene, as will the occasional IDH-wild–type case (16). Because these genetic defects nearly always lead to loss of ATRX protein expression, they are conveniently identify using ATRX antibodies (Figure 3-25). Nonneoplastic endothelia, microglia, and astrocytes, all of which express ATRX, provide an internal positive control for the immunostain. In cases with sparse tumor cells, these background cells can make it difficult to ascertain the tumor cell status. Loss of ATRX immunostaining is very rare in 1p/19q-deleted oligodendrogliomas and provides strong evidence that an IDH-mutant glioma is an astrocytoma.

The vast majority of IDH-mutant astrocytomas also have mutations in the *TP53* gene. Many of those mutations interfere with the normal traffic of the p53 protein from the nucleus into the cytosol, causing accumulation.

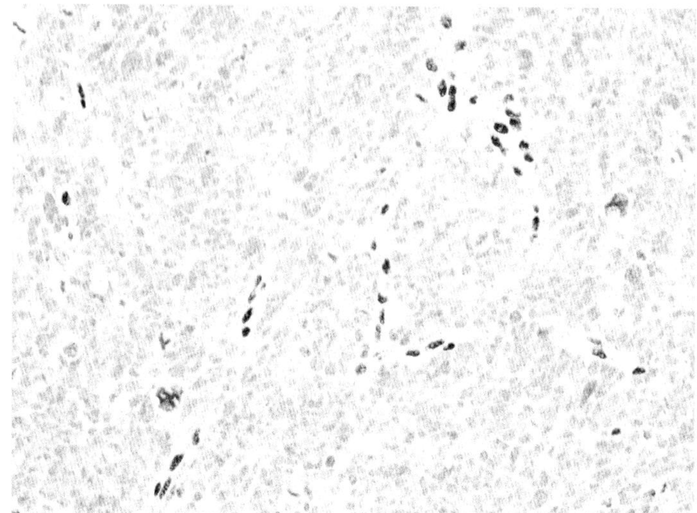

FIGURE 3-25 ATRX immunostaining is a reliable way to identify loss of ATRX expression as a surrogate for *ATRX* mutation and/or deletion.

This nuclear accumulation correlates well with *TP53* mutation and, when strongly and diffusely positive, provides an immunohistochemical marker for neoplastic astrocytes (Figure 3-26). Although some p53 staining has been described in a variety of reactive lesions, it is usually only in scattered cells and mild to moderate in intensity, which is typical of wild-type p53 (69,70). Rarely, a *TP53* mutation can eliminate the antigenicity of the p53

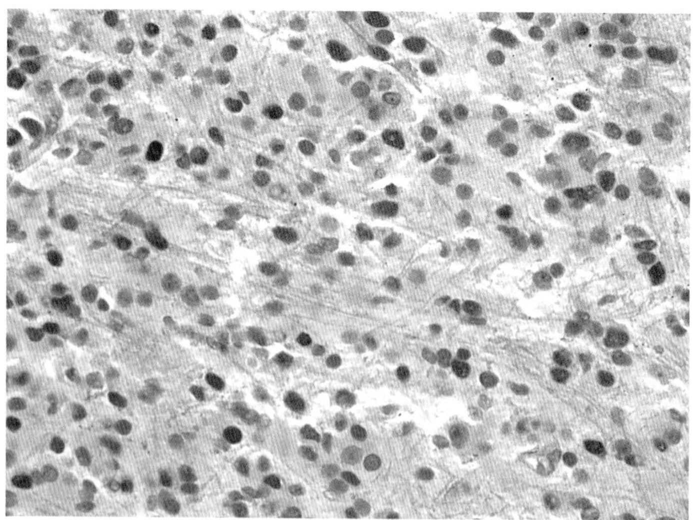

FIGURE 3-26 Strong nuclear p53 reactivity strongly favors that a population of astrocytes is neoplastic.

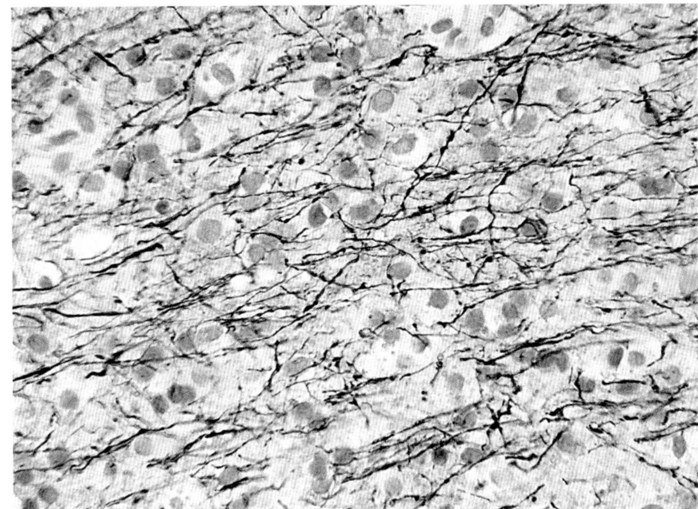

FIGURE 3-27 Neurofilament immunohistochemistry highlights native axons infiltrated by astrocytoma cells.

protein and result in a complete absence of immunostaining in tumor cells. Because it is much lower incidence with 1p/19q codeletion, strong and diffuse (mutation pattern) p53 immunostaining suggests astrocytic differentiation in an infiltrating glioma.

Neurofilament, though not expressed by tumor cells, serves to mark the native axons of the white matter as they are infiltrated by individual tumor cells, indicating the diffuse nature of the lesion (Figure 3-27). In addition to IDH mutation status, chromosome arms 1p and 19q must be intact to render a diagnosis of IDH-mutant astrocytoma. Many cases, probably most, are evaluated for 1p19q codeletion by FISH, which is a well-established and generally reliable method. However, the codeletion associated with oligodendrogliomas results in whole arm losses, and the FISH probes will occasionally (~5%) give a false positive when smaller interstitial deletions only eliminate the probe loci. In such cases, astrocytoma-pattern p53 and ATRX immunostaining will usually suggest that a more comprehensive evaluation of the chromosome arms is needed, for instance by SNP microarray or array CGH.

Glioblastoma, IDH Mutant (WHO Grade IV)

IDH mutations are present in only about 5% to 10% of glioblastomas, those representing what previously were frequently called "secondary" glioblastomas, or those that arose from lower-grade infiltrating astrocytomas. In most cases there is a previously biopsied lower-grade lesion, yet there are certainly also documented cases of de novo IDH-mutant glioblastoma. The differences between IDH-mutant and IDH-wild–type glioblastomas parallel those of the lower-grade infiltrating astrocytomas; those with IDH mutations occur in younger patients, have better prognosis, and respond better to therapy (4,71). In fact, IDH-mutant glioblastomas have exhibited better survival than lower histologic grade IDH-wild–type astrocytomas in at least one series (72). Compared to IDH-wild–type glioblastomas, IDH-mutant cases have a survival around twice as long, 31 months versus 15 months in one series (4). Whereas survival differences between grade II and grade III IDH-mutant astrocytomas are modest, there is a significant decrease in survival rates with grade IV histology (73).

In addition to having a lower median age, one series showed IDH-mutant glioblastomas to have a greater tendency to arise in the frontal lobes and to be incompletely contrast enhancing on MRI when compared to IDH-wild–type cases (74). IDH mutations are rare in glioblastoma patients over the age of 55 (75).

Histologically, IDH-mutant glioblastomas are generally indistinguishable from IDH-mutant ones. One large series showed lower amounts of necrosis, particularly of the palisading type, in mutant cases (74).

Conceptually, IDH-mutant glioblastoma is merely a higher histologic grade of IDH-mutant astrocytoma and shares the cardinal genetic features of the lower-grade tumors. Specifically, most IDH-mutant glioblastomas also have inactivating *TP53* and *ATRX* mutations (76). However, IDH-mutant glioblastomas usually have additional genetic features that correlate with their higher-grade histology, the most consistent of which is deletion of 10q, which contains the PTEN gene (see IDH-wild–type glioblastoma) (73). Deletion of 9p (*CDKN2A/B*) and gains involving EGFR may also be seen, though at lower rates than in IDH-wild–type glioblastoma (71).

IDH-WILD–TYPE INFILTRATING GLIOMAS

Diffuse Astrocytoma, IDH Wild Type (WHO Grade II) and Anaplastic Astrocytoma, IDH Wild Type (WHO Grade III)

The clinical and neuroimaging context of IDH-wild–type infiltrating astrocytomas overlaps with that of IDH-mutant cases, except that the IDH-wild–type patients are older and have a worse prognosis. Of astrocytomas that are IDH wild type, most of those are glioblastomas. Of those remaining, approximately 80% are histologically grade III. However, the converse is not true; given a grade III anaplastic astrocytoma, only about 20% of those will be IDH wild type. IDH-wild–type grade II astrocytomas are rare and many times reflect nonrepresentative sampling of the lesion.

Extensive infiltration of the brain, including three or more lobes, justifies the use of the term "**gliomatosis cerebri**," a clinicopathologic diagnosis that more reflects the wide distribution of tumor rather than a distinct tumor type. Although many glioblastomas would technically meet criteria for affecting three lobes, gliomatosis cerebri is generally taken to mean a subtle infiltration without a distinct mass. IDH mutations are found in cases of "gliomatosis cerebri" with a solid component (77). Imaging by computed tomography (CT) often fails to identify the process, but the edema evoked by the invading tumor cells can usually be identified on T2/FLAIR MR sequences.

IDH-wild–type infiltrating astrocytomas are morphologically indistinguishable from IDH-mutant ones. Differences in immunohistochemical profiles reflect the genetic differences between IDH-wild–type and mutant astrocytomas. In addition to lacking mutant IDH expression, the vast majority of IDH-wild–type infiltrating astrocytomas show a pattern of weak p53 expression (wild type) and retention of nuclear ATRX staining. Infiltrating astrocytomas in children and young adults that involve midline structures such as the thalami, brain stem, and spinal cord usually express the K27M-mutant form of the histone H3 protein, in which case they are diagnosed as "diffuse midline glioma, H3 K27M mutant (WHO grade IV)."

To limit redundancy, and because IDH-wild–type infiltrating astrocytomas are genetically and clinically more similar to IDH-wild–type glioblastomas, the specific histologic and genetic variations of those two diagnoses are discussed together in the following section.

Because they lack consistent expression of specific immunohistochemical markers, IDH-wild–type astrocytomas can be more challenging to identify when cells are sparse. Most cases are histologically high grade and for that reason not problematic from a morphology standpoint.

Glioblastoma, IDH Wild Type (WHO Grade IV)

GENERAL. The general concept of IDH-wild–type glioblastoma is essentially that of the classic, archetypal, primary glioblastoma that affects older adults, arises de novo in the hemispheres, and is inexorably aggressive, causing death in around 1 year. Such classic cases are the vast majority of IDH-wild–type glioblastomas, yet there is a good deal of genetic heterogeneity among those cases, and even among small subgroups with very different clinical and genetic profiles. Although the histopathology of these groups overlaps to a high degree, important differences in their biology continue to be discovered and may result in further subdivisions being incorporated into clinical practice.

CLINICAL CONTEXT. IDH-wild–type glioblastoma is one of the most common surgical neuropathology specimens, constituting almost half of primary intra-axial neoplasms (10). There is a bimodal age distribution of IDH-wild–type glioblastomas, with most occurring after 60 years of age and a smaller number arising in childhood, although the two groups are genetically distinct outside of having no IDH mutations (4,10).

One established risk factor for developing glioblastoma, nearly all of which are IDH wild type, is exposure to ionizing radiation. Many such patients receive radiotherapy for other intracranial processes, such as craniopharyngioma, medulloblastoma, or acute lymphoblastic leukemia. In the past, a tragically large number of radiation-associated glioblastomas occurred in patients who had received scalp irradiation for treatment of tinea capitis, a practice now abandoned (78). The resulting astrocytomas generally occur several years after radiation and have a clinical and genetic profile similar to other de novo glioblastomas (79).

Patients with DNA mismatch repair enzyme defects and hereditary nonpolyposis colon cancer (HNPCC) may be at higher risk than the general population for developing glioblastoma (80). This association of colorectal neoplasia and brain tumors is the Turcot clinical syndrome, the majority of which represent *APC* gene mutations with polyposis and medulloblastoma. The minority, with *MLH1*, *MSH2/6*, or *PMS2* gene mutations (microsatellite instability) and fewer polyps, tend to develop glioblastoma.

Although most IDH-wild–type glioblastomas arise in the cerebral hemispheres, they may occur anywhere in the neuraxis. Hemispheric lesions are usually situated in the subcortical white matter, with extension into the adjacent cortex and spread along white matter tracts. In some instances, multiple discrete lesions will be present, suggesting metastatic disease. These "multifocal" glioblastomas most likely represent growth of tumor cells that have already migrated away from the tumor epicenter and not multiple independent processes. The diagnosis of glioblastoma in this situation is sometimes unanticipated by the clinical team who are expecting metastatic disease. Brainstem and spinal cord locations are more common in children, where they are likely to belong to the new WHO category of malignant glioma, "diffuse midline glioma, H3 K27M mutant," some of which have glioblastoma histology. Occasionally, glioblastomas will show roughly symmetric bilateral masses that are bridged by infiltrated white matter, classically referred to as a butterfly glioma, due to the outline of the lesion when sectioned or on neuroimaging.

The classic radiologic description of glioblastoma is that of a ring-enhancing mass, referring to the irregular rim of contrast enhancement that surrounds the nonenhancing, necrotic tumor core (Figure 3-28).

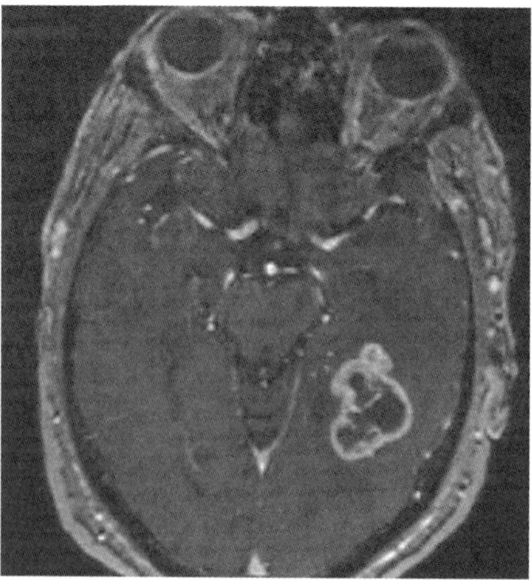

FIGURE 3-28 T1-weighted, contrast-enhanced magnetic resonance imaging (MRI) shows an irregular rim of enhancement around the necrotic core of this typical glioblastoma.

TABLE 3-2 Diagnostic Considerations: Ring-Enhancing Lesion on Neuroimaging

Diagnosis	Distinguishing Feature(s)
Glioblastoma	Infiltrative, palisading necrosis, tumor cells fibrillar on smear
Metastasis	Sharp tumor-brain interface, cohesive polygonal cells on smear
Lymphoma	Perivascular distribution, noncohesive nonfibrillar tumor cells on smear
Demyelinating lesion	Macrophages plus perivascular lymphoplasmacytic infiltrate
Abscess, bacterial	Neutrophils, firm wall with fibroblastic cells
Abscess, toxoplasma	Hypocellular necrosis, occasional pseudocysts filled with bradyzoites
Radiation necrosis	Hyalinized vessels and hemosiderin in background of hypocellular necrosis and reactive astrocytosis

Although there are subtle differences in appearance, a ring-enhancing lesion raises the differential diagnosis of glioblastoma, metastasis, lymphoma, abscess, or demyelinating lesion (Table 3-2). If the lesion has an infiltrative border, extensive surrounding edema, and extension along, or enlargement of white matter tracts, glioblastoma is strongly favored. Multifocality and superficial location favor a metastatic process, whereas an incomplete ring of enhancement is characteristic of a demyelinating lesion. Abscesses usually display "restricted diffusion" of their core material on diffusion-weighted images by MRI, meaning that the water molecules in that area undergo less Brownian motion than the surrounding tissue, that is, their diffusion is restricted. This finding is present in many abscesses but is not specific, being also seen in occasional metastases and acute demyelinating lesions (81). Primary CNS lymphoma (PCNSL) does not have any findings that necessarily differentiate it from glioblastoma, although it is more often multifocal and periventricular. None of the above imaging findings is specific; glioblastoma will occasionally be suspected to be each of the other entities on the radiologic examination and vice versa.

Extracranial metastases from glioblastoma are rare, occurring in less than 1% of cases. Most reported examples arise postsurgically, possibly due to contamination of the dural or scalp lymphatics, with viable tumor. The most common recipients of metastatic glioblastoma are the cervical lymph nodes, although a variety of target organs have been reported, including small intestine (82), liver (83), lung, and bone marrow (84). It is extremely rare, but a handful of glioblastomas have been reported to spontaneously metastasize without surgical manipulation. Gliosarcomas may have a higher rate of extracranial metastasis than other glioblastoma patterns (85). Occasional cases of peritoneal gliomatosis due to metastatic seeding through a ventriculoperitoneal shunt have been reported and may be more common in children (86).

Leptomeningeal dissemination follows surgical intervention in a fraction of intraparenchymal glioblastomas, but rare patients may present with a primary leptomeningeal tumor with no identifiable intraparenchymal component (87,88). Imaging shows a plaque-like or diffuse meningeal thickening that is contrast enhancing.

Pediatric glioblastomas are uncommon, only representing about 3% of all primary CNS neoplasms in children (10). The clinical features of specific varieties of IDH-wild–type glioblastomas in children are discussed further below in the section on genetics and ancillary studies.

Glioblastoma patients are at greatly increased risk for developing venous thromboses and thromboemboli when compared with patients with other brain tumors, and these conditions create significant morbidity and mortality among malignant glioma patients (89).

TREATMENT AND SURVIVAL. The current standard therapy for glioblastomas includes ionizing external beam radiation and chemotherapy with temozolomide. Although numerous other approaches have been taken, none have shown consistent improvement in survival. Those patients whose tumors display MGMT promoter methylation (see below) may have a better prognosis following treatment with temozolomide. Some promising emerging therapies make use of the immune system to attack the tumor, for example through tumor vaccines and immune checkpoint inhibitors.

Survival for patients with IDH-wild–type glioblastoma is dismal, with median survival of a year or less and a survival rate of about 3% at 3 years (54,71). Although the vast majority of people die within 2 years of diagnosis, exceptional cases with bona fide glioblastoma may survive 10 years or more, although the IDH mutation status of those cases is unknown (90). One series of long-term glioblastoma survivors showed a low rate of IDH mutations, raising the possibility that other factors, such as immune response, may have a role in some cases (91).

Age was once the most important and consistent prognostic factor in glioblastoma survival. It is now believed that most of this effect is due to the association of older age of patients with IDH-wild–type glioblastomas. It is unclear whether age has much of an impact on the prognosis among IDH-wild–type glioblastomas.

HISTOPATHOLOGY. Glioblastoma, IDH wild type is a malignant, infiltrative astrocytoma that, by diagnostic criteria, must contain necrosis and/or microvascular proliferation. Beyond these criteria, the other histologic characteristics of glioblastoma are extremely variable, both from case to case and, often, within the same tumor. Because the different histologic aspects of glioblastoma are so variable, each is discussed separately below, as are specific patterns that have diagnostic and/or prognostic relevance.

CELLULAR FEATURES. In general, glioblastoma cells are pleomorphic and overtly malignant, although some cases are uniform and relatively bland, especially those with a small-cell pattern. Many cells may lack concrete astrocytic differentiation ("naked nuclei"), but astrocytic forms (fibrillar eosinophilic cytoplasm) are usually scattered throughout. In smear preparations, even epithelioid cells retain a small amount of cytoplasmic fibrillarity. Most of the other cytologic features of glioblastoma are so variable as to frustrate description.

NECROSIS. The classic form of necrosis in glioblastoma is multifocal and composed of pockets and serpiginous strips of nucleus-poor necrosis trimmed by bands of hypercellularity (Figure 3-29). The descriptive term "pseudopalisading," or "palisading" as termed in the 2016 WHO classification, reflects the radial orientation of many tumor cells on the perimeter of these structures, possibly migrating away from zones of hypoxia (92). The center often holds scattered pyknotic nuclear debris and liquefied tissue but can be smooth and felt like neuropil that hardly appears necrotic. The presence of a thrombotically occluded blood vessel at the core of some foci perhaps suggests a cause for the necrosis and an explanation for its often irregular and perivascular distribution (92).

The other form of necrosis common in glioblastoma is widespread and confluent, represented on MRI by the nonenhancing center of the lesion. Confluent necrosis can constitute the vast majority of the tumor mass, leaving only a flimsy mantle of viable malignant cells at the edges. Recognizable palisading can be wholly absent. Diagnosis based on needle

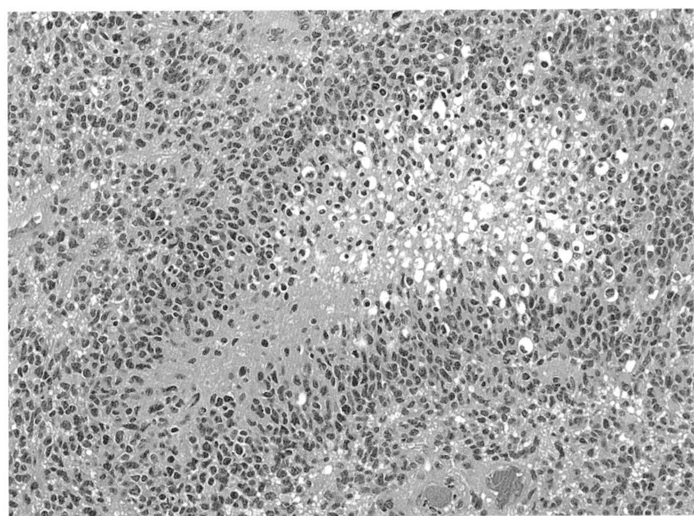

FIGURE 3-29 Palisading necrosis, with a rim of radially oriented cells around a hypocellular center with scattered pyknotic nuclear debris, is the hallmark feature of glioblastoma, though not always present.

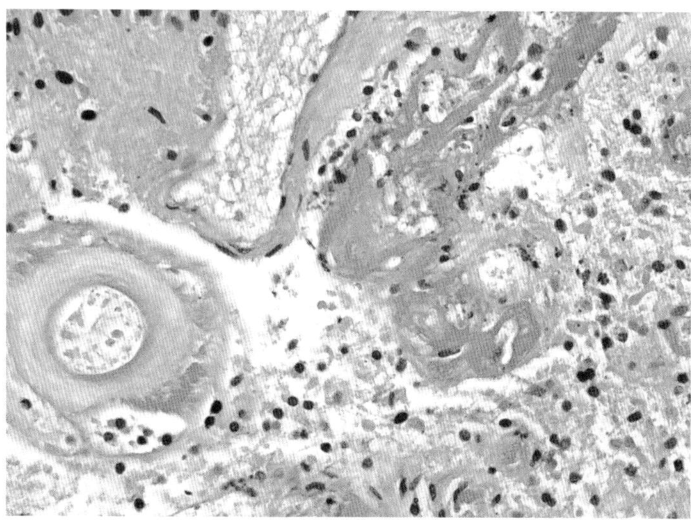

FIGURE 3-30 Necrosis from radiation therapy usually has thickened and hyalinized vessels in a background of necrosis, pyknotic debris, and hemosiderin and should not be used to diagnose glioblastoma unless other features indicate that.

biopsy specimens from such lesions can be difficult, with nothing but traces of suitable tissue available for identification.

Care must be taken to prevent interpretation of treatment-related necrosis of a lower-grade astrocytoma as spontaneous necrosis, precipitating a diagnosis of glioblastoma. Lower-grade diffuse gliomas are frequently biopsied after treatment with radiation because imaging shows development or expansion of contrast enhancement, which can be seen in either tumor progression or radiation necrosis. Radiated brain and glioma tissue show thickening and hyalinization of blood vessel walls, reactive astrocytosis, scattered macrophages, and coagulative necrosis (Figure 3-30). Familiarity with the patient's history of radiation therapy and recognition of the histologic features of radiation effects will protect against this mistake.

VASCULAR PROLIFERATION. Microvascular proliferation does not refer to the density of individual blood vessels within a lesion but rather to the reduplication of individual vessels into complex nodular structures, or as concentric multilayering of endothelial cells along vessel walls. The more nodular structures are composed of convoluted knots with abundant endothelial cells and other vascular components that form multiple lumens, resembling renal glomeruli when round. Not limited to glomeruloid configuration, these structures can also be elongated or irregular in outline. Occasionally, the nodules of proliferating vessels can overshadow the neoplastic cells (Figure 3-31). These proliferations are not specific to glioblastoma, or even neoplastic processes, and can be misleading in the wrong context. Low-grade tumors, such as pilocytic astrocytoma and ganglioglioma, can show nodular microvascular proliferation, typically in long arcing arrays.

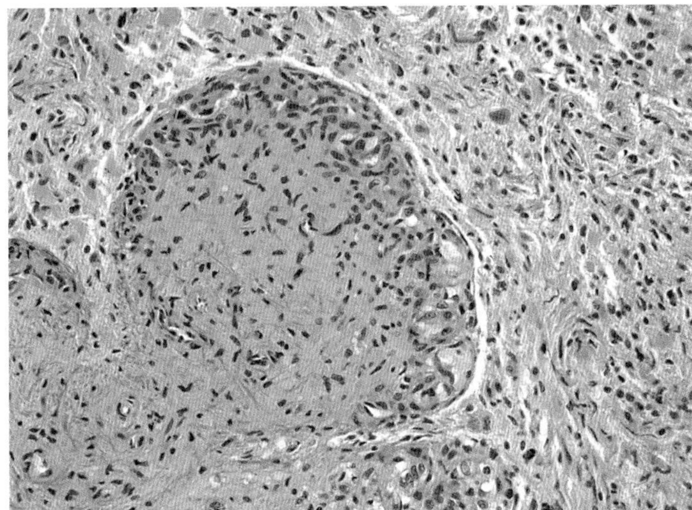

FIGURE 3-31 Microvascular proliferation can be florid and nodular, with knots of endothelial cells apparently growing toward hypoxic necrotic areas.

Vascular tufts can also be seen as postoperative changes in the brain, although the endothelial nuclei tend to be smaller and more quiescent.

Less striking, but just as diagnostically relevant, is the appearance of vessels that retain their single-lumen configuration but are lined by activated and hyperplastic endothelial cells that overlap and form multiple layers (Figure 3-32). Although endothelial nuclei may enlarge and activate

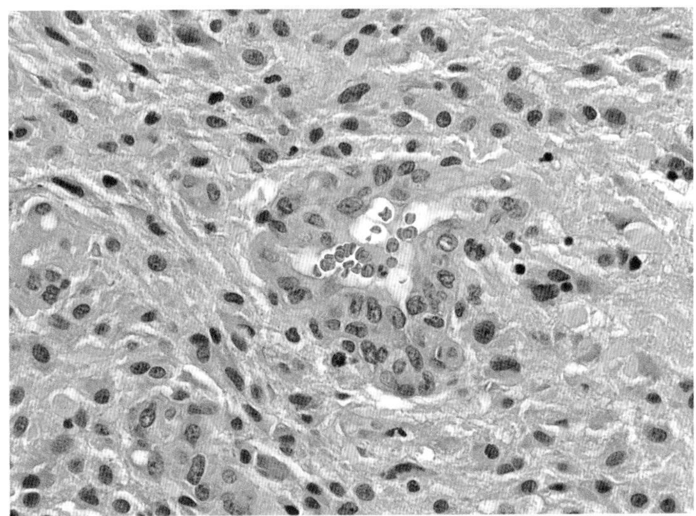

FIGURE 3-32 Concentric hyperplasia and overlap of endothelial cells is another manifestation of microvascular proliferation that is more specific to glioblastoma.

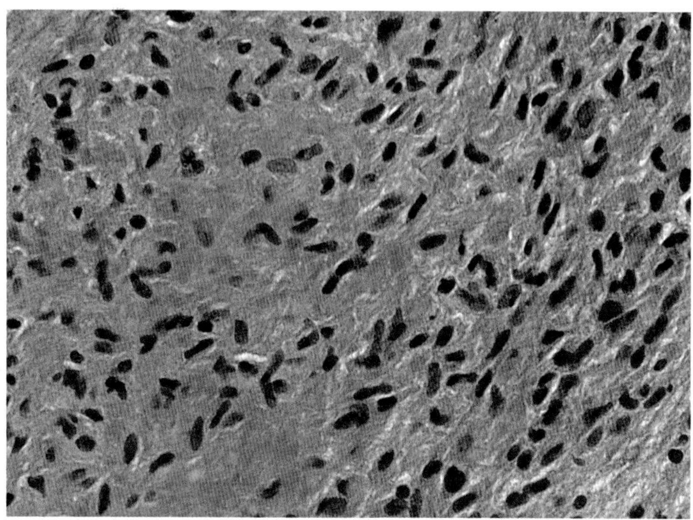

FIGURE 3-33 Glioblastomas sometimes produce a chondromyxoid ground substance that dilutes the cellularity and gives a mesenchymal appearance while the cells retain an astrocytic phenotype.

(endothelial hypertrophy) as a prelude to endothelial hyperplasia, a nonoverlapping monolayer of such cells is considered by some to be insufficient to qualify as microvascular proliferation in glioblastomas, which should show at least focal multilayering of endothelial cells.

DIVERGENT DIFFERENTIATION. In a small number of glioblastomas, some tumor cells exchange their glial identities for those of other cell types. Mesenchymal elements are probably the most common nonglial component, and can be fibroblastic, chondromatous, osseous, or muscular. Epithelial elements can also be present, even producing a glandular, or adenoid, appearance (93). Some glioblastoma secrete a rich, ground substance that gives them a mesenchymal appearance (Figure 3-33), yet the tumor cells retain their fibrillarity and GFAP immunoreactivity.

INFLAMMATION. A minority of glioblastomas have a prominent inflammatory cell infiltrate that varies in composition, most often seen in the giant, gemistocytic, and granular cell types. Lymphocytic infiltrates are mostly cytotoxic T cells distributed perivascularly, with a few B cells present. Evidence as to whether lymphocytic infiltrates influence patient outcome is inconclusive. Macrophages are generally indicative of nonneoplastic lesions but can occasionally be prominent within the necrotic parts of glioblastoma. Neutrophils also intermittently respond to necrotic glioblastoma and can simulate the appearance of an abscess, potentially distracting from the correct diagnosis.

RHABDOID CHANGE. Some glioblastomas have focal rhabdoid morphology, that is, the cells are discrete and epithelioid with eccentric, eosinophilic cytoplasm and have pale nuclei with prominent nucleoli. These cells may show monosomy of chromosome 22 and loss of *SMARCB1/INI1* immunostaining, but should not be interpreted as being malignant rhabdoid tumors (94). The diagnosis of atypical teratoid rhabdoid tumor (AT/RT) requires these findings throughout.

GIANT CELL GLIOBLASTOMA. This pattern is characterized clinically by its relative circumscription and slightly better overall survival than more typical glioblastomas. Grossly, the tumor is less infiltrative than other glioblastomas, lending itself to more complete surgical resection, which may explain the improved survival. Giant cell glioblastomas occur at a younger median age than regular glioblastomas, which could also explain some of the difference in prognosis (95). Pediatric giant cell glioblastomas are rare but have been reported and do not appear to have a better prognosis than other pediatric glioblastomas (96).

Histologically, the defining feature of this lesion is very large tumor cells with marked cellular pleomorphism and bizarre nuclear features (Figure 3-34). The giant cells can be enlarged to many times the diameter of nonneoplastic cells, spanning hundreds of microns. Such cells can be seen in small numbers in many glioblastomas, but they must dominate the histology for a lesion to be considered "giant cell." Stromal reticulin fibrosis and perivascular lymphocytic infiltrates are also present in most cases.

The histologic features of giant cell glioblastoma are similar to those of pleomorphic xanthoastrocytoma (PXA), WHO grade II, and the consideration that one should necessarily raise the possibility of the other. Distinguishing features of PXA are that it tends to occur in the temporal lobe of

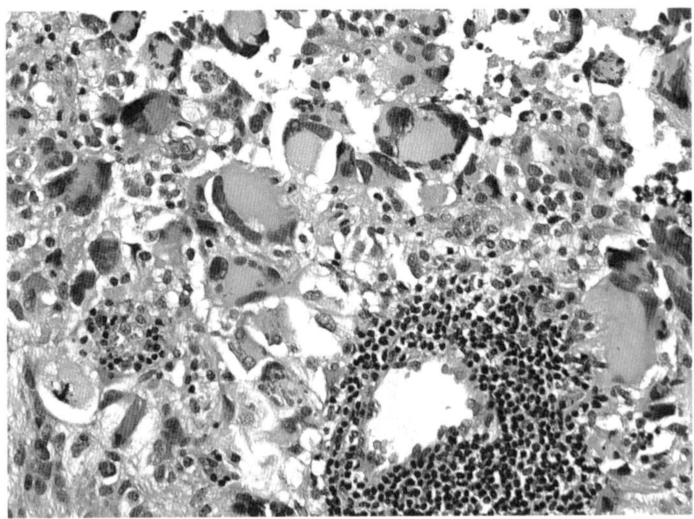

FIGURE 3-34 Giant cell glioblastomas are less infiltrative than other glioblastomas and have bizarre cytologic atypia and perivascular lymphocytic infiltrates.

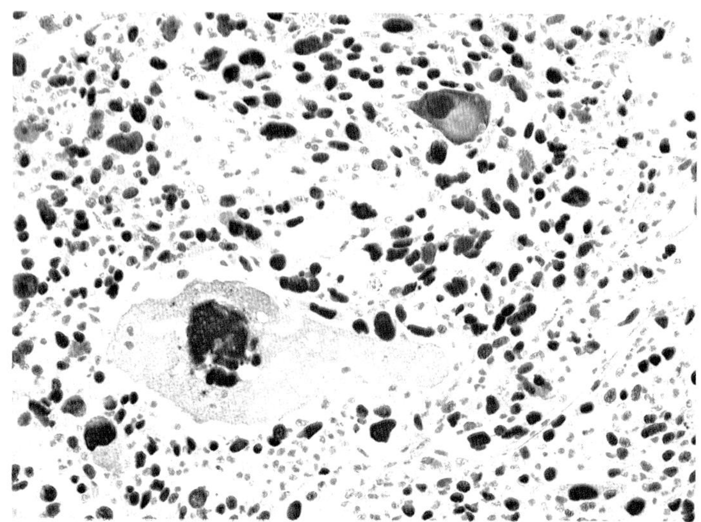

FIGURE 3-35 Giant cell glioblastomas usually express p53 immunohistochemically, setting them apart from pleomorphic xanthoastrocytoma.

children, has EGBs, few mitoses, and does not show nuclear p53 immunoreactivity. In contrast, giant cell glioblastomas have a median age of about 50 years, lack EGBs, are mitotically active, and usually display strong positivity for p53 (Figure 3-35). Although giant cell glioblastoma can show widespread reticulin staining, it is less pervasive than that of PXA and will envelop groups of cells instead of individual cells (Figure 3-36).

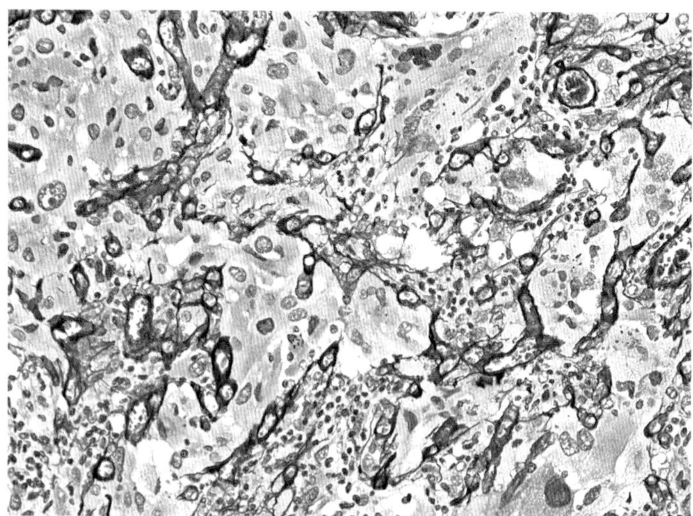

FIGURE 3-36 In giant cell glioblastoma, reticulin staining outlines clusters and large nests of tumor cells.

One may now also use molecular genetic features to decide between giant cell glioblastoma and PXA. Giant cell glioblastomas have high rates of *TP53* mutations (~80%), deletion of 10q (~50%), deletions of 19q (~40%), and mutations of *PTEN* (~30%), all of which are not characteristic of PXAs (97). In contrast, PXAs exhibit *BRAF* V600E mutations (~50% to 60%) and high rates of *CDKN2A/B* (p16) homozygous deletion (~90%) (98,99) The former is never seen in giant cell glioblastoma, and the latter is rare (~3%).

GLIOSARCOMA. Occasionally, the neoplastic cells of a glioblastoma divergently differentiate into spindle-shaped collagen-producing mesenchymal cells that form fascicles of sarcoma-like tissue interspersed with pockets of more glial tumor cells, creating a distinct biphasic appearance (Figure 3-37). This biphasic pattern can be subtle on H&E staining but is obvious after reticulin staining or GFAP, the former marking the collagenous mesenchymal elements and the latter creating the inverse pattern (Figure 3-38). The sarcomatous cells are often less pleomorphic and anaplastic than their glial component, sometimes appearing low grade. Because the glial element may be largely overrun by the sarcomatous element, an intra-axial apparently sarcomatous neoplasm should be sampled thoroughly to rule out gliosarcoma. Other tissue types, such as cartilage and bone, are more frequent in gliosarcoma than in glioblastoma.

To the surgeon, gliosarcoma will have a gross appearance much more similar to a fibrotic metastasis or meningioma than to glioblastoma, with distinct borders and a tough, fibrous texture. For this reason, the diagnosis may not be expected before histologic examination.

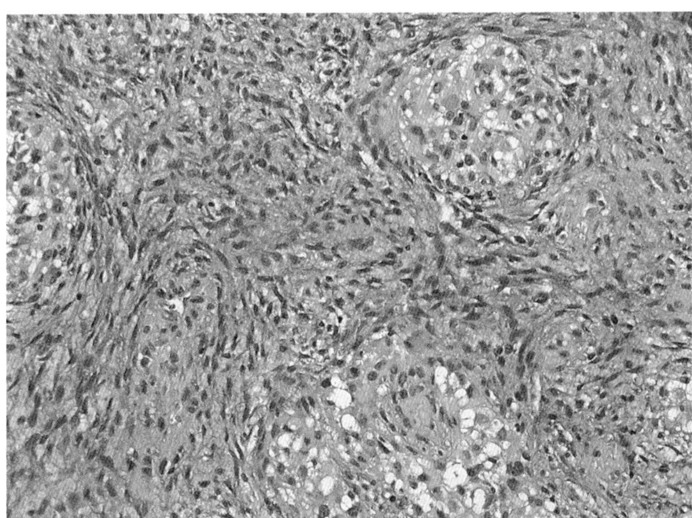

FIGURE 3-37 Gliosarcomas are biphasic tumors with spindle-cell sarcoma elements and scattered islands of residual fibrillar pink astrocytoma.

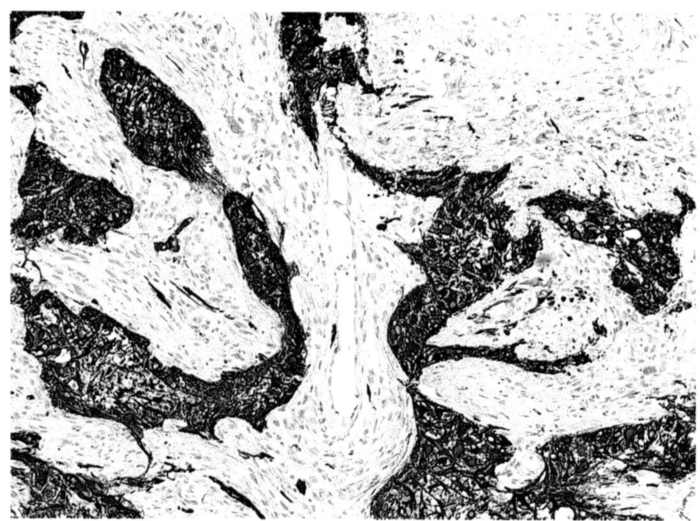

FIGURE 3-38 GFAP immunostaining marks nests of astrocytoma and accentuates the biphasic nature of gliosarcoma.

Although the histology can be strikingly different from a classic glioblastoma, gliosarcomas are essentially the same as other IDH-wild–type glioblastomas in clinical characteristics and behavior. Furthermore, gliosarcomas are genetically similar to other IDH-wild–type glioblastomas, except that they only rarely have amplifications of EGFR (97,100). The sarcomatous elements were originally thought to be a second malignant neoplasm arising from the perivascular fibroblasts in proliferating vessels, but they have been shown to have the same *TP53* and *PTEN* point mutations as the glial components, suggesting a common origin (100).

SMALL-CELL GLIOBLASTOMA. This pattern was of more importance when classification of gliomas was more based on histologic features because it would mimic the significantly less aggressive anaplastic oligodendroglioma (101,102). However, such lesions now depend on objective demonstration of genetic features, essentially eliminating the once significant diagnostic overlap between the two. Small-cell glioblastomas are composed of a densely hypercellular and monotonous population of infiltrating tumor cells with oval, mildly hyperchromatic nuclei, small perinuclear haloes, and minimal cytoplasm. Arcades of "chicken-wire" capillaries, perineuronal satellitosis, and calcifications are also common (Figure 3-39). The presence of an IDH mutation and 1p/19q codeletion rules out small-cell glioblastoma and supports the diagnosis of oligodendroglioma. Small-cell morphology is strongly associated with IDH-wild–type status, EGFR amplification, and deletion of 10q (PTEN) (101,103).

EPITHELIOID GLIOBLASTOMA. Epithelioid morphology (Figure 3-40) has long been recognized to occur in glioblastoma occasionally, and more

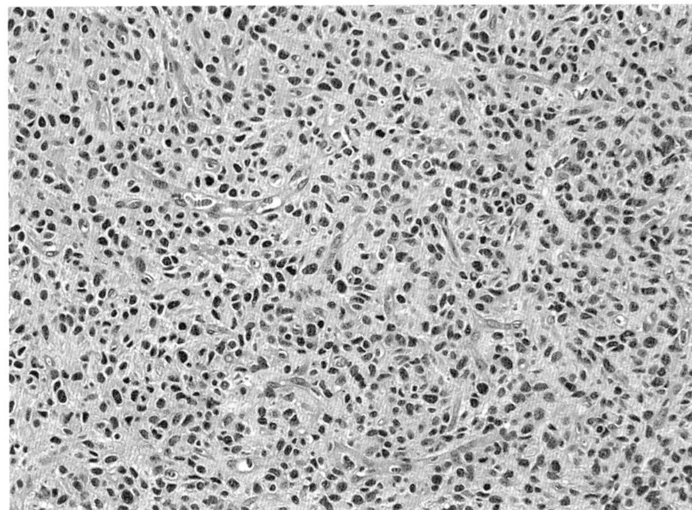

FIGURE 3-39 Small-cell glioblastomas have monotonous cells with oval and round nuclei among a capillary-rich vasculature, resembling oligodendroglioma but with genetic findings typical of IDH-wild–type glioblastoma.

recent observations suggest that those cases with a predominant epithelioid component are a genetically distinct variant with a high rate of *BRAF* V600E mutations and occurring in younger patients (mean ~30 years; range 2 to 79) (94,104). Epithelioid glioblastoma is thought to have better survival than other IDH-wild–type glioblastomas, though experience with this entity is still limited.

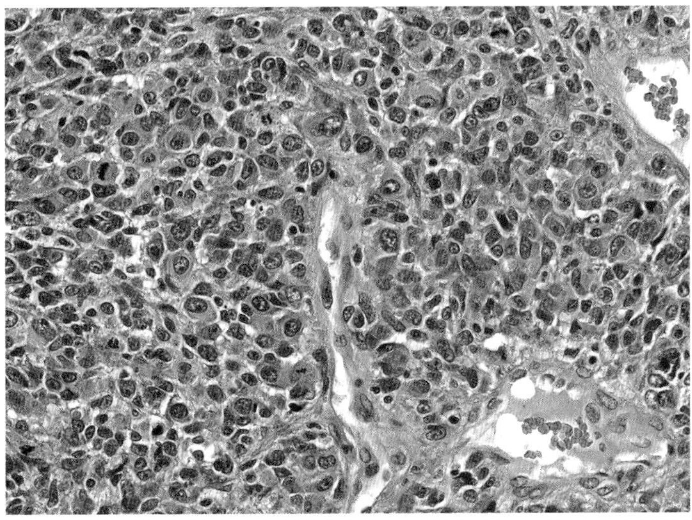

FIGURE 3-40 Epithelioid areas in some glioblastomas can closely mimic metastatic carcinoma or melanoma, but are rarely the sole histologic pattern.

About half of epithelioid glioblastomas will have a *BRAF* V600E mutation, and epithelioid changes have been noted in anaplastic PXAs, so those entities may be pathogenetically related (104). Other than *BRAF* mutations and wild-type IDH, there are no consistent genetic findings yet described in this entity. The discrete, polygonal cells of the epithelioid component remain glial in differentiation and are not the same as epithelial metaplasia, where the tumor cells differentiate into a fully epithelial phenotype.

PRIMITIVE NEURONAL (FORMERLY PNET-LIKE) COMPONENT. An uncommon subset of diffuse, high-grade gliomas contains a component of poorly differentiated, primitive neuronal cells similar to medulloblastoma or neuroblastoma (Figure 3-41) (105). Not only do such components show morphologic similarities to primitive neuronal tumors, which include neuroblastic (Homer Wright) rosettes, they also display similar expression of neuronal markers and genetic amplifications of *MYC* or *MYCN* oncogenes. It appears that they also resemble embryonal neuroblastic tumors in their proclivity to disseminate through the cerebrospinal fluid (CSF). Immunohistochemistry creates sharp contrasts in staining for synaptophysin, MIB1, and GFAP between the glial and PNET components (Figure 3-42). A small number of these, around one-fifth, are IDH mutant and thus may have a better prognosis than the typical IDH-wild–type glioblastoma.

Another small set of IDH-wild–type glioblastomas in children have a strong tendency to develop an embryonal component, one that frequently overshadows the glial elements and may be the only tissue present in surgical specimens (106). Mutations in the *H3F3A* gene in codon 34

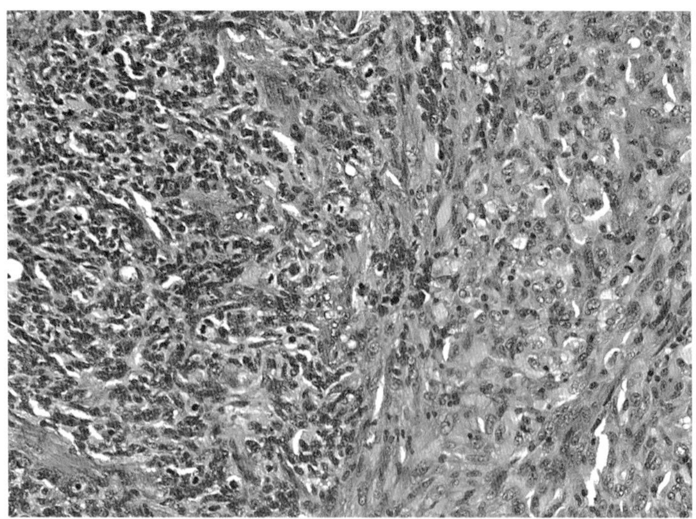

FIGURE 3-41 Glioblastoma with a primitive neuronal component has distinctly separate areas of typical glioblastoma (right) and PNET (left).

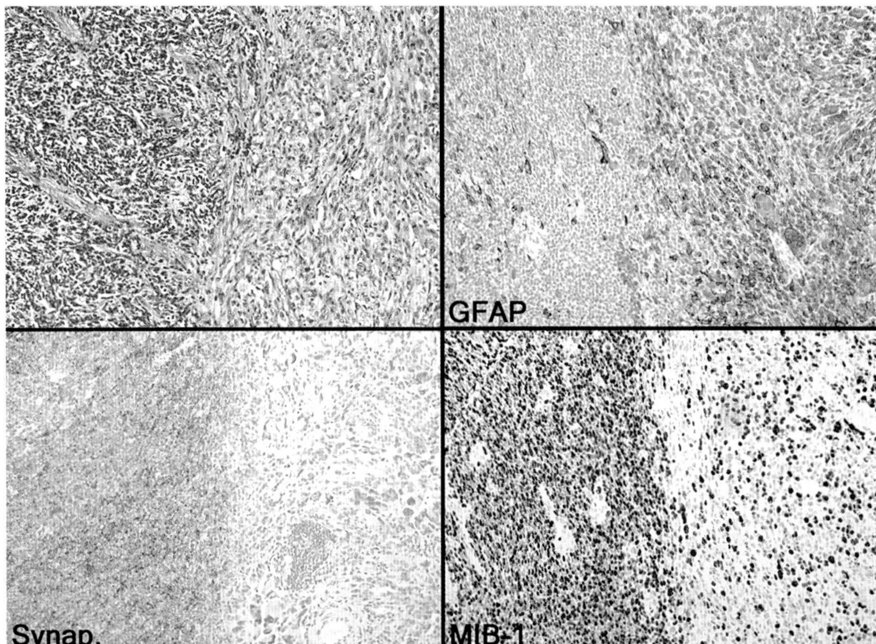

FIGURE 3-42 The separate elements of glioblastoma with primitive neuronal, or neuroblastic, component show the immunophenotypes of their respective histologies (glioblastoma on right, primitive neuronal on left).

(G34R or G34V), *TP53* mutations, and *ATRX* loss characterize these mostly pediatric, hemispheric glioblastomas. It has been suggested that, unlike adult glioblastomas with primitive neuronal components, the H3.3 G34R/V cases do not have a tendency to metastasize and should not be diagnosed as embryonal/neuroblastic tumors, even when a glial component is not present (107). This distinction is important because glioblastoma and neuroblastic tumors (formerly CNS-PNET) have completely different treatment regimens.

GRANULAR CELL ASTROCYTOMA/GLIOBLASTOMA. A rare subset of infiltrating astrocytomas possesses an overabundance of lysosomes in many tumor cells, giving the cytoplasm a distinct granular appearance. Similar to gemistocytic astrocytomas, the proportion of cells with the namesake feature varies from a minority to an overwhelming majority. The defining series for this entity used a minimum cutoff of 30% granular cells as an inclusion criterion (108). Relative to conventional diffuse astrocytomas, granular cell cases have a lower MIB1 index, lower mitotic count, and higher male:female ratio. The literature contains only single cases that occurred outside of the cerebral hemispheres, one in the cerebellum (109) and the other in the spinal cord (110). Although they are graded using the same WHO criteria as other infiltrating astrocytomas, granular cell astrocytomas are

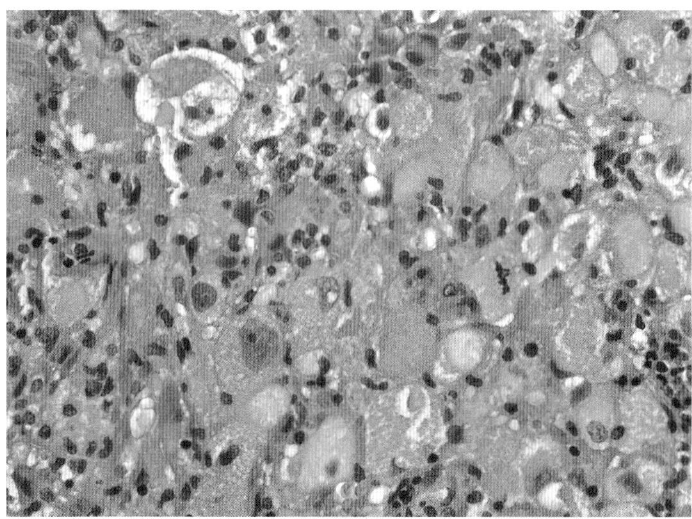

FIGURE 3-43 Granular cell astrocytomas simulate macrophage-rich lesions because of large tumor cells with ample granular cytoplasm filled with lysosomes, although the nuclei are large and atypical.

consistently associated with a highly aggressive course, even when histologically grade II. The vast majority of reported cases where survival is mentioned died within 1 year of diagnosis, thus behave in a WHO grade IV manner.

Histologically, the tumor cells have abundant, lightly eosinophilic, granular cytoplasm (Figure 3-43). The granules are PAS positive and either distributed diffusely or as a thick peripheral band within the circumference of the plasma membrane. Lymphocytes surround the blood vessels in most cases (Figure 3-44). By immunohistochemistry, the granular cells are positive for GFAP, S100, and CD68. GFAP staining is variable among the granular cells, usually marking only a minority of them. Epithelial membrane antigen (EMA) is expressed in most cases and is cytoplasmic, not membranous, in pattern.

Distinguishing granular cell astrocytoma from macrophage-rich, nonneoplastic processes, such as multiple sclerosis, progressive multifocal leukoencephalopathy (PML), and infarct, is the main diagnostic consideration. A lesion of discrete, large cells with ample cytoplasm and perivascular lymphocytic infiltrates can give a strong impression of demyelinating lesion at low power. This false impression can be fostered by immunostaining for CD68, a lysosomal protein. CD163 is a newer marker that is nonlysosomal and more exclusive to histiocytes, but remains untested in granular cell astrocytomas. Olig-2 is a reliable glial marker in granular cell astrocytomas (111). Systematic examination of the typical IDH, p53, and ATRX status has been limited, yet one series of three showed no IDH1 R132H, p53, or ATRX abnormalities by immunohistochemistry (112). In another series, no consistent pattern of allelic losses was found in a select number

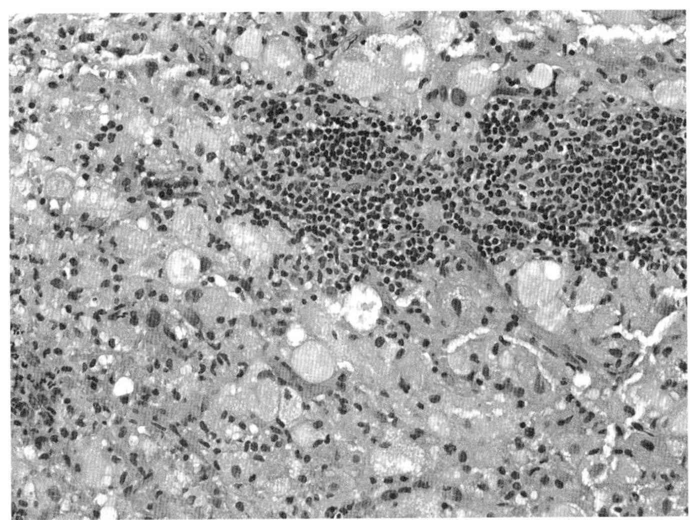

FIGURE 3-44 Granular cell astrocytomas also typically have lymphocytic perivascular infiltrates that add to the illusion of a demyelinating lesion.

of loci, yet 9 of 10 cases had at least one loss on chromosome arm 10q and 2 of 10 had a *TP53* mutation (113).

OLIGODENDROGLIOMA COMPONENT. Some glioblastomas have elements of classic oligodendroglial morphology and were recognized as a distinct subset for a time, although they are now understood to be a part of the histologic variability of glioblastoma. Such cases have a similar distribution of genetic findings as morphologically defined glioblastomas as a whole, including a small percentage of IDH-mutant cases (114). There is some evidence that, despite genetic similarities with other morphologically defined glioblastomas as a whole, those with an oligodendroglial component have somewhat better survival (115).

IMMUNOHISTOCHEMISTRY. IDH-wild–type glioblastomas retain immunohistochemical expression of ATRX, providing a useful adjunct to IDH1 R132H immunostaining in ruling out IDH mutations. However, strong p53 immunostaining, although present in almost all IDH-mutant cases, is also seen in up to 30% of IDH-wild–type glioblastomas. If DNA-based molecular testing is not routinely performed to rule out non-R132H and IDH2 mutations in glioblastomas, loss of ATRX immunostaining in tumor cells is an important prompt to further investigate for less common IDH mutations, even in patients older than 55 (116).

True to their astrocytic nature, the vast majority of glioblastomas express GFAP, at least focally. Staining for this cytoskeletal protein is most prominent in fibrillary processes and varies in abundance with the amount of cytoplasm, with small-cell examples showing only modest tendrils of positivity. Because GFAP is negative in virtually all metastases, a positive

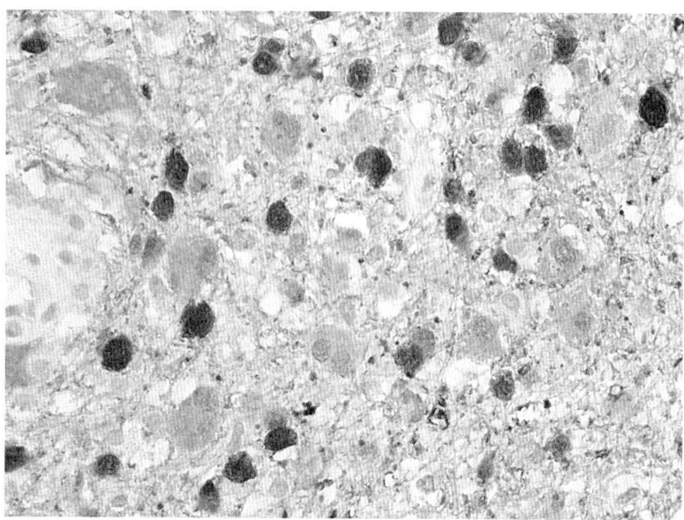

FIGURE 3-45 Some glioblastomas show surprising reactivity for AE1/3 cytokeratin antibodies, although usually only focally.

GFAP stain will reliably rule out carcinoma, melanoma, and lymphoma when faced with a malignant intracerebral tumor; however, lack of GFAP reactivity does not completely rule out glioblastoma. Reactivity can rarely be entirely absent, either by tissue processing that destroys the target epitopes or by innate loss of GFAP expression. In the former case, vimentin immunostaining can be used to assess tissue integrity.

Broad-spectrum cytokeratin antibodies, particularly AE1/3, often show reactivity in both neoplastic and nonneoplastic astrocytes, complicating the use of those antibodies in differentiating malignant astrocytomas from carcinomas (Figure 3-45). Other keratin stains, specifically CAM 5.2, show less cross-reactivity, but should always be accompanied by GFAP if the aim is differentiating metastatic carcinoma from glioblastoma (117).

Because glioblastomas express S100 protein, other markers of melanocytic differentiation, such as HMB45, microphthalmia transcription factor (MITF), MART 1/melan A, and tyrosinase, should be used to distinguish them from melanoma.

GENETICS AND ANCILLARY STUDIES

IDH TESTING. Ruling out an IDH mutation is definitional for IDH-wild–type glioblastoma and the most important aspect of any diagnostic genetic workup. IDH1 R132H immunostaining is sufficient in most cases, and reactivity can be taken as evidence for the mutation's presence. However, given the importance of identifying IDH mutations in all diffuse gliomas, glioblastomas should all have some additional assessment beyond IDH R132H immunostaining. A minimal, yet generally effective, approach is ATRX immunostaining (116). DNA-based methods such as sequencing or allele-specific PCR may be employed to confirm alternate IDH mutations in immunohistochemically suspicious cases.

MGMT TESTING. Temozolomide is currently the first-line chemotherapy for glioblastoma and causes alkylation (addition of a methyl group) of guanine nucleotides at the O6 position, precipitating numerous transition point mutations in all subsequent daughter strands of DNA. This alkylation is reversed by the DNA repair enzyme MGMT (O6-methylguanine-DNA methyltransferase) (118,119). Thus, tumors with low levels of MGMT expression should be less able to repair alkylation damage and be more sensitive to temozolomide. The expression level of MGMT is regulated by methylation of the gene's promoter, which prevents it from being transcribed. This epigenetic silencing of MGMT occurs in around 75% of IDH-mutant glioblastomas and around 20% of IDH-wild–type glioblastomas and can be assessed by PCR-based tests of genomic tumor DNA. Epigenetic silencing of MGMT in IDH-wild–type glioblastoma is correlated with a longer survival among patients treated with temozolomide and radiotherapy. Antibodies are available for the detection of the MGMT protein, but the correlation of MGMT immunoreactivity with promoter methylation and response to therapy or survival is poor (120). Because temozolomide has become a standard of care for the treatment of glioblastoma, testing for MGMT methylation status is now a necessary component of a complete diagnostic workup.

EGFR AMPLIFICATION. Amplifications of EGFR occur in around 40% of all glioblastomas and roughly 70% of small-cell examples; however, such amplifications are rare in giant cell glioblastomas and gliosarcomas. EGFR amplification is generally restricted to primary glioblastomas and is not seen in lower-grade astrocytomas and secondary glioblastomas. Roughly half of cases with EGFR amplification express a mutated form lacking exons 2 to 7, which results in a truncated protein with constitutive tyrosine kinase activity (EGFRvIII). Neither EGFR amplification nor EGFRvIII rearrangement appears to be independently associated with survival in patients with glioblastoma (121).

EGFR amplifications are useful diagnostically because their presence is strongly associated with IDH-wild–type glioblastoma and rare or absent in other high-grade gliomas (101,102).

DELETION OF CHROMOSOME 10. Genetic losses on chromosome 10, whether detected by microarray, LOH studies, or by FISH, are the most frequent genetic alterations in glioblastoma, present in around 80% of cases, including many IDH-mutant examples. Most cases, primary and secondary, have distal deletions of the long arm that include the locus for the tumor suppressor gene *PTEN*. Complete loss of 10 may also be seen but is generally less common than loss at 10q. Isolated deletion of 10p is present in a small minority of glioblastomas and may be incidental. Losses on chromosome 10 are much less common among oligodendrogliomas, making them useful diagnostic markers for high-grade astrocytomas. Mutations of PTEN are also common, identified in around 30% of glioblastomas (122).

TERT PROMOTER MUTATIONS. Like oligodendrogliomas, most glioblastomas have activating mutations in the promoter for TERT, or telomerase reverse transcriptase, albeit at a slightly lower rate in the latter (34). Although potentially useful diagnostically in lower-grade diffuse gliomas, the presence of TERT promoter mutations in glioblastoma makes them less useful for that in high-grade infiltrating gliomas.

CDKN2A/B DELETIONS. Loss of chromosome 9p, which is usually homozygous and includes the *CDKN2A/B* locus that encodes the tumor suppressor p16, is present in a little more than half of IDH-wild–type glioblastomas (122). This finding is also common in pediatric high-grade gliomas that otherwise have different genetic profiles.

OTHER GENETIC FINDINGS. IDH-wild–type glioblastomas also display lower rates of the following: *TP53* mutation (~35%), *PDGFRA* amplification (~13%), *NF1* mutation or homozygous deletion (~15%), and *PIK3CA* mutations (~15%).

DIFFERENTIAL DIAGNOSIS. Metastatic lesions can radiologically and histologically resemble glioblastoma, but several morphologic cues differentiate the two well. Glioblastomas invade the surrounding brain as individual cells, whereas metastases have pushing borders with sharp delineation. Staining for neurofilament illuminates the infiltrative quality of glioblastoma by labeling the overrun axons of native neurons, which are altogether absent among the cells of metastases. Most of the cells seen in glioblastoma also lack the sharp cell–cell borders and polygonal shape of melanomas and carcinomas, instead being more syncytial and fibrillary, the former being especially apparent on cytologic preparations. Although vascular proliferation can be seen in metastases, it is not florid or nodular as in glioblastoma. Beyond morphologic features, expression of GFAP rules out the possibility of metastases except in a few cases.

PCNSL is perivascular in distribution and formed from large, round, poorly cohesive cells with open chromatin and large nucleoli, leaving it and glioblastoma with little in common, morphologically. However, on small specimens, the angiocentric nature can be obscured and infiltration by individual lymphoma cells can give a strong impression of a glial malignancy, especially on frozen section where cytologic details are distorted. Smear preparations are helpful in this situation to assess for the fibrillar cytoplasmic processes seen in glioblastoma.

Pilocytic astrocytoma and PXA, two low-grade, poorly infiltrative astrocytomas, can be difficult to distinguish from glioblastoma in some circumstances. Differentiating glioblastoma from PXA and pilocytic astrocytoma is discussed with those lesions in the section on Giant Cell Glioblastoma and in the next chapter, respectively.

A constant threat to accurate diagnosis is sampling of tissue that is away from tumor bulk, but infiltrated by neoplastic cells, giving the appearance of a lower-grade glioma. Awareness of the imaging characteristics of the intended biopsy target is paramount.

CNS infections due to toxoplasma can cause a necrotizing encephalitis that is coagulative, lacks macrophage infiltrates, and destroys blood vessels, making it similar to the necrosis seen in some glioblastomas. Because of a degree of overlap in the imaging findings of these two entities, biopsy of toxoplasma abscesses happens occasionally when a patient's impaired immunity is unrecognized before surgery. Awareness of this potential situation and restraint from diagnosing based on necrotic tissue safeguard against this mistake.

Recent cerebral infarcts are rarely biopsied on suspicion of a neoplastic process and can appear vaguely similar to glioblastoma, with blood vessels proliferating in response to hypoxia and increased cellularity due to macrophage infiltrates. The absence of atypia in macrophages and their well-delineated foamy cytoplasm make the resemblance superficial. Smear preparations at intraoperative consultation are more ideally suited to identifying macrophages than frozen sections.

Diffuse Midline Glioma, H3 K27M Mutant (WHO Grade IV)

CLINICAL CONTEXT. Children and young adults have a propensity to develop diffuse gliomas (in the ventral brain stem, thalamus, and spinal cord) that are rapidly fatal, even when histologically grade II. Clinically, ventral brain stem cases are known as diffuse intrinsic pontine gliomas (DIPG). When these tumors contain K27M point mutations in one of the genes encoding the histone H3 protein, *H3F3A*, *HIST1H3B*, or *HIST1H3C*, they meet criteria for the diagnosis "diffuse midline glioma, H3 K27M mutant, WHO grade IV." Such mutations are present in about 70% of DIPGs and thalamic infiltrating gliomas in young patients.

The mean age at diagnosis is around 10 to 14 years when adult cases are included, although most cases occur in the first two decades of life (123,124). These patients typically present with cranial nerve deficits, spasticity, and/or obstructive hydrocephalus. Imaging shows expansion and T2 abnormalities, with contrast enhancement in cases with higher histologic grade. There is no reliable imaging finding that can distinguish H3 K27M-mutant gliomas from H3 wild-type ones in the midline (125). Imaging is considered sufficient for diagnosis in many cases of brain stem glioma, partially due to the high risk associated with brainstem biopsy (Figure 3-46). However, now that biological markers are being increasingly used for classification, biopsy rates may be increasing. The low rate of brainstem biopsies may also result in an overrepresentation of thalamic H3 K27M-mutant cases in the literature.

Radiation is the cornerstone of treatment for DIPG and prolongs progression-free survival, but overall survival is unaffected, averaging less than 12 months (126). Standard chemotherapy has little effect on these lesions.

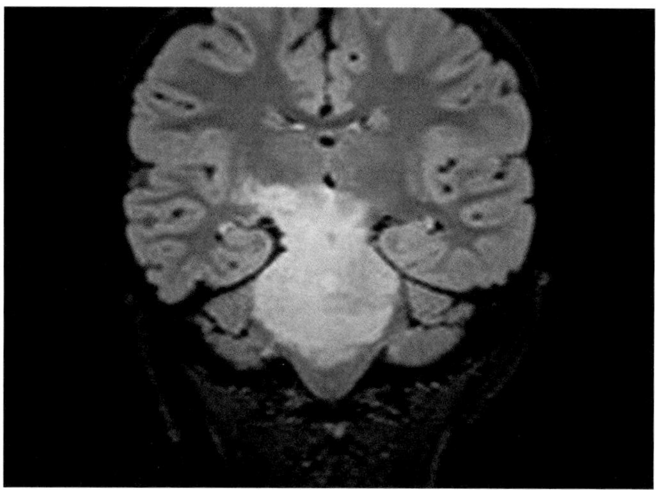

FIGURE 3-46 Many midline gliomas in children and young adults, particularly those of the pons, seen here, and thalamus exhibit H3 K27M histone mutations and now constitute a separate WHO category of infiltrating glioma.

HISTOPATHOLOGY AND GENETICS. Histologically, H3 K27M-mutant diffuse midline gliomas show the same variability in morphology as other infiltrating gliomas, the vast majority having an astrocytic appearance (123). About half are histologically grade IV, and the other half split between histologic grades II and III. An antibody to the K27M-mutant protein can reliably identify these cases, regardless of whether the protein results from mutations in *H3F3A* or *HIST1H3B* (Figure 3-47) (127).

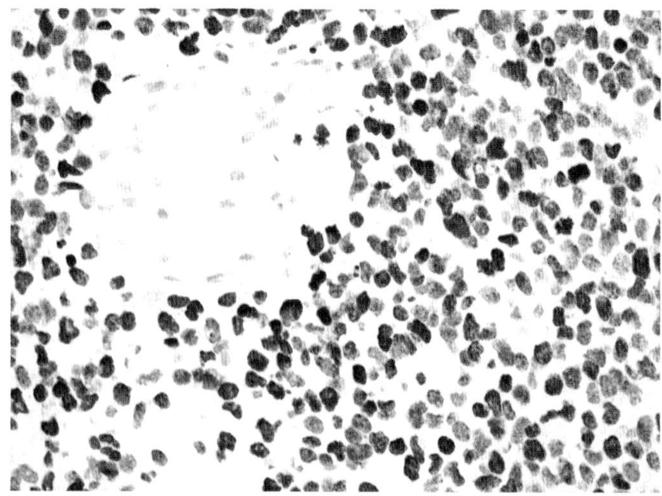

FIGURE 3-47 The H3 K27M antibody can detect the mutant protein from either the *H3F3A* or *HIST1H3B* gene.

Other genetic features in H3 K27M-mutant diffuse midline gliomas are heterogeneous. There are *TP53* mutations in around half and lower frequency mutations in *ACVR1, PPM1D, NF1,* and *ATRX*. Around half also have copy-number gains, including high-level amplifications, of *PDGFRA*. Other copy-number changes include amplifications or low-level gains of MYCN, as well as losses of 10q (PTEN) and 17p (TP53) (128). Around 5% of H3 K27M-mutant midline gliomas also have BRAF V600E mutations (123,124), which is important because the drug vemurafenib can be used to target the mutant protein, possibly prolonging survival.

REFERENCES

1. Louis DN, Ohgaki H, Wiestler OD, et al. WHO Classification of Tumours of the Central Nervous System. 4th, revised ed. Lyon, France: IARC Press; 2016.
2. Waitkus MS, Diplas BH, Yan H. Isocitrate dehydrogenase mutations in gliomas. *Neuro Oncol.* 2016;18(1):16–26.
3. Parsons DW, Jones S, Zhang X, et al. An integrated genomic analysis of human glioblastoma multiforme. *Science.* 2008;321(5897):1807–1812.
4. Yan H, Parsons DW, Jin G, et al. IDH1 and IDH2 mutations in gliomas. *N Engl J Med.* 2009;360(8):765–773.
5. Dang L, White DW, Gross S, et al. Cancer-associated IDH1 mutations produce 2-hydroxyglutarate. *Nature.* 2009;462(7274):739–744.
6. Struys EA. 2-Hydroxyglutarate is not a metabolite; D-2-hydroxyglutarate and L-2-hydroxyglutarate are! *Proc Natl Acad Sci USA.* 2013;110(51):E4939.
7. Napier CE, Huschtscha LI, Harvey A, et al. ATRX represses alternative lengthening of telomeres. *Oncotarget.* 2015;6(18):16543–16558.
8. Arita H, Narita Y, Fukushima S, et al. Upregulating mutations in the TERT promoter commonly occur in adult malignant gliomas and are strongly associated with total 1p19q loss. *Acta Neuropathol.* 2013;126(2):267–276.
9. Ostrom QT, Gittleman H, Xu J, et al. CBTRUS statistical report: primary brain and other central nervous system tumors diagnosed in the United States in 2009–2013. *Neuro Oncol.* 2016;18(suppl 5):v1–v75.
10. Ostrom QT, Gittleman H, Fulop J, et al. CBTRUS Statistical Report: primary brain and central nervous system tumors diagnosed in the United States in 2008–2012. *Neuro Oncol.* 2015;17 Suppl 4:iv1–iv62.
11. Mork SJ, Lindegaard KF, Halvorsen TB, et al. Oligodendroglioma: incidence and biological behavior in a defined population. *J Neurosurg.* 1985;63(6):881–889.
12. Nauen D, Haley L, Lin MT, et al. Molecular analysis of pediatric oligodendrogliomas highlights genetic differences with adult counterparts and other pediatric gliomas. *Brain Pathol.* 2016;26(2):206–214.
13. Shaw EG, Scheithauer BW, O'Fallon JR, et al. Oligodendrogliomas: the Mayo Clinic experience. *J Neurosurg.* 1992;76(3):428–434.
14. Perry A. Oligodendroglial neoplasms: current concepts, misconceptions, and folklore. *Adv Anat Pathol.* 2001;8(4):183–199.
15. Jenkinson MD, du Plessis DG, Smith TS, et al. Histological growth patterns and genotype in oligodendroglial tumours: correlation with MRI features. *Brain.* 2006;129 (Pt 7):1884–1891.
16. Cancer Genome Atlas Research Network, Brat DJ, Verhaak RG, et al. Comprehensive, integrative genomic analysis of diffuse lower-grade gliomas. *N Engl J Med.* 2015;372(26): 2481–2498.

17. Leeper HE, Caron AA, Decker PA, et al. IDH mutation, 1p19q codeletion and ATRX loss in WHO grade II gliomas. *Oncotarget.* 2015;6(30):30295–30305.
18. van den Bent MJ, Taphoorn MJ, Brandes AA, et al. Phase II study of first-line chemotherapy with temozolomide in recurrent oligodendroglial tumors: the European Organization for Research and Treatment of Cancer Brain Tumor Group Study 26971. *J Clin Oncol.* 2003;21(13):2525–2528.
19. Intergroup Radiation Therapy Oncology Group T, Cairncross G, Berkey B, et al. Phase III trial of chemotherapy plus radiotherapy compared with radiotherapy alone for pure and mixed anaplastic oligodendroglioma: Intergroup Radiation Therapy Oncology Group Trial 9402. *J Clin Oncol.* 2006;24(18):2707–2714.
20. Coons SW, Johnson PC, Scheithauer BW, et al. Improving diagnostic accuracy and interobserver concordance in the classification and grading of primary gliomas. *Cancer.* 1997;79(7):1381–1393.
21. Gupta M, Djalilvand A, Brat DJ. Clarifying the diffuse gliomas: an update on the morphologic features and markers that discriminate oligodendroglioma from astrocytoma. *Am J Clin Pathol.* 2005;124(5):755–768.
22. Yoshida T, Nakazato Y. Characterization of refractile eosinophilic granular cells in oligodendroglial tumors. *Acta Neuropathol.* 2001;102(1):11–19.
23. Perry A, Scheithauer BW, Macaulay RJ, et al. Oligodendrogliomas with neurocytic differentiation. A report of 4 cases with diagnostic and histogenetic implications. *J Neuropathol Exp Neurol.* 2002;61(11):947–955.
24. Herpers MJ, Budka H. Glial fibrillary acidic protein (GFAP) in oligodendroglial tumors: gliofibrillary oligodendroglioma and transitional oligoastrocytoma as subtypes of oligodendroglioma. *Acta Neuropathol.* 1984;64(4):265–272.
25. Kros JM, Van Eden CG, Stefanko SZ, et al. Prognostic implications of glial fibrillary acidic protein containing cell types in oligodendrogliomas. *Cancer.* 1990;66(6): 1204–1212.
26. Vyberg M, Ulhøi BP, Teglbjaerg PS. Neuronal features of oligodendrogliomas–an ultrastructural and immunohistochemical study. *Histopathol.* 2007;50(7):887–896.
27. Wharton SB, Chan KK, Hamilton FA, et al. Expression of neuronal markers in oligodendrogliomas: an immunohistochemical study. *Neuropathol App Neurobiol.* 1998;24(4):302–308.
28. Okamoto Y, Di Patre PL, Burkhard C, et al. Population-based study on incidence, survival rates, and genetic alterations of low-grade diffuse astrocytomas and oligodendrogliomas. *Acta Neuropathol.* 2004;108(1):49–56.
29. Cairncross JG, Ueki K, Zlatescu MC, et al. Specific genetic predictors of chemotherapeutic response and survival in patients with anaplastic oligodendrogliomas. *J Nat Can Inst.* 1998;90(19):1473–1479.
30. Perry A, Fuller CE, Banerjee R, et al. Ancillary FISH analysis for 1p and 19q status: preliminary observations in 287 gliomas and oligodendroglioma mimics. *Front Biosci.* 2003;8:a1–a9.
31. Louis DN, Ohgaki H, Wiestler OD, et al. WHO Classification of Tumours of the Central Nervous System. Revised 4th ed. Lyon, France: IARC Press; 2016.
32. Jenkins RB, Blair H, Ballman KV, et al. A t(1;19)(q10;p10) mediates the combined deletions of 1p and 19q and predicts a better prognosis of patients with oligodendroglioma. *Cancer Res.* 2006;66(20):9852–9861.
33. Koelsche C, Sahm F, Capper D, et al. Distribution of TERT promoter mutations in pediatric and adult tumors of the nervous system. *Acta Neuropathol.* 2013;126(6): 907–915.
34. Eckel-Passow JE, Lachance DH, Molinaro AM, et al. Glioma groups based on 1p/19q, IDH, and TERT promoter mutations in tumors. *N Engl J Med.* 2015;372(26):2499–2508.

35. Jeon YK, Park K, Park CK, et al. Chromosome 1p and 19q status and p53 and p16 expression patterns as prognostic indicators of oligodendroglial tumors: a clinicopathological study using fluorescence in situ hybridization. *Neuropathology.* 2007;27(1):10–20.
36. Aihara K, Mukasa A, Nagae G, et al. Genetic and epigenetic stability of oligodendrogliomas at recurrence. *Acta Neuropathol Commun.* 2017;5(1):18.
37. Giannini C, Scheithauer BW, Weaver AL, et al. Oligodendrogliomas: reproducibility and prognostic value of histologic diagnosis and grading. *J Neuropathol Exp Neurology.* 2001;60(3):248–262.
38. Qaddoumi I, Orisme W, Wen J, et al. Genetic alterations in uncommon low-grade neuroepithelial tumors: BRAF, FGFR1, and MYB mutations occur at high frequency and align with morphology. *Acta Neuropathologica.* 2016;131(6):833–845.
39. Kakkar A, Majumdar A, Kumar A, et al. Alterations in BRAF gene, and enhanced mTOR and MAPK signaling in dysembryoplastic neuroepithelial tumors (DNTs). *Epilepsy Res.* 2016;127:141–151.
40. Korshunov A, Meyer J, Capper D, et al. Combined molecular analysis of BRAF and IDH1 distinguishes pilocytic astrocytoma from diffuse astrocytoma. *Acta Neuropathologica.* 2009;118(3):401–405.
41. Preusser M, Laggner U, Haberler C, et al. Comparative analysis of NeuN immunoreactivity in primary brain tumours: conclusions for rational use in diagnostic histopathology. *Histopathology.* 2006;48(4):438–444.
42. Rodriguez FJ, Mota RA, Scheithauer BW, et al. Interphase cytogenetics for 1p19q and t(1;19)(q10;p10) may distinguish prognostically relevant subgroups in extraventricular neurocytoma. *Brain Pathol.* 2009;19(4):623–629.
43. Rodriguez FJ, Perry A, Rosenblum MK, et al. Disseminated oligodendroglial-like leptomeningeal tumor of childhood: a distinctive clinicopathologic entity. *Acta Neuropathol.* 2012;124(5):627–641.
44. Schniederjan MJ, Alghamdi S, Castellano-Sanchez A, et al. Diffuse leptomeningeal neuroepithelial tumor: 9 pediatric cases with chromosome 1p/19q deletion status and IDH1 (R132H) immunohistochemistry. *Am J Surg Pathol.* 2013;37(5):763–771.
45. Rodriguez FJ, Schniederjan MJ, Nicolaides T, et al. High rate of concurrent BRAF-KIAA1549 gene fusion and 1p deletion in disseminated oligodendroglioma-like leptomeningeal neoplasms (DOLN). *Acta Neuropathol.* 2015;129(4):609–610.
46. Zhang J, Wu G, Miller CP, et al. Whole-genome sequencing identifies genetic alterations in pediatric low-grade gliomas. *Nature Genet.* 2013;45(6):602–612.
47. Ramkissoon LA, Horowitz PM, Craig JM, et al. Genomic analysis of diffuse pediatric low-grade gliomas identifies recurrent oncogenic truncating rearrangements in the transcription factor MYBL1. *Proc Natl Acad Sci USA.* 2013;110(20):8188–8193.
48. Huse JT, Diamond EL, Wang L, et al. Mixed glioma with molecular features of composite oligodendroglioma and astrocytoma: a true "oligoastrocytoma"? *Acta Neuropathol.* 2015;129(1):151–153.
49. Qu M, Olofsson T, Sigurdardottir S, et al. Genetically distinct astrocytic and oligodendroglial components in oligoastrocytomas. *Acta Neuropathol.* 2007;113(2):129–136.
50. Kim YH, Nobusawa S, Mittelbronn M, et al. Molecular classification of low-grade diffuse gliomas. *Am J Pathol.* 2010;177(6):2708–2714.
51. Reuss DE, Mamatjan Y, Schrimpf D, et al. IDH mutant diffuse and anaplastic astrocytomas have similar age at presentation and little difference in survival: a grading problem for WHO. *Acta Neuropathol.* 2015;129(6):867–873.
52. Iwama T, Yamada H, Sakai N, et al. Correlation between magnetic resonance imaging and histopathology of intracranial glioma. *Neurol Res.* 1991;13(1):48–54.
53. Wessels PH, Weber WE, Raven G, et al. Supratentorial grade II astrocytoma: biological features and clinical course. *Lancet Neurol.* 2003;2(7):395–403.

54. Ohgaki H, Kleihues P. Population-based studies on incidence, survival rates, and genetic alterations in astrocytic and oligodendroglial gliomas. *J Neuropathol Exp Neurol.* 2005;64(6):479–489.
55. Rao RD, Krishnan S, Fitch TR, et al. Phase II trial of carmustine, cisplatin, and oral etoposide chemotherapy before radiotherapy for grade 3 astrocytoma (anaplastic astrocytoma): results of North Central Cancer Treatment Group trial 98-72-51. *Int J Radiat Oncol Biol Phys.* 2005;61(2):380–386.
56. Suzuki H, Aoki K, Chiba K, et al. Mutational landscape and clonal architecture in grade II and III gliomas. *Nat Genet.* 2015;47(5):458–468.
57. Reis RM, Hara A, Kleihues P, et al. Genetic evidence of the neoplastic nature of gemistocytes in astrocytomas. *Acta Neuropathol.* 2001;102(5):422–425.
58. Watanabe K, Peraud A, Gratas C, et al. p53 and PTEN gene mutations in gemistocytic astrocytomas. *Acta Neuropathol.* 1998;95(6):559–564.
59. Krouwer HG, Davis RL, Silver P, et al. Gemistocytic astrocytomas: a reappraisal. *J Neurosurg.* 1991;74(3):399–406.
60. Elvidge AR, Martinez-Coll A. Long-term follow-up of 106 cases of astrocytoma, 1928–1939. *J Neurosurg.* 1956;13(4):230–243.
61. Martins DC, Malheiros SM, Santiago LH, et al. Gemistocytes in astrocytomas: are they a significant prognostic factor? *J Neuro Oncol.* 2006;80(1):49–55.
62. Yang HJ, Kim JE, Paek SH, et al. The significance of gemistocytes in astrocytoma. *Acta Neurochir (Wien).* 2003;145(12):1097–1103; discussion 1103.
63. Ohta T, Kim YH, Oh JE, et al. Alterations of the RRAS and ERCC1 genes at 19q13 in gemistocytic astrocytomas. *J Neuropathol Exp Neurol.* 2014;73(10):908–915.
64. Tihan T, Vohra P, Berger MS, et al. Definition and diagnostic implications of gemistocytic astrocytomas: a pathological perspective. *J Neuro Oncol.* 2006;76(2):175–183.
65. Prayson RA, Estes ML. MIB1 and p53 immunoreactivity in protoplasmic astrocytomas. *Pathol Int.* 1996;46(11):862–866.
66. Prayson RA, Estes ML. Protoplasmic astrocytoma. A clinicopathologic study of 16 tumors. *Am J Clin Pathol.* 1995;103(6):705–709.
67. Huse JT, Nafa K, Shukla N, et al. High frequency of IDH-1 mutation links glioneuronal tumors with neuropil-like islands to diffuse astrocytomas. *Acta Neuropathol.* 2011; 122(3):367–369.
68. Capper D, Weissert S, Balss J, et al. Characterization of R132H mutation-specific IDH1 antibody binding in brain tumors. *Brain Pathol.* 2010;20(1):245–254.
69. Yaziji H, Massarani-Wafai R, Gujrati M, et al. Role of p53 immunohistochemistry in differentiating reactive gliosis from malignant astrocytic lesions. *Am J Surg Pathol.* 1996;20(9):1086–1090.
70. Kurtkaya-Yapicier O, Scheithauer BW, Hebrink D, et al. p53 in nonneoplastic central nervous system lesions: an immunohistochemical and genetic sequencing study. *Neurosurgery.* 2002;51(5):1246–1254; discussion 1254–1255.
71. Nobusawa S, Watanabe T, Kleihues P, et al. IDH1 mutations as molecular signature and predictive factor of secondary glioblastomas. *Clin Can Res.* 2009;15(19):6002–6007.
72. Hartmann C, Hentschel B, Wick W, et al. Patients with IDH1 wild type anaplastic astrocytomas exhibit worse prognosis than IDH1-mutated glioblastomas, and IDH1 mutation status accounts for the unfavorable prognostic effect of higher age: implications for classification of gliomas. *Acta Neuropathol.* 2010;120(6):707–718.
73. Cohen A, Sato M, Aldape K, et al. DNA copy number analysis of grade II-III and grade IV gliomas reveals differences in molecular ontogeny including chromothripsis associated with IDH mutation status. *Acta Neuropathol Commun.* 2015;3:34.
74. Lai A, Kharbanda S, Pope WB, et al. Evidence for sequenced molecular evolution of IDH1 mutant glioblastoma from a distinct cell of origin. *J Clin Oncol.* 2011;29(34): 4482–4490.

75. Chen L, Voronovich Z, Clark K, et al. Predicting the likelihood of an isocitrate dehydrogenase 1 or 2 mutation in diagnoses of infiltrative glioma. *Neuro Oncol.* 2014;16(11):1478–1483.
76. Liu XY, Gerges N, Korshunov A, et al. Frequent ATRX mutations and loss of expression in adult diffuse astrocytic tumors carrying IDH1/IDH2 and TP53 mutations. *Acta Neuropathol.* 2012;124(5):615–625.
77. Seiz M, Tuettenberg J, Meyer J, et al. Detection of IDH1 mutations in gliomatosis cerebri, but only in tumors with additional solid component: evidence for molecular subtypes. *Acta Neuropathol.* 2010;120(2):261–267.
78. Salvati M, D'Elia A, Melone GA, et al. Radio-induced gliomas: 20-year experience and critical review of the pathology. *J Neuro Oncol.* 2008;89(2):169–177.
79. Brat DJ, James CD, Jedlicka AE, et al. Molecular genetic alterations in radiation-induced astrocytomas. *Am J Pathol.* 1999;154(5):1431–1438.
80. Hamilton SR, Liu B, Parsons RE, et al. The molecular basis of Turcot's syndrome. *N Eng J Med.* 1995;332(13):839–847.
81. Hartmann M, Jansen O, Heiland S, et al. Restricted diffusion within ring enhancement is not pathognomonic for brain abscess. *AJNR Am J Neuroradiol.* 2001;22(9):1738–1742.
82. Mujic A, Hunn A, Taylor AB, et al. Extracranial metastases of a glioblastoma multiforme to the pleura, small bowel and pancreas. *J Clin Neurosci.* 2006;13(6):677–681.
83. Widjaja A, Mix H, Golkel C, et al. Uncommon metastasis of a glioblastoma multiforme in liver and spleen. *Digestion.* 2000;61(3):219–222.
84. Kleinschmidt-DeMasters BK. Diffuse bone marrow metastases from glioblastoma multiforme: the role of dural invasion. *Hum Pathol.* 1996;27(2):197–201.
85. Han SJ, Yang I, Tihan T, et al. Primary gliosarcoma: key clinical and pathologic distinctions from glioblastoma with implications as a unique oncologic entity. *J Neuro Oncol.* 2010;96(3):313–320.
86. Narayan A, Jallo G, Huisman TA. Extracranial, peritoneal seeding of primary malignant brain tumors through ventriculo-peritoneal shunts in children: case report and review of the literature. *Neuroradiol J.* 2015;28(5):536–539.
87. Trivedi RA, Nichols P, Coley S, et al. Leptomeningeal glioblastoma presenting with multiple cranial neuropathies and confusion. *Clin Neurol Neurosurg.* 2000;102(4):223–226.
88. Wakabayashi K, Shimura T, Mizutani N, et al. Primary intracranial solitary leptomeningeal glioma: a report of 3 cases. *Clinical Neuropathol.* 2002;21(5):206–213.
89. Semrad TJ, O'Donnell R, Wun T, et al. Epidemiology of venous thromboembolism in 9489 patients with malignant glioma. *J Neurosurg.* 2007;106(4):601–608.
90. Sperduto CM, Chakravarti A, Aldape K, et al. Twenty-year survival in glioblastoma: a case report and molecular profile. *Int J Radiat Oncol Biol Phys.* 2009;75(4):1162–1165.
91. Sarmiento JM, Mukherjee D, Black KL, et al. Do long-term survivor primary glioblastoma patients harbor IDH1 mutations? *J Neurol Surg A Cent Eur Neurosurg.* 2016;77(3):195–200.
92. Rong Y, Durden DL, Van Meir EG, et al. 'Pseudopalisading' necrosis in glioblastoma: a familiar morphologic feature that links vascular pathology, hypoxia, and angiogenesis. *J Neuropathol Exp Neurol.* 2006;65(6):529–539.
93. Rodriguez FJ, Scheithauer BW, Giannini C, et al. Epithelial and pseudoepithelial differentiation in glioblastoma and gliosarcoma: a comparative morphologic and molecular genetic study. *Cancer.* 2008;113(10):2779–2789.
94. Kleinschmidt-DeMasters BK, Aisner DL, Birks DK, et al. Epithelioid GBMs show a high percentage of BRAF V600E mutation. *Am J Surg Pathol.* 2013;37(5):685–698.
95. Kozak KR, Moody JS. Giant cell glioblastoma: a glioblastoma subtype with distinct epidemiology and superior prognosis. *Neuro Oncol.* 2009;11(6):833–841.

96. Karremann M, Butenhoff S, Rausche U, et al. Pediatric giant cell glioblastoma: new insights into a rare tumor entity. *Neuro Oncol.* 2009;11(3):323–329.
97. Oh JE, Ohta T, Nonoguchi N, et al. Genetic alterations in gliosarcoma and giant cell glioblastoma. *Brain Pathol.* 2016;26(4):517–522.
98. Vaubel RA, Caron AA, Yamada S, et al. Recurrent copy number alterations in low-grade and anaplastic pleomorphic xanthoastrocytoma with and without BRAF V600E mutation. *Brain Pathol.* 2017. doi: 10.1111/bpa.12495 [Epub ahead of print].
99. Dias-Santagata D, Lam Q, Vernovsky K, et al. BRAF V600E mutations are common in pleomorphic xanthoastrocytoma: diagnostic and therapeutic implications. *PloS One.* 2011;6(3):e17948.
100. Reis RM, Konu-Lebleblicioglu D, Lopes JM, et al. Genetic profile of gliosarcomas. *Am J Pathol.* 2000;156(2):425–432.
101. Perry A, Aldape KD, George DH, et al. Small cell astrocytoma: an aggressive variant that is clinicopathologically and genetically distinct from anaplastic oligodendroglioma. *Cancer.* 2004;101(10):2318–2326.
102. Burger PC, Pearl DK, Aldape K, et al. Small cell architecture–a histological equivalent of EGFR amplification in glioblastoma multiforme? *J Neuropathol Exp Neurol.* 2001; 60(11):1099–1104.
103. Takeuchi H, Kitai R, Hosoda T, et al. Clinicopathologic features of small cell glioblastomas. *J Neuro Oncol.* 2016;127(2):337–344.
104. Alexandrescu S, Korshunov A, Lai SH, et al. Epithelioid glioblastomas and anaplastic epithelioid pleomorphic xanthoastrocytomas–same entity or first cousins? *Brain Pathol.* 2016;26(2):215–223.
105. Perry A, Miller CR, Gujrati M, et al. Malignant gliomas with primitive neuroectodermal tumor-like components: a clinicopathologic and genetic study of 53 cases. *Brain Pathol.* 2009;19(1):81–90.
106. Sturm D, Orr BA, Toprak UH, et al. New brain tumor entities emerge from molecular classification of CNS-PNETs. *Cell.* 2016;164(5):1060–1072.
107. Korshunov A, Capper D, Reuss D, et al. Histologically distinct neuroepithelial tumors with histone 3 G34 mutation are molecularly similar and comprise a single nosologic entity. *Acta Neuropathol.* 2016;131(1):137–146.
108. Brat DJ, Scheithauer BW, Medina-Flores R, et al. Infiltrative astrocytomas with granular cell features (granular cell astrocytomas): a study of histopathologic features, grading, and outcome. *Am J Surg Pathol.* 2002;26(6):750–757.
109. Saad A, Mo J, Miles L, et al. Granular cell astrocytoma of the cerebellum: report of the first case. *Am J Clin Pathol.* 2006;126(4):602–607.
110. Rodriguez Y, Baena R, Di Ieva A, et al. Intramedullary astrocytoma with granular cell differentiation. *Neurosurg Rev.* 2007;30(4):339–343; discussion 343.
111. Joseph NM, Phillips J, Dahiya S, et al. Diagnostic implications of IDH1-R132H and OLIG2 expression patterns in rare and challenging glioblastoma variants. *Mod Pathol.* 2013;26(3):315–326.
112. Senetta R, Mellai M, Manini C, et al. Mesenchymal/radioresistant traits in granular astrocytomas: evidence from a combined clinical and molecular approach. *Histopathology.* 2016;69(2):329–337.
113. Castellano-Sanchez AA, Ohgaki H, Yokoo H, et al. Granular cell astrocytomas show a high frequency of allelic loss but are not a genetically defined subset. *Brain Pathol.* 2003;13(2):185–194.
114. Hinrichs BH, Newman S, Appin CL, et al. Farewell to GBM-O: genomic and transcriptomic profiling of glioblastoma with oligodendroglioma component reveals distinct molecular subgroups. *Acta Neuropathol Commun.* 2016;4:4.

115. Laxton RC, Popov S, Doey L, et al. Primary glioblastoma with oligodendroglial differentiation has better clinical outcome but no difference in common biological markers compared with other types of glioblastoma. *Neuro Oncol.* 2013;15(12):1635–1643.

116. Robinson C, Kleinschmidt-DeMasters BK. IDH1-mutation in diffuse gliomas in persons age 55 years and over. *J Neuropathol Exp Neurol.* 2017;76(2):151–154.

117. Oh D, Prayson RA. Evaluation of epithelial and keratin markers in glioblastoma multiforme: an immunohistochemical study. *Arch Pathol Lab Med.* 1999;123(10):917–920.

118. Hegi ME, Diserens AC, Gorlia T, et al. MGMT gene silencing and benefit from temozolomide in glioblastoma. *N Engl J Med.* 2005;352(10):997–1003.

119. Stupp R, Mason WP, van den Bent MJ, et al. Radiotherapy plus concomitant and adjuvant temozolomide for glioblastoma. *N Engl J Med.* 2005;352(10):987–996.

120. Rodriguez FJ, Thibodeau SN, Jenkins RB, et al. MGMT immunohistochemical expression and promoter methylation in human glioblastoma. *Appl Immunohistochem Mol Morphol.* 2008;16(1):59–65.

121. Liu L, Backlund LM, Nilsson BR, et al. Clinical significance of EGFR amplification and the aberrant EGFRvIII transcript in conventionally treated astrocytic gliomas. *J Mol Med.* 2005;83(11):917–926.

122. Cancer Genome Atlas Research Network. Comprehensive genomic characterization defines human glioblastoma genes and core pathways. *Nature.* 2008;455(7216): 1061–1068.

123. Solomon DA, Wood MD, Tihan T, et al. Diffuse midline gliomas with histone h3-k27m mutation: a series of 47 cases assessing the spectrum of morphologic variation and associated genetic alterations. *Brain Pathology.* 2016;26(5):569–580.

124. Sturm D, Witt H, Hovestadt V, et al. Hotspot mutations in H3F3A and IDH1 define distinct epigenetic and biological subgroups of glioblastoma. *Cancer Cell.* 2012;22(4): 425–437.

125. Aboian MS, Solomon DA, Felton E, et al. Imaging characteristics of pediatric diffuse midline gliomas with histone H3 K27M mutation. *AJNR Am J Neuroradiol.* 2017;38(4):795–800.

126. Frazier JL, Lee J, Thomale UW, et al. Treatment of diffuse intrinsic brainstem gliomas: failed approaches and future strategies. *J Neurosurg Pediatr.* 2009;3(4):259–269.

127. Venneti S, Santi M, Felicella MM, et al. A sensitive and specific histopathologic prognostic marker for H3F3A K27M mutant pediatric glioblastomas. *Acta Neuropathol.* 2014;128(5):743–753.

128. Buczkowicz P, Hoeman C, Rakopoulos P, et al. Genomic analysis of diffuse intrinsic pontine gliomas identifies three molecular subgroups and recurrent activating ACVR1 mutations. *Nat Genet.* 2014;46(5):451–456.

4

OTHER ASTROCYTOMAS

PILOCYTIC ASTROCYTOMA (WHO GRADE I)

Clinical Context

GENERAL. Pilocytic astrocytomas are the most common primary CNS neoplasms in childhood, accounting for about 17% of all such lesions (1). No significant sex predilection exists. The incidence of pilocytic astrocytomas remains level through childhood and tapers to occasional cases after the age of 30 years (2). Rare examples are found in the elderly, up to 85 years old (3). Patients with neurofibromatosis type 1 (NF1) have a predisposition to develop gliomas, which are most often pilocytic astrocytomas (4). Although many cases present classically as a circumscribed posterior fossa lesion, pilocytic astrocytomas can occur anywhere in the neuraxis. Other common sites include the optic chiasm/hypothalamus, thalamus, cerebral hemisphere, and brainstem. Although the histology of pilocytic astrocytomas has a large degree of overlap between all anatomic sites, their clinical contexts are distinct and discussed separately below.

CEREBELLAR. The vast majority of astrocytomas that occur in the cerebellum are pilocytic and occur in children, the remaining minority being diffusely infiltrative and nonpilocytic in older patients (5). Patients present with signs and symptoms similar to other cerebellar neoplasms, with incoordination/ataxia and increased intracranial pressure. The vast majority of cerebellar cases are cystic with about half of those being the classic cyst with mural nodule. Treatment consists of simple surgical resection in most cases. Long-term survival is good, almost 80% at 20 years from diagnosis in one series (5).

OPTIC PATHWAY. The optic nerves, chiasm, and tracts are common sites for pilocytic astrocytomas in infants and young children and are sometimes referred to as *optic gliomas* or *optic pathway gliomas*. About 60% of cases occur in the setting of NF1. Unlike in other locations, optic pathway pilocytic astrocytomas infiltrate the native substance of the optic apparatus and extend longitudinally within the nerve, forming a tapered, fusiform outline. Radiology may also show a characteristic "buckling" of the optic nerve (6). Many patients present with decreased visual acuity or nystagmus, but those with NF1 are frequently diagnosed when asymptomatic, as part of clinical workup of their syndrome (7). Cases that are bilateral or involve the optic nerve proper are more characteristic of patients with NF1, whereas sporadic cases tend to be centered on the chiasm (8,9). Chiasmatic lesions frequently involve the superjacent hypothalamus and for that reason cannot be completely resected.

Optic gliomas in patients with NF1 most often present with decreased visual acuity, but are also found incidentally in the clinical workup for NF1. Two large series found a significant female majority (~3:2, female:male) among optic glioma patients with NF1 (10,11). The clinical approach to, and natural history of, optic pathway gliomas depends heavily on the patient's NF1 status. Syndromic lesions are indolent and tend to stabilize around puberty, whereas sporadic cases are more likely to continually progress. Observation with surveillance imaging is the initial approach for many NF1 patients, reserving more aggressive care for the minority of cases that progress. Sporadic optic pathway gliomas and NF1-related cases that progress are treated with multiagent chemotherapy. Radiation is less commonly used due to long-term complications, especially in NF1 patients (12).

Because of the intimate association of the tumor to optic nerve axons, surgical resection is avoided in favor of a small diagnostic biopsy. Debulking surgery can be undertaken when vision is already severely compromised, when the tumor grows exophytically from the chiasm, or to relieve hydrocephalus, but is no longer considered a primary treatment option for most optic pathway gliomas.

Long-term (10-year) overall survival for optic pathway gliomas is high, approaching 98% in one large series (7). Both NF1-associated and sporadic cases have been documented to regress spontaneously in rare instances (13).

CEREBRAL HEMISPHERES. Only a few percent of supratentorial gliomas are pilocytic astrocytomas, but recognition of those few is essential because of their drastically different biology from infiltrating gliomas. Age of incidence in cerebral cases parallels that of cerebellar pilocytic astrocytomas and greatly overlaps that of infiltrating gliomas, making the prospect of having to distinguish the two likely. Most cases localize to the temporal and parieto-occipital lobes. Circumscription, strong contrast enhancement, and cystic spaces strongly favor pilocytic astrocytoma over diffuse glioma (14). Among published cases of cerebral pilocytic astrocytomas, long-term survival is high after surgical resection, about 80% of 102 cases with mean follow-up of around 15 years (14,15). The major risk factor for recurrence was subtotal resection in both of those studies.

BRAINSTEM. A small subset of pilocytic astrocytomas occur in the brainstem, where they are often dorsally exophytic from the medulla or midbrain (16). Formerly classified among other brainstem gliomas, pilocytic astrocytoma is recognized to have a much better prognosis than the more common diffuse brainstem gliomas, which occur mostly in the ventral

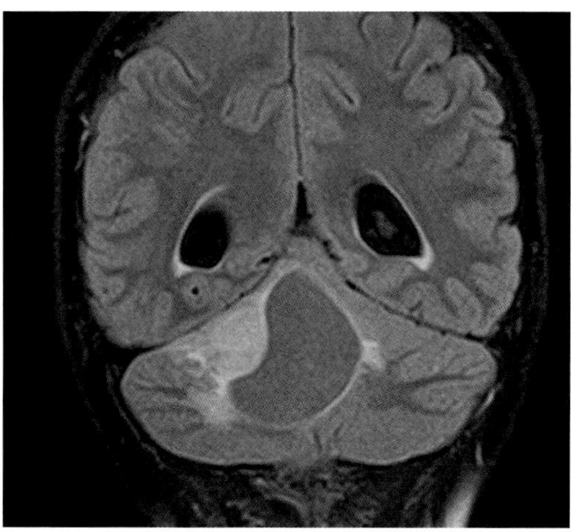

FIGURE 4-1 Pilocytic astrocytomas usually present as "cyst with mural nodule" lesions in children, as shown in this T2-weighted/FLAIR magnetic resonance imaging (MRI).

pons (17). Progression-free survival in brainstem pilocytic astrocytomas is favorable with complete surgical resection, 74% at 5 years versus 20% for incompletely resected lesions (18). Imaging characteristics are similar to pilocytic astrocytomas occurring elsewhere.

RADIOLOGIC FEATURES. Neuroimaging shows a circumscribed round or oval lesion that usually contains cystic areas and produces little edema in surrounding tissue. The "cyst with mural nodule" configuration is typical of cerebellar pilocytic astrocytomas (Figure 4-1). The solid portions of tumor are hypo- to isointense on CT scan and exhibit widespread contrast enhancement. On MRI, pilocytic astrocytomas are hypointense in T1-weighted sequences and hyperintense on T2 (19). Circumscription, cyst formation, and bright contrast enhancement help to separate pilocytic astrocytomas from infiltrating (grades II to IV) astrocytomas radiologically.

MENINGEAL DISSEMINATION. Leptomeningeal dissemination, either as diffuse or discrete lesions, occurs in a small number of patients with pilocytic astrocytoma. Hypothalamic/chiasmatic lesions account for about 70% of those patients (20). Many cases of dissemination result from mobilization of tumor cells into the CSF at the time of resection, but a few present with this finding: 5 out of 126 in one large institutional review (21). Patients will often show signs and symptoms of increased intracranial pressure and hydrocephalus, possibly due to clogging of the arachnoid villi by tumor cells. The clinical significance of dissemination is not completely understood, but it has a generally favorable outcome (20,22).

PILOMYXOID ASTROCYTOMA. Pilomyxoid astrocytoma is a variant subcategory of pilocytic astrocytoma that until the 2016 WHO update was considered grade II due to its reportedly more aggressive clinical course (23). They are most common in the first 3 years of life, and, like pilocytic astrocytomas, occur in progressively lower frequencies as age increases. Rare examples have been described in adults (24,25). Most cases are centered in the chiasmatic/hypothalamic area, yet pilomyxoid astrocytoma can be found anywhere in the neuraxis. It has been suggested that this tendency for hypothalamic location prevents their complete excision, thus explaining the less favorable outcomes, rather than it being due to the inherent biology of the tumor. Several cases from the spinal cord have been described (25,26). Neuroimaging fails to reveal any consistent differences between pilocytic and pilomyxoid astrocytomas (27). Several series have shown that the pilomyxoid variant is more aggressive and has a higher rate of recurrence and lower rate of survival, although the effect is difficult to separate from that of location (28–30). Nevertheless, evidence does at least seem to indicate that pilomyxoid astrocytoma has a higher rate of leptomeningeal dissemination, supporting a more intrinsically aggressive nature (31,32).

HEMORRHAGE. A recently recognized tendency of pilocytic astrocytomas is to develop intracranial hemorrhage at the site of the tumor. Two large series found the rate of clinically apparent hemorrhage to be about 8% to 11%, higher than any other category of glial neoplasm within the same time period (33,34). Cerebellar cases are much less likely to hemorrhage than those in other locations. The tendency to hemorrhage may be linked to the abnormally proliferating vasculature seen in these lesions.

Histopathology

No one description captures the spectrum of appearances in pilocytic astrocytomas, but several features remain constant through the vast majority. A *biphasic* pattern (Figure 4-2) of loose myxoid glial tissue alternating

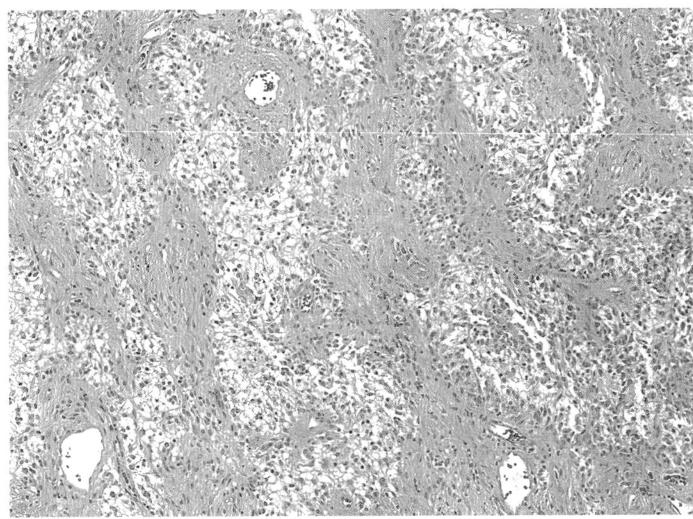

FIGURE 4-2 Pilocytic astrocytomas are usually biphasic at low magnification, with dense fibrillar areas and looser myxoid areas.

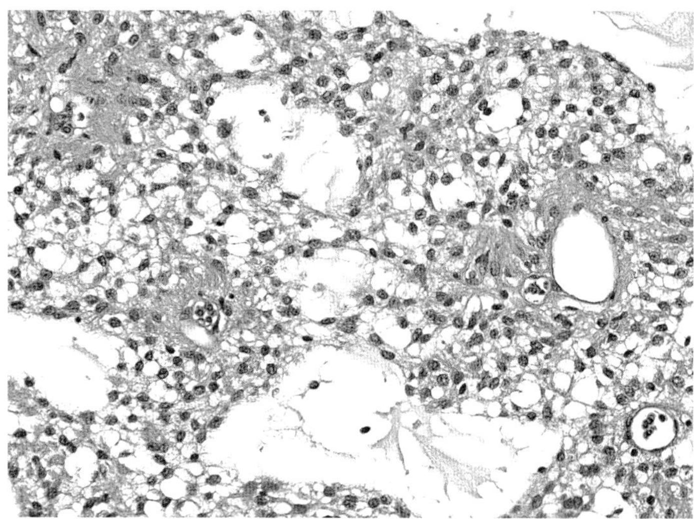

FIGURE 4-3 The loose areas in pilocytic astrocytomas are generally rich in myxoid material that frequently pools into microcysts.

with areas of densely fibrillar tissue is present at least subtly in the most cases. The loose areas contain monotonous round to oval nuclei with a few processes suspended in a mucoid material, creating a spongy microcystic look (Figure 4-3). The compact areas of fibrillar tissue are composed of elongate cells with thick fibrillar processes (Figure 4-4) that give the impression of matted hair, the origin of the tumor's name (Latin: pilus—hair). The

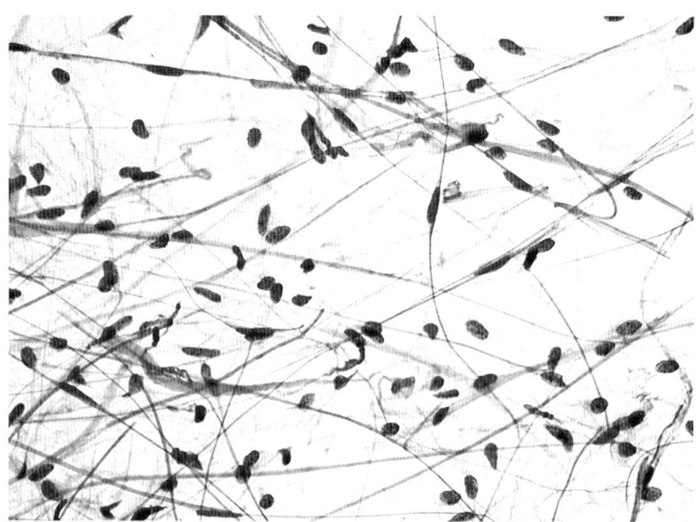

FIGURE 4-4 Smear preparations of pilocytic astrocytoma show oval to elongate, bipolar glial cells, many of which contain a single prominent eosinophilic thread through the cytoplasm.

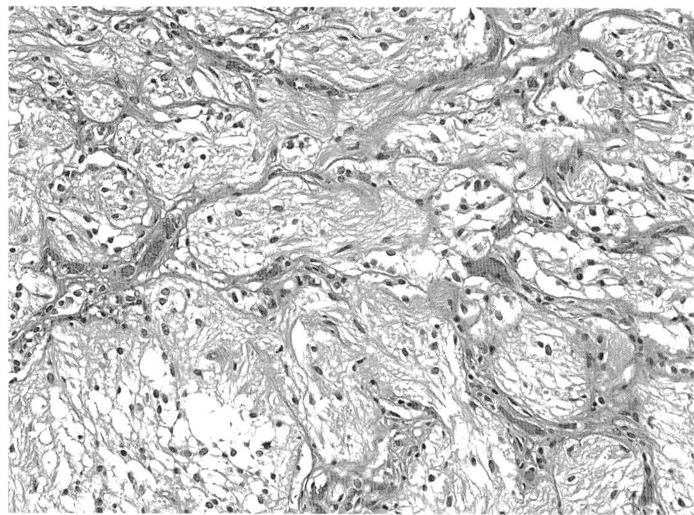

FIGURE 4-5 Pilocytic astrocytomas grow in a nested, fibrotic pattern in superficial areas involving the leptomeninges.

nuclei in fibrillar areas are uniform and oval to elongate. Calcifications and vascular hyalinization, common in low-grade lesions, are seen, but the former is uncommon. However, calcification may be more common in cases that spontaneously hemorrhage (33). Large parts of some pilocytic astrocytomas show a nodular nested pattern in superficial areas (Figure 4-5).

Some cases of pilocytic astrocytoma display a resemblance to oligodendrogliomas, with apparently infiltrative elements containing uniform cells with round nuclei and perinuclear haloes (Figure 4-6). When such tissue comes from a cystic cerebellar mass in a child, the diagnosis is straightforward, but in the cerebrum of older children and young adults, cautious review of all available evidence, including genetic characterization, should guide this distinction. Some have noted an increased incidence of recurrence in cerebellar cases with this feature (35).

Eosinophilic granular bodies (EGBs) may be seen in the microcystic portions of pilocytic astrocytomas and provide histologic evidence of the lesion's low-grade nature. EGBs are brightly eosinophilic, spherical protein droplets that occur in aggregates (Figure 4-7) or as larger single globules. Also seen in pleomorphic xanthoastrocytomas (PXAs) and gangliogliomas, EGBs develop intracytoplasmically within astrocytes and are composed of ubiquitinated alpha-1 chymotrypsin and alpha-1 antitrypsin (36). As with Rosenthal fibers, EGBs are neither specific nor sufficient for a diagnosis of pilocytic astrocytoma and can rarely be seen in higher-grade lesions, even glioblastoma (37). Like the hepatocellular inclusions of mutant alpha-1 antitrypsin in alpha-1 antitrypsin deficiency, EGBs are accentuated by PAS staining.

Rosenthal fibers are intensely eosinophilic, wormlike cords of aggregated protein that originate, like EGBs, within the cytoplasm of astrocytes

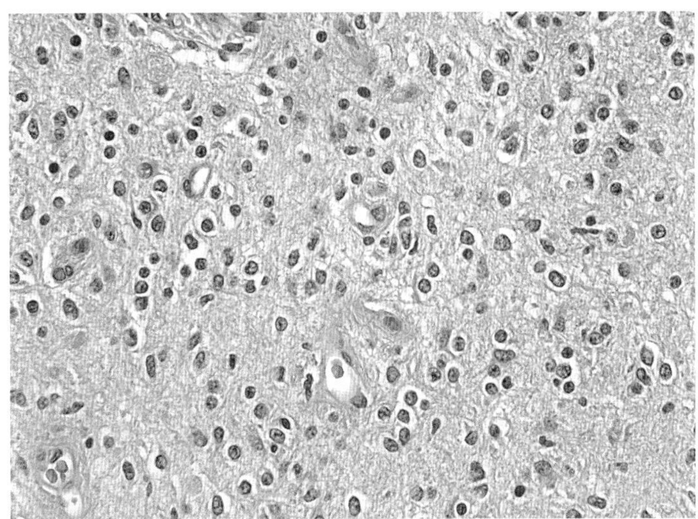

FIGURE 4-6 Some posterior fossa pilocytic astrocytomas have areas with a monotonous population of haloed cells with round regular nuclei, imitating the appearance of oligodendrogliomas.

(Figure 4-8). Although Rosenthal fibers are a consistent feature of pilocytic astrocytomas, these structures are also typical components of the reactive *piloid gliosis* in compressed brain tissue around indolent mass lesions, such as a craniopharyngioma, hemangioblastoma, or syrinx. In pilocytic astrocytomas, Rosenthal fibers are generally restricted to the dense regions and can range in quantity from zero to numerous. Rosenthal fibers have

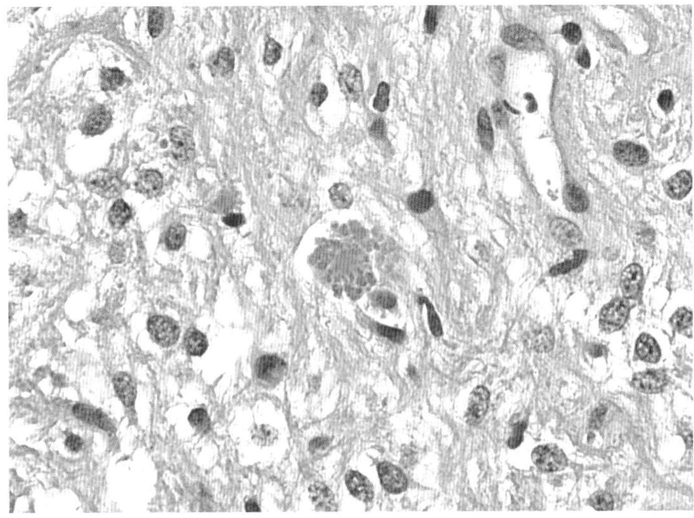

FIGURE 4-7 Eosinophilic granular bodies (EGBs) are common in the loose areas of pilocytic astrocytomas and in several other low-grade CNS neoplasms.

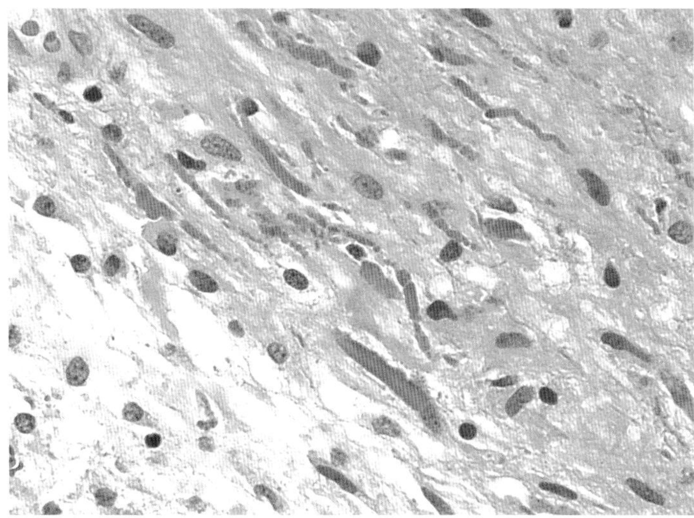

FIGURE 4-8 Rosenthal fibers are intensely eosinophilic vermiform structures that are seen in the dense areas of pilocytic astrocytomas.

also been described in malignant CNS tumors but are extremely unusual in that setting (38).

The circumscription of pilocytic astrocytomas on neuroimaging sometimes belies the extent of infiltration seen histologically (39). Mature nonneoplastic neurons can be entrapped well into the tumor, creating a potential nosologic crisis between pilocytic astrocytoma entrapping neurons and ganglioglioma with a piloid glial component. Fortunately, location separates most of these cases, and the consequences of misidentifying entrapped neurons as neoplastic are minimal.

PILOMYXOID FEATURES. The pilomyxoid variant is architecturally monomorphic, lacking the densely fibrillar element and biphasic appearance of classic pilocytic astrocytoma, instead demonstrating a loose myxoid pattern throughout. Pilomyxoid astrocytoma also has a distinctive perivascular orientation of tumor cells (Figure 4-9), similar to the perivascular pseudorosettes of ependymomas. Rosenthal fibers are lacking, but rare EGBs are allowable (23). Infiltration of surrounding tissue is limited but reported to exceed that of classic pilocytic astrocytoma (40). To suffice for a diagnosis of pilomyxoid astrocytoma, the vast majority of the tumor should show typical pilomyxoid features. The significance of focal pilomyxoid features is unknown, and their presence can be communicated either in comment form, or as an appendage to the diagnosis of pilocytic astrocytoma. Pilomyxoid astrocytoma will recur with a more typical, classic pilocytic growth pattern (41).

ANAPLASIA. Anaplastic change is remarkably rare in pilocytic astrocytomas, occurring in less than 2% in one large series (42). That same series

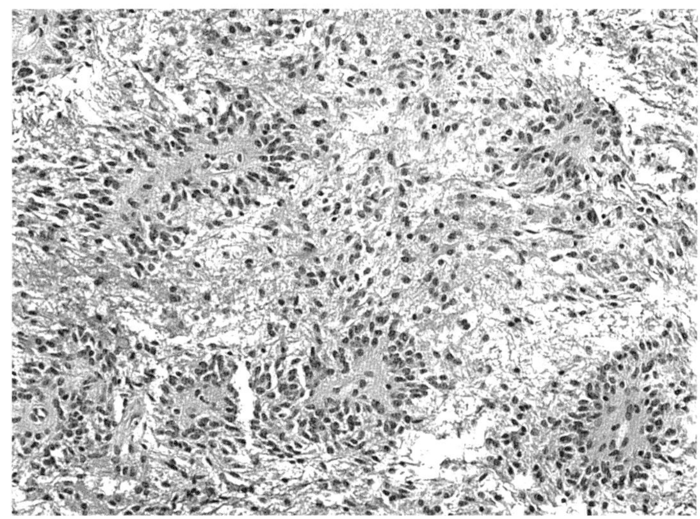

FIGURE 4-9 The pilomyxoid variant of pilocytic astrocytoma is characterized by prominent perivascular orientation of tumor cells in a monophasic myxoid background that generally lacks Rosenthal fibers.

also showed radiation to be a risk factor for anaplasia, although accounting for a smaller fraction of anaplastic tumors than what had been reported in the literature (42–45). The cases in that study, and most other reported cases were morphologically defined, so it's unclear if those that developed anaplasia were genetically distinct or had any molecular risk factor for progression. Anaplastic pilocytic astrocytomas are generally considered WHO grade III and not equivalent to a diagnosis of glioblastoma. Histologic criteria associated with poor outcome include ≥4 mitotic figures in 10 (400×) fields and necrosis (42). The criterion of mitotic activity does not apply in cases of optic pathway glioma in the setting of NF1, as it has not been shown to convey increased risk (4).

The features of necrosis, nuclear atypia, and vascular proliferation, characteristic of high grade in diffuse gliomas, can be disturbing but inconsequential components when noted in pilocytic astrocytomas (Figures 4-10 and 4-11). Necrosis is focally present in about 10% of cases, with a coagulative and infarct-like appearance, possibly resulting from either compression or occlusion of effete, hyalinized vessels (46). On the other hand, necrosis in the context of high mitotic activity, i.e., anaplastic histology, has been associated with poor outcomes (42). Vascular proliferation typically manifests as florid glomeruloid tufts or as long arcs of clustered capillaries in the walls of cystic cavities. Nuclear atypia can be prominent, similar to the symplastic "ancient change" common to schwannomas, sometimes forming multinucleate tumor cells.

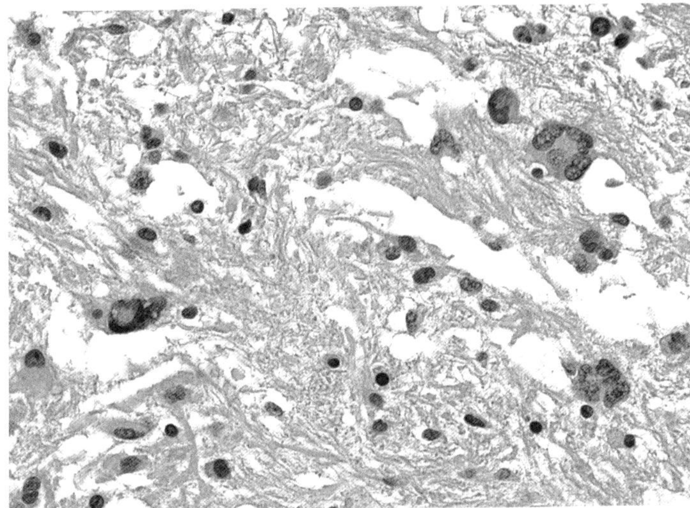

FIGURE 4-10 Nuclear atypia and multinucleate tumor cells are most likely due to degeneration and have no special significance in pilocytic astrocytoma.

Immunohistochemistry

The fibrillar processes in pilocytic astrocytomas predictably stain with GFAP, but this finding merely confirms the fibrillarity of the H&E-stained slide. Fewer than 10% of pilocytic astrocytomas show mildly increased nuclear staining for p53, a finding that correlates with higher rates of MIB1

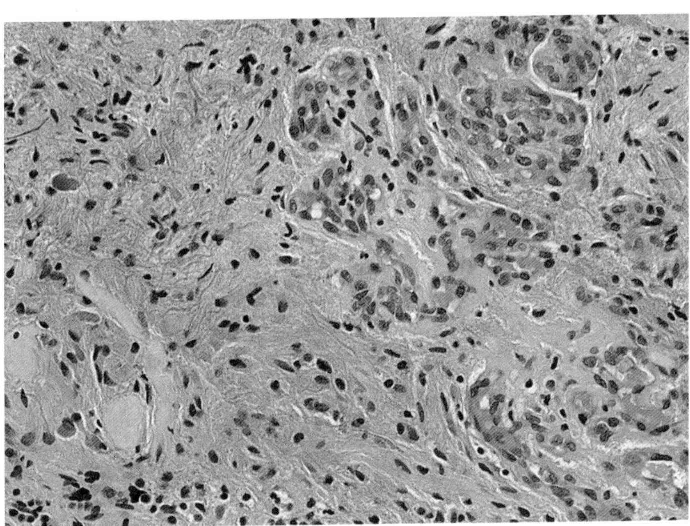

FIGURE 4-11 Microvascular proliferation, which is usually nodular and glomeruloid, holds no prognostic significance in pilocytic astrocytoma.

positivity and higher apoptotic rates but does not impact clinical outcome (47). Ki-67/MIB1 rates range as high as 20%, but are usually below 3%. Neurofilament staining shows varying gradients of infiltrated native axons in biopsied tumor fragments. Some cerebellar cases show surprising amounts of infiltration.

Genetics

The unifying genetic theme of pilocytic astrocytomas is activation of the MAP kinase pathway, generally through increased activity of the B-Raf protein. The frequency of specific genetic abnormalities varies based on the location of the tumor, the most common overall being a tandem duplication–fusion event between the *BRAF* and *KIAA1549* genes on chromosome 7 (48). These are present in about 80% of classic posterior fossa cases, 60% of non–NF1-related, chiasmatic/hypothalamic cases, and around 15% in hemispheric ones (49). *BRAF* V600E mutations are more common in hemispheric cases, accounting for about 13% of those and around 33% of diencephalic ones (50). Other alterations that may be seen include other fusions involving *BRAF*, *FGFR1* mutations, *KRAS* mutations, and losses of *NF1* in syndromic cases (48).

There is not yet any specific genetic finding used routinely to stratify pilocytic astrocytomas by risk, although gain of chromosome 7 seems to be associated with higher rates of recurrence (22). Pilomyxoid examples are as a group distinct from other pilocytic astrocytomas, yet have not shown any consistent, specific differences (41,51).

The above genetic alterations are useful in some cases to confirm the diagnosis of pilocytic astrocytoma; however, caution must be exercised to interpret the genetic findings in the context of all available histologic and neuroimaging data, as well as other genetic findings. *KIAA1549-BRAF* fusions were found in almost 15% of other types of pediatric brain tumors, including a variety of malignant ones (52).

Differential Diagnosis

The crucial distinction to make is between a diffuse glioma and pilocytic astrocytoma, the latter being highly curable by surgery and the former being incurable despite surgery, chemotherapy, and radiation. Review of the patient's neuroimaging should resolve doubt in most cases, showing circumscription, cyst formation, diffuse contrast enhancement, and minimal peripheral edema in pilocytic astrocytoma. Immunohistochemistry is useful in two ways: neurofilament staining shows a relatively broad infiltrative gradient in diffuse gliomas compared with the often steep gradient in pilocytic astrocytomas, and mutant IDH1 staining essentially rules out a pilocytic astrocytoma.

Mistaking a pilocytic astrocytoma for glioblastoma, or vice versa, has potentially disastrous implications. Although the age and anatomic distributions of the two tumors mostly overlap at the fringes, malignant infiltrating gliomas are not uncommon in the pediatric population and may present a diagnostic challenge. Glioblastomas usually show at least moderate peritumoral edema on T2-weighted MRI, whereas pilocytic astrocytomas have minimal or mild edema. Pilocytic astrocytomas occasionally show necrosis, but only rarely is there even vague palisading. Both may show florid vascular proliferation and intravascular thrombi. *EGFR* amplification, polysomy 7, deletion 10q, and *TP53* mutations are all seen in large subsets of adult GBM but not often in pediatric cases. Markers of pediatric malignant gliomas include histone mutations (H3 K27M or G34), *CDKN2A/B* deletions, *TP53* mutations, ATRX loss, and *PDGFRA* amplification, among others. Again, review of the lesion's imaging characteristics is necessary. Detection of the characteristic *KIAA1549-BRAF* fusion gene offers another tool to identify pilocytic astrocytoma in elusive cases, yet it should be interpreted in the context of all available information (53).

PLEOMORPHIC XANTHOASTROCYTOMA (WHO GRADE II) AND ANAPLASTIC PLEOMORPHIC XANTHOASTROCYTOMA (WHO GRADE III)

Clinical Context

PXA is most common in the first three decades of life; however, cases out into the 8th decade have been described (46,54). Males and females are equally affected. A majority of patients present with a long-term history of intractable seizures. A little more than a third of PXAs arise within the temporal lobe, with most of the remainder occurring elsewhere in the cerebral hemispheres. In these locales, the tumor maintains a superficial cortical position, often abutting and extending into the leptomeninges. PXAs rarely arise in other locations, including the cerebellum (55), spinal cord (56), pineal gland (57), and even in the retina (58).

Neuroimaging shows a circumscribed tumor that is isointense to gray matter on T1-weighted sequences, mildly hyperintense on T2, and intensely contrast enhancing (59). The pattern of contrast enhancement is typically heterogeneous within the solid tumor. Most contain cystic areas that sometimes form the "cyst with mural nodule" configuration. Edema surrounds most cases of PXA and ranges from mild to severe (60,61). As with other superficial, low-grade tumors, scalloping of the inner table of the skull may be seen.

The principle treatment for PXA is surgical resection, but many cases in the literature also received radiation and chemotherapy in varying doses and regimens. Giannini et al. identified extent of surgical resection (as estimated by the neurosurgeon) as the single most important factor in progression-free survival, with atypical mitoses and ≥5 mitoses/10 hpf also significantly correlated in univariate analysis (46). Progression-free survival was about 65% to 70% at 5 years and 55% to 60% at 10 years when cases with anaplastic features were included (46,54). Overall survival seems to be most associated with mitotic rate (≥5/10 hpf), thus providing the justification for a separate diagnosis of anaplastic PXA in such cases (54). When separated by grade, 5-year survival for grade II PXAs is almost 90% versus around 55% for anaplastic PXAs. Necrosis correlates with survival, but only insofar as it also correlates highly with increased mitotic activity, outside of which context its significance is unknown (54).

For cases with *BRAF* V600E mutations (see below under Genetics), there exists a specific inhibitor molecule, vemurafenib, that targets the mutant protein and is used to treat other tumor types with the same mutation, such as papillary thyroid carcinoma and melanoma. For anaplastic and recurrent cases of PXA, vemurafenib may provide an additional treatment strategy beyond traditional chemotherapy (62).

Histopathology

At its most fundamental level, PXA is a circumscribed astrocytoma with large cells that are almost always pleomorphic with multinucleate tumor giant cells (Figure 4-12). These bizarre elements overshadow the background of less atypical tumor cells that tend to be elongated and arranged in vague to distinct fascicles (Figure 4-13). Lymphocytes infiltrate the tissue near blood vessels. Mitotic figures and necrosis may be seen and are associated with a worse prognosis (see Grading). Vascular proliferation should not be a component of initial resection specimens but can occur as a reactive change after surgical manipulation. Calcifications are not common.

Despite the name, the histologic picture of PXA is not usually dominated by xanthic cells, that is, lipidized tumor cells with vacuolated cytoplasm, but they can be found in most cases if searched for.

As in ganglioglioma, most PXAs show varying forms of protein aggregates scattered throughout. Aggregates mirror the forms in ganglioglioma,

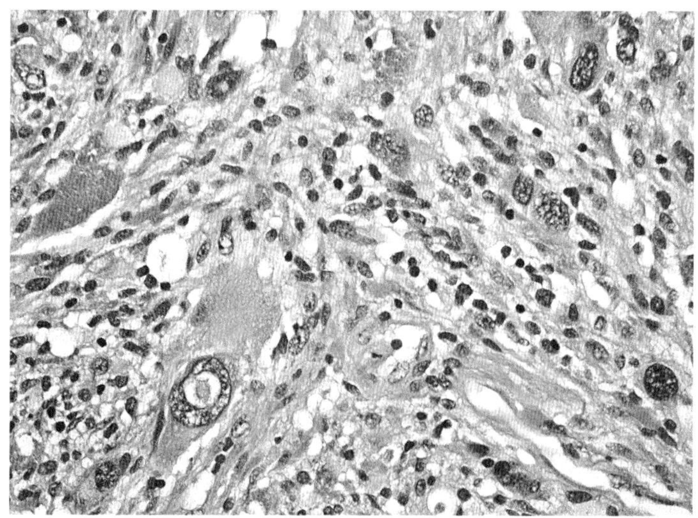

FIGURE 4-12 Pleomorphic xanthoastrocytomas have striking cytologic atypia that is out of proportion to their low rates of proliferation and generally indolent behavior.

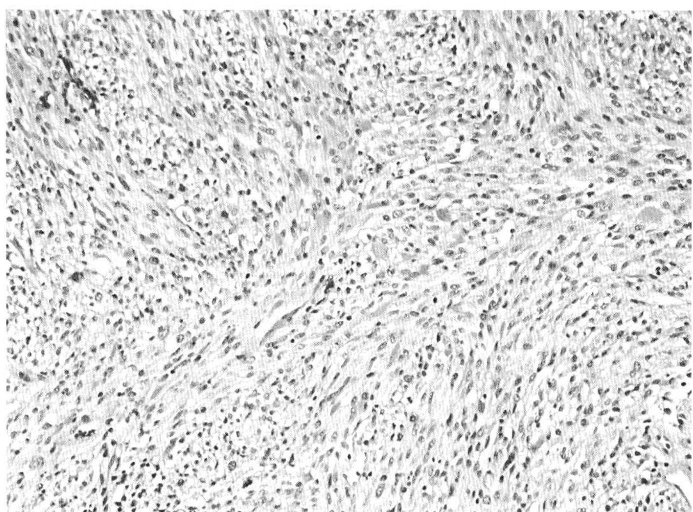

FIGURE 4-13 Pleomorphic xanthoastrocytoma may be vaguely fascicular and contain areas that are less pleomorphic. Note the scattered EGBs.

with intensely eosinophilic spheres that appear in clusters or as single round globes (see Figure 4-13), and others are more pale and finely granular, inspiring the term "pale granular bodies." Rosenthal fibers are present in a minority of PXAs.

Reticulin staining marks the pervasive network of basal lamina that surrounds each of the individual cells in PXA (Figure 4-14) and distinguishes it from the giant cell pattern of glioblastoma, which has sheets and clusters of cells within reticulin.

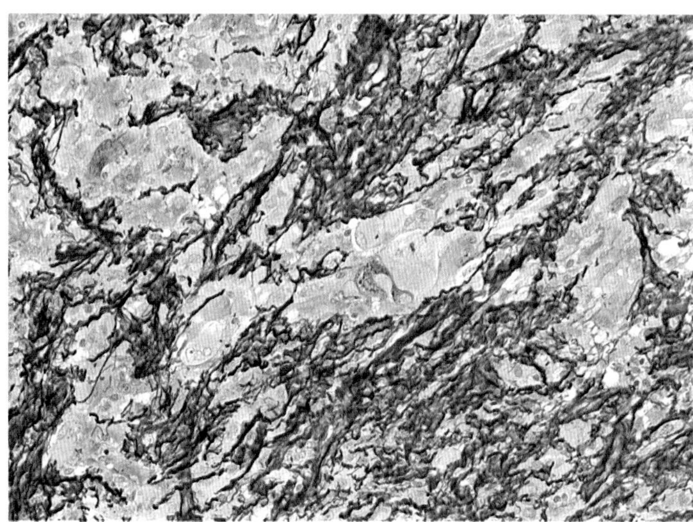

FIGURE 4-14 Reticulin staining demonstrates the dense network of collagen that envelops individual cells in pleomorphic xanthoastrocytoma.

PXA overlaps with ganglioglioma in location, age distribution, clinical presentation, and imaging features. The similarities extend into the microscopic realm, where both show a loosely fascicular architecture of glial cells, reticulin background, protein aggregates, and perivascular lymphocytes. Both tumor types also have significant rates of *BRAF* V600E mutations. In view of those things, it should not be surprising that PXA and ganglioglioma occasionally occur as distinct regions within the same tumor mass, and that otherwise typical PXAs sometimes contain a ganglion cell component (63–65).

Immunohistochemistry

The immunophenotype of PXA generally follows expectations for an astrocytic neoplasm, with diffuse positivity for S100 and GFAP, although GFAP expression can be focal, weak, or absent (66). Neuronal markers, including synaptophysin, neurofilament, and microtubule-associated protein 2 (MAP2), can be positive in a small number of PXA cells in a minority of cases (63). MIB1/Ki-67 labeling indices are generally below 3% in grade II PXAs and elevated in anaplastic cases. As in meningiomas, MIB1 staining can indicate the best places for counting mitotic figures. Mutations in the *TP53* gene are rare in PXA, and staining for p53 should be limited to low levels in scattered cells (67). Neurofilament staining should show modest infiltration, although focal single-cell infiltration may be seen around the edges in some cases.

The VE1 antibody clone against the mutant BRAF V600E protein offers a rapid and inexpensive assay for the mutation, yet can display high levels of nonspecific staining in some neuropathology cases, making it difficult to interpret. Nevertheless, this antibody has been used successfully in PXAs, where it is apparently expressed at high levels, as a reliable surrogate for DNA-based molecular testing (68).

Some PXAs express melanocytic markers, and even overt pigmentation, that can occasionally obscure the correct diagnosis (69–73). Morphology and GFAP staining are present in most cases, but in cases where GFAP staining is less prominent or focal, the diagnosis of melanoma should be excluded (66).

Grading

Most PXAs are WHO grade II. Increased mitosis (≥5/10 hpf) is sufficient for a diagnosis of anaplastic pleomorphic xanthoastrocytoma, WHO grade III (74). Necrosis is usually in the setting of increased mitotic activity and is of uncertain importance in the unusual cases where it occurs on a background of low proliferation. Likewise, microvascular proliferation is typically coincident with increased mitotic activity and necrosis.

Genetics

Two genetic findings typify PXAs and anaplastic PXAs: *BRAF* V600E mutations and homozygous deletions of *CDKN2A/B* on chromosome arm 9p. Mutations in *BRAF* are present in 50% to almost 80% of PXAs and do not seem to have an impact on tumor aggressiveness (50,68,75,76). Although not specific to the tumor type, the presence of a *BRAF* mutation can support the diagnosis of PXA over other entities in which it is rare, such as giant cell glioblastoma. Homozygous loss of *CDKN2A/B* is present in 80% to 90% of PXAs, regardless of grade or *BRAF* mutation status, suggesting that it is important in PXA tumorigenesis (77).

Differential Diagnosis

The most important and commonly encountered distinction is between PXA and giant cell glioblastoma. Both are generally circumscribed, with marked pleomorphism and lymphocytic infiltrates histologically. The marks of a PXA that are not seen in giant cell glioblastoma include a fascicular architecture, EGBs, and extensive intercellular reticulin deposition. Mitosis and necrosis are uncommon in PXAs and are very common in giant cell glioblastoma, but do not rule out the possibility of anaplastic PXA. Immunohistochemically, p53 is expressed diffusely in the majority of giant cell glioblastomas and only focally in a minority of PXA, making it a useful diagnostic tool. *BRAF* mutations are not expected in giant cell glioblastoma, although homozygous *CDKN2A/B* loss is occasionally seen.

Ganglioglioma overlaps with PXA on many different levels (see above in Histopathology), with some cases defying distinct categorization. *CDKN2A/B* deletions are rare in gangliogliomas and are present in the vast majority of PXAs.

SUBEPENDYMAL GIANT CELL ASTROCYTOMA (WHO GRADE I)

Clinical Context

Few primary CNS neoplasms have a more stereotyped clinical setting than that of subependymal giant cell astrocytoma (SEGA). The vast majority of SEGA are thought to occur in the context of tuberous sclerosis (78); however, because of variable expression, some SEGA patients will not show clinically apparent signs of the syndrome (facial angiofibromas, cortical tubers, intractable seizures, subungual fibromas, "ash-leaf spots," and shagreen patches) until later, if at all (79,80). The age at tumor diagnosis extends from in utero (81) to 75 years (38), with most cases presenting in the first two decades. Males and females are affected at similar rates. Resected cases are only seen in less than 10% of tuberous sclerosis patients (78) but may be detected by imaging in around 20% (82). Almost all SEGAs occur in the lateral or third ventricles, many of those centered near the foramina of Monro (Figure 4-15). Because of the proximity to this conduit of CSF flow, some patients will present with signs and symptoms of CSF obstruction. The onset of seizures may also precipitate the discovery of SEGA. CT shows a partially calcified nodule on the medial wall of the lateral ventricle that is T1 isointense and T2 hyperintense by MR (83). Contrast material intensely enhances the lesion. Other

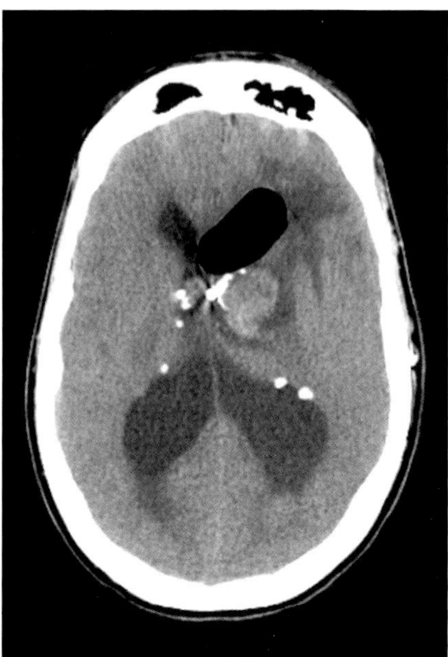

FIGURE 4-15 Subependymal giant cell astrocytomas (SEGAs) arise around the foramina of Monro and frequently block CSF flow, as seen in this nonenhanced CT image. White areas of calcification are present within tumor and subependymal "candle gutterings."

findings may include smaller subependymal nodules ("candle gutterings"), cortical tubers, and curvilinear white matter abnormalities (84).

Treatment consists of gross total resection in symptomatic cases, or when a lesion progresses during surveillance (85). Metastases have been described in rare cases (86,87). Everolimus, which inhibits mTOR, the target of the mutated proteins in tuberous sclerosis, has been shown in controlled trials to be effective for treating SEGA and may offer a lower-risk alternative to surgical intervention (88).

Histopathology

Sheetlike growth of large polygonal cells is seen in most cases of SEGA. The cells are large with eccentric, smooth, eosinophilic cytoplasm and one or two neuron-like nuclei with open chromatin and prominent central nucleoli (Figure 4-16). Cytoplasmic processes produce a fibrillar background, giving an overall appearance resembling large, reactive astrocytes. Alternatively, some examples contain streaming and fascicular arrangements of elongate cells. It is not uncommon to have perivascular fibrillar areas that resemble the pseudorosettes seen in ependymomas (Figure 4-17). Although SEGA contains rather large cells, truly giant cells are an uncommon component. Microcalcifications are common and can occasionally overshadow the tumor cells (89). Mitosis and necrosis have been described in cases with benign courses, suggesting that they are not worrisome observations (90).

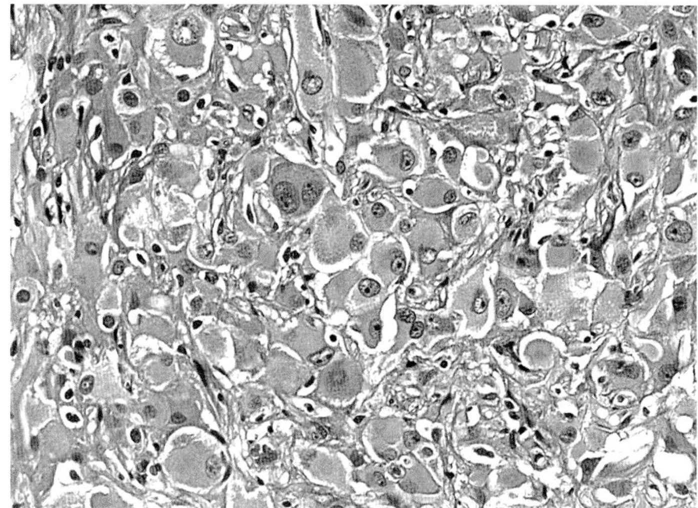

FIGURE 4-16 SEGAs are formed of large ovoid cells with eccentric pink cytoplasm and nuclei with pale chromatin and prominent nucleoli.

Circumscription is the rule in SEGA and infiltration should not be present. Scattered mast cells are common, as they are in hemangioblastoma and secretory meningioma.

Immunohistochemistry

Most SEGAs express both glial and neuronal antigens, with varying mixtures of GFAP, S100, neurofilament, class III beta-tubulin, synaptophysin, neuron-specific enolase, and MAP2 in most examples (89,91). This

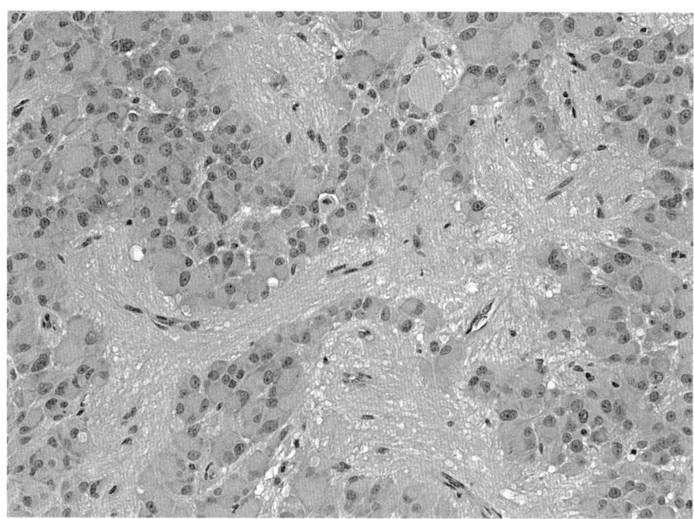

FIGURE 4-17 SEGAs can have fibrillar perivascular pseudorosette-like areas, similar to an ependymoma.

biphenotypic profile, supported by ultrastructural evidence, has led some to suggest reclassification of this tumor as glioneuronal in nature (89). The other tumors seen in the tuberous sclerosis complex, such as renal angiomyolipoma and cardiac rhabdomyoma, react with the monoclonal antibody HMB45, but this feature is not seen in SEGA (79,92). Almost all SEGAs express thyroid transcription factor-1 (TTF-1), which may be related to their anatomic distribution (93). Another series showed consistent expression of TTF-1 in SEGAs and little or no staining in other tumors that may mimic SEGA (94).

Differential Diagnosis

Gemistocytic astrocytoma probably bears the closest resemblance to SEGA, but it is an infiltrative lesion that does not form an intraventricular mass, a feature easily assessed by neuroimaging. Immunohistochemistry can eliminate the possibility of gemistocytic astrocytoma by showing a lack of infiltration (neurofilament) and mixed glial and neuronal staining in SEGA. Immunoreactivity for TTF-1 and BRAF V600E essentially rules out the possibility of gemistocytic astrocytoma, as does IDH1 R132H staining essentially rule out the possibility of SEGA.

Cases with elongate cells can vaguely simulate an ependymoma, especially if anucleate fibrillar zones surround blood vessels. Ependymomas also tend to have smaller nuclei with condensed chromatin and inapparent nucleoli and express dot- and ring-like cytoplasmic positivity for EMA. Ependymomas also lack immunostaining for TTF-1 and should not harbor BRAF mutations.

Central neurocytomas occur around the foramina of Monro and can show significant overlap in immunostaining for neuronal markers with SEGA, including NeuN. Central neurocytomas can also show weak to moderate immunostaining for TTF-1 (94). Nevertheless, the histologic overlap between central neurocytoma and SEGA is minimal. The cells of central neurocytomas are monotonous and contain round nuclei that usually have perinuclear clearing like oligodendrogliomas.

REFERENCES

1. Ostrom QT, Gittleman H, Xu J, et al. CBTRUS Statistical Report: primary brain and other central nervous system tumors diagnosed in the United States in 2009–2013. *Neuro Oncol.* 2016;18(suppl 5):v1–v75.
2. Bell D, Chitnavis BP, Al-Sarraj S, et al. Pilocytic astrocytoma of the adult–clinical features, radiological features and management. *Br J Neurosurg.* 2004;18(6):613–616.
3. Burkhardt K, Heuberger F, Delavelle J. Pilocytic astrocytoma in the elderly. *Clin Neuropathol.* 2007;26(6):306–310.
4. Rodriguez FJ, Perry A, Gutmann DH, et al. Gliomas in neurofibromatosis type 1: a clinicopathologic study of 100 patients. *J Neuropathol Exp Neurol.* 2008;67(3):240–249.
5. Hayostek CJ, Shaw EG, Scheithauer B, et al. Astrocytomas of the cerebellum. A comparative clinicopathologic study of pilocytic and diffuse astrocytomas. *Cancer.* 1993;72(3): 856–869.

6. Hollander MD, FitzPatrick M, O'Connor SG, et al. Optic gliomas. *Radiol Clin North Am.* 1999;37(1):59–71, ix.
7. Nicolin G, Parkin P, Mabbott D, et al. Natural history and outcome of optic pathway gliomas in children. *Pediatr Blood Cancer.* 2009;53(7):1231–1237.
8. Chateil JF, Soussotte C, Pedespan JM, et al. MRI and clinical differences between optic pathway tumours in children with and without neurofibromatosis. *Br J Radiol.* 2001; 74(877):24–31.
9. Singhal S, Birch JM, Kerr B, et al. Neurofibromatosis type 1 and sporadic optic gliomas. *Arch Dis Child.* 2002;87(1):65–70.
10. Czyzyk E, Jóźwiak S, Roszkowski M, et al. Optic pathway gliomas in children with and without neurofibromatosis 1. *J Child Neurol.* 2003;18(7):471–478.
11. Listernick R, Charrow J, Greenwald M, et al. Natural history of optic pathway tumors in children with neurofibromatosis type 1: a longitudinal study. *J Pediatr.* 1994;125(1):63–66.
12. Grill J, Couanet D, Cappelli C, et al. Radiation-induced cerebral vasculopathy in children with neurofibromatosis and optic pathway glioma. *Ann Neurol.* 1999;45(3):393–396.
13. Piccirilli M, Lenzi J, Delfinis C, et al. Spontaneous regression of optic pathways gliomas in three patients with neurofibromatosis type I and critical review of the literature. *Childs Nerv Syst.* 2006;22(10):1332–1337.
14. Forsyth PA, Shaw EG, Scheithauer BW, et al. Supratentorial pilocytic astrocytomas. A clinicopathologic, prognostic, and flow cytometric study of 51 patients. *Cancer.* 1993; 72(4):1335–1342.
15. Palma L, Guidetti B. Cystic pilocytic astrocytomas of the cerebral hemispheres. Surgical experience with 51 cases and long-term results. *J Neurosurg.* 1985;62(6):811–815.
16. Khatib ZA, Heideman RL, Kovnar EH, et al. Predominance of pilocytic histology in dorsally exophytic brain stem tumors. *Pediatr Neurosurg.* 1994;20(1):2–10.
17. Fisher PG, Breiter SN, Carson BS, et al. A clinicopathologic reappraisal of brain stem tumor classification. Identification of pilocystic astrocytoma and fibrillary astrocytoma as distinct entities. *Cancer.* 2000;89(7):1569–1576.
18. Kestle J, Townsend JJ, Brockmeyer DL, et al. Juvenile pilocytic astrocytoma of the brainstem in children. *J Neurosurg.* 2004;101(1 Suppl):1–6.
19. Lee YY, Van Tassel P, Bruner JM, et al. Juvenile pilocytic astrocytomas: CT and MR characteristics. *AJR Am J Roentgenol.* 1989;152(6):1263–1270.
20. Buschmann U, Gers B, Hildebrandt G. Pilocytic astrocytomas with leptomeningeal dissemination: biological behavior, clinical course, and therapeutical options. *Childs Nerv Syst.* 2003;19(5–6):298–304.
21. Hukin J, Siffert J, Velasquez L, et al. Leptomeningeal dissemination in children with progressive low-grade neuroepithelial tumors. *Neuro Oncol.* 2002;4(4):253–260.
22. Roth JJ, Fierst TM, Waanders AJ, et al. Whole chromosome 7 gain predicts higher risk of recurrence in pediatric pilocytic astrocytomas independently from KIAA1549-BRAF fusion status. *J Neuropathol Exp Neurol.* 2016;75(4):306–315.
23. Tihan T, Fisher PG, Kepner JL, et al. Pediatric astrocytomas with monomorphous pilomyxoid features and a less favorable outcome. *J Neuropathol Exp Neurol.* 1999;58(10): 1061–1068.
24. Omura T, Nawashiro H, Osada H, et al. Pilomyxoid astrocytoma of the fourth ventricle in an adult. *Acta Neurochir(Wien).* 2008;150(11):1203–1206; discussion 1206.
25. Sajadi A, Janzer RC, Lu TL, et al. Pilomyxoid astrocytoma of the spinal cord in an adult. *Acta Neurochir (Wien).* 2008;150(7):729–731.
26. Komotar RJ, Carson BS, Rao C, et al. Pilomyxoid astrocytoma of the spinal cord: report of three cases. *Neurosurgery.* 2005;56(1):191.

27. Linscott LL, Osborn AG, Blaser S, et al. Pilomyxoid astrocytoma: expanding the imaging spectrum. *AJNR Am J Neuroradiol.* 2008;29(10):1861–1866.
28. Komotar RJ, Burger PC, Carson BS, et al. Pilocytic and pilomyxoid hypothalamic/chiasmatic astrocytomas. *Neurosurg.* 2004;54(1):72–79; discussion 79–80.
29. Johnson MW, Eberhart CG, Perry A, et al. Spectrum of pilomyxoid astrocytomas: intermediate pilomyxoid tumors. *Am J Surg Pathol.* 2010;34(12):1783–1791.
30. Colin C, Padovani L, Chappe C, et al. Outcome analysis of childhood pilocytic astrocytomas: a retrospective study of 148 cases at a single institution. *Neuropathol Appl Neurobiol.* 2013;39(6):693–705.
31. Lee IH, Kim JH, Suh YL, et al. Imaging characteristics of pilomyxoid astrocytomas in comparison with pilocytic astrocytomas. *Eur J Radiol.* 2011;79(2):311–316.
32. Alkonyi B, Nowak J, Gnekow AK, et al. Differential imaging characteristics and dissemination potential of pilomyxoid astrocytomas versus pilocytic astrocytomas. *Neuroradiol.* 2015;57(6):625–638.
33. White JB, Piepgras DG, Scheithauer BW, et al. Rate of spontaneous hemorrhage in histologically proven cases of pilocytic astrocytoma. *J Neurosurg.* 2008;108(2):223–226.
34. Kondziolka D, Bernstein M, Resch L, et al. Significance of hemorrhage into brain tumors: clinicopathological study. *J Neurosurg.* 1987;67(6):852–857.
35. Horbinski C, Hamilton RL, Lovell C, et al. Impact of morphology, MIB-1, p53 and MGMT on outcome in pilocytic astrocytomas. *Brain Pathol.* 2010;20(3):581–588.
36. Katsetos CD, Krishna L, Friedberg E, et al. Lobar pilocytic astrocytomas of the cerebral hemispheres: II. Pathobiology–morphogenesis of the eosinophilic granular bodies. *Clin Neuropathol.* 1994;13(6):306–314.
37. Sasaki A, Yoshida T, Kurihara H, et al. Glioblastoma with large numbers of eosinophilic hyaline droplets in neoplastic astrocytes. *Clin Neuropathol.* 2001;20(4):156–162.
38. Takei H, Adesina AM, Powell SZ. Solitary subependymal giant cell astrocytoma incidentally found at autopsy in an elderly woman without tuberous sclerosis complex. *Neuropathol.* 2009;29(2):181–186.
39. Coakley KJ, Huston J, 3rd, Scheithauer BW, et al. Pilocytic astrocytomas: well-demarcated magnetic resonance appearance despite frequent infiltration histologically. *Mayo Clin Proceed.* 1995;70(8):747–751.
40. Fernandez C, Figarella-Branger D, Girard N, et al. Pilocytic astrocytomas in children: prognostic factors–a retrospective study of 80 cases. *Neurosurgery.* 2003;53(3):544–553; discussion 554–545.
41. Kleinschmidt-DeMasters BK, Donson AM, Vogel H, et al. Pilomyxoid astrocytoma (PMA) shows significant differences in gene expression vs. pilocytic astrocytoma (PA) and variable tendency toward maturation to PA. *Brain Pathol.* 2015;25(4):429–440.
42. Rodriguez FJ, Scheithauer BW, Burger PC, et al. Anaplasia in pilocytic astrocytoma predicts aggressive behavior. *Am J Surg Pathol.* 2010;34(2):147–160.
43. Ellis JA, Waziri A, Balmaceda C, et al. Rapid recurrence and malignant transformation of pilocytic astrocytoma in adult patients. *J Neuro Oncol.* 2009;95(3):377–382.
44. Tomlinson FH, Scheithauer BW, Hayostek CJ, et al. The significance of atypia and histologic malignancy in pilocytic astrocytoma of the cerebellum: a clinicopathologic and flow cytometric study. *J Child Neurol.* 1994;9(3):301–310.
45. Parsa CF, Givrad S. Juvenile pilocytic astrocytomas do not undergo spontaneous malignant transformation: grounds for designation as hamartomas. *Br J Ophthalmol.* 2008; 92(1):40–46.
46. Giannini C, Scheithauer BW, Burger PC, et al. Pleomorphic xanthoastrocytoma: what do we really know about it?*Cancer.* 1999;85(9):2033–2045.
47. Haapasalo H, Sallinen S, Sallinen P, et al. Clinicopathological correlation of cell proliferation, apoptosis and p53 in cerebellar pilocytic astrocytomas. *Neuropathol Appl Neurobiol.* 1999;25(2):134–142.

48. Collins VP, Jones DT, Giannini C. Pilocytic astrocytoma: pathology, molecular mechanisms and markers. *Acta Neuropathol.* 2015;129(6):775–788.
49. Jacob K, Albrecht S, Sollier C, et al. Duplication of 7q34 is specific to juvenile pilocytic astrocytomas and a hallmark of cerebellar and optic pathway tumours. *Br J Cancer.* 2009;101(4):722–733.
50. Schindler G, Capper D, Meyer J, et al. Analysis of BRAF V600E mutation in 1,320 nervous system tumors reveals high mutation frequencies in pleomorphic xanthoastrocytoma, ganglioglioma and extra-cerebellar pilocytic astrocytoma. *Acta Neuropathol.* 2011;121(3):397–405.
51. Jeon YK, Cheon JE, Kim SK, et al. Clinicopathological features and global genomic copy number alterations of pilomyxoid astrocytoma in the hypothalamus/optic pathway: comparative analysis with pilocytic astrocytoma using array-based comparative genomic hybridization. *Mod Pathol.* 2008;21(11):1345–1356.
52. Antonelli M, Badiali M, Moi L, et al. KIAA1549:BRAF fusion gene in pediatric brain tumors of various histogenesis. *Pediatr Blood Cancer.* 2015;62(4):724–727.
53. Sievert AJ, Jackson EM, Gai X, et al. Duplication of 7q34 in pediatric low-grade astrocytomas detected by high-density single-nucleotide polymorphism-based genotype arrays results in a novel BRAF fusion gene. *Brain Pathol.* 2009;19(3):449–458.
54. Ida CM, Rodriguez FJ, Burger PC, et al. Pleomorphic xanthoastrocytoma: natural history and long-term follow-up. *Brain Pathol.* 2015;25(5):575–586.
55. Hamlat A, Le Strat A, Guegan Y, et al. Cerebellar pleomorphic xanthoastrocytoma: case report and literature review. *Surg Neurol.* 2007;68(1):89–94; discussion 94–95.
56. Nakamura M, Chiba K, Matsumoto M, et al. Pleomorphic xanthoastrocytoma of the spinal cord. Case report. *J Neurosurg Spine.* 2006;5(1):72–75.
57. Thakar S, Sai Kiran NA, Ghosal N, et al. Pleomorphic xanthoastrocytoma: a new differential diagnosis for a pediatric pineal neoplasm. *Brain Tumor Pathol.* 2012;29(3): 168–171.
58. Zarate JO, Sampaolesi R. Pleomorphic xanthoastrocytoma of the retina. *Am J Surg Pathol.* 1999;23(1):79–81.
59. Tien RD, Cardenas CA, Rajagopalan S. Pleomorphic xanthoastrocytoma of the brain: MR findings in six patients. *AJR Am J Roentgenol.* 1992;159(6):1287–1290.
60. Yu S, He L, Zhuang X, et al. Pleomorphic xanthoastrocytoma: MR imaging findings in 19 patients. *Acta Radiol.* 2011;52(2):223–228.
61. Moore W, Mathis D, Gargan L, et al. Pleomorphic xanthoastrocytoma of childhood: MR imaging and diffusion MR imaging features. *AJNR Am J Neuroradiol.* 2014;35(11):2192–2196.
62. Lee EQ, Ruland S, LeBoeuf NR, et al. Successful treatment of a progressive BRAF V600E-mutated anaplastic pleomorphic xanthoastrocytoma with vemurafenib monotherapy. *J Clin Oncol.* 2016;34(10):e87–e89.
63. Giannini C, Scheithauer BW, Lopes MB, et al. Immunophenotype of pleomorphic xanthoastrocytoma. *Am J Surg Pathol.* 2002;26(4):479–485.
64. Perry A, Giannini C, Scheithauer BW, et al. Composite pleomorphic xanthoastrocytoma and ganglioglioma: report of four cases and review of the literature. *Am J Surg Pathol.* 1997;21(7):763–771.
65. Powell SZ, Yachnis AT, Rorke LB, et al. Divergent differentiation in pleomorphic xanthoastrocytoma. Evidence for a neuronal element and possible relationship to ganglion cell tumors. *Am J Surg Pathol.* 1996;20(1):80–85.
66. Gelpi E, Popovic M, Preusser M, et al. Pleomorphic xanthoastrocytoma with anaplastic features presenting without GFAP immunoreactivity: implications for differential diagnosis. *Neuropathol.* 2005;25(3):241–246.
67. Giannini C, Hebrink D, Scheithauer BW, et al. Analysis of p53 mutation and expression in pleomorphic xanthoastrocytoma. *Neurogenetics.* 2001;3(3):159–162.

68. Ida CM, Vrana JA, Rodriguez FJ, et al. Immunohistochemistry is highly sensitive and specific for detection of BRAF V600E mutation in pleomorphic xanthoastrocytoma. *Acta Neuropathol Commun.* 2013;1:20.
69. Kanzawa T, Takahashi H, Hayano M, et al. Melanotic cerebral astrocytoma: case report and literature review. *Acta Neuropathol.* 1997;93(2):200–204.
70. Sharma MC, Arora R, Khanna N, et al. Pigmented pleomorphic xanthoastrocytoma: report of a rare case with review of the literature. *Arch Pathol Lab Med.* 2001;125(6): 808–811.
71. Soffer D, Lach B, Constantini S. Melanotic cerebral ganglioglioma: evidence for melanogenesis in neoplastic astrocytes. *Acta Neuropathol.* 1992;83(3):315–323.
72. Chapman EM, Ranger A, Lee DH, et al. A 15 year old boy with a posterior fossa tumor. *Brain Pathol.* 2009;19(2):349–352.
73. Krossnes BK, Mella O, Wester K, et al. Pigmented astrocytoma with suprasellar location: case report and literature review. *Acta Neuropathol.* 2004;108(5):461–466.
74. Louis DN, Ohgaki H, Wiestler OD, et al., eds. WHO Classification of Tumours of the Central Nervous System. 4th, revised ed. Lyon, France: IARC Press; 2016.
75. Dias-Santagata D, Lam Q, Vernovsky K, et al. BRAF V600E mutations are common in pleomorphic xanthoastrocytoma: diagnostic and therapeutic implications. *PloS One.* 2011;6(3):e17948.
76. Koelsche C, Sahm F, Wohrer A, et al. BRAF-mutated pleomorphic xanthoastrocytoma is associated with temporal location, reticulin fiber deposition and CD34 expression. *Brain Pathol.* 2014;24(3):221–229.
77. Vaubel RA, Caron AA, Yamada S, et al. Recurrent copy number alterations in low-grade and anaplastic pleomorphic xanthoastrocytoma with and without BRAF V600E mutation. *Brain Pathol.* 2017. doi:10.1111/bpa.12495.
78. Shepherd CW, Scheithauer BW, Gomez MR, et al. Subependymal giant cell astrocytoma: a clinical, pathological, and flow cytometric study. *Neurosurgery.* 1991;28(6):864–868.
79. Gyure KA, Prayson RA. Subependymal giant cell astrocytoma: a clinicopathologic study with HMB45 and MIB-1 immunohistochemical analysis. *Mod Pathol.* 1997;10(4): 313–317.
80. Sharma M, Ralte A, Arora R, et al. Subependymal giant cell astrocytoma: a clinicopathological study of 23 cases with special emphasis on proliferative markers and expression of p53 and retinoblastoma gene proteins. *Pathology.* 2004;36(2):139–144.
81. Hussain N, Curran A, Pilling D, et al. Congenital subependymal giant cell astrocytoma diagnosed on fetal MRI. *Arch Dis Child.* 2006;91(6):520.
82. Goh S, Butler W, Thiele EA. Subependymal giant cell tumors in tuberous sclerosis complex. *Neurology.* 2004;63(8):1457–1461.
83. Inoue Y, Nemoto Y, Murata R, et al. CT and MR imaging of cerebral tuberous sclerosis. *Brain Dev.* 1998;20(4):209–221.
84. Iwasaki S, Nakagawa H, Kichikawa K, et al. MR and CT of tuberous sclerosis: linear abnormalities in the cerebral white matter. *AJNR Am J Neuroradiol.* 1990;11(5): 1029–1034.
85. Clarke MJ, Foy AB, Wetjen N, et al. Imaging characteristics and growth of subependymal giant cell astrocytomas. *Neurosurg Focus.* 2006;20(1):E5.
86. Aguilera D, Flamini R, Mazewski C, et al. Response of subependymal giant cell astrocytoma with spinal cord metastasis to everolimus. *J Pediatr Hematol/Oncol.* 2014;36(7): e448–e451.
87. Telfeian AE, Judkins A, Younkin D, et al. Subependymal giant cell astrocytoma with cranial and spinal metastases in a patient with tuberous sclerosis. Case report. *J Neurosurg.* 2004;100(5 Suppl Pediatrics):498–500.

88. Franz DN, Belousova E, Sparagana S, et al. Efficacy and safety of everolimus for subependymal giant cell astrocytomas associated with tuberous sclerosis complex (EXIST-1): a multicentre, randomised, placebo-controlled phase 3 trial. *Lancet.* 2013;381(9861):125–132.
89. Buccoliero AM, Franchi A, Castiglione F, et al. Subependymal giant cell astrocytoma (SEGA): is it an astrocytoma? morphological, immunohistochemical and ultrastructural study. *Neuropathology.* 2009;29(1):25–30.
90. Chow CW, Klug GL, Lewis EA. Subependymal giant-cell astrocytoma in children. An unusual discrepancy between histological and clinical features. *J Neurosurg.* 1988;68(6): 880–883.
91. Lopes MB, Altermatt HJ, Scheithauer BW, et al. Immunohistochemical characterization of subependymal giant cell astrocytomas. *Acta Neuropathol.* 1996;91(4):368–375.
92. Sharma MC, Ralte AM, Gaekwad S, et al. Subependymal giant cell astrocytoma–a clinicopathological study of 23 cases with special emphasis on histogenesis. *Pathol Oncol Res.* 2004;10(4):219–224.
93. Hewer E, Vajtai I. Consistent nuclear expression of thyroid transcription factor 1 in subependymal giant cell astrocytomas suggests lineage-restricted histogenesis. *Clin Neuropathol.* 2015;34(3):128–131.
94. Hang JF, Hsu CY, Lin SC, et al. Thyroid transcription factor-1 distinguishes subependymal giant cell astrocytoma from its mimics and supports its cell origin from the progenitor cells in the medial ganglionic eminence. *Mod Pathol.* 2017;30(3):318–328.

5

EPENDYMAL TUMORS

GENERAL

Ependymomas are glial tumors that display morphologic, immunophenotypic, and ultrastructural similarities to the ependymal cells lining the cerebral ventricular system. As a group, ependymomas have recently undergone extensive genetic and epigenetic examination which has subcategorized them into nine distinct genetic groups (1). Although four of these groups involve WHO grade I myxopapillary ependymomas and subependymomas and are not necessarily relevant to clinical management, the other five groups represent clinically meaningful entities among classic ependymomas, or what previously was in essence one category with two histologic grades. The 2016 WHO classification is a snapshot of the as yet incomplete transition from histologically defined classic ependymomas to a more genetically based scheme, in which the future relevance of histologic grading is unclear. It retains the general morphologic categories and histologic grading of the previous system while adding a category of supratentorial ependymoma defined by the presence of *RELA* gene fusions in the context of ependymoma morphology (2). Although the grade I entities are unlikely to change, the grade II and III ependymomas will likely undergo further subcategorization by genetic features in future editions. Here I present the morphologic categories of ependymoma and include the separate, genetically defined WHO diagnostic entity of "Ependymoma, *RELA* fusion–positive" among classic (grade II and III) ependymomas.

EPENDYMOMA (WHO GRADE II), ANAPLASTIC EPENDYMOMA (WHO GRADE III), AND EPENDYMOMA, *RELA* FUSION–POSITIVE

Clinical Context

Classic ependymomas occur primarily in children and young adults, and may arise anywhere along the neuraxis within the ventricles, spinal cord, or the cerebral hemispheres (3–6). As a whole, ependymal tumors peak in incidence in children ages 1 to 4 years where the rate is about a third higher than in infancy and twice as high as from 5 to 18 years (7). Most of those cases are in the posterior fossa and the rest are supratentorial or, rarely, spinal (1). Ependymoma incidence decreases with increasing age, decreasing to rare events after the age of 35 (8). A second, smaller peak of ependymomas occurs in older children and adolescents, in whom the supratentorial compartment in the lateral ventricles and hemispheres is the most common site. Spinal cord ependymomas occur most often in adults (30 to 40 years) and are most frequent in the cervical and cervicothoracic regions.

The clinical symptoms of ependymomas necessarily depend on patient age and tumor location (9,10). Posterior fossa masses in infants may present with an enlarging head due to increased intracranial pressure with incompletely fused cranial sutures, whereas slightly older children will often present with increased intracranial pressure and hydrocephalus with headaches, nausea, vomiting, dizziness, and ataxia. Spinal ependymomas present clinically with sensory and motor deficits that correspond to the spinal level involved.

By neuroimaging, ependymomas are generally solid, well circumscribed, and contrast enhancing (Figure 5-1). They push aside adjacent nervous system rather than diffusely invading it. In the posterior fossa, ependymomas typically fill the fourth ventricle and displace the cerebellum posteriorly. It is often difficult to determine if a posterior fossa tumor arises from the cerebellum and extends into the fourth ventricle (as expected for medulloblastoma) or if the tumor arises in the ventricle and extends into the cerebellum (typical of ependymoma). Ependymomas in this location may extend into the adjacent subarachnoid space by exiting through the foramina of Luschka. Although ependymomas are contrast-enhancing tumors, the degree of enhancement is variable and the pattern is often heterogeneous.

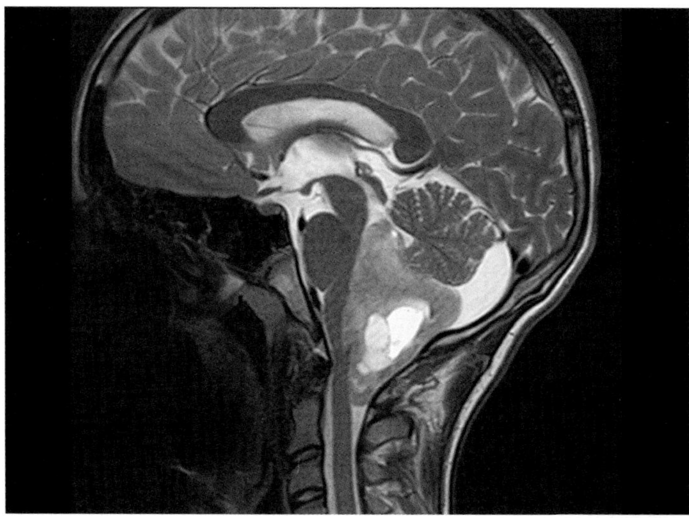

FIGURE 5-1 Sagittal, T2-weighted, noncontrast magnetic resonance imaging of a typical fourth ventricular ependymoma with cystic spaces.

The only known consistent risk factor for ependymomas is neurofibromatosis type 2 (NF2), in which patients are also predisposed to developing vestibular schwannomas and meningiomas. The ependymomas in NF2 usually occur in the spinal cord, particularly the cervical segment, and have an indolent clinical course compared to intracranial examples.

Prognostic Factors

AGE AND LOCATION. Patient age is one of the major prognostic features for ependymomas (11–13). The effect of age, though, is difficult to separate from location and extent of resection, because the vast majority of ependymomas occurring before 4 years are in the posterior fossa where they are many times impossible to dissect free of the floor of the fourth ventricle without severely harming the patient. Nevertheless, these tumors appear to have a poorer prognosis compared with ependymomas that occur in adults when adjusting for those factors. In contrast, ependymomas arising in adults, most of which are in the spinal cord, have a relatively good prognosis following resection.

EXTENT OF RESECTION. Gross total resection has been shown to be an important and often the statistically strongest prognostic indicator for ependymomas, and numerous studies have shown a survival benefit from total versus subtotal resection. Given their generally circumscribed margins, at least in comparison to the diffuse gliomas, this makes some intuitive sense. However, extension of fourth ventricular tumors into the subarachnoid space to involve brainstem structures and cranial nerves may preclude complete resection.

GENETIC CLASSIFICATION. Evidence from DNA methylation profiling and copy number studies has supported the idea that tumor location is a major determinant of ependymoma biology and that there are subgroups within each anatomic segment that have significant prognostic impacts. In brief, posterior fossa ependymomas can be divided into two groups; the majority are "group A," and the rest are "group B." Group A, posterior fossa ependymomas occur in younger children, mostly <4 years, and have significantly lower survival (Table 5-1). Group B tumors have better outcomes and occur in older children and young adults. Similarly, supratentorial ependymomas can be placed in two clusters along genetic lines, one group with fusions of the *RELA* gene and poor survival and others with *YAP1* gene fusions and better survival (Table 5-1). Spinal cord ependymomas form their own genetic group among classic ependymomas and have a much better outcome than intracranial cases. These five groups are discussed further below.

GAINS OF 1q. Gain of the long arm of chromosome 1 may be seen in any posterior fossa ependymoma or in *RELA* fusion–positive supratentorial ependymomas and is associated with decreased survival and/or increased recurrence rates when assessed in aggregate with all intracranial

TABLE 5-1 Intracranial Classic Ependymomas: Genetic Groups

Location	Genetic Group	Characteristics
Posterior fossa	Group A	Age: peak 1–4 yrs, rare after 18 Genetic feature: balanced genome Prognosis: good, 5-yr OS: ~70%
	Group B	Age: Mostly adults, some older children Genetic feature: unstable genome, chromosome 6 del Prognosis: good, 5-yr OS: ~100%
Supratentorial	*RELA* fusion	Age: broad range, peaks 4–18 yrs Genetic feature: *RELA* fusion, chromothripsis on 11q Prognosis: good, 5-yr OS: ~75%
	YAP1 fusion	Age: peak 1–4 yrs, some in older adults Genetic feature: *YAP1* gene fusion Prognosis: good, 5-yr OS: ~100%

ependymomas (14,15). However, when separated by molecular groups, decreases in overall survival were only noted among group A posterior fossa tumors, not *RELA* fusion or group B cases, although the latter did show increased recurrence (1).

TUMOR GRADE. Much effort has been made to construct a prognostically relevant, reproducible histologic grading scheme for classic ependymomas, and the results have been mixed. DNA methylation profiling shows no meaningful biological differences between grade II and anaplastic grade III ependymomas (1,16). Large series conducted by experienced neuropathologists have not shown significant differences in overall survival based on histologic grade, although there does appear to be differences in recurrence rates (17,18). The current consensus statement from an international group of pediatric brain tumor researchers recommends histologic grading not be used alone for stratifying clinical trials or clinical decision making, rather that it be integrated with molecular subgrouping routinely (19).

Treatment

Because they have shown consistent positive effects, both surgical resection and postoperative local irradiation of the tumor bed are the mainstays of current therapy for intracranial ependymomas. Chemotherapy has shown inconsistent results and does not have an established role in the treatment of ependymoma. Spinal cord ependymomas are usually treated with surgical resection alone.

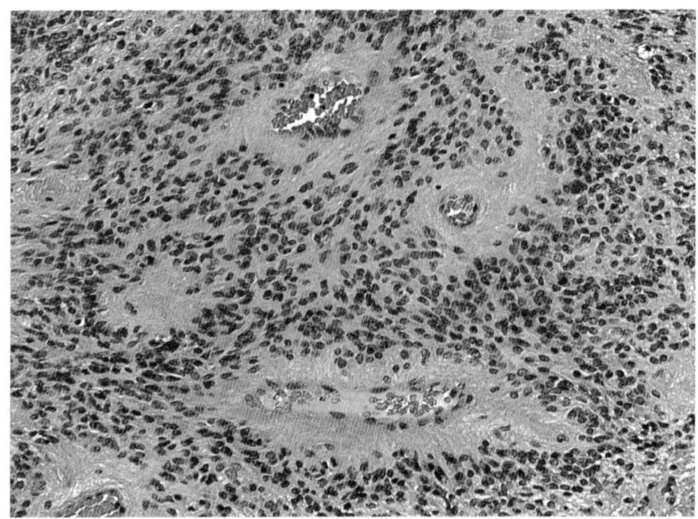

FIGURE 5-2 The perivascular pseudorosette is the hallmark of ependymomas, although similar structures can be seen in several other lesions.

Histopathology

Classic ependymomas are characterized by tumor cells that form pseudorosettes around central blood vessels and "true" ependymal rosettes. Pseudorosettes consist of ependymal tumor cells oriented around a central blood vessel with long fibrillar processes that extend radially from the vessel and give a pinwheel appearance (Figures 5-2 and 5-3). True rosettes

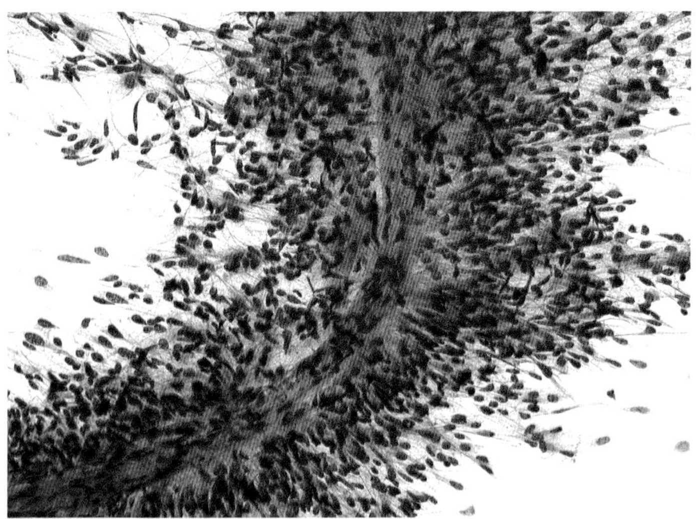

FIGURE 5-3 In smear preparations, the pseudorosettes of ependymomas form fibrillar pseudopapillary structures.

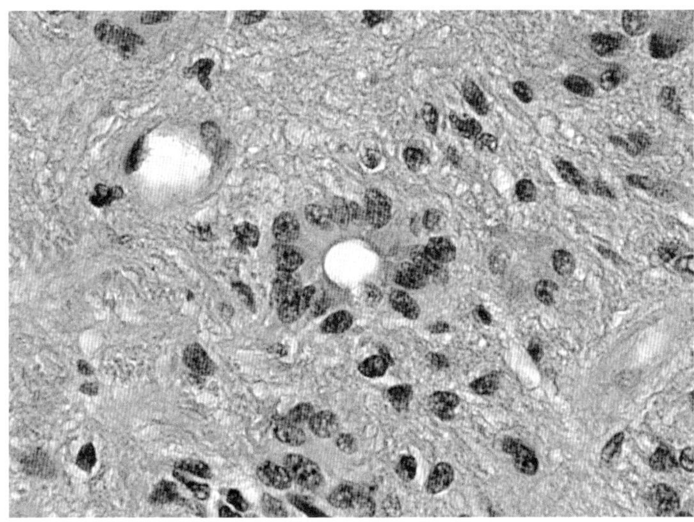

FIGURE 5-4 True ependymal rosettes exhibit a sharply defined central lumen and are only present in a minority of ependymomas.

(or canals), on the other hand, form a lumen centrally, reminiscent of the central canal of the spinal cord (Figure 5-4). One may also see epithelioid surfaces lined by ependymal tumor cells recapitulating their function of lining the ventricular system (Figure 5-5). Ependymomas show a wide range of cellularity and degrees of fibrillarity. Other features that can be seen in ependymoma include intratumoral hemorrhage, foci of necrosis,

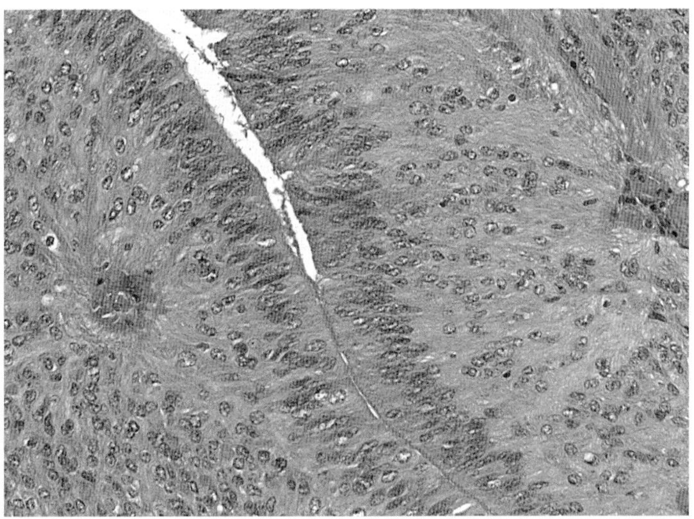

FIGURE 5-5 Ependyma-lined canals are ependymal rosettes on a larger scale.

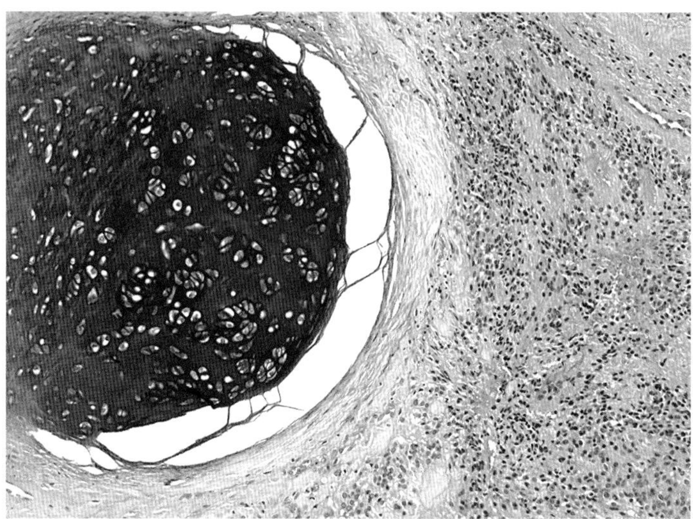

FIGURE 5-6 Although many types of heterotopic tissue can be seen in ependymomas, cartilage is among the most common.

cartilaginous and osseous metaplasia (20), calcification, and hyalinization of blood vessels (Figure 5-6).

Cytologic smear preparations can be helpful in diagnosing ependymomas intraoperatively. The tumor cells maintain their angiocentric arrangement, forming separate gliovascular units with fibrillar cytoplasm splayed out from the vessel, freeing many of the intervening nuclei onto the slide surface. The nuclear features of ependymoma are helpful in distinguishing them from medulloblastomas, which are a common diagnostic consideration in pediatric posterior fossa tumors. The nuclei of ependymomas are elliptical and usually regular with rigid nuclear membranes that contain coarsely granular chromatin, versus those of medulloblastoma, which are delicate, naked nuclei that contain fine chromatin that ruptures out and streams in smears.

HISTOLOGIC PATTERNS

TANYCYTIC EPENDYMOMA. Named for their supposed origin from tanycytes (*tanyos*—Greek word meaning stretched), tanycytic ependymomas are rare and differ from classic ependymomas in that they are less cellular, more fibrillar, and often have only vague perivascular pseudorosettes in a somewhat fascicular architecture (Figure 5-7). This lesion has a better prognosis than classic ependymoma, most likely because it occurs in the spinal cord of young adults, where all types of ependymomas have better outcomes. Although it is important to recognize the tanycytic pattern to prevent misdiagnosis as a schwannoma, specific mention of this histologic pattern in the diagnostic line of the pathology report is not necessary, as it usually does not influence the decision making of the treating physician.

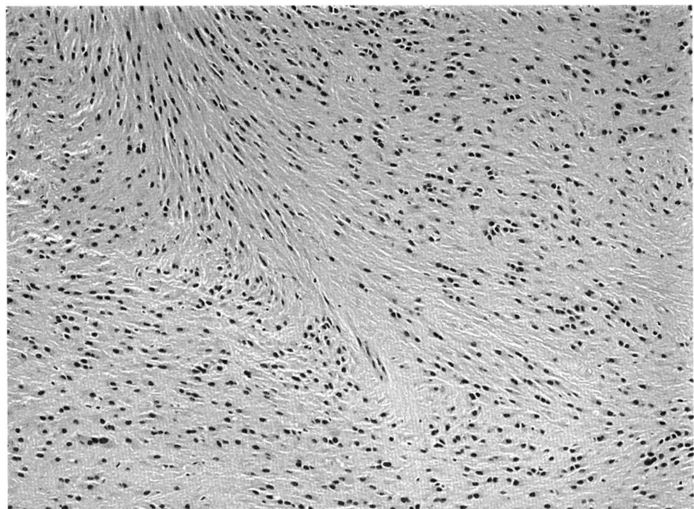

FIGURE 5-7 Tanycytic ependymomas may be fascicular and have only vague perivascular pseudorosettes.

CLEAR CELL EPENDYMOMA. The rare clear cell pattern of ependymoma is similar in concept to the clear cell meningioma in that its cells have clear, glycogen-rich cytoplasm and that they tend to be more aggressive. The lesion is composed of cells with small round nuclei and a modest amount of clear, halo-like cytoplasm and rich, branching capillary networks, imitating the histology of oligodendroglioma and central neurocytoma (Figure 5-8) (21,22).

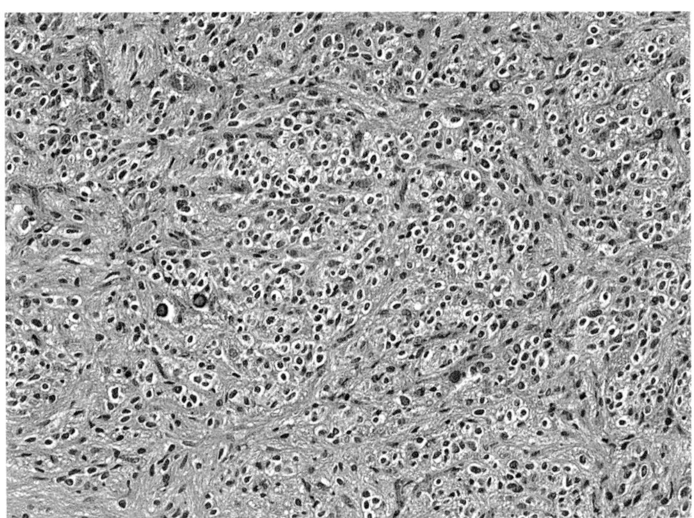

FIGURE 5-8 The round, regular, and haloed cells of the clear cell ependymoma can bear resemblance to neurocytomas and oligodendrogliomas.

Immunohistochemistry helps to eliminate neurocytomas from consideration if there is no synaptophysin or NeuN reactivity. Demonstrating absence of either IDH mutations or 1p/19q codeletion effectively rules out oligodendroglioma in adults.

PAPILLARY EPENDYMOMA. This rare pattern may have an appearance similar to a choroid plexus tumor because a smooth ependymal lining that coats branching fibrovascular cores, the cells tethered down to the vessel surface by GFAP-positive cytoplasmic extensions. This pattern has only been reported as individual cases and is very rare, so little is known about its clinical behavior overall.

Genetic Categories

There are five relevant categories of classic ependymomas, each having a specific set of clinical characteristics and being essentially restricted to one anatomic compartment of the central nervous system (CNS).

POSTERIOR FOSSA: GROUP A. If there were an archetypal representative of ependymomas, it would likely be from the genetic "group A" of posterior fossa cases, which constitute a majority of all ependymomas. Group A ependymomas only arise in the posterior fossa and overwhelmingly affect children under the age of 10 where they have a poor prognosis. One large series revealed a 56% recurrence rate at 5 years and 35% 5-year mortality, compared to 25% and 5% for group B cases, respectively (23). This group is defined by gene expression, DNA methylation, and copy number analysis, which reveal an overarching theme of genomic/chromosomal stability, evident in the relative lack of chromosomal abnormalities in group A tumors. Group A ependymomas are difficult to identify using traditional means and have no standardized criteria for clinical diagnosis. By age, the vast majority of posterior fossa ependymomas under 4 years will be group A, and they become rare after 18 years (1,23). An immunostain for the LAMA2 protein, which is expressed in group A but not group B ependymomas, has been suggested as a clinical biomarker for the former, although it is not in wide use (23).

POSTERIOR FOSSA: GROUP B. These ependymomas are a minority of those occurring in the posterior fossa and are more common in older children and adults, where they have a better prognosis than those of group A. Group B cases are characterized by genomic instability and have numerous chromosomal abnormalities on average. The most common abnormalities are loss of 22 and 6q, each being observed in about half of cases. Even though these losses are uncommon in group A cases, they cannot be used to reliably diagnose group B cases. Reactivity for NELL2 protein characterizes group B ependymomas and can potentially be used in conjunction with LAMA2 to clinically diagnose posterior fossa molecular groups (23).

SUPRATENTORIAL: *RELA* GENE FUSIONS. Supratentorial ependymomas make up about a quarter to a third of intracranial cases, and most, or about three-quarters of those have a rearrangement on chromosome 11 of the *RELA* gene resulting in overexpression via fusion, usually with the gene *C11ORF95* (24,25). These fusions nearly always result from a process called *chromothripsis* in which numerous DNA breaks and faulty repairs in a chromosomal region lead to what is essentially a random shuffling of DNA sequences. This shuffling results in a complex pattern of duplications, deletions, and fusions. *RELA* fusion–associated ependymomas are restricted to the supratentorial compartment and have a 25% mortality rate at 5 years versus 0% for *YAP1* fusion cases in the same cohort. This more aggressive behavior in the context of a clinically testable, defining genetic feature has led to this group being classified as a separate WHO entity: *Ependymoma, RELA fusion–positive* (2). FISH probes for *RELA* can assess for rearrangements clinically, or an immunostain for L1CAM may be used as a surrogate, it being positive in the vast majority of *RELA* fusion ependymomas. These are understood to behave in a high-grade fashion, yet are still histologically graded as either grade II or grade III for an integrated genetic–histopathologic diagnosis, a practice that may eventually be abandoned.

SUPRATENTORIAL: YAP1 GENE FUSIONS. Many of the remaining supratentorial ependymomas have fusions of the *YAP1* gene on chromosome 11 and exhibit a highly favorable clinical course, with a 5-year overall survival rate of 100% in one series, although those results remain to be replicated in other cohorts (1). Because of its good prognosis and tumor-defining genetic change, this group will likely also become a separate WHO entity once more experience with them is gained.

SPINAL. Classic, nonmyxopapillary ependymomas arising in the spinal cord are predominantly in adults and frequently occur in the context of NF2. Both sporadic and syndromic cases have similar high rates of loss of chromosome 22 (~90%) and mutations in the NF2 gene, suggesting a consistent pathogenetic theme among spinal cord ependymomas (26,27), which is supported by DNA methylation profiling (1).

Immunohistochemistry

GFAP immunostaining can be very useful in highlighting the typical pattern of thin cytoplasmic processes radiating from blood vessels in the center of perivascular pseudorosettes. EMA staining is variable, but when present it is usually seen along the surfaces formed by ependymal cells, either in linear arrays or around the lumens of ependymal rosettes. More helpful in less differentiated examples is a dot-like and ring-like pattern of intracytoplasmic staining, corresponding to the intracytoplasmic lumens seen on electron microscopy (Figure 5-9). Ring-like intracytoplasmic EMA reactivity showed

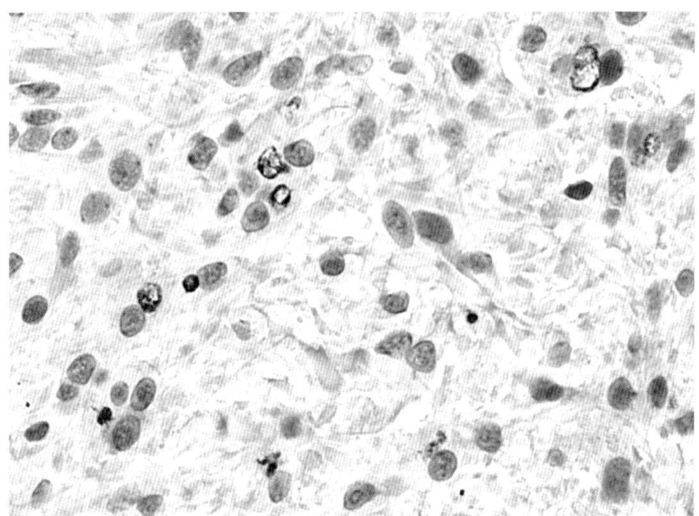

FIGURE 5-9 EMA staining reveals cytoplasmic dot-like and ring-like structures in ependymomas, except for myxopapillary cases.

100% specificity for ependymal lesions when compared with other primary CNS tumors, although the sensitivity was low, especially among myxopapillary ependymomas where they are absent (28). Similar EMA-positive structures are seen in other tumors of putative ependymal origin, such as chordoid glioma. As with many other CNS tumors, a neurofilament stain can be invaluable in determining whether a lesion is infiltrative in nature.

The immunostains LAMA2 and NELL2 have been suggested as effective surrogate markers for categorizing posterior fossa ependymomas into group A or group B, although this is not yet in widespread use, nor has it been yet replicated in other series (23). Similarly, L1CAM immunohistochemistry has been suggested as a marker for *RELA* fusion–positive ependymomas and is also not yet in widespread use (24).

Grading

The consensus is that histopathologic grading is neither a meaningful measure of ependymoma biology nor a useful tool for predicting tumor-related mortality and should not be used for clinical decision making or trial stratification (2,19). Nevertheless, the WHO system separates grade II and grade III ependymomas into different entities and provides vague guidelines for distinguishing them. High mitotic activity, microvascular proliferation, palisading necrosis, and hypercellularity are all factors that have been used for assigning anaplasia.

Differential Diagnosis

The differential diagnosis of a posterior fossa mass in a child includes medulloblastoma, ependymoma, pilocytic astrocytoma, and atypical

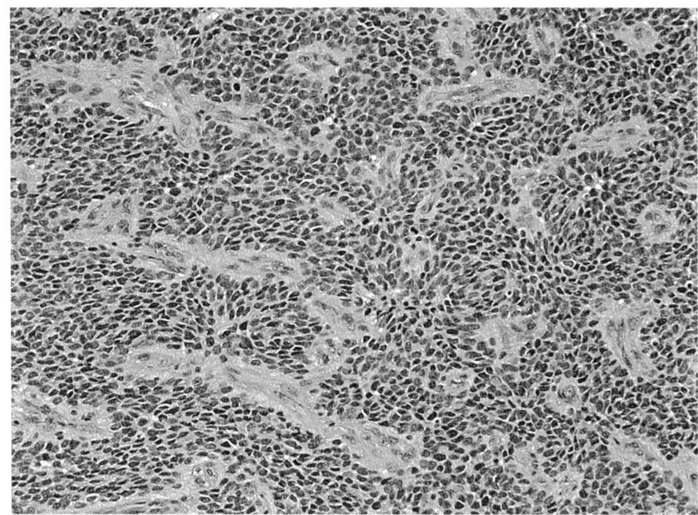

FIGURE 5-10 Anaplastic ependymomas can have scant perivascular fibrillarity and dense cellularity that may give a false impression of primitive neuroectodermal tumor or other embryonal neoplasm.

teratoid/rhabdoid tumor (AT/RT), with other tumors occurring less commonly. Anaplastic ependymomas that are highly cellular and poorly differentiated can have a high degree of morphologic overlap with medulloblastomas and other embryonal tumors in some instances. In these uncommon cases, anaplastic ependymomas are composed by a high density of tumor cells that show only a vague perivascular orientation without the high degree of perivascular pseudorosettes (Figure 5-10) that are present in well-differentiated cases. Medulloblastomas can also have a pattern of perivascular orientation, which can make the distinction between anaplastic ependymoma and medulloblastoma difficult. In most cases of anaplastic ependymoma, a well-differentiated component will be present at least focally in tissue sections. In other cases, immunohistochemistry can be helpful. Medulloblastomas are usually strongly positive for neuronal markers, such as synaptophysin or, less commonly, neurofilament. Some medulloblastomas may be focally positive for GFAP. Ependymomas, even those that are poorly differentiated, will usually show moderate to strong and diffuse GFAP staining but are generally negative for neuronal markers.

Astroblastomas may, at low magnification, appear very similar to ependymomas because both are well circumscribed and composed of a solid configuration and numerous pseudorosettes. Astroblastomas, however, are defined by astroblastic pseudorosettes, which contain elongated, columnar cells with stout, epithelioid cellular processes that extend to central vessels. They differ from ependymal rosettes, which show a high degree of fibrillarity. Indeed, the overall degree of fibrillarity noted in ependymoma is not seen in astroblastoma. A second prominent feature of astroblastomas is their high degree of perivascular hyalinization and regional hyaline changes within the tumor stroma. Tumor cells are strongly immunoreactive for S-100 protein, GFAP, and vimentin, while staining for EMA is strong in the pseudorosettes.

MYXOPAPILLARY EPENDYMOMA (WHO GRADE I)

Clinical Context

Myxopapillary ependymomas have a distinctive histologic pattern and a preferential localization to the region of the cauda equina, where they often arise from the filum terminale (Figure 5-11). Rarely, they occur in other CNS locations and can also present as sacrococcygeal tumors involving subcutaneous soft tissue. Myxopapillary ependymomas may occur at any age and are most common in young adults (median age: ~36 years). There is no strong predilection for either sex. Tumors generally grow as circumscribed, sausage-shaped masses extending down from the cauda equina and filling the intradural sac. They present clinically with low back pain and lower extremity symptoms.

The prognosis for patients with myxopapillary ependymoma is generally good from the perspective of mortality; rates of tumor-related mortality are less than 10% at 10 years. On the other hand, almost one-third of patients experience treatment failure, usually in the form of local recurrence (29). As with many other lesions in the CNS, completeness of resection is

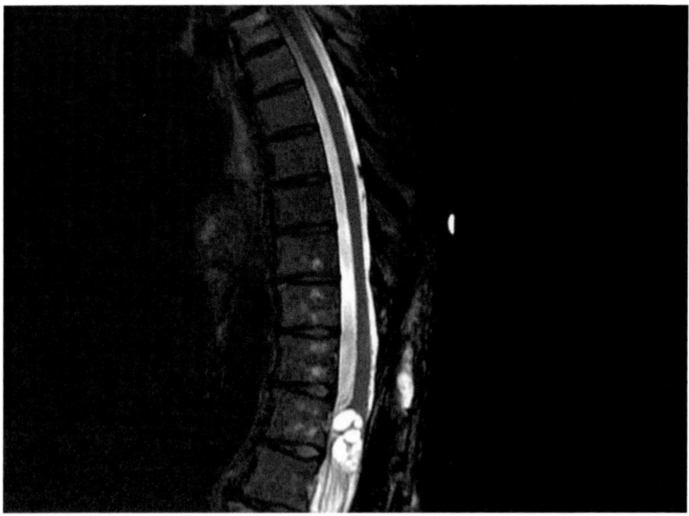

FIGURE 5-11 T2-weighted magnetic resonance imaging of myxopapillary ependymoma arising in the conus medullaris.

a key determinant of outcome. Younger patients (<35 years) have a more variable course and are more likely to experience poor outcomes. It is unusual for WHO grade I tumors to receive radiotherapy in addition to surgery, yet myxopapillary ependymomas seem to have improved control and fewer recurrences when the surgical site is radiated (29). Although metastases from such lesions are reported, they are rare (30–33). No histologic criteria for predicting metastatic or locally aggressive behavior of these lesions exist.

Histopathology

Myxopapillary ependymoma are frequently not overtly papillary under the microscope. Instead, they often will have a microcystic, almost cribriform, appearance with numerous pools of mucinous material among a monomorphic population of fibrillar glial cells and thickly hyalinized blood vessels (Figures 5-12 and 5-13). Alternatively, other cases may be composed of fibrillar cuboidal-to-columnar cells surrounding a central vessel and connective tissue stroma, giving a distinctly papillary architecture (Figure 5-14). The presence of a rim of hyaline or mucin surrounding the central blood vessel and separating it from the circumferential ependymal tumor cells is a classic, yet inconstant feature. The resulting distinctive histology of myxopapillary ependymoma comes from this pattern of degenerative, myxoid change and the production of mucin by tumor cells. Occasionally, the hyaline deposition around blood vessels almost completely replaces the original lesion,

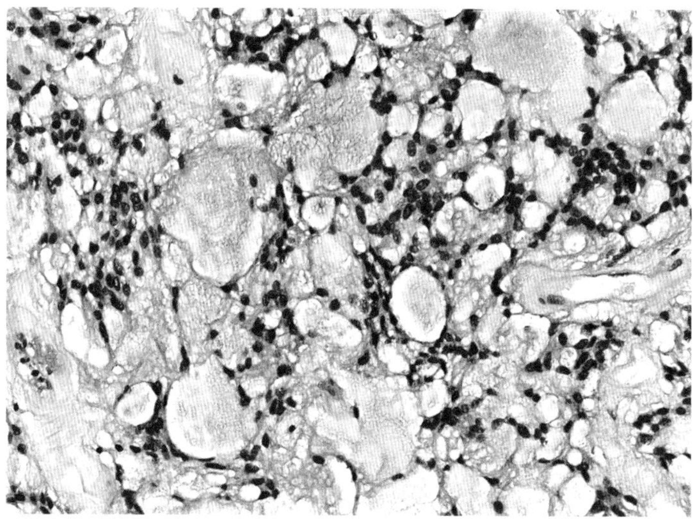

FIGURE 5-12 One of the most common features seen in myxopapillary ependymoma: pools of mucin in a field of fibrillar glial cells.

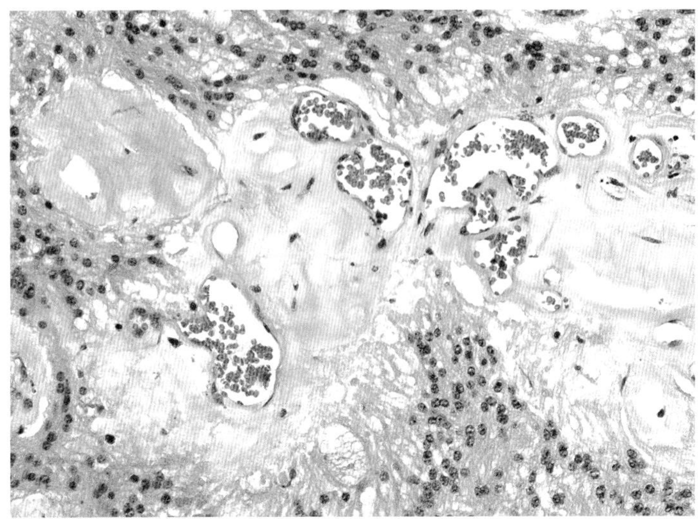

FIGURE 5-13 The vasculature of myxopapillary ependymomas is typically hyalinized.

leaving little recognizable as myxopapillary ependymoma (Figure 5-15). Like more typical ependymomas, the myxopapillary type is positive for GFAP, S-100 protein, vimentin, and CD99. Dot-like and ring-like immunoreactivity for EMA, which is present in other ependymomas, is not seen in the myxopapillary type.

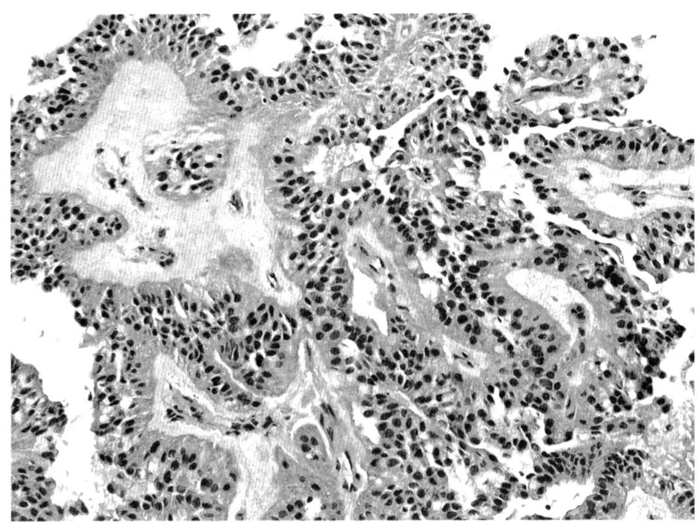

FIGURE 5-14 Less often, myxopapillary ependymomas have distinct papillae with perivascular mucin surrounded by columnar epithelioid cells.

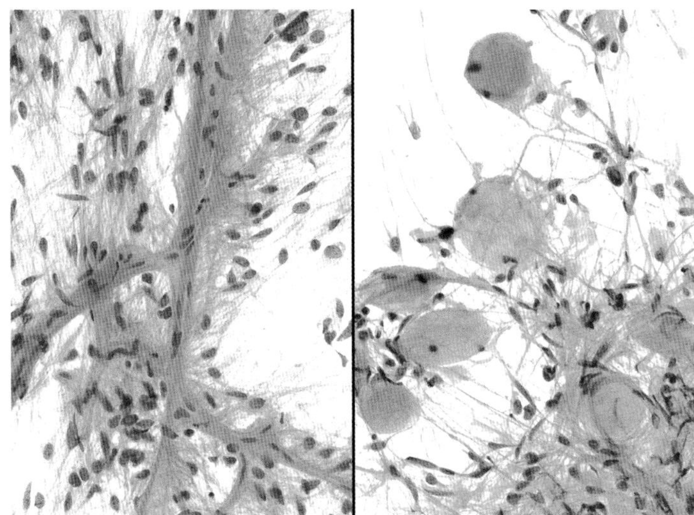

FIGURE 5-15 Crush preparations separate myxopapillary ependymomas into fibrillar pseudopapillary structures (**left**) that may contain inspissated spheroids of mucin (**right**).

SUBEPENDYMOMA (WHO GRADE I)

Clinical Context

Subependymomas are slowly growing tumors that are related to ependymomas in that they are solid, intraventricular glial tumors derived from ependymal cells. They are typically benign in their behavior and thus designated as WHO grade I. Subependymomas are often asymptomatic and are detected as incidental lesions by neuroimaging. They occasionally present incidentally at postmortem examination. They occur most often in adults, generally in an older population and more frequently in males. Subependymomas occur with greatest frequency in the fourth ventricle (50% to 60%) and in the lateral ventricles (30% to 40%) and can also occur in other ventricular sites. Spinal subependymomas occur centrally in the spinal cord, are well demarcated, and grow slowly.

Subependymomas are typically either observed or treated with surgical excision, after which few recur. Long-term, overall survival rates for subependymoma are around 100%.

Histopathology

Subependymomas are grossly lobulated tumors composed of clusters of monotonous, low-grade ependymal cells that are embedded in a densely fibrillar "astrocyte-like" glial matrix (Figures 5-16 and 5-17). The extent of the fibrillar zones is typically in excess to the cellular zones, and the overall cellularity is low. In some instances, tumor cells form rosettes or pseudorosettes, similar to those in classic ependymoma. In fact, cases of mixed

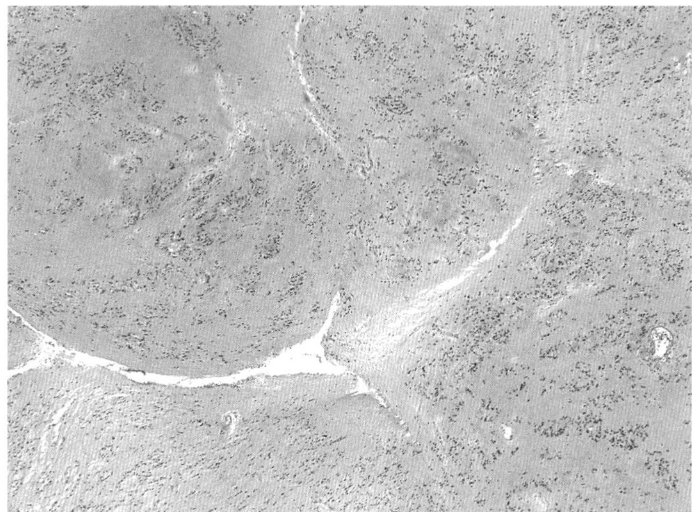

FIGURE 5-16 Subependymomas are vaguely lobular with clusters of banal glial cells in an otherwise acellular fibrillar matrix.

subependymoma–ependymoma are well recognized although it is unclear whether such cases have any worse outcomes than histologically pure subependymomas. Because of their slow growth, many subependymomas contain degenerative or secondary changes, such as cysts, hemosiderin deposition, vascular thickening, myxoid change, and calcification. Neither anaplastic features nor significant mitotic activity is seen.

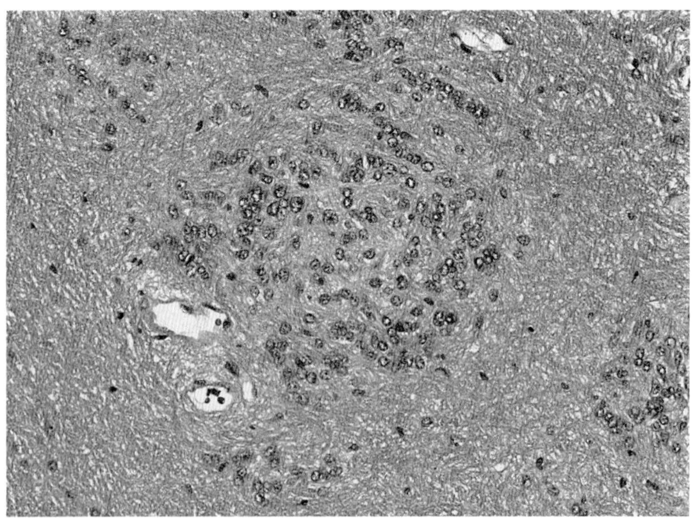

FIGURE 5-17 Subependymoma nuclei are bland and monomorphic and rest in a dense fibrillar background.

REFERENCES

1. Pajtler KW, Witt H, Sill M, et al. Molecular classification of ependymal tumors across all cns compartments, histopathological grades, and age groups. *Cancer Cell.* 2015;27(5): 728–743.
2. Louis DN, Ohgaki H, Wiestler OD, et al., eds. WHO Classification of Tumours of the Central Nervous System. 4th revised ed. Lyon, France: IARC Press; 2016.
3. Figarella-Branger D, Civatte M, Bouvier-Labit C, et al. Prognostic factors in intracranial ependymomas in children. *J Neurosurg.* 2000;93(4):605–613.
4. Ho DM, Hsu CY, Wong TT, et al. A clinicopathologic study of 81 patients with ependymomas and proposal of diagnostic criteria for anaplastic ependymoma. *J Neurooncol.* 2001;54(1):77–85.
5. Korshunov A, Golanov A, Sycheva R, et al. The histologic grade is a main prognostic factor for patients with intracranial ependymomas treated in the microneurosurgical era: an analysis of 258 patients. *Cancer.* 2004;100(6):1230–1237.
6. Merchant TE, Jenkins JJ, Burger PC, et al. Influence of tumor grade on time to progression after irradiation for localized ependymoma in children. *Int J Radiat Oncol Biol Phys.* 2002;53(1):52–57.
7. Ostrom QT, de Blank PM, Kruchko C, et al. Alex's lemonade stand foundation infant and childhood primary brain and central nervous system tumors diagnosed in the united states in 2007-2011. *Neuro Oncol.* 2015;16(suppl 10):x1–x36.
8. Ostrom QT, Gittleman H, Xu J, et al. CBTRUS statistical report: primary brain and other central nervous system tumors diagnosed in the united states in 2009-2013. *Neuro Oncol.* 2016;18(suppl 5):v1–v75.
9. Foreman NK, Love S, Thorne R. Intracranial ependymomas: analysis of prognostic factors in a population-based series. *Pediatr Neurosurg.* 1996;24(3):119–125.
10. Smyth MD, Horn BN, Russo C, et al. Intracranial ependymomas of childhood: current management strategies. *Pediatric neurosurgery.* 2000;33(3):138–150.
11. Paulino AC, Wen BC, Buatti JM, et al. Intracranial ependymomas: an analysis of prognostic factors and patterns of failure. *Am J Clin Oncol.* 2002;25(2):117–122.
12. Robertson PL, Zeltzer PM, Boyett JM, et al. Survival and prognostic factors following radiation therapy and chemotherapy for ependymomas in children: a report of the Children's Cancer Group. *J Neurosurg.* 1998;88(4):695–703.
13. van Veelen-Vincent ML, Pierre-Kahn A, Kalifa C, et al. Ependymoma in childhood: prognostic factors, extent of surgery, and adjuvant therapy. *J Neurosurg.* 2002;97(4): 827–835.
14. Mendrzyk F, Korshunov A, Benner A, et al. Identification of gains on 1q and epidermal growth factor receptor overexpression as independent prognostic markers in intracranial ependymoma. *Clin Cancer Res.* 2006;12(7 Pt 1):2070–2079.
15. Kilday JP, Mitra B, Domerg C, et al. Copy number gain of 1q25 predicts poor progression-free survival for pediatric intracranial ependymomas and enables patient risk stratification: a prospective European clinical trial cohort analysis on behalf of the Children's Cancer Leukaemia Group (CCLG), Societe Francaise d'Oncologie Pediatrique (SFOP), and International Society for Pediatric Oncology (SIOP). *Clin Cancer Res.* 2012;18(7):2001–2011.
16. Rogers HA, Kilday JP, Mayne C, et al. Supratentorial and spinal pediatric ependymomas display a hypermethylated phenotype which includes the loss of tumor suppressor genes involved in the control of cell growth and death. *Acta Neuropathol.* 2012;123(5): 711–725.
17. Ellison DW, Kocak M, Figarella-Branger D, et al. Histopathological grading of pediatric ependymoma: reproducibility and clinical relevance in European trial cohorts. *J Negat Results Biomed.* 2011;10:7.

18. Tihan T, Zhou T, Holmes E, et al. The prognostic value of histological grading of posterior fossa ependymomas in children: a Children's Oncology Group study and a review of prognostic factors. *Modern Pathol.* 2008;21(2):165–177.
19. Pajtler KW, Mack SC, Ramaswamy V, et al. The current consensus on the clinical management of intracranial ependymoma and its distinct molecular variants. *Acta Neuropathol.* 2017;133(1):5–12.
20. Mridha AR, Sharma MC, Sarkar C, et al. Anaplastic ependymoma with cartilaginous and osseous metaplasia: report of a rare case and review of literature. *J Neuro Oncol.* 2007; 82(1):75–80.
21. Jain D, Sharma MC, Arora R, et al. Clear cell ependymoma: a mimicker of oligodendroglioma—report of three cases. *Neuropathol.* 2008;28(4):366–371.
22. Koperek O, Gelpi E, Birner P, et al. Value and limits of immunohistochemistry in differential diagnosis of clear cell primary brain tumors. *Acta Neuropathol.* 2004;108(1): 24–30.
23. Witt H, Mack SC, Ryzhova M, et al. Delineation of two clinically and molecularly distinct subgroups of posterior fossa ependymoma. *Cancer Cell.* 2011;20(2):143–157.
24. Parker M, Mohankumar KM, Punchihewa C, et al. C11orf95-RELA fusions drive oncogenic NF-kappaB signalling in ependymoma. *Nature.* 2014;506(7489):451–455.
25. Pietsch T, Wohlers I, Goschzik T, et al. Supratentorial ependymomas of childhood carry C11orf95-RELA fusions leading to pathological activation of the NF-kappaB signaling pathway. *Acta Neuropathol.* 2014;127(4):609–611.
26. Rubio MP, Correa KM, Ramesh V, et al. Analysis of the neurofibromatosis 2 gene in human ependymomas and astrocytomas. *Cancer Res.* 1994;54(1):45–47.
27. Ebert C, von Haken M, Meyer-Puttlitz B, et al. Molecular genetic analysis of ependymal tumors. NF2 mutations and chromosome 22q loss occur preferentially in intramedullary spinal ependymomas. *Am J Pathol.* 1999;155(2):627–632.
28. Hasselblatt M, Paulus W. Sensitivity and specificity of epithelial membrane antigen staining patterns in ependymomas. *Acta Neuropathol.* 2003;106(4):385–388.
29. Weber DC, Wang Y, Miller R, et al. Long-term outcome of patients with spinal myxopapillary ependymoma: treatment results from the MD Anderson Cancer Center and institutions from the Rare Cancer Network. *Neuro Oncol.* 2015;17(4):588–595.
30. Davis C, Barnard RO. Malignant behavior of myxopapillary ependymoma. Report of three cases. *J Neurosurg.* 1985;62(6):925–929.
31. Jatana KR, Jacob A, Slone HW, et al. Spinal myxopapillary ependymoma metastatic to bilateral internal auditory canals. *Ann Otol Rhinol Laryngol.* 2008;117(2):98–102.
32. Mridha AR, Sharma MC, Sarkar C, et al. Myxopapillary ependymoma of lumbosacral region with metastasis to both cerebellopontine angles: report of a rare case. *Child's Nerv Sys.* 2007;23(10):1209–1213.
33. Woesler B, Moskopp D, Kuchelmeister K, et al. Intracranial metastasis of a spinal myxopapillary ependymoma. A case report. *Neurosurg Rev.* 1998;21(1):62–65.

6

OTHER GLIOMAS

ASTROBLASTOMA

Clinical Context

The sum of knowledge of this rare glial neoplasm encompasses fewer than 300 cases, many of those known only through large tumor registry databases such as surveillance, epidemiology, end results (SEER) taken over the course of more than 35 years (1). A literature review in 2011 revealed only 116 cases, the many of which were individual case reports (2). In one large review, most of the patients were younger than 18 years, and the distribution was bimodal with a second peak in the third decade and a female predominance of around 2.5:1 (2). The population characteristics of other cases reported in the literature, however, differ from those in the large SEER database, which show a broad age distribution and an even sex distribution (1). These differences could possibly reflect changes in diagnostic practices during the long period covered by SEER and the absence of peer review for SEER diagnoses. In contrast, most other reported astroblastomas are from 1989 or later, when more restrictive histopathologic criteria were suggested (3). No familial predisposition or other disease associations have been described.

Magnetic resonance imaging (MRI) and computed tomography (CT) studies most often reveal a circumscribed supratentorial mass that is calcified, well circumscribed, and heterogeneously enhancing (4,5). The vast majority of cases have been in the cerebral hemispheres, with rare examples arising elsewhere (2). An identifying feature of astroblastoma on postcontrast, T1-weighted images is a "bubbly" appearance created by multiple intratumoral cysts (4). The extent of surrounding edema is highly variable.

Although two general categories of histologic aggressiveness are recognized, well-differentiated and malignant, definitive WHO grading remains to be established. Treatment for these lesions usually consists of surgical excision that is followed by radiation therapy in malignant cases. In the former, recurrence-free survival in reported cases with gross total resection has been favorable, around 85% at 5 years (2). One recent series showed statistically significant decreases in survival associated with mitotic index of ≥5/10 hpf, but not with overall grade (high vs. low), patient age, or sex (6).

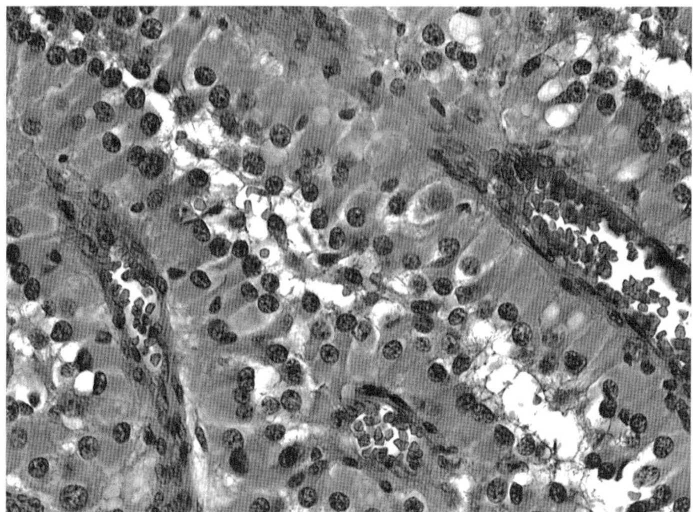

FIGURE 6-1 Astroblastomas invariably contain pseudorosettes of glial cells with broad columnar foot processes planted on vascular cores.

Histopathology

Although several series describe its characteristics, the exact criteria defining this entity are not universally agreed upon. The unifying histologic feature of astroblastoma is perivascular pseudorosettes similar to those of ependymoma, but with broad column-like foot processes that extend from the vessel surface (Figure 6-1). The perivascular cells in astroblastoma are relatively distinct with well-defined cell borders, whereas the fibrillar processes in ependymoma blend together and obscure the borders of perivascular tumor cells. The stout bands of cytoplasm terminate in an uneven layer of nuclei that have little or no cytoplasm on their outer aspect.

The other cardinal features of astroblastoma are circumscription and vascular hyalinization. The vast majority of astroblastomas show thickening and sclerosis of blood vessels, with a minority also containing regional hyalinization. They are, as a rule, circumscribed histologically, with pushing borders and little intermingling with surrounding brain parenchyma. Although focal infiltration can be seen, the significance of this is unknown.

The remaining features of astroblastoma are variable. The cells are usually elongated with small, oval to round nuclei but can be polygonal with other nuclear patterns. Focal rhabdoid change with peripheral cytoplasmic clearing is common (Figure 6-2). Necrosis is seen more often in cases with multiple malignant features but can be present in otherwise low-grade examples (5). Pseudopalisading of tumor cells around necrosis can be seen and is similar to that seen in glioblastoma.

Histologically malignant features in astroblastoma include elevated mitotic rates (>5/10 hpf), vascular proliferation, nuclear atypia, loss of

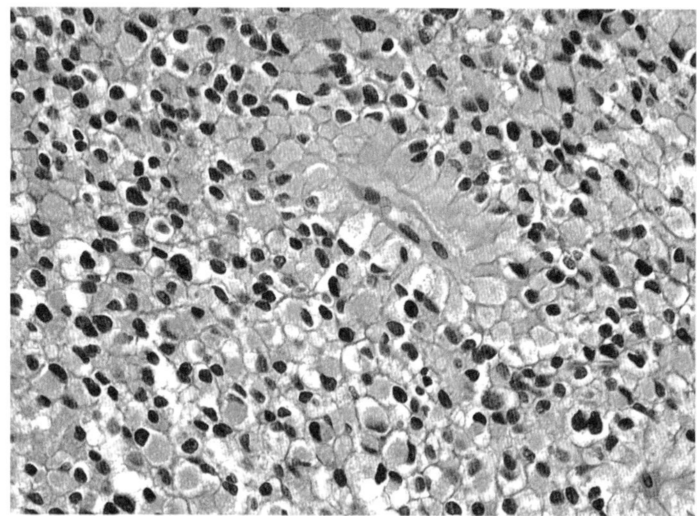

FIGURE 6-2 Solid sheets of cells between pseudorosettes and rhabdoid change are common in astroblastoma.

architecture, and palisading necrosis; however, the boundary between malignant and low-grade astroblastoma is not a universally accepted one.

Immunohistochemistry and Genetics

Immunoreactivity for vimentin, S100, and GFAP, all in a cytoplasmic pattern, is typical of astroblastoma, albeit focal in some cases. Cytoplasmic EMA reactivity is present in some cases, and it is usually focal and lacks the ring-like positivity seen in ependymomas. The glial marker Olig2 is expressed in the vast majority of astroblastomas, and expression of ATRX and SMARCB1/INI1 are retained (6).

Comparative genomic hybridization in a set of seven astroblastomas showed an absence of chromosomal abnormalities that are common in astrocytomas and ependymomas and no consistent specific copy number changes (5). *BRAF* V600E mutations were detected in DNA from 38% of another set of astroblastomas, opening the possibility for targeted therapy in some cases, should they recur (6).

Differential Diagnosis

Ependymomas are histologically similar to astroblastomas; however, most astroblastomas occur in adulthood and are almost exclusively found in the cerebral hemispheres. Nevertheless, ependymomas can occur in the cerebral hemispheres of adults perhaps as frequently as the rare astroblastoma. The hallmark of astroblastoma that is not seen in ependymoma is the broad, column like cytoplasm in perivascular tumor cells. Perivascular hyaline is also more suggestive of astroblastoma.

Papillary glioneuronal tumor has some histologic overlap with astroblastoma at low magnification but lacks broad cytoplasmic processes and has a biphasic pattern of GFAP and synaptophysin staining.

CHORDOID GLIOMA (WHO GRADE II)

Clinical Context

This rare entity was first described by Brat et al. in 1998 and added to the WHO classification in 2000. Only a few dozen cases have been described, and understanding of its biology is still evolving as cases accumulate. Most cases arise in adults at a mean age of around 46 years, but the range is broad and extends from 5 to 71 years (7,8). Almost twice as many females have been reported with chordoid glioma than males (7). No associations with other diseases have been observed. Suggested to derive from the organum vasculosum of the lamina terminalis (OVLT) (9,10), the vast majority of chordoid gliomas originate in the anterior third ventricle, with the exception of a single substantiated case from near the occipital horn of the lateral ventricle (11). Presenting symptoms and signs are variable, but similar to other third-ventricular/hypothalamic tumors, with headache, visual problems, and hydrocephalus being common (8,12,13).

MR images show a circumscribed third-ventricular/hypothalamic mass that is ovoid and not contiguous with the pituitary gland. The tumor is typically isointense in T1-weighted sequences, slightly hyperintense on T2/FLAIR, and brightly and homogeneously contrast enhancing. CT images are hyperdense relative to gray matter (13). Calcification is not seen.

Resection is the treatment of choice. The anatomic complexity and importance of surrounding structures preclude complete removal in many cases, resulting in a significant rate of recurrence. Radiation therapy has been attempted in a few cases with mixed results, but the numbers are too small to draw firm conclusions (7).

Histopathology

Chordoid gliomas resemble chordomas in that they are composed of cords and nests of eosinophilic, epithelioid cells in a vacuolated background of basophilic myxoid material (Figure 6-3). The tumor edges may adhere to the surroundings but are noninfiltrative and sharply delineated. The component cells have a moderate amount of eosinophilic cytoplasm and contain monotonous round-to-ovoid nuclei. Lymphoplasmacytic infiltrates are present in varying amounts and usually contain spherical aggregates of immunoglobulin (Russell bodies) (Figure 6-4).

Immunohistochemistry

Antibodies to GFAP and vimentin react in a cytoplasmic pattern in essentially every case (12). Immunostaining for CD34 is present in the many cases (14). Expression of thyroid transcription factor-1 (TTF-1) is consistently

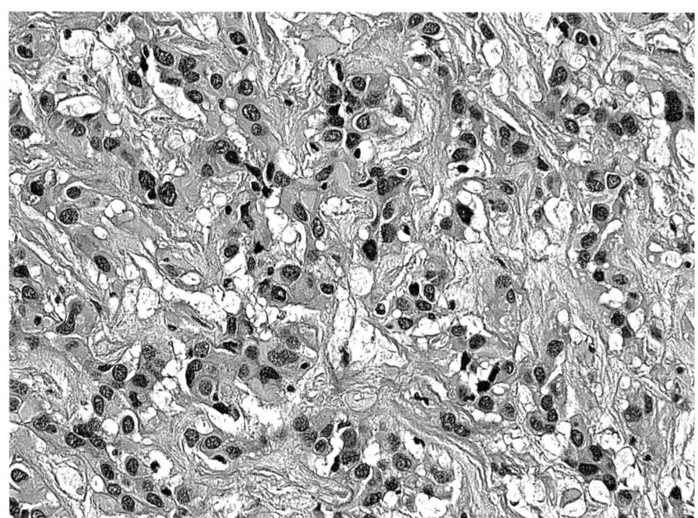

FIGURE 6-3 Chordoid gliomas comprise cords and nests of polygonal glial cells with lightly eosinophilic cytoplasm in a basophilic myxoid background.

present in chordoid gliomas and has been suggested as evidence that the tumor arises from the OVLT and may be related to TTF-1-expressing tumors in the pituitary gland such as pituicytoma and granular cell tumor (10,15). Similar to ependymomas, and in concert with the ultrastructural finding of intracytoplasmic lumina containing microvilli, EMA may show a pattern of scattered dot- and ring-like structures in some cases.

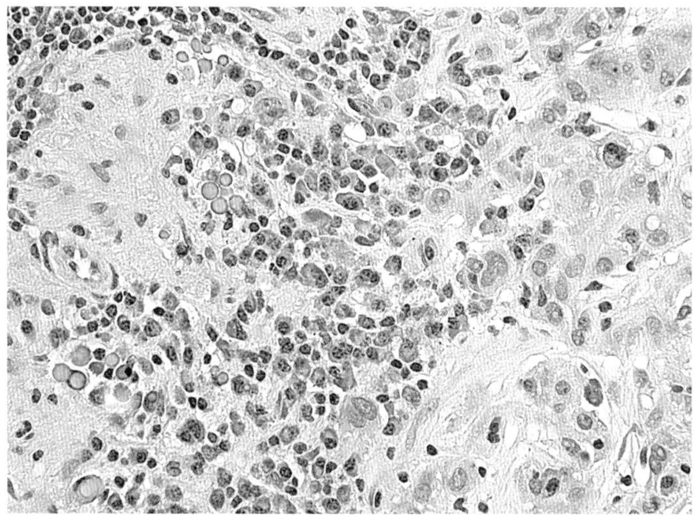

FIGURE 6-4 Lymphoplasmacytic infiltrates surround the perimeter of chordoid gliomas and frequently contain Mott cells with multiple Russell bodies.

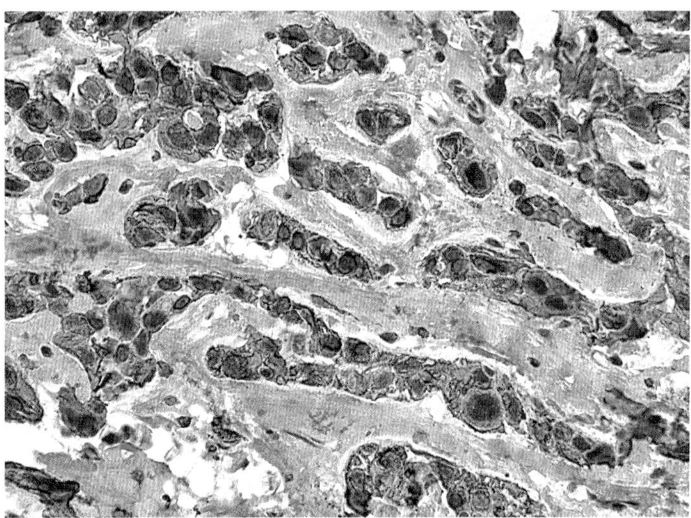

FIGURE 6-5 Glial fibrillary acidic protein reactivity is always present in chordoid glioma and essentially rules out other chordoid lesions in the differential diagnosis.

Differential Diagnosis

The diagnostic considerations include other neoplasms with a chordoid appearance, such as chordoid meningioma and chordoma, although location in the anterior third ventricle is highly unlikely in either case. Immunostaining for GFAP also essentially rules out chordoma and chordoid meningioma (Figure 6-5). TTF-1 immunoreactivity is also not seen in other chordoid lesions.

ANGIOCENTRIC GLIOMA (WHO GRADE I)

Clinical Context

Of established tumors of the central nervous system, angiocentric glioma is among the least common and least reported. Only a few dozen are documented, yet the clinical and pathologic findings are distinct and consistent enough to warrant inclusion into the WHO nomenclature. Along with ganglioglioma and dysembryoplastic neuroepithelial tumor, angiocentric glioma is a low-grade tumor strongly associated with long-standing, drug-resistant partial epilepsy. Males and females are equally affected, with onset of seizures in childhood or adolescence (16–21).

Neuroimaging of angiocentric glioma shows a unitary, superficial, cortical area of T2/FLAIR hyperintensity that usually does not enhance with contrast administration. T1-weighted sequences may show a thin rim of cortical hyperintensity (16,17). All cases have been supratentorial, except one case from the midbrain (22). There is no obvious predilection for any specific lobe, as there is for temporal lobe in ganglioglioma.

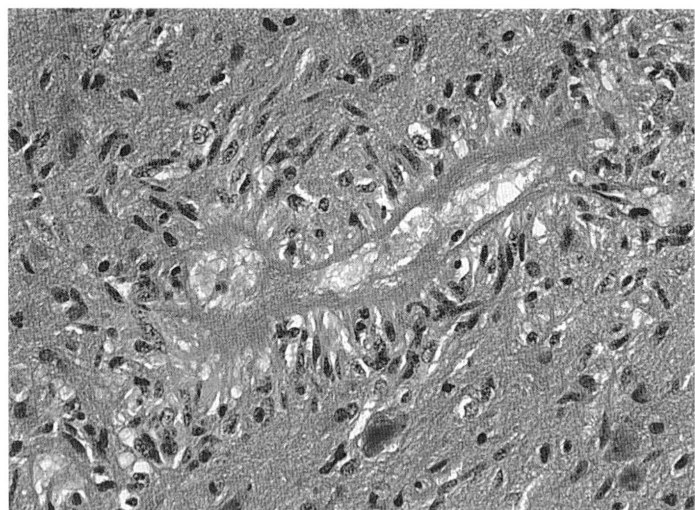

FIGURE 6-6 Angiocentric gliomas may show tapered glial cells radiating from blood vessels that travel through otherwise normal brain.

The vast majority of reported cases have maintained an indolent course, except for one case in which onset of seizures was during adulthood and the patient died of disease. Most patients are cured of their epilepsy after removal of the tumor, unless it is subtotally resected.

Histopathology

To say that angiocentric gliomas are infiltrative may be implying motion to an essentially static process, yet the cells of this lesion are unquestionably intermingled with brain parenchyma in an infiltrative pattern (Figure 6-6). Other areas may exhibit a more solid growth pattern, but the lesion lacks the pushing border of many other low-grade neoplasms. Individual cells and fascicles stream through the affected area and arrange around small and large blood vessels radially, longitudinally, or concentrically (Figures 6-7 and 6-8). The radial arrays of tumor cells resemble the perivascular pseudorosettes in ependymomas and astroblastomas. Similar arrangements may be formed along the subpial surface, with the bipolar tumor cells either parallel or perpendicular to the pia.

The tumor cells are uniform and mostly bipolar with cigar-shaped nuclei and thick glial cytoplasmic processes. A small nucleolus may be apparent. Some cells contain an eosinophilic structure within the cytoplasm that corresponds to microlumens seen by electron microscopy (19). Mitoses should be absent or very rare.

Immunohistochemistry and Genetics

GFAP is generally positive but can be variable or weak. Cytoplasmic microlumens appear as solid, round, or irregular points of reactivity on

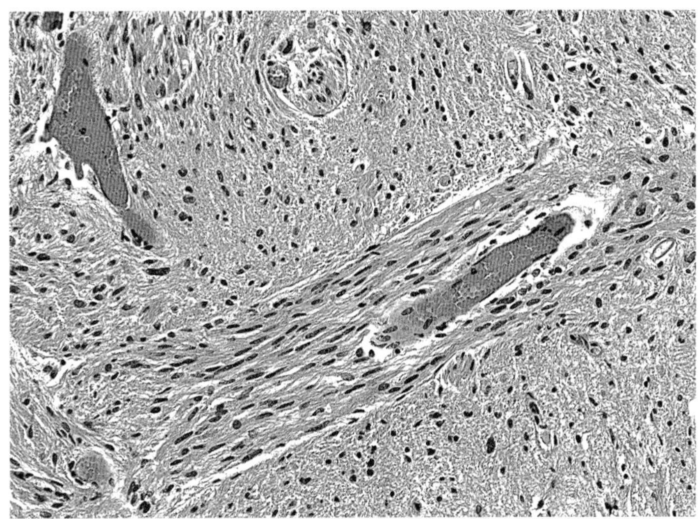

FIGURE 6-7 Angiocentric glioma cells may also travel in parallel with blood vessels, creating a fascicular appearance.

EMA staining (Figure 6-9). EMA also labels membranes and cytoplasm in an inconsistent manner. MIB rates for angiocentric glioma are generally very low, around 1% to 2% (16). Rare cases may have elevated markers of proliferation, the significance of which is unknown, although one case proved ultimately fatal (19,23,24).

The vast majority of angiocentric gliomas contain a fusion of the *MYB* and *QKI* genes on chromosome 6q (25–27). This fusion has also

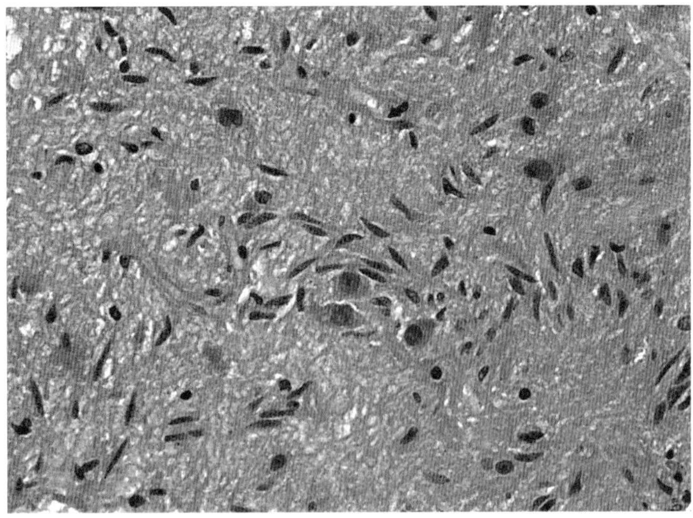

FIGURE 6-8 Although angiocentric glioma cells can be intimately admixed with normal brain, this static lesion is not progressively infiltrative.

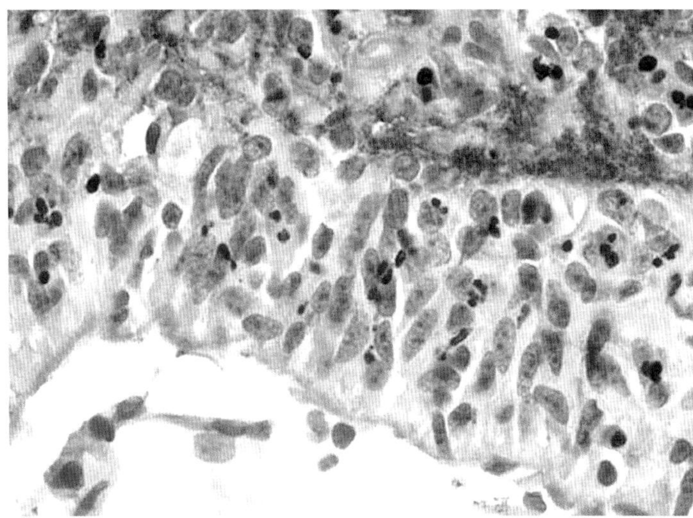

FIGURE 6-9 Epithelial membrane antigen immunohistochemistry shows cytoplasmic dots and rings, similar to classic ependymomas.

been observed in DNTs and pediatric diffuse astrocytomas, albeit at lower frequencies. It is unclear from the literature to date whether the diffuse gliomas with this finding behave more like angiocentric gliomas or adult-type diffuse astrocytomas.

Differential Diagnosis

The dispersion of tumor cells through brain in angiocentric glioma can create concern for an infiltrating astrocytoma. Both may present with a history of seizures, but in the case of the former, the history is generally protracted, sometimes spanning decades. Although perivascular "secondary structures" can be seen in infiltrating gliomas, they lack the organization, symmetry, and extent of those formed by angiocentric glioma. The nuclei in angiocentric glioma, although they can show some variability, tend to be uniform and elongated. In suspected cases of angiocentric glioma, it is crucial to rule out adult-type infiltrating astrocytomas at least with immunohistochemical surrogates of molecular findings such as IDH1 and p53 mutations and ATRX loss.

Ependymoma and astroblastoma also have radial perivascular cells but are both circumscribed and discreet, whereas angiocentric gliomas are infiltrative in distribution. Angiocentric glioma also usually occurs in the setting of long-standing partial epilepsy, which is unusual for the other two.

REFERENCES

1. Ahmed KA, Allen PK, Mahajan A, et al. Astroblastomas: a surveillance, epidemiology, and end results (SEER)-based patterns of care analysis. *World Neurosurg.* 2014;82(1–2): e291–297.

2. Sughrue ME, Choi J, Rutkowski MJ, et al. Clinical features and post-surgical outcome of patients with astroblastoma. *J Clin Neurosci*. 2011;18(6):750–754.
3. Bonnin JM, Rubinstein LJ. Astroblastomas: a pathological study of 23 tumors, with a postoperative follow-up in 13 patients. *Neurosurgery*. 1989;25(1):6–13.
4. Bell JW, Osborn AG, Salzman KL, et al. Neuroradiologic characteristics of astroblastoma. *Neuroradiology*. 2007;49(3):203–209.
5. Brat DJ, Hirose Y, Cohen KJ, et al. Astroblastoma: clinicopathologic features and chromosomal abnormalities defined by comparative genomic hybridization. *Brain Pathol*. 2000;10(3):342–352.
6. Lehman NL, Hattab EM, Mobley BC, et al. Morphological and molecular features of astroblastoma, including BRAFV600E mutations, suggest an ontological relationship to other cortical-based gliomas of children and young adults. *Neuro Oncol*. 2017;19(1):31–42.
7. Vanhauwaert DJ, Clement F, Van Dorpe J, et al. Chordoid glioma of the third ventricle. *Acta Neurochir (Wien)*. 2008;150(11):1183–1191.
8. Desouza RM, Bodi I, Thomas N, et al. Chordoid glioma: ten years of a low-grade tumor with high morbidity. *Skull Base*. 2010;20(2):125–138.
9. Leeds NE, Lang FF, Ribalta T, et al. Origin of chordoid glioma of the third ventricle. *Arch Pathol Lab Med*. 2006;130(4):460–464.
10. Bielle F, Villa C, Giry M, et al. Chordoid gliomas of the third ventricle share TTF-1 expression with organum vasculosum of the lamina terminalis. *Am J Surg Pathol*. 2015; 39(7):948–956.
11. Jain D, Sharma MC, Sarkar C, et al. Chordoid glioma: report of two rare examples with unusual features. *Acta Neurochir (Wien)*. 2008;150(3):295–300; discussion 300.
12. Brat DJ, Scheithauer BW, Staugaitis SM, et al. Third ventricular chordoid glioma: a distinct clinicopathologic entity. *J Neuropathol Exp Neurol*. 1998;57(3):283–290.
13. Pomper MG, Passe TJ, Burger PC, et al. Chordoid glioma: a neoplasm unique to the hypothalamus and anterior third ventricle. *AJNR Am J Neuroradiol*. 2001;22(3):464–469.
14. Reifenberger G, Weber T, Weber RG, et al. Chordoid glioma of the third ventricle: immunohistochemical and molecular genetic characterization of a novel tumor entity. *Brain Pathol*. 1999;9(4):617–626.
15. Hewer E, Beck J, Kellner-Weldon F, et al. Suprasellar chordoid neoplasm with expression of thyroid transcription factor 1: evidence that chordoid glioma of the third ventricle and pituicytoma may form part of a spectrum of lineage-related tumors of the basal forebrain. *Hum Pathol*. 2015;46(7):1045–1049.
16. Lellouch-Tubiana A, Boddaert N, Bourgeois M, et al. Angiocentric neuroepithelial tumor (ANET): a new epilepsy-related clinicopathological entity with distinctive MRI. *Brain Pathol*. 2005;15(4):281–286.
17. Preusser M, Hoischen A, Novak K, et al. Angiocentric glioma: report of clinico-pathologic and genetic findings in 8 cases. *Am J Surg Pathol*. 2007;31(11):1709–1718.
18. Shakur SF, McGirt MJ, Johnson MW, et al. Angiocentric glioma: a case series. *J Neurosurg Pediatr*. 2009;3(3):197–202.
19. Wang M, Tihan T, Rojiani AM, et al. Monomorphous angiocentric glioma: a distinctive epileptogenic neoplasm with features of infiltrating astrocytoma and ependymoma. *J Neuropathol Exp Neurol*. 2005;64(10):875–881.
20. Ni HC, Chen SY, Chen L, et al. Angiocentric glioma: a report of nine new cases, including four with atypical histological features. *Neuropathol Appl Neurobiol*. 2015;41(3):333–346.
21. Buccoliero AM, Castiglione F, Degl'innocenti DR, et al. Angiocentric glioma: clinical, morphological, immunohistochemical and molecular features in three pediatric cases. *Clin Neuropathol*. 2013;32(2):107–113.
22. Covington DB, Rosenblum MK, Brathwaite CD, et al. Angiocentric glioma-like tumor of the midbrain. *Pediatr Neurosurg*. 2009;45(6):429–433.

23. Pokharel S, Parker JR, Parker JC, Jr, et al. Angiocentric glioma with high proliferative index: case report and review of the literature. *Ann Clin Lab Sci*. 2011;41(3):257–261.
24. Li JY, Langford LA, Adesina A, et al. The high mitotic count detected by phospho-histone H3 immunostain does not alter the benign behavior of angiocentric glioma. *Brain Tumor Pathol*. 2012;29(1):68–72.
25. Qaddoumi I, Orisme W, Wen J, et al. Genetic alterations in uncommon low-grade neuroepithelial tumors: BRAF, FGFR1, and MYB mutations occur at high frequency and align with morphology. *Acta Neuropathol (Berl)*. 2016;131(6):833–845.
26. Tatevossian RG, Tang B, Dalton J, et al. MYB upregulation and genetic aberrations in a subset of pediatric low-grade gliomas. *Acta Neuropathol (Berl)*. 2010;120(6):731–743.
27. Bandopadhayay P, Ramkissoon LA, Jain P, et al. MYB-QKI rearrangements in angiocentric glioma drive tumorigenicity through a tripartite mechanism. *Nat Genet*. 2016;48(3):273–282.

7

NEURONAL AND MIXED GLIONEURONAL NEOPLASMS

GANGLIOGLIOMA/GANGLIOCYTOMA (WHO GRADE I) AND ANAPLASTIC GANGLIOGLIOMA (WHO GRADE III)

Clinical Context

Ganglioglioma is probably the most common of the neuronal and glioneuronal tumors, with hundreds reported in the literature (1–5), whereas pure gangliocytomas are rare. Anaplastic gangliogliomas are uncommon, approximately 8% of gangliogliomas in one large series (6).

The usual site for gangliogliomas is the temporal lobe, the location accounting for over three-quarters of all cases (1). The frontal lobe produces most of the remaining cases, with the last few percent occurring elsewhere in the CNS, primarily the cerebral hemispheres, but also rarely including the cerebellum (7), brainstem (8), and spinal cord (9). Males are slightly more prone to developing gangliogliomas in some series, making up from two-thirds of cases (1,10) to just less than half (11). Gangliogliomas can be identified in a wide range of patient ages, with most occurring in the second to fifth decades.

Even more consistent than their tendency to localize to the temporal lobes is the tendency of gangliogliomas to be associated with long-standing partial seizures of greater than 1 year, approaching a rate of 100% in one large series (3). Those not associated with epilepsy do not present with any specific signs or symptoms. No known consistent associations exist between ganglion cell tumors and familial tumor syndromes.

The radiologic appearance of gangliogliomas, aside from location, is variable and nonspecific. Neuroimaging of gangliogliomas shows two general patterns of growth, solid and "cyst with mural nodule," each that represents about half of all cases (Figure 7-1). A small minority appears entirely cystic on imaging, but diminutive mural nodules can be missed between tomographic slices (5,12). The solid examples tend to be larger, but both are well circumscribed with scant to moderate surrounding edema. Calcification, density on computed tomography (CT), T1 and T2 signal intensity on MR, and contrast enhancement are not consistent in pattern or extent in ganglioglioma (5,12). CT may show erosion of the

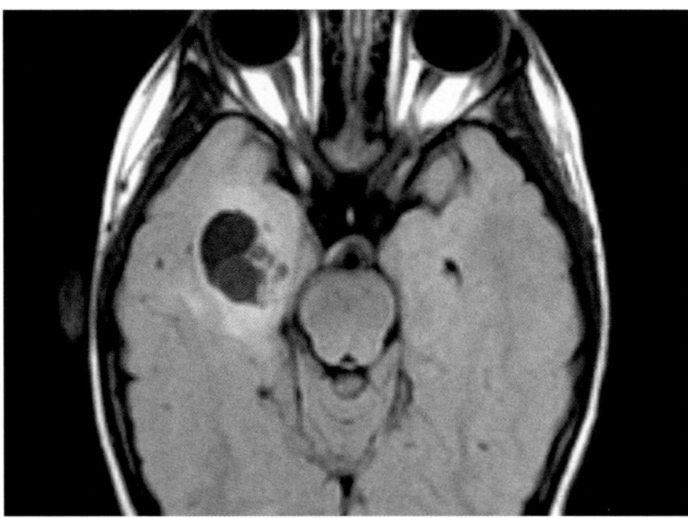

FIGURE 7-1 A majority of gangliogliomas present in the temporal lobe, either as cysts with a mural nodule or as a solid mass.

skull overlying more superficial lesions (12). A large amount of edema surrounding a ganglioglioma can be associated with more aggressive clinical course.

The clinical outcome for the vast majority of gangliogliomas is favorable, as reflected by their WHO grade I status, with a 7.5-year recurrence-free survival rate of more than 90% (3). Anaplastic, WHO grade III gangliogliomas have dismal clinical outcomes, with median overall survivals of 24.7 and 27 months in two large series (6,13). It is unclear whether these anaplastic cases have a different genetic profile, or have other markers of anaplasia that are nonmorphologic. The presence of BRAF V600E mutations in gangliogliomas presents the opportunity to use targeted inhibitors such as vemurafenib to treat inoperable cases (14,15).

Histopathology

Gangliocytomas contain neuronal cells that vary from large polyhedral ganglion cells with large vesicular nuclei and prominent nucleoli to inconspicuous, small granule neurons. In contrast to the neurons of normal cerebral cortex, those of gangliocytomas and gangliogliomas are more variable in size and shape and have no recognizable architectural organization (Figure 7-2). In contrast to those in gangliogliomas, normal cortical pyramidal neurons are arranged into somewhat distinct layers with their triangular cell bodies all oriented in the same direction like arrowheads pointing to the cortical surface. However, in assessing the architecture of biopsy tissue, it is important to recognize that there is no guarantee that sections will be perpendicular to the cortical surface, or areas that do not have isocortical architecture, such as the amygdala, will be excluded. Tumor

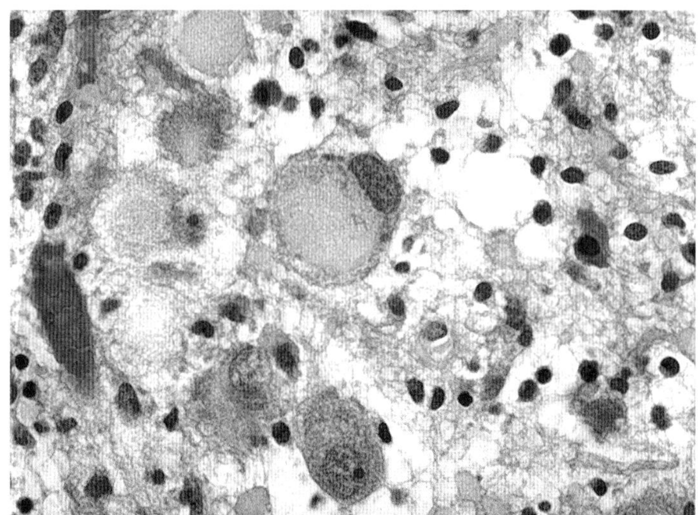

FIGURE 7-2 Neoplastic ganglion cells form disorganized clusters and display abnormal cytologic features.

neurons can have multiple nuclei in about half of ganglion cell tumors, a finding that is specific but not sensitive (Figure 7-3). Neurofibrillary tangles are occasionally seen in neoplastic ganglion cells in older patients. The cellular density ranges from very high with back-to-back cells to low, approaching that of normal cerebral cortex. A variable perivascular lymphocytic infiltrate is commonly present, as are eosinophilic granular bodies

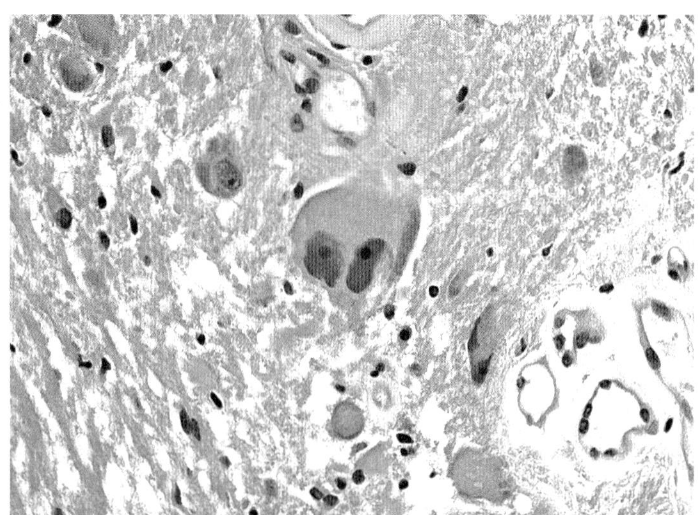

FIGURE 7-3 Binucleation, although usually difficult to find or absent, is helpful in establishing the neoplastic nature of neurons in ganglioglioma.

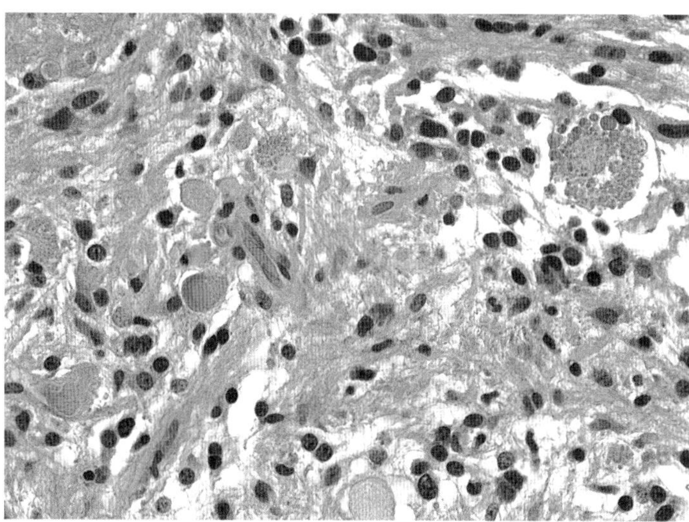

FIGURE 7-4 Spherical protein aggregates, either in the form of eosinophilic granular bodies (upper right) or single droplets (left center), are common in gangliogliomas and suggest the lesion's chronicity.

(EGBs). EGBs are focal, sometimes intracellular, collections of glassy, eosinophilic spheroids of protein and are found typically in slowly growing, low-grade, primary lesions in the CNS (Figure 7-4). Single, spherical, eosinophilic protein droplets are also common.

The fundamental histologic finding in gangliogliomas is a biphasic tumor cell population with neuronal and glial elements, but the forms of these two elements and the patterns in which they combine are truly diverse. The neuronal element reflects the cytologic features of neurons in gangliocytomas and can range from obvious to subtle, depending mostly on the amount and distribution of the cells. Although neuronal proliferation has been reported in in vitro cell culture of gangliogliomas (16), the neuronal population has not been shown to proliferate in vivo. The glial population is the actively dividing component of gangliogliomas and is the part of the tumor that can recur after excision. The glial cells are also more variable and can display features of fibrillar or pilocytic astrocytoma, or even appear oligodendroglial.

The architecture of ganglioglioma is generally sheetlike or vaguely fascicular and streaming (Figure 7-5), but microcystic myxoid areas similar to dysembryoplastic neuroepithelial tumor (DNT) and pilocytic astrocytoma can be seen (Figure 7-6). The background stroma shows areas of desmoplasia with an extensive network of delicate, reticular collagen fibers. Masson trichrome or reticulin staining highlights this feature when subtle. As with gangliocytoma, a perivascular lymphocytic infiltrate is present in a majority of cases. Vascular proliferation, rare mitoses, and degenerative nuclear atypia are permissible in ganglioglioma, but necrosis

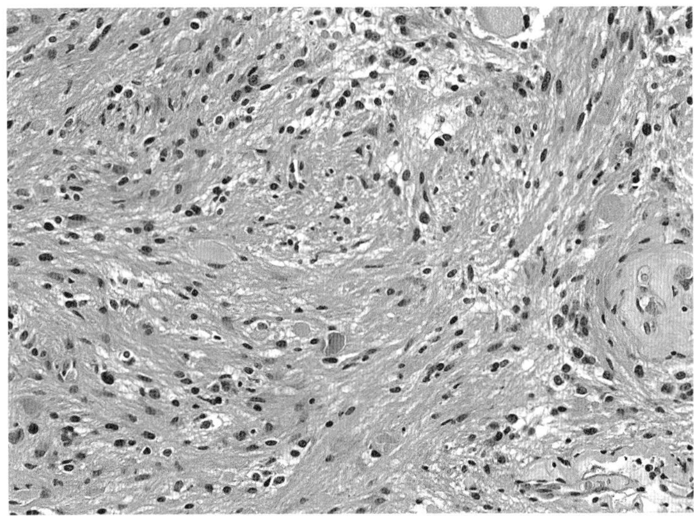

FIGURE 7-5 The glial element in ganglioglioma is frequently arranged in a vaguely fascicular pattern. Also note scattered eosinophilic granular bodies and hyalinized blood vessels.

is generally absent, except in anaplastic cases. EGBs are commonplace and Rosenthal fibers can sometimes be seen, yet these also appear in other lesions within the differential diagnosis of ganglioglioma. Small "satellite lesions" of tumor may be present around the edges of the main tumor bulk, but the interface between the lesion and surrounding brain should be well delineated and not show significant infiltration.

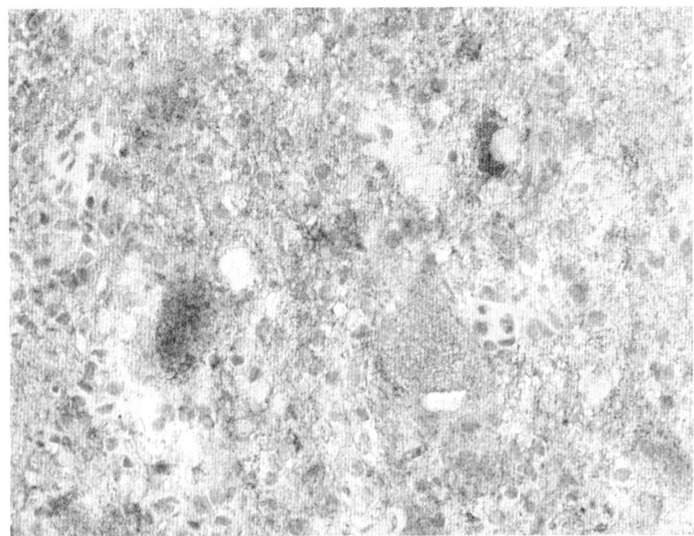

FIGURE 7-6 When the mutation is present, immunostaining for the BRAF V600E mutant protein is typically more prominent in the ganglion cells of ganglioglioma.

Immunohistochemistry

Tumor neurons stain similarly to their nonneoplastic counterparts, with reactivity for synaptophysin, chromogranin, neurofilament, class III beta tubulin, MAP2, and NeuN reported (2,4). Neoplastic glial cells show immunoreactivity for GFAP. Any significant immunostaining for p53 is unusual in gangliogliomas and when present, is most often noted in the glial component of recurrent tumors with high rates of MIB1 reactivity (>20%) (2). Other studies have not confirmed significant p53 staining in ganglioglioma (4). MIB1 staining is an important supplement to histology in cases where atypical or anaplastic features are suspected; it is discussed in the following section. CD34 staining is common in the neuronal component in gangliogliomas and could be helpful, if positive, to rule out a nonneoplastic population of entrapped neurons (1) The VE1 antibody to BRAF V600E mutant protein can detect the mutation in gangliogliomas. The typical pattern is strong staining in the neuronal component and weak expression in the glial component (Figure 7-7) (17,18).

Grading

The current WHO classification allows for two grades, grade I for most gangliogliomas and grade III for those that are histologically malignant (anaplastic ganglioglioma). Around 8% to 10% of all gangliogliomas will be diagnosed as anaplastic (1,6). Anaplastic cases are associated with a higher MIB1 proliferation index (>5%) compared with grade I gangliogliomas, which are generally around 1% to 3% (2). Histologically, the WHO criteria are not very explicitly defined and include increased mitosis, hypercellularity, and nuclear anaplasia, with microvascular proliferation and

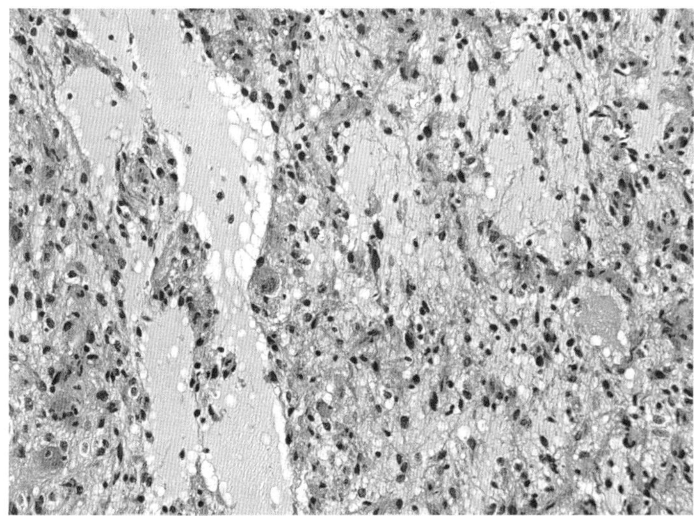

FIGURE 7-7 Mucinous microcysts similar to those in pilocytic astrocytoma and dysembryoplastic neuroepithelial tumor can also appear in ganglioglioma.

necrosis also mentioned (19). These changes are typically only seen in the glial component. Of the few dozen anaplastic reported gangliogliomas, patient survival has been poor, around a median of about 2 years. Some of the reported cases have been shown to exhibit p53 overexpression, loss of ATRX, H3 K27M mutations and *hTERT* promoter mutations, perhaps suggesting genetic overlap with other entities (6).

Formerly, a WHO grade II designation was recognized for gangliogliomas that showed increased cellularity, prominent vascular proliferation, and glial nuclear anaplasia. Although the grade II designation is no longer in use, the term atypical ganglioglioma can still be used to communicate the unusual appearance to the treating physician and perhaps prompt closer follow-up.

Genetics

Depending on location, gangliogliomas may have BRAF V600E point mutations in 18% to 60% of cases, with those in the temporal lobe and posterior fossa having the highest rates (Table 7-1) (8,17,20,21). Because brainstem gangliogliomas are frequently inoperable, the targeted inhibitor vemurafenib can be used successfully to treat progressions of those lesions. Other common genetic features in gangliogliomas include gains of chromosomes 7 (~20%), or 5 (~15%) and losses on 22q (~20%) (22).

Differential Diagnosis

Because of their innate tendency to infiltrate among native neurons, diffuse gliomas can give the impression of ganglioglioma on histology. In contrast to the high surgical cure rate for gangliogliomas, infiltrating gliomas are incurable with multiple treatment modalities and progress over time. The importance of distinguishing these two processes from one another cannot be overstated. The first defense against mistaking these two entities is a familiarity with the patient's clinical history, especially imaging findings. A circumscribed, solid, or solid-cystic mass in the mesial temporal lobe of a patient with a long history of epilepsy would strongly argue

TABLE 7-1 Most Common Genetic Findings in Neuronal and Glioneuronal Tumors

Tumor Type	Genetic Finding(s)
Dysembryoplastic neuroepithelial tumor	FGFR1 duplications, fusions, mutations
Papillary glioneuronal tumor	*SLC44A1-PRKCA* fusion
Rosette-forming glioneuronal tumor	*PIK3CA* mutation
Desmoplastic infantile ganglioglioma/ astrocytoma	No consistent changes
Diffuse leptomeningeal glioneuronal tumor	*KIAA1549-BRAF* fusion, deletion 1p

against an infiltrating glioma. Contrast enhancement almost rules out a grade II infiltrating glioma. Histologic features that favor ganglioglioma are multinucleate neurons, clustered or disorganized neurons, fascicular architecture, EGBs, and discreet circumscription. Diffuse gliomas do not show a rich background of reticulin fibers. Because higher grade, IDH wild type diffuse gliomas are unlikely to appear like grade I gangliogliomas, assessment of IDH mutation status, ATRX expression, and 1p/19q deletion will prevent any mischaracterizations.

Of the lesions on the differential diagnosis with ganglioglioma, pleomorphic xanthoastrocytoma (PXA) can be the most indistinguishable due to its overlap in age group, symptoms, location, imaging characteristics, histology, and immunohistochemistry. However, the most important difference between them necessitates their diagnostic separation; PXAs are more aggressive. All of the histologic features of ganglioglioma are seen in PXA, including neoplastic cells resembling dysmorphic neurons, and the genetic feature of BRAF V600E mutations is shared also. Immunohistochemistry and special staining are most useful if the lesion in question is a PXA without ganglionic differentiation. The hallmark of PXA is the presence of large, atypical tumor cells, which should not be present in ganglioglioma. Rarely, PXA and ganglioglioma occur in combination, either as separate foci within the same tumor or as dysmorphic ganglion cells within an otherwise typical PXA. Deletions of *CDKN2A/B* on 9q are much more common in PXAs than gangliogliomas.

Native nonneoplastic ganglion cells can become entrapped within the substance of pilocytic astrocytomas, imitating the histology of ganglioglioma. Add to that the occasional occurrence of pilocytic astrocytomas in the temporal lobe, the association with epilepsy in this location, overlapping imaging characteristics, and a confusing diagnostic picture can develop. Myxoid microcystic change, EGBs, and Rosenthal fibers are seen in both, so they do not necessarily distinguish. *KIAA1549-BRAF* fusions strongly favor pilocytic astrocytoma, although BRAF mutations can be seen in either.

DNTs also overlap with ganglioglioma in clinical presentation, location, mixed glial, and neuronal components. The presence of prominent, microcystic, myxoid areas and oligodendroglia-like cells favors DNT, whereas the presence of EGBs, reticular collagen, and lymphocytic infiltrates favors ganglioglioma. The distinction is not of high importance clinically and may be a subjective judgment. Indeed, one may even find examples of composite ganglioglioma/DNT (23).

DYSEMBRYOPLASTIC NEUROEPITHELIAL TUMOR (WHO GRADE I)

Clinical Context

This low-grade tumor with limited growth potential is strongly associated with drug-resistant, complex partial seizures and was first identified in

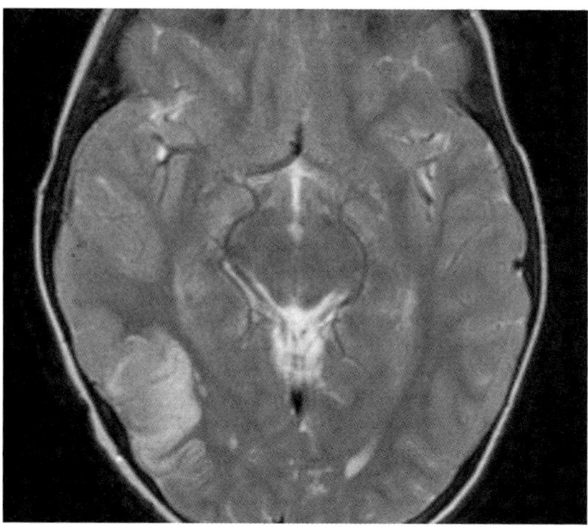

FIGURE 7-8 Right parietal dysembryoplastic neuroepithelial tumor showing typical T2-hyperintense expansion of the cortical ribbon and 2-minute satellite nodules.

temporal lobe specimens removed for seizure control (24). Most patients present with a long history of refractory epilepsy beginning in childhood but can have onset well into adulthood. DNTs have a generally even distribution between the sexes (25–28).

The classic location for DNT is supratentorial within the cortex of the temporal lobe, often mesially situated, but a large minority of them arises in other areas of cortex and ventricles (29,30). Other noncortical examples have been reported in the cerebellum and brainstem (31,32). Because of their unusual location, ventricular examples arising from the septum pellucidum are frequently misdiagnosed as gliomas, potentially leading to unnecessary treatment (30,33).

On neuroimaging, DNT expands the cortex without showing mass effect or edema (Figure 7-8). Multiple small cystic or pseudocystic structures may be present. T1-weighted MRI shows hypo- or isointensity, while T2-weighted images are hyperintense. Indentation and thinning of overlying calvarium, testament to the slow growth of the lesions, is common. Contrast enhancement is unusual but nodular or ringlike when present. Calcifications are common on CT examination (34). Extracortical cases show similar radiologic features, with the obvious exception of location (Figure 7-9). There is no correlation between radiologic features and histologic type (35).

Histopathology

The calling card of DNT is the *specific glioneuronal element*, an arrangement of axons clustered in columns that run perpendicular to the cortical surface and are flanked by oligodendroglia-like cells and microcystic pools of acidic mucopolysaccharide material (Figure 7-10). The microcysts

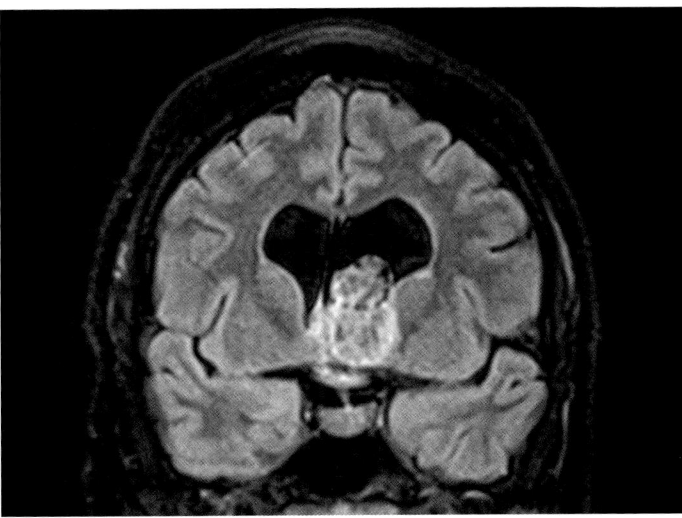

FIGURE 7-9 FLAIR-MRI: Dysembryoplastic neuroepithelial tumors are usually unexpected when arising from the septum and often misdiagnosed as gliomas.

occasionally contain "floating neurons," a unique characteristic of DNT (Figure 7-11). The oligodendroglia-like cells are monomorphic with round regular nuclei, dark closed chromatin, and prominent perinuclear halos. Fibrillar astrocytes dot the background (24). The larger architecture and configuration of DNT is highly variable and has three general patterns.

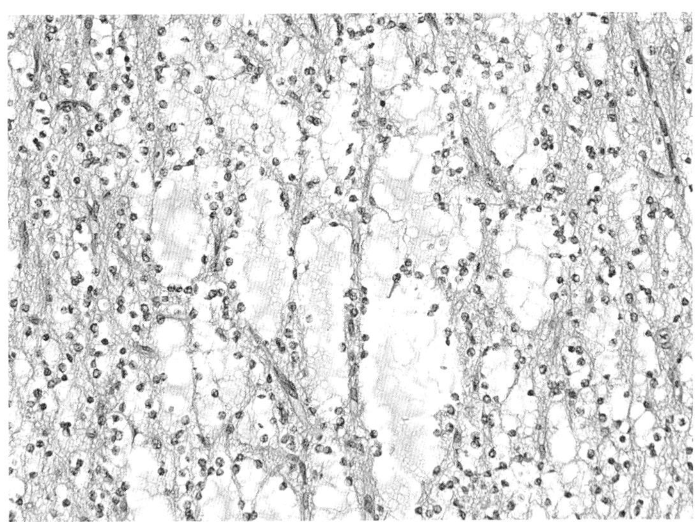

FIGURE 7-10 The "specific glioneuronal element" in dysembryoplastic neuroepithelial tumor consists of axon clusters surrounded by oligodendroglioma-like cells and mucinous microcysts.

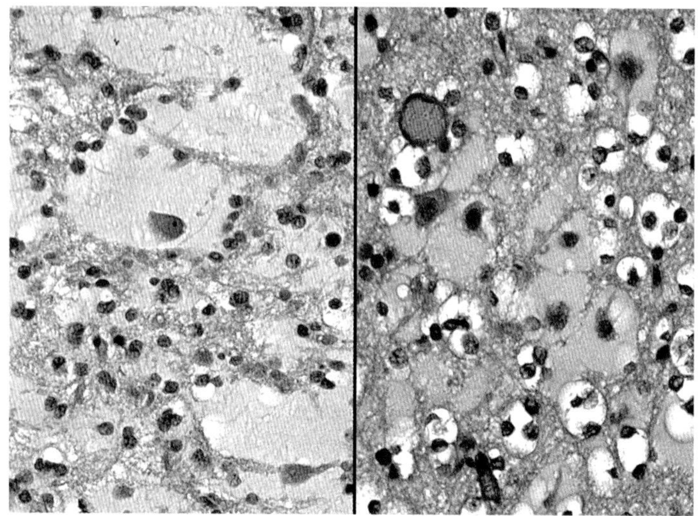

FIGURE 7-11 "Floating neurons" are a distinguishing feature of dysembryoplastic neuroepithelial tumor and can occur in large microcysts lined with oligo-like cells (left) or in smaller and less cellular ones (right).

These patterns do not have any specific clinical correlations and are more important for the sake of recognition and preventing them from being diagnosed as something else.

SIMPLE PATTERN. When the tumor is composed entirely of the specific glioneuronal element, it is termed the "simple" pattern of DNT. The lesion may be unitary, or may have multiple patches with intervening normal cortex. This is the least common pattern of DNT (35).

COMPLEX PATTERN. These DNTs additionally contain "glial nodules" that create a distinctly multinodular appearance on histologic sections. Most glial nodules are formed of the same oligodendroglia-like cells seen in the specific glioneuronal element, but they may have a highly variable appearance that can resemble pilocytic astrocytoma, diffuse astrocytoma, ganglioglioma, or others. The specific glioneuronal element is present focally in most cases with this pattern.

NONSPECIFIC/DIFFUSE PATTERN. This pattern is somewhat controversial because it more often lacks the specific element and has a broad spectrum of potential histologic features that overlap substantially with diffuse gliomas, pilocytic astrocytomas, angiocentric gliomas, gangliogliomas, and others (36). Because this pattern can be purely infiltrative in appearance on biopsy, the most crucial thing to rule out is a diffuse glioma, discussed below (Figure 7-12). One series suggests that, regardless of histology, the diagnosis of DNT should be considered if the following clinical criteria are met: (1) partial seizures that begin before age 20 (2) no neurologic deficit, (3) cortical topography seen on MRI, and (4) no mass effect on imaging (36).

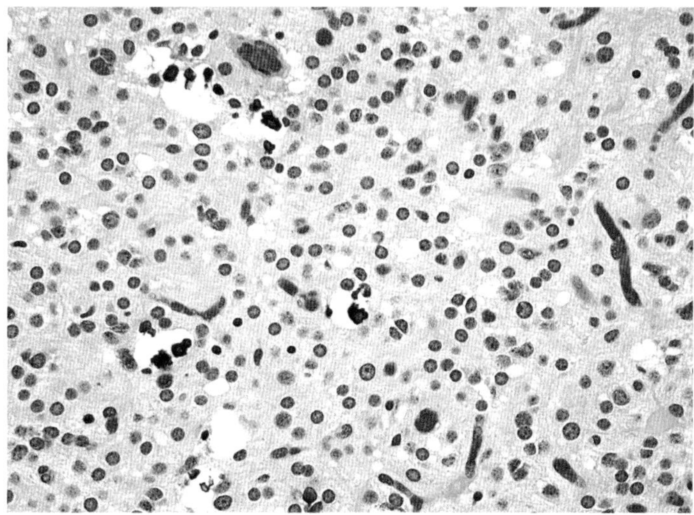

FIGURE 7-12 Some DNTs have little or no myxoid background and can appear similar to an oligodendroglioma.

Microvascular proliferation, necrosis, rare mitosis, and nuclear atypia can all be seen and have no impact on the status of the lesion as benign (37). The vascular proliferation can be florid and form glomeruloid structures or long arcing rims of redundant vessels, usually in association with the wall of a cystic area (Figure 7-13). Some reports have identified architectural and cytologic disarray consistent with cortical dysplasia in the brain adjacent from most cases of DNT (36,38).

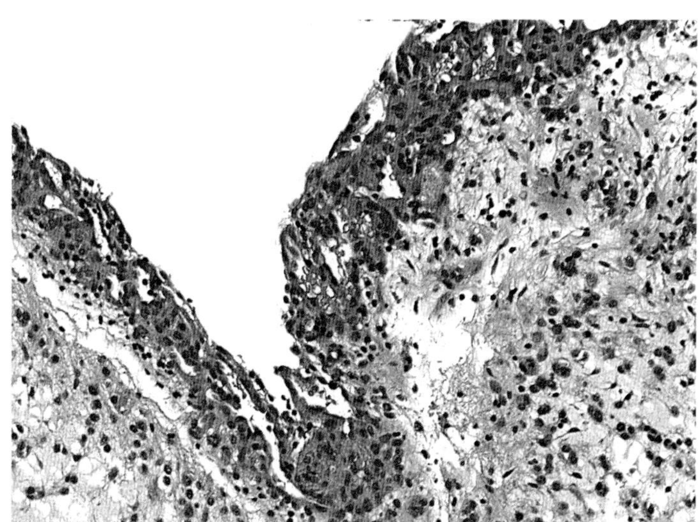

FIGURE 7-13 Microvascular proliferation is usually seen along the cyst lining in dysembryoplastic neuroepithelial tumor as long arrays of glomeruloid capillary proliferation.

The cells of DNT yield little helpful information upon immunohistochemical interrogation. The oligodendroglia-like cells show consistent S100 positivity but are only sporadically positive for synaptophysin, neurofilament, and class III beta tubulin (39). Otherwise, the cells of DNT show staining profiles that reflect their morphologic differentiation. MIB1 may be the most useful antibody in distinguishing DNT, with a positivity rate below 1% in most cases (40). Patchy CD34 immunostaining is present in most complex and nonspecific pattern DNTs (35).

Genetics

The morphologic findings of DNT being diverse and diagnostic interpretation of them somewhat subjective, it might not be surprising that different institutions with different customs in diagnosing DNT would find different rates of specific genetic abnormalities in their cases. Indeed, that seems to be what is recorded in the literature. BRAF V600E mutations have been reported at widely varying rates in DNTs, from 0% (21,41) to 51% (42). Taken together, it seems that BRAF mutations are uncommon in DNTs, particularly when centrally reviewed by expert neuropathologists. Alterations in the *FGFR1* gene, which include activating mutations, internal tandem duplications of the tyrosine kinase region, and gene fusions, have been identified in a majority of DNTs and not in other similar tumors (41,43). However, there is a recently described series of tumors that morphologically and immunohistochemically overlap with nonspecific DNTs and have *BRAF* mutations, or *FGFR2* or *FGFR3* fusions (44).

Differential Diagnosis

Because they both may have a monotonous population of cells with round, regular nuclei and perinuclear halos, often with a microcystic myxoid background, an infiltrative distribution of cells and nodular areas of growth, DNT and oligodendroglioma must both be considered when confronted with a lesion with these characteristics. Although this morphologic overlap is substantial, there are several features that differ. DNTs are centered in the cortex and show a profile of nodular cortical expansion when viewed in cross section, whereas oligodendrogliomas generally involve both the white matter and the cortex. Oligodendrogliomas also tend to have a delicate but extensive network of fine capillaries that are usually lacking in DNT. The nuclear details of the oligodendroglia-like cells in DNT are also more innocent appearing, with condensed chromatin and smaller size. Perineuronal satellitosis by tumor cells is seen frequently in oligodendrogliomas but not as much as in DNT. Although there is no set point at which MIB1 staining becomes indicative of oligodendroglioma, a rate below 1% favors DNT.

In ruling out an oligodendroglioma, assessment of molecular features is mandatory. The presence of an IDH mutation in a DNT-like lesion equals diffuse glioma, and oligodendroglioma if it is also 1p/19q deleted. Some would argue that the absence of those features does not rule out oligodendroglioma in pediatric patients. However, such "oligodendrogliomas" have excellent clinical courses and have the same *FGFR1* alterations seen in the vast majority of DNTs (41,45,46).

Distinguishing DNT from pilocytic astrocytoma, which can show monotonous round haloed cells and mucinous microcysts, can sometimes be difficult histologically but is usually less clinically relevant than ruling out an oligodendroglioma. Although BRAF mutations have been described in both, *FGFR1* mutations and duplications are much more typical of DNTs.

CENTRAL NEUROCYTOMA (WHO GRADE II), EXTRAVENTRICULAR NEUROCYTOMA (WHO GRADE II), AND ATYPICAL NEUROCYTOMA

Although discussed as separate entities in the 2016 WHO, central neurocytoma and extraventricular neurocytoma are essentially the same lesion from the morphologic standpoint and are discussed together here. Atypical cases of both central and extraventricular neurocytomas are recognized in the 2016 WHO classification, yet no explicit grade is assigned (19).

Clinical Context

Neurocytomas are conceptually tumors composed of cells that are intermediate in maturity between embryonal neuronal precursors (neuroblasts) and ganglion cells. These are divided into two groups based on their anatomic site. Central neurocytomas by definition occur within the ventricles, usually around the foramen of Monro, whereas extraventricular neurocytomas arise intraparenchymally. Approximately equal fractions of males and females between the ages of 20 and 50 together account for over three-quarters of central neurocytomas (47–49).

Presenting complaints are typically headache, nausea, vomiting, and other signs and symptoms of increased intracranial pressure, probably due to the occlusion of cerebrospinal fluid (CSF) flow by lesions near the foramen of Monro in the case of central neurocytomas. By magnetic resonance imaging (MRI), central neurocytomas are well circumscribed, hypo-to isointense on T1, hyperintense on T2, and variably contrast enhancing (50). A "soap bubble" appearance has been described on T2-weighted MR, meaning there are multiple internal cysts that resemble suds (51). CT scan may show calcifications. Similar radiologic characteristics describe extraventricular neurocytomas, except that they are more apt to form cystic cavities and take on a "cyst with mural nodule" configuration.

Central neurocytomas reported to date show a generally indolent clinical course, with long-term cure affected by gross total resection in patients with "typical" histology (52,53). Extent of resection and mitotic activity (atypical histology) affect recurrence and overall survival rates. Outcomes and risk factors arc similar for extraventricular neurocytomas (54). For cases with atypical features and/or subtotal resection, radiotherapy seems to improve outcomes (53).

Histopathology

Neurocytomas are characterized by consistently monotonous and dense populations of small cells with round regular nuclei and perinuclear clearing in a finely fibrillar background with frequent calcifications (Figure 7-14). Nuclei contain granular chromatin and small nucleoli. Neurocytomas may also possess a rich network of capillaries around which a small area of cortex-like granular neuropil may extend, occasionally resembling the perivascular pseudorosettes seen in ependymomas. These nucleus-free patches of neuropil also occur without any association with blood vessels (Figure 7-15). Except in atypical cases, mitotic figures should be difficult to find, and necrosis or microvascular proliferation should be absent. Neurocytomas are poorly infiltrative and one should not see a gradual transition from tumor to brain at the lesion edges. A minority of neurocytomas show slightly elongated nuclei arranged in a streaming pattern. Fully mature ganglion cells may also be seen.

Immunohistochemistry shows strong and diffuse positivity for synaptophysin in the neuropil and cell bodies. Whereas oligodendrogliomas can also express synaptophysin (55), the neuronal nuclear transcription factor NeuN is often widely positive in the nuclei of neurocytomas and negative or focal in oligodendrogliomas, making it useful in differentiating these two tumors when it is positive (56). GFAP expression can be surprisingly widespread, but it is typically from entrapped nonneoplastic astrocytes (Figure 7-16), although its expression has been demonstrated in some neurocytoma cells (57). Neurofilament, the intermediate filament of neurons, is usually negative but can be seen focally where tumor cells

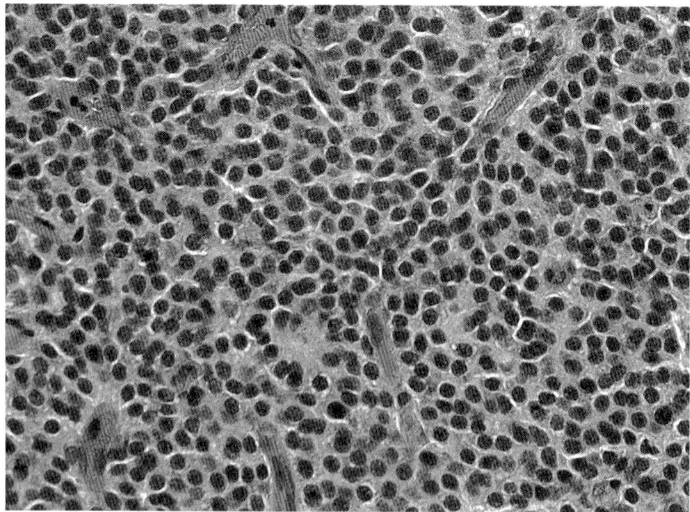

FIGURE 7-14 Central neurocytoma: monotonous cells with granular chromatin, rich capillary vasculature, and fine, homogeneous cytoplasm.

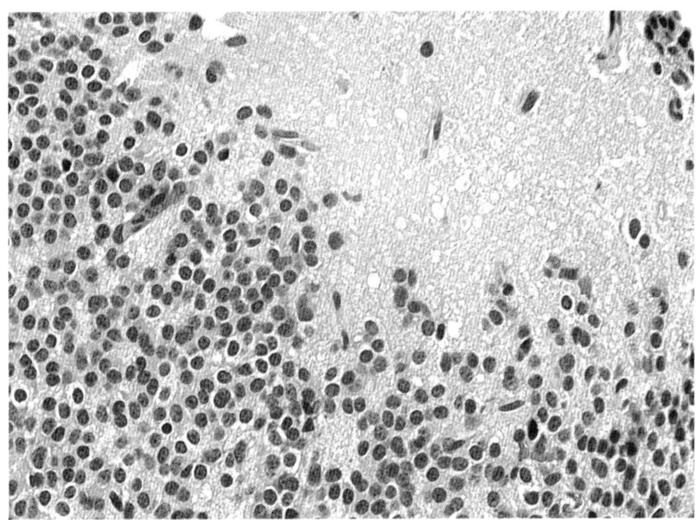

FIGURE 7-15 Patches of nucleus-poor, cortex-like neuropil are a distinguishing feature of neurocytomas.

have developed into mature ganglion cells (49). Neurofilament staining should highlight only entrapped axons around the tumor edges, and should not demonstrate a diffusely infiltrative pattern such as that of oligodendroglioma. IDH immunostaining is always negative in neurocytomas by definition.

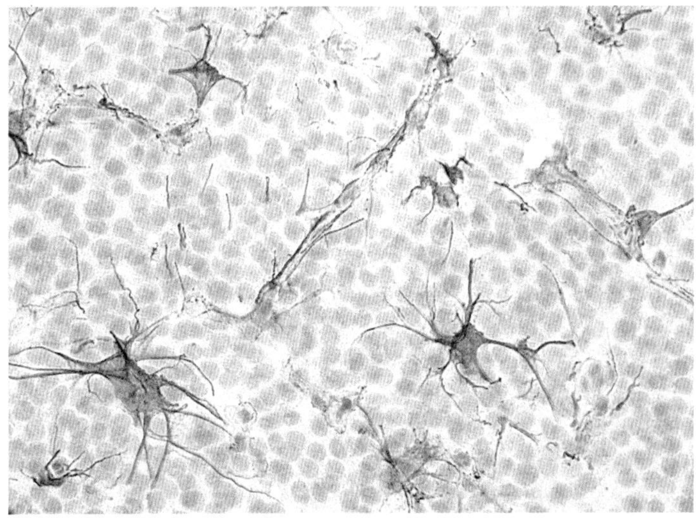

FIGURE 7-16 GFAP-positive nonneoplastic astrocytes scaffold the capillaries and neurocytoma cells and can be more numerous than pictured here.

Differential Diagnosis

Before their description, central neurocytomas were called "intraventricular oligodendrogliomas," reflecting the close histologic resemblance between the two (Figure 7-17). Oligodendrogliomas may even be frankly neurocytic, making the task of distinguishing the two by morphology and immunohistochemistry truly daunting (58). Fortunately, now that oligodendrogliomas are defined by IDH mutations and 1p/19q codeletion, that task is straightforward. If something that looks and stains like a neurocytoma has an IDH mutation, it is not a neurocytoma. Codeletion of 1p and 19q has been reported in extraventricular neurocytomas and associated with a worse prognosis (58,59). These reports are from before IDH testing was available and likely represent oligodendrogliomas with neurocytic differentiation.

DNT-like tumors of the septum pellucidum occur in the same area as central neurocytomas and also have monotonous oligodendroglia-like cells. In contrast to neurocytomas, they typically also have microcystic myxoid areas and lower overall cellularity. DNTs of the septum pellucidum do not show staining for NeuN in the oligodendroglia-like cell component.

Intraoperative recognition of this tumor can be difficult because the haloed nuclei are not produced by frozen sections. The dense growth of small cells can raise concerns for glioblastoma or metastatic malignancy, especially when the nuclei are distorted into an angular, dark, and pleomorphic appearance by the freezing process. Areas of nucleus-free neuropil can also suggest foci of necrosis. Cytologic smear preparations prove their worth in such situations by demonstrating the neurocytoma's banal

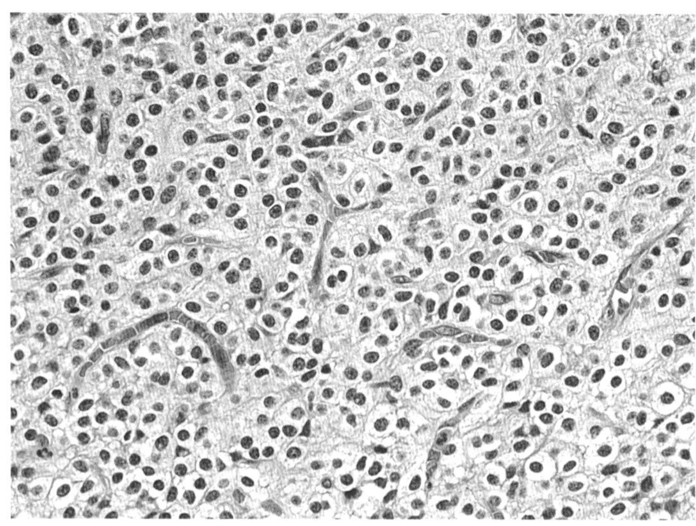

FIGURE 7-17 Perinuclear halos give many neurocytomas a strong resemblance to oligodendrogliomas.

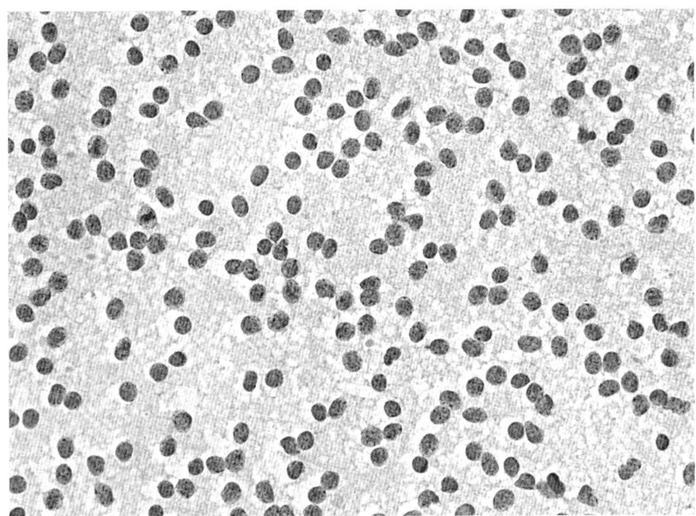

FIGURE 7-18 Squash preparations reveal the finely granular background of neurocytoma and complete lack of cytoplasmic processes on tumor cells.

uniform nuclei, tame granular chromatin, and general lack of coarse fibrillar processes extending from tumor cells (Figure 7-18).

Grading

Although neurocytomas are relatively uncommon, enough cases have been published to generalize their clinical behavior. According to one large series, the two most important factors associated with recurrence and survival are completeness of resection and the presence of atypical histologic features (52). Another series found that mitotic activity was prognostic, but extent of resection was not (60). Atypical histologic features include frequent mitotic figures, microvascular proliferation, and necrosis. Atypical status for central neurocytomas has been suggested for cases surpassing 2% MIB1 positivity (48), whereas extraventricular cases have been called atypical for having mitotic activity of ≥3/10 hpf (61).

DYSPLASTIC CEREBELLAR GANGLIOCYTOMA (LHERMITTE–DUCLOS DISEASE) (WHO GRADE I)

Clinical Context

Arising most frequently in adults, this rare nonneoplastic lesion is a pathognomonic clinical diagnostic criterion for the Cowden syndrome (62), an inherited predisposition to a variety of benign and malignant tumors due to an autosomal dominant mutation in the *PTEN* gene on the long arm of chromosome 10. One case has been reported with wild type *PTEN* and an activating, germline mutation in the *EGFR* gene, the protein from which is inhibited by PTEN (63). Occurring by definition in the cerebellum, most patients with this lesion present between the third and fifth decades with headache, nausea, vomiting, vertigo, and other signs of increased intracranial pressure (64). No sex or race predilection has been shown.

The radiologic findings of Lhermitte–Duclos disease (LDD) are characteristic: nonenhancing unilateral enlargement of the cerebellum that is T1 hypointense and T2 hyperintense and shows parallel striations, or "tiger stripes" in axial images (65), although younger patients may have MRI findings similar to medulloblastoma (66).

Most cases of LDD occur in the context of Cowden syndrome, yet only a minority of patients with Cowden syndrome has evidence of LDD. In a series of 35 patients with the syndrome confirmed by criteria other than LDD, a little more than a third had some evidence of focal cerebellar expansion (67). LDD appears to arise from the extant cerebellar granular neurons and has a limited growth potential with essentially no proliferation (64,68), arguing against a neoplastic process, but can "recur" both at the site of excision (69) and in noncontiguous cerebellum (70). Whether this "recurrence" represents dysplastic or ongoing hypertrophic change of previously normal granular neurons remains to be demonstrated. Because this condition is caused by the enlargement of normal cells, it is probably best categorized as hypertrophic in nature and not neoplastic or hamartomatous. Most patients with LDD enjoy long-term recurrence-free survival.

Histopathology

Granular neurons in the affected area are transformed into ganglionic cells with large centrally placed nuclei that show open vesicular chromatin and prominent nucleoli. This change occurs along a gradient, with the interface of the lesion and normal cerebellum being a mixture of normal granular neurons and swollen lesional neurons that range from just slightly larger than normal to almost the size of Purkinje cells (Figure 7-19). The enlarged cells become more dominant farther away from normal cerebellum where residual normal granular neurons are nearly absent (Figure 7-20). The white matter is not involved. Prominent vacuolation is often present and has been suggested as the cause for striations on T2-weighted MRI (64). Calcification is sometimes present, especially within the walls of blood vessels (Figure 7-21). Immunohistochemically, the signature-enlarged neurons express NeuN and synaptophysin and should not show any significant proliferation by MIB1.

Differential Diagnosis

The identification of this process is important because patients with Cowden syndrome require increased surveillance for breast and thyroid carcinomas, and it may be confused with more sinister entities that result in unnecessary treatment for the patient. Other ganglion cell tumors, such as ganglioglioma and gangliocytoma, only rarely appear in the cerebellum and do not demonstrate the undulating pattern that follows the contour of

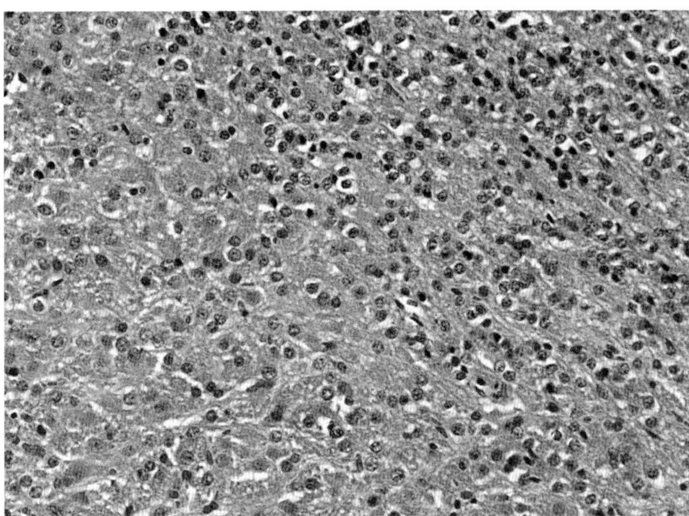

FIGURE 7-19 The transition from normal granular neurons (upper right) to dysplastic ones (lower left) creates a pseudoinfiltrative pattern at the edges of dysplastic cerebellar gangliocytomas.

cerebellar folia and respects the white matter. Infiltrating astrocytomas are uncommon in the cerebellum and can create an expansile appearance in cerebellar folia, but they are composed of smaller cells that intermingle with granular neurons and permeate the white matter. Immunoreactivity of atypical cells for synaptophysin and NeuN and not for GFAP should steer one away from infiltrating astrocytoma.

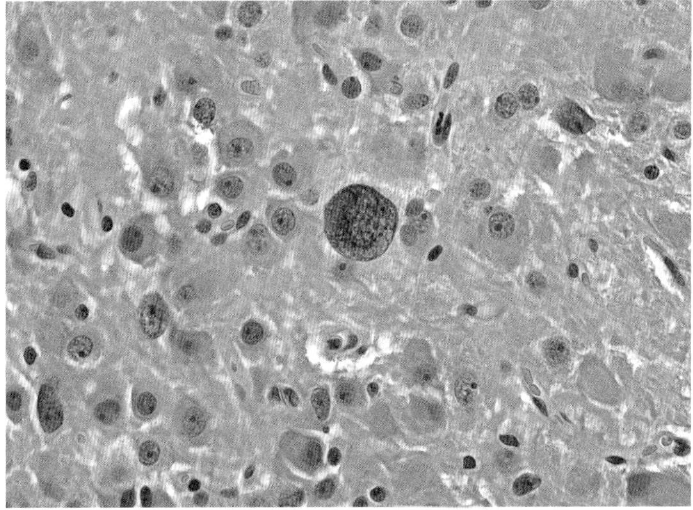

FIGURE 7-20 Dysplastic cerebellar gangliocytoma is formed of bland-appearing neurons, but some atypia (enlarged nucleus) is permissible.

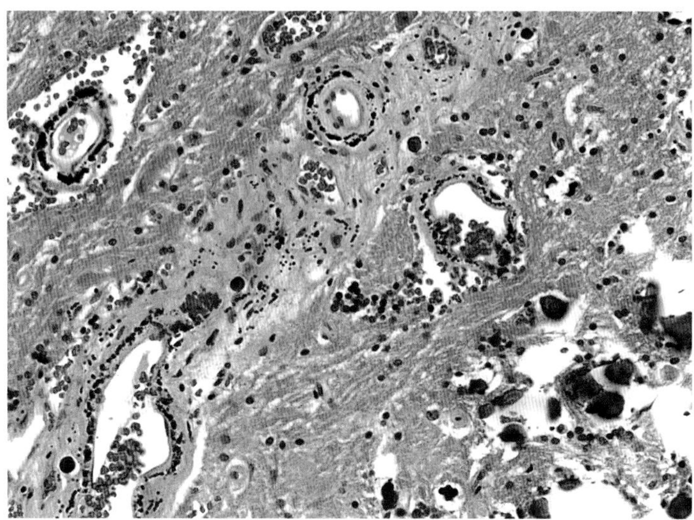

FIGURE 7-21 Older dysplastic cerebellar gangliocytomas accumulate vascular and parenchymal calcifications.

DESMOPLASTIC INFANTILE GANGLIOGLIOMA AND ASTROCYTOMA (WHO GRADE I)

Clinical Context

As the name would indicate, this tumor chiefly occurs in infants, having a mean and median age at presentation of around 6 months (71,72), although more than 15 cases from later in childhood have been reported (73,74). Males are affected more than females at a ratio of 1.5:1, with a greater disparity among older patients (75). Infant patients present with bulging of the fontanelle, increased head size, and stupor. Neuroimaging shows a large heterogeneous and partially cystic mass compressing a cerebral hemisphere and abutting the dura (Figure 7-22). The lesion usually has a contrast-enhancing T1-isointense solid component that lies more superficially and a cystic T2-hyperintense portion centrally. Edema, calcifications, and bone remodeling are variable (76). Desmoplastic infantile ganglioglioma/astrocytoma (DIG/A) has not been described outside of the supratentorial compartment to date. Despite the typically striking image of DIG/A on MRI, the patients respond well to surgical excision without adjunct therapies. Patients with complete resection of their tumor can expect long-term cure, as can most of those with incomplete removal (77). Instances of aggressive DIG/A with high MIB1 rates and metastases have been reported, but are rare (78). One review suggests that DIAs are generally more aggressive than DIGs (79).

Histopathology

Most DIG/As show two main patterns of growth within the same lesion. The solid part near the surface comprises an astroglial population dispersed

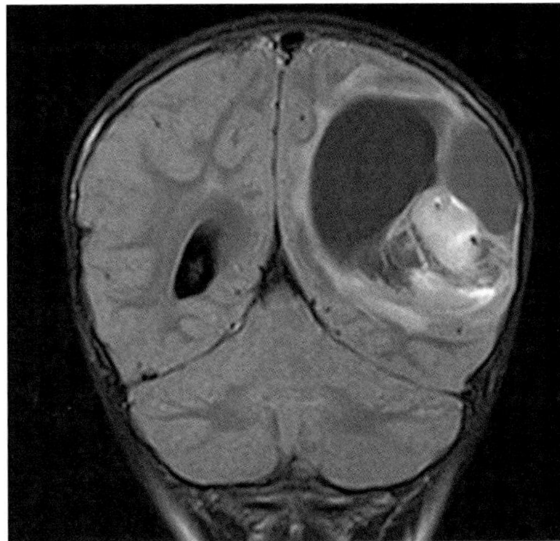

FIGURE 7-22 FLAIR-MRI of a desmoplastic infantile ganglioglioma showing a large, superficial, multicystic, heterogeneous, hemispheric mass that is often suspected to be malignant preoperatively.

throughout a background of wavy dense collagen fibrils and spindle-shaped fibroblasts in a storiform pattern with short fascicles (72). The ratio of tumor cells to collagen can vary widely, even within the same tumor, being sclerotic and hypocellular in areas (Figure 7-23). Neurons, which are currently viewed as the sole difference between DIA and DIG, may be found in this component most often as small polygonal cells with little obvious neuronal differentiation and less often as overt ganglion cells. The collagen

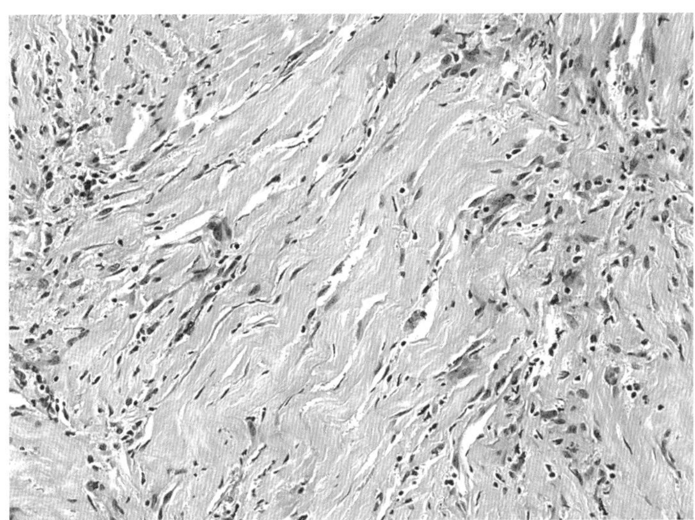

FIGURE 7-23 Dense sclerosis masks the neuroglial nature of desmoplastic infantile ganglioglioma/astrocytoma.

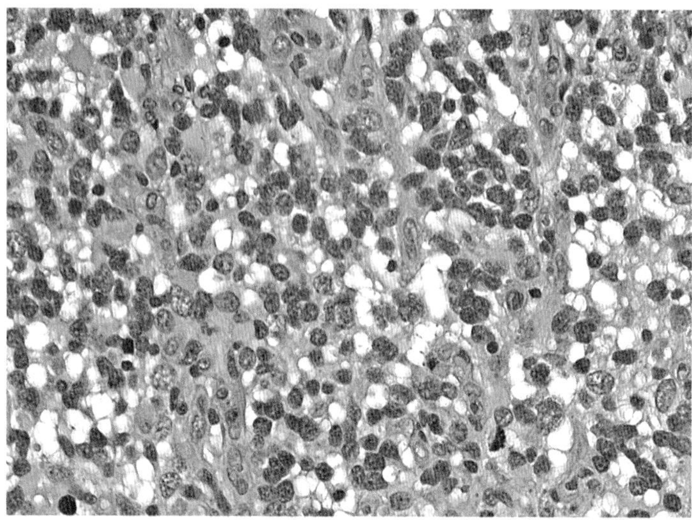

FIGURE 7-24 Aggressive-appearing small-cell areas are common in desmoplastic infantile ganglioglioma and do not predict a poorer outcome.

fibrils are intimately deposited between the tumor cells and can be clearly displayed by reticulin staining, similar in concept to the collagen background of hemangiopericytoma. An immature or embryonal component is usually present focally, composed of small basophilic cells with scant cytoplasm and little morphologic differentiation (Figure 7-24). This component lacks a dense collagen background and can occasionally contain mitosis and/or necrosis that may be worrisome for, but not indicative of, a more aggressive neoplasm. Indeed, the prognostic impact of these hypercellular areas is surprisingly little (71,75). Although DIG is a circumscribed tumor, invasion into its surroundings along perivascular spaces is common (Figure 7-25).

Immunohistochemistry is helpful for demonstrating the glial and, if present, neuronal components of this neoplasm (Figure 7-26). GFAP reactivity illuminates the sometimes subtle astrocytes embedded in desmoplasia. Because hematoxylin and eosin (H&E) staining may also fail to show clear neuronal differentiation, synaptophysin is helpful to reveal any neoplastic neurons. MIB1 labeling should generally be seen in 5% or fewer tumor nuclei.

There is no specific genetic signature for DIG/A. A few cases have had BRAF V600E mutations, but they represent only a minute fraction of the total cases.

Differential Diagnosis

The clinical context in which this lesion occurs is almost stereotyped: a large, heterogeneous, superficial, contrast-enhancing, partially cystic mass

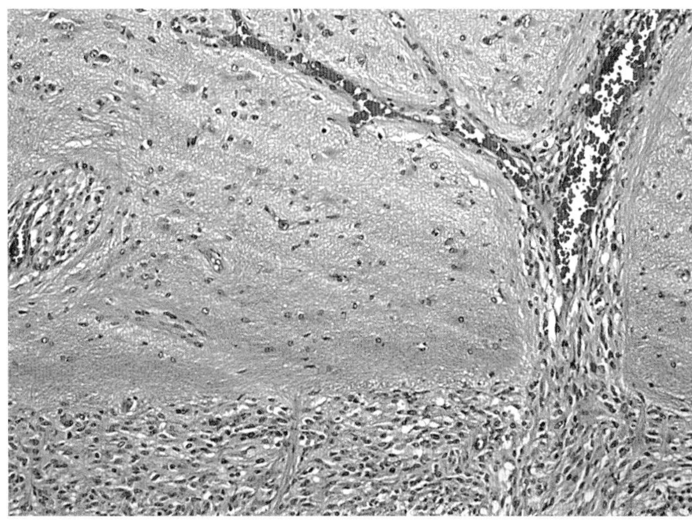

FIGURE 7-25 Sharp circumscription with perivascular extension is common in desmoplastic infantile ganglioglioma/astrocytoma.

in the supratentorial compartment of an infant. DIG/A should be strongly suspected in such cases and regarded as less likely when these elements are not present. Because DIG/A is a WHO grade I lesion, it is imperative to separate it from more malignant lesions that receive aggressive chemo- and radiotherapeutic treatment. Circumspection and restraint should be exercised in the face of this benign lesion that can appear malignant.

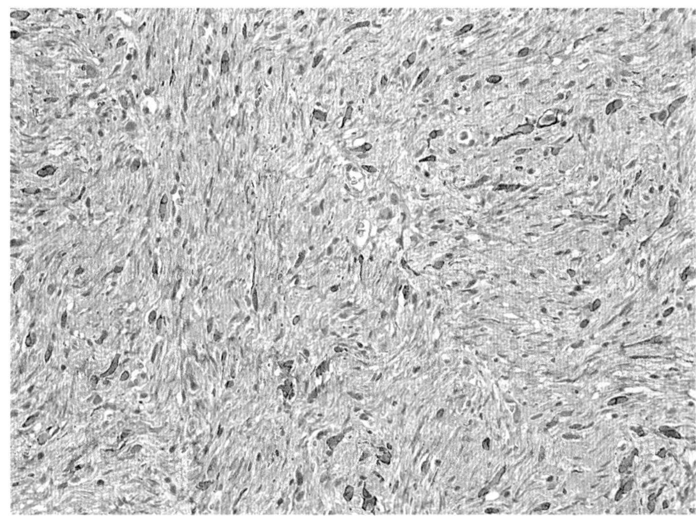

FIGURE 7-26 Immunohistochemistry for GFAP highlights the glial component of this DIG against a collagenous background.

An infantile glioblastoma or gliosarcoma could also enter the differential with DIG/A. Although the embryonal component of DIG/A may show necrosis and vascular proliferation, it does not permeate the surrounding brain parenchyma as single cells or show the intertwined fascicles of sarcomatous and gliomatous elements. A neurofilament stain can help in this situation by demonstrating whether the tumor is infiltrative or not. DIG/A is also not prone to mutations in *TP53* or immunohistochemical staining for p53 (80,81), whereas pediatric and infantile glioblastomas are (82,83).

Other CNS lesions with extensive fibrosis may enter the differential based on histologic similarity, but none are likely in the clinical and radiologic context of DIG/A. Among these are fibrous meningioma, solitary fibrous tumor, and fibrosarcoma, all of which can be ruled out by positive GFAP staining. PXA would also express GFAP and contain fine collagen, but it is generally more pleomorphic and usually lacks the dense sclerotic collagen of DIG.

DIFFUSE LEPTOMENINGEAL GLIONEURONAL TUMOR (GRADE UNASSIGNED)

This new addition to the 2016 WHO nomenclature has been described in the literature as leptomeningeal oligodendrogliomatosis and several other names since the early 1940s. Diffuse leptomeningeal glioneuronal tumor (DLGT) is rare, with only several dozen cases described in the literature.

Clinical Context

DLGT occurs mostly in children, the vast majority in the first decade, although cases in young adults have been reported (84,85). The typical presentation is that of obstructive hydrocephalus, with symptoms of headache, nausea, vomiting, and ataxia being among the most common complaints. Neuroimaging shows diffuse thickening and contrast enhancement of the leptomeninges, sometimes with a discrete spinal cord tumor, and possibly with small cystic structures around the cerebellum and brainstem. The appearance is often mistaken for dissemination of a high grade tumor, or as meningitis, although CSF studies are typically negative for anything except elevated protein (84).

Due to the rare occurrence of DLGT, there is no consensus on what the best therapy is. Most cases receive chemotherapy, at least upon progression, and some cases undergo radiation therapy. The outcome in most cases is generally good, with many cases achieving stable disease following treatment (84,86). There is a subset of DLGTs that have glomeruloid microvascular proliferation and/or increased proliferation, defined as presence of mitosis, MIB1 staining >4%, and progress with a significant mortality rate (87).

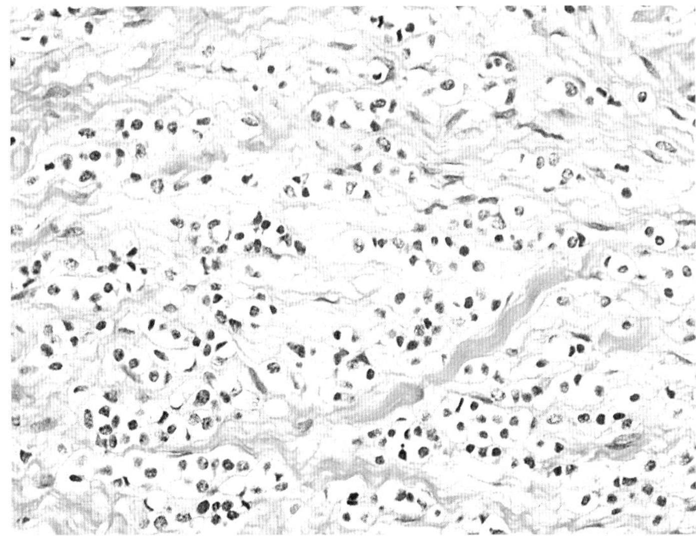

FIGURE 7-27 Diffuse leptomeningeal glioneuronal tumor (DLGT) typically has an oligodendroglial morphology in a background of fibrosis in leptomeningeal biopsies.

Histopathology and Immunohistochemistry

Biopsy of DLGT can be difficult and initial attempts may be nondiagnostic. Microscopically, the fibrotic meninges contain nests and cords of monotonous cells with round, hyperchromatic nuclei and perinuclear clearing, similar to oligodendrogliomas (Figure 7-27). Myxoid material may be present (Figure 7-28), and may form microcysts in some cases.

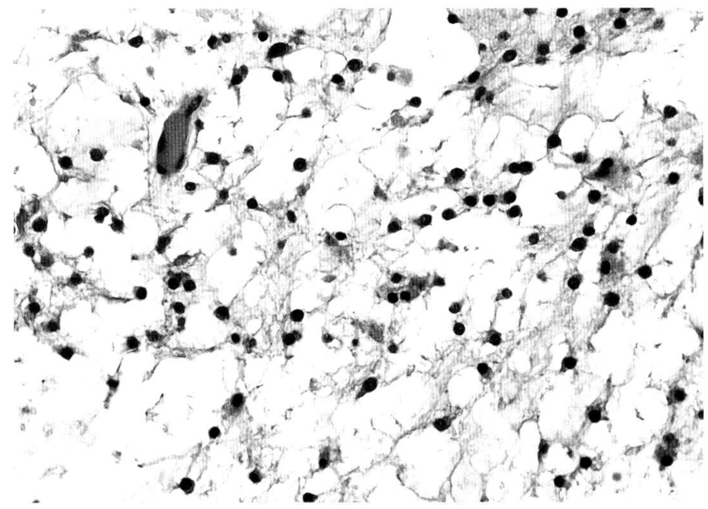

FIGURE 7-28 Some cases of DLGT may have a more myxoid background.

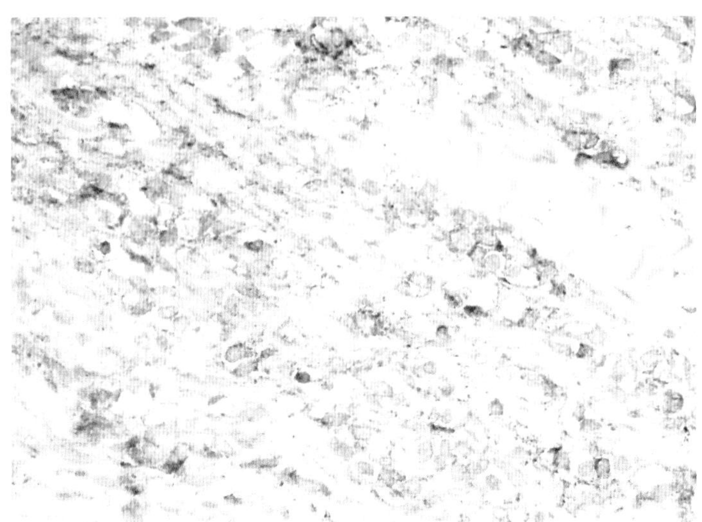

FIGURE 7-29 Most DLGTs will express synaptophysin (seen here) as well as S100 and Olig2.

Ganglion cells have been described in a few cases. Extension along the subpial surface is occasionally present in biopsied material.

Nearly all DLGTs express S100 protein, and most also express synaptophysin (Figure 7-29) and the glial marker Olig2. Almost half of DLGTs express GFAP.

Genetics

The genetic background in DLGT is somewhat heterogeneous, yet a few findings are common in this tumor type. About two-thirds to three-quarters of DLGTs have a *KIAA1549-BRAF* duplication similar to pilocytic astrocytomas (85). Though unlike pilocytic astrocytomas, DLGTs also have deletions of 1p in a similar proportion of cases and deletion of 19q in a minority (84,85,87). Those deletions were mostly detected by FISH, so it is unknown how many have the whole-arm deletions seen in oligodendrogliomas. At least one case was documented to have the typical t(1;19)(q10;p10) (88). *IDH1* R132H mutations have not been found in DLGTs. The *BRAF* V600E mutation has been described in at least one case (86).

PAPILLARY GLIONEURONAL TUMOR (WHO GRADE I)

Clinical Context

Fewer than 100 cases of this rare neoplasm have been reported in the literature to date, but a reasonably clear picture of its typically indolent nature has developed. Most cases have occurred in the second and third decades of life, with the range of patient ages spanning from 4 to 75 years (89,90). Males and females represent similar numbers of cases. There are

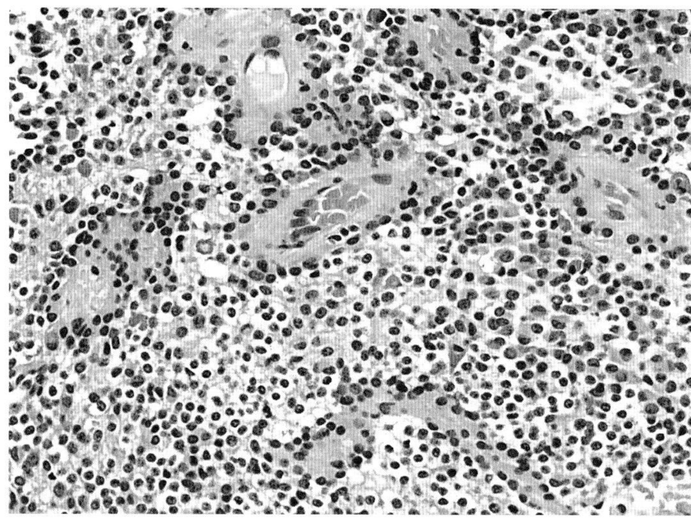

FIGURE 7-30 Papillary glioneuronal tumor usually with biphasic population of perivascular glial pseudopapillae in a background of monotonous neurocytic cells.

no specific symptoms or signs associated with papillary glioneuronal tumor (PGNT), and many examples are discovered incidentally. When symptoms do occur, headaches and seizures are the most common (91,92). Neuroimaging shows a circumscribed contrast-enhancing supratentorial mass that is sometimes cystic and borders one of the lateral ventricles. Little surrounding edema is seen, and a minority are calcified (92). Most reported cases of PGNTs have been cured by excision without any additional treatment. Several cases with dissemination, local extension, or high-grade histology have been reported, and may expand the concept of this entity (93,94).

Histopathology

Two distinct populations of cells occur in this tumor, glial and neuronal. The glial component is essentially astrocytic in morphology, with fibrillar eosinophilic cytoplasm and more smoothly hyperchromatic chromatin than the neuronal element. These glial cells form a monolayer that lines the outside of prominent fibrovascular cores (Figure 7-30). The glia-lined vessels are separated from each other by the neuronal component, which is a heterogeneous population of neuronal cells in various modes of differentiation, mostly small and neurocytic with scattered larger ganglioid cells and intermediate forms, although mature forms can predominate (Figure 7-31). The neurocytes have round regular nuclei that are distributed in various densities in a finely fibrillar neuropil matrix. Artifactual perinuclear halos may be present. Although not truly papillary, the hyalinized vessels can tear free of the intervening neuronal cells and form characteristic pseudopapillary structures. Degenerative changes, such as

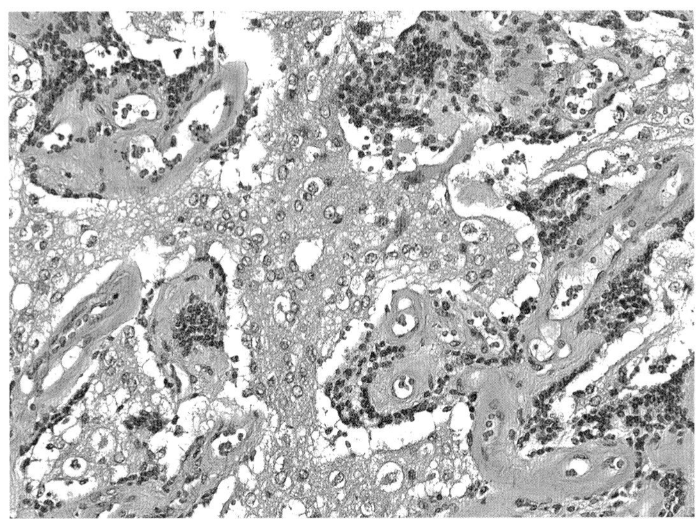

FIGURE 7-31 The neuronal component of papillary glioneuronal tumor can show ganglionic maturity and fibrillarity, and vessels are often hyalinized.

hemosiderin deposition, macrophages, and punctate calcifications, may occasionally be seen, as may rare EGBs and Rosenthal fibers (92).

Immunohistochemical staining for GFAP and synaptophysin creates a unique pattern of GFAP-positive perivascular glia, and an inversely synaptophysin-positive neuronal population (Figure 7-32). Neurofilament highlights the more mature ganglioid cells (92).

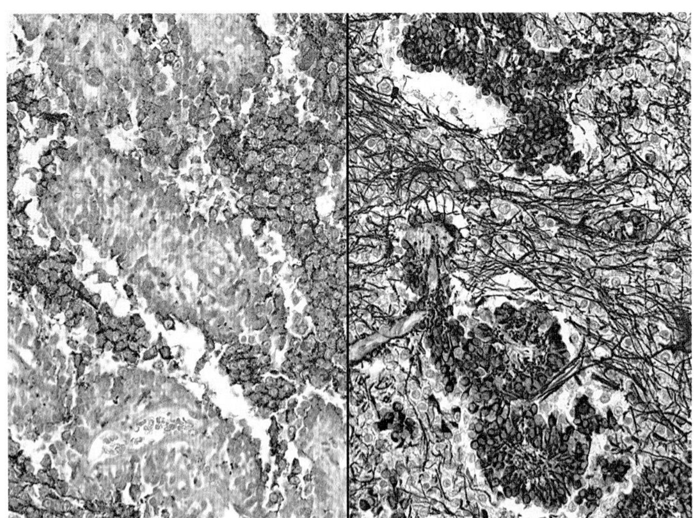

FIGURE 7-32 Immunohistochemistry for synaptophysin is positive in the neurocytic cells and negative in perivascular cells, whereas GFAP highlights the perivascular cells and non-neoplastic astrocytes among the neurocytic component.

Genetics

PGNTs have been shown to have high rates of a translocation between chromosomes 9 and 17 involving fusion of the genes *SLC44A1* on 9q31 and *PRKCA* on 17q24, usually in the absence of any other identified abnormalities (95–97). This translocation has not been identified in other brain tumors and has been suggested as the primary pathogenetic event in the formation of PGNTs, thus a suitable diagnostic feature (96).

ROSETTE-FORMING GLIONEURONAL TUMOR (WHO GRADE I)

Clinical Context

This entity was initially described as a DNT-like neoplasm that occurred in the fourth ventricle and was later described elsewhere, such as in the chiasm, spinal cord, and cerebellum (98–100). Fewer than 75 cases have been reported, and most of those have occurred within the second to fourth decades of life with no significant sex predilection. Headache and ataxia, along with other symptoms of increased intracranial pressure, are common in rosette-forming glioneuronal tumor (RGNT) due to obstruction of the cerebral aqueduct and are seen in about half of reported cases. However, the onset of symptoms is slow, often lasting for months before the mass lesion is discovered.

Although not all cases are within the fourth ventricle, MRI of typical cases does show a solid and partially cystic circumscribed midline mass that is hyperintense on T2 sequences and hypointense on T1. Administration of contrast material shows at least focal nodular enhancement in most instances (101). Calcification is present in about half of reported cases.

In keeping with the histologically low-grade appearance of this lesion, RGNT has been treated primarily by surgical resection without adjuvant chemotherapy or radiation. Many patients with RGNT have had lasting neurologic deficits after treatment, but this may reflect the difficulty of resecting tumors in and around the fourth ventricle (102,103). Most RGNTs do not recur following resection.

Histopathology

Although distinct, RGNT shares some features with DNT. Like DNT, the major cellular component is monotonous with small, round, hyperchromatic nuclei and scant fibrillar cytoplasm. These monotonous cells line areas of granular neuropil that forms columns, perivascular pseudorosettes, and small fibrillar rosettes in a background of myxoid material (Figure 7-33). Similar to pilocytic astrocytomas and DNT, the cells can also grow in sheets of oligodendroglia-like cells. Mucinous microcysts with "floating neurons" are occasionally noted and overall cellularity is low. Fibrillar astrocytic cells form another component and may appear piloid.

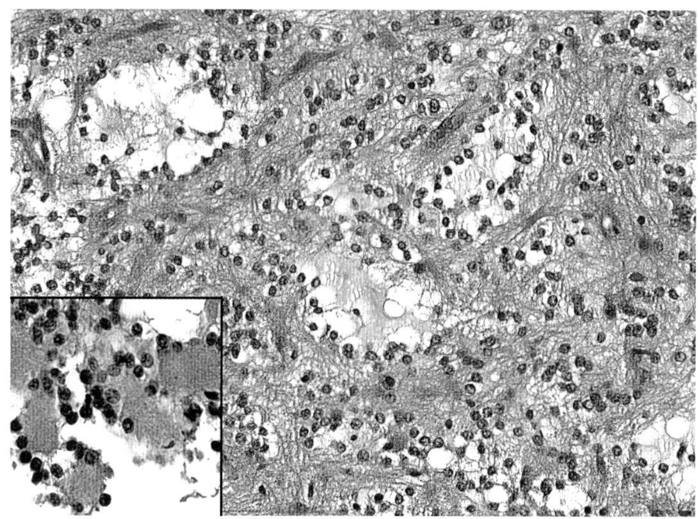

FIGURE 7-33 Rosette-forming glioneuronal tumor with fibrillar rosettes and perivascular pseudorosettes.

Immunohistochemistry shows synaptophysin reactivity around vessels and within rosettes and diffuse GFAP staining among more piloid astroglial cells. A MIB1 proliferation index should be below 2% to 3%.

Genetics

Activating point mutations in the *PIK3CA* gene are a recurring genetic finding in RGNT and were observed in three of four tested cases (104). Such mutations are not specific to RGNT and occur infrequently in other brain tumors, both malignant and benign. However, in RGNT they typically occur in absence of other mutations or chromosomal changes. Another series found *FGFR1* point mutations in two of eight RGNTs (105). Similar mutations have been seen in a small number of pilocytic astrocytomas, and it some posit that this may be a pathogenetic link between these two morphologically similar tumors. The most common abnormalities in pilocytic astrocytomas, KIAA1549-BRAF fusions and BRAF V600 mutations, have not been identified in RGNTs (106).

CEREBELLAR LIPONEUROCYTOMA (WHO GRADE II)

Clinical Context

Originally called "lipomatous medulloblastoma," this exceptionally rare tumor actually bears little clinical resemblance to medulloblastoma. Cerebellar liponeurocytomas are generally tumors of adults (mean and median age ~50 years) and occur in the cerebellum (107–112), although five liponeurocytomas have been described in the lateral ventricles (113). Men and women are equally affected.

The clinical presentation mirrors that of other posterior fossa tumors, with headache and cerebellar symptoms being common. MRI shows a circumscribed lesion that is heterogeneous on T1- and T2-weighted images due to its pattern of lipid deposition. Contrast enhancement is moderate (114).

Due to the rarity of this lesion, its long-term prognosis is difficult to determine, but recurrences are common among those with long follow-up. About half of reported cases survive at least 5 years after diagnosis (107,115). Described pediatric cases of lipidized/lipomatous medulloblastoma have behaved much more aggressively than cerebellar liponeurocytoma, have higher proliferative indices, and are fundamentally medulloblastomas with lipid accumulation (116).

Histopathology

At low power, cerebellar liponeurocytoma has a biphasic appearance with geographic foci of vacuolated, lipidized cells separated by sheets of monotonous, small neurocytes with round, regular nuclei and a small to moderate amount of cytoplasm (Figure 7-34). Tumor cell nuclei contain speckled chromatin and inconspicuous nucleoli and are ringed by perinuclear halos in some cases. Lipidized cells have a single large cytoplasmic vacuole and a small nucleus compressed at the periphery. Anaplasia, necrosis, and vascular proliferation should not be seen in this lesion. Mitotic figures are rare.

Tumor cells express neuronal antigens such as synaptophysin and MAP2 by immunostaining, but focal positivity for GFAP is common. No differences in staining profiles are noted between the neurocytic and lipidized components, indicating that the vacuolated cells are not metaplastic adipocytes but tumor cells with accumulation of lipid. MIB1

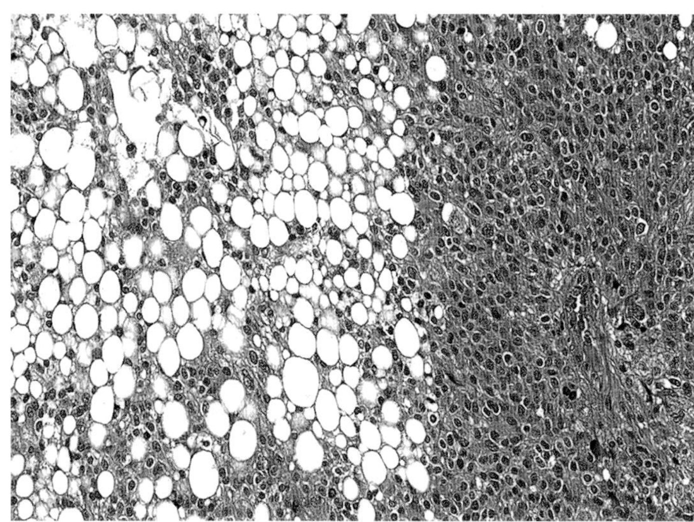

FIGURE 7-34 Cerebellar liponeurocytomas contain typical neurocytic tumor cells (right) and patches of lipidized tumor cells (left).

staining is important in distinguishing liponeurocytoma from medulloblastoma, with rates less than 5% strongly favoring the former.

Because there is overlap in location, histologic appearance, and immunostaining, the main differential diagnosis is between cerebellar liponeurocytoma and medulloblastoma. Liponeurocytomas have a much older age at presentation than medulloblastoma, allowing suspicions to be appropriately set before the lesion is examined histologically. Lipidized cells in liponeurocytomas cluster together to form fat-like patches, whereas they are more diffusely distributed and individually disposed in lipidized medulloblastoma.

SPINAL PARAGANGLIOMA (PARAGANGLIOMA OF THE FILUM TERMINALE) (WHO GRADE I)

General

Although this tumor is not strictly neuronal in origin, instead deriving from neuroendocrine epithelium, it is discussed here among truly neuronal and glioneuronal tumors.

Clinical Context

The filum terminale, conus medullaris, and nerves of the cauda equina produce paragangliomas similar to those seen in other parts of the body, such as the carotid body. Most cases arise within the filum terminale, cauda equina, and conus medullaris, all of which are at the levels of vertebrae L1 to L3. Because of overlap (the filum terminale is part of the cauda equina) and vagueness in terminology ("lumbar region"), it is difficult to determine exactly which structure is affected in many reports. Spinal paragangliomas occur mostly in adults, with a mean age of about 46 years, and show a male predominance of about 1.5:1 (117). Lower back pain is the most common presenting complaint, often occurring with sciatica over the course of several months before diagnosis. The primary treatment for spinal paraganglioma is surgical excision, which is effective for long-term cure in almost all cases with complete removal, and in most cases with incomplete resection. Adjuvant chemotherapy and radiation are not generally used. Recurrences usually happen years after initial surgery and are amenable to reexcision.

HISTOPATHOLOGY. H&E-stained sections show a solid tumor with a monomorphic cell population that is arranged in clusters (*Zellballen*) separated by an extensive network of small delicate vascular channels (Figure 7-35). The dominant tumor cells, the chief cells, are generally polygonal, round, or somewhat columnar with a moderate amount of cytoplasm and monotonous nuclei with finely granular chromatin and inconspicuous nucleoli. The cytoplasm is most often lightly eosinophilic with very fine granular particles. Occasional cells may be clear. A smaller, more-subtle population of spindle-shaped and stellate sustentacular cells is scattered individually around the edges of the *Zellballen*. Mitoses and necroses are not seen. Mature ganglion cells are commonly seen in spinal

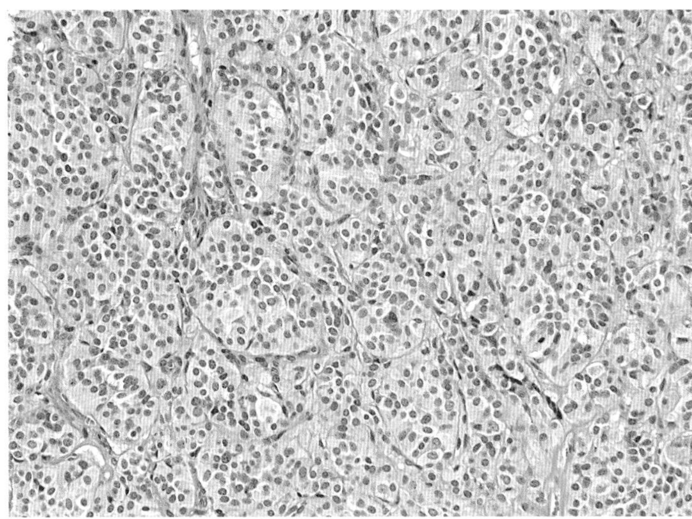

FIGURE 7-35 The nested *Zellballen* pattern of spinal paraganglioma is similar to that of paragangliomas elsewhere.

paragangliomas and, when prominent, have inspired the name "gangliocytic paraganglioma," which is not necessary to mention in the diagnostic line, but may be appropriate for a comment.

The chief cells of spinal paragangliomas stain similarly to paragangliomas elsewhere in the body, showing synaptophysin, chromogranin, and neuron-specific enolase reactivity. Spinal cases are unique in that they also express cytokeratin (Figure 7-36). One should bear this in mind and not

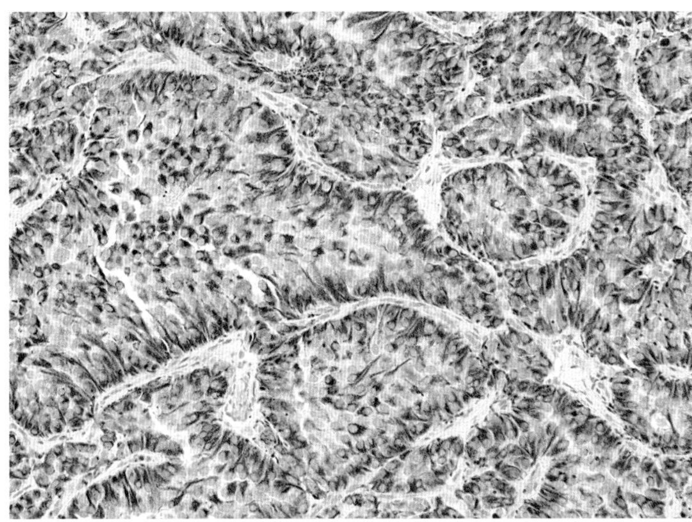

FIGURE 7-36 Strong staining for cytokeratin (AE1/3) is not seen in paragangliomas outside of the spinal cord and should not be mistaken as evidence of metastatic carcinoma.

mistake the cytokeratin staining as evidence of a metastatic carcinoid or carcinoma. The sustentacular cells uniformly show S100 positivity and may also express GFAP. Reticulin staining outlines the circumference of the cellular clusters.

The only entity that is usually considered in the differential with spinal paraganglioma is myxopapillary ependymoma, mostly because of the overlap in location. Histologically, paragangliomas lack mucin production and are overtly epithelioid, whereas myxopapillary ependymomas are fibrillar with readily identifiable mucin in round pools and ensheathing vessels. Well-differentiated metastatic neuroendocrine carcinomas are also within the differential of spinal paraganglioma, at least hypothetically. The low-grade histology and long history of progressive symptoms will almost always separate the two.

REFERENCES

1. Blumcke I, Wiestler OD. Gangliogliomas: an intriguing tumor entity associated with focal epilepsies. *J Neuropathol Exp Neurol*. 2002;61(7):575–584.
2. Hirose T, Scheithauer BW, Lopes MB, et al. Ganglioglioma: an ultrastructural and immunohistochemical study. *Cancer*. 1997;79(5):989–1003.
3. Luyken C, Blumcke I, Fimmers R, et al. Supratentorial gangliogliomas: histopathologic grading and tumor recurrence in 184 patients with a median follow-up of 8 years. *Cancer*. 2004;101(1):146–155.
4. Wolf HK, Muller MB, Spanle M, et al. Ganglioglioma: a detailed histopathological and immunohistochemical analysis of 61 cases. *Acta Neuropathol (Berl)*. 1994;88(2):166–173.
5. Zentner J, Wolf HK, Ostertun B, et al. Gangliogliomas: clinical, radiological, and histopathological findings in 51 patients. *J Neurol Neurosurg Psychiatry*. 1994;57(12): 1497–1502.
6. Zanello M, Pages M, Tauziede-Espariat A, et al. Clinical, imaging, histopathological and molecular characterization of anaplastic ganglioglioma. *J Neuropathol Exp Neurol*. 2016;75(10):971–980.
7. Puget S, Alshehri A, Beccaria K, et al. Pediatric infratentorial ganglioglioma. *Child's Nerv Syst*. 2015;31(10):1707–1716.
8. Donson AM, Kleinschmidt-DeMasters BK, Aisner DL, et al. Pediatric brainstem gangliogliomas show BRAF(V600E) mutation in a high percentage of cases. *Brain Pathol*. 2014;24(2):173–183.
9. Gessi M, Dorner E, Dreschmann V, et al. Intramedullary gangliogliomas: histopathologic and molecular features of 25 cases. *Hum Pathol*. 2016;49:107–113.
10. Prayson RA, Khajavi K, Comair YG. Cortical architectural abnormalities and MIB1 immunoreactivity in gangliogliomas: a study of 60 patients with intracranial tumors. *J Neuropathol Exp Neurol*. 1995;54(4):513–520.
11. Johnson JH, Jr, Hariharan S, Berman J, et al. Clinical outcome of pediatric gangliogliomas: ninety-nine cases over 20 years. *Pediatr Neurosurg*. 1997;27(4):203–207.
12. Zhang D, Henning TD, Zou LG, et al. Intracranial ganglioglioma: clinicopathological and MRI findings in 16 patients. *Clin Radiol*. 2008;63(1):80–91.
13. Terrier LM, Bauchet L, Rigau V, et al. Natural course and prognosis of anaplastic gangliogliomas: a multicenter retrospective study of 43 cases from the French Brain Tumor Database. *Neuro Oncol*. 2017;19(5):678–688.

14. Rush S, Foreman N, Liu A. Brainstem ganglioglioma successfully treated with vemurafenib. *J Clin Oncol.* 2013;31(10):e159–e160.
15. Aguilera D, Janss A, Mazewski C, et al. Successful retreatment of a child with a refractory brainstem ganglioglioma with vemurafenib. *Pediatr Blood Cancer.* 2016;63(3): 541–543.
16. Miller DC, Lang FF, Epstein FJ. Central nervous system gangliogliomas. Part 1: pathology. *J Neurosurg.* 1993;79(6):859–866.
17. Koelsche C, Wohrer A, Jeibmann A, et al. Mutant BRAF V600E protein in ganglioglioma is predominantly expressed by neuronal tumor cells. *Acta Neuropathol (Berl).* 2013; 125(6):891–900.
18. Blumcke I, Giencke K, Wardelmann E, et al. The CD34 epitope is expressed in neoplastic and malformative lesions associated with chronic, focal epilepsies. *Acta Neuropathol (Berl).* 1999;97(5):481–490.
19. Louis DN, Ohgaki H, Wiestler OD, et al., eds. WHO Classification of Tumours of the Central Nervous System. 4th ed. Lyon, France: IARC Press; 2016.
20. Chappe C, Padovani L, Scavarda D, et al. Dysembryoplastic neuroepithelial tumors share with pleomorphic xanthoastrocytomas and gangliogliomas BRAF(V600E) mutation and expression. *Brain Pathol.* 2013;23(5):574–583.
21. Schindler G, Capper D, Meyer J, et al. Analysis of BRAF V600E mutation in 1,320 nervous system tumors reveals high mutation frequencies in pleomorphic xanthoastrocytoma, ganglioglioma and extra-cerebellar pilocytic astrocytoma. *Acta Neuropathol (Berl).* 2011;121(3):397–405.
22. Hoischen A, Ehrler M, Fassunke J, et al. Comprehensive characterization of genomic aberrations in gangliogliomas by CGH, array-based CGH and interphase FISH. *Brain Pathol.* 2008;18(3):326–337.
23. Prayson RA, Napekoski KM. Composite ganglioglioma/dysembryoplastic neuroepithelial tumor: a clinicopathologic study of 8 cases. *Hum Pathol.* 2012;43(7):1113–1118.
24. Daumas-Duport C, Scheithauer BW, Chodkiewicz JP, et al. Dysembryoplastic neuroepithelial tumor: a surgically curable tumor of young patients with intractable partial seizures. Report of thirty-nine cases. *Neurosurgery.* 1988;23(5):545–556.
25. Bilginer B, Yalnizoglu D, Soylemezoglu F, et al. Surgery for epilepsy in children with dysembryoplastic neuroepithelial tumor: clinical spectrum, seizure outcome, neuroradiology, and pathology. *Child's Nerv Syst.* 2009;25(4):485–491.
26. Chan CH, Bittar RG, Davis GA, et al. Long-term seizure outcome following surgery for dysembryoplastic neuroepithelial tumor. *J Neurosurg.* 2006;104(1):62–69.
27. Honavar M, Janota I, Polkey CE. Histological heterogeneity of dysembryoplastic neuroepithelial tumour: identification and differential diagnosis in a series of 74 cases. *Histopathology.* 1999;34(4):342–356.
28. Campos AR, Clusmann H, von Lehe M, et al. Simple and complex dysembryoplastic neuroepithelial tumors (DNT) variants: clinical profile, MRI, and histopathology. *Neuroradiology.* 2009;51(7):433–443.
29. Altinörs N, Calisaneller T, Gül en S, et al. Intraventricular dysembryoplastic neuroepithelial tumor: case report. *Neurosurgery.* 2007;61(6):E1332–E1333; discussion E1333.
30. Baisden BL, Brat DJ, Melhem ER, et al. Dysembryoplastic neuroepithelial tumor-like neoplasm of the septum pellucidum: a lesion often misdiagnosed as glioma: report of 10 cases. *Am J Surg Pathol.* 2001;25(4):494–499.
31. Fujimoto K, Ohnishi H, Tsujimoto M, et al. Dysembryoplastic neuroepithelial tumor of the cerebellum and brainstem. Case report. *J Neurosurg.* 2000;93(3):487–489.
32. Kuchelmeister K, Demirel T, Schlorer E, et al. Dysembryoplastic neuroepithelial tumour of the cerebellum. *Acta Neuropathol (Berl).* 1995;89(4):385–390.

33. Gessi M, Hattingen E, Dorner E, et al. Dysembryoplastic neuroepithelial tumor of the septum pellucidum and the supratentorial midline: histopathologic, neuroradiologic, and molecular features of 7 cases. *Am J Surg Pathol.* 2016;40(6):806–811.
34. Stanescu Cosson R, Varlet P, Beuvon F, et al. Dysembryoplastic neuroepithelial tumors: CT, MR findings and imaging follow-up: a study of 53 cases. *J Neuroradiol.* 2001; 28(4):230–240.
35. Thom M, Toma A, An S, et al. One hundred and one dysembryoplastic neuroepithelial tumors: an adult epilepsy series with immunohistochemical, molecular genetic, and clinical correlations and a review of the literature. *J Neuropathol Exp Neurol.* 2011; 70(10):859–878.
36. Daumas-Duport C, Varlet P, Bacha S, et al. Dysembryoplastic neuroepithelial tumors: nonspecific histological forms – a study of 40 cases. *J Neurooncol.* 1999;41(3):267–280.
37. Daumas-Duport C. Dysembryoplastic neuroepithelial tumours. *Brain Pathol.* 1993; 3(3):283–295.
38. Takahashi A, Hong SC, Seo DW, et al. Frequent association of cortical dysplasia in dysembryoplastic neuroepithelial tumor treated by epilepsy surgery. *Surg Neurol.* 2005; 64(5):419–427.
39. Hirose T, Scheithauer BW, Lopes MB, et al. Dysembryoplastic neuroeptihelial tumor (DNT): an immunohistochemical and ultrastructural study. *J Neuropathol Exp Neurol.* 1994;53(2):184–195.
40. Prayson RA, Morris HH, Estes ML, et al. Dysembryoplastic neuroepithelial tumor: a clinicopathologic and immunohistochemical study of 11 tumors including MIB1 immunoreactivity. *Clin Neuropathol.* 1996;15(1):47–53.
41. Rivera B, Gayden T, Carrot-Zhang J, et al. Germline and somatic FGFR1 abnormalities in dysembryoplastic neuroepithelial tumors. *Acta Neuropathol (Berl).* 2016;131(6):847–863.
42. Lee D, Cho YH, Kang SY, et al. BRAF V600E mutations are frequent in dysembryoplastic neuroepithelial tumors and subependymal giant cell astrocytomas. *J Surg Oncol.* 2015;111(3):359–364.
43. Fina F, Barets D, Colin C, et al. Droplet digital PCR is a powerful technique to demonstrate frequent FGFR1 duplication in dysembryoplastic neuroepithelial tumors. *Oncotarget.* 2017;8(2):2104–2113.
44. Huse JT, Snuderl M, Jones DT, et al. Polymorphous low-grade neuroepithelial tumor of the young (PLNTY): an epileptogenic neoplasm with oligodendroglioma-like components, aberrant CD34 expression, and genetic alterations involving the MAP kinase pathway. *Acta Neuropathol (Berl).* 2017;133(3):417–429.
45. Qaddoumi I, Orisme W, Wen J, et al. Genetic alterations in uncommon low-grade neuroepithelial tumors: BRAF, FGFR1, and MYB mutations occur at high frequency and align with morphology. *Acta Neuropathol (Berl).* 2016;131(6):833–845.
46. Zhang J, Wu G, Miller CP, et al. Whole-genome sequencing identifies genetic alterations in pediatric low-grade gliomas. *Nat Genet.* 2013;45(6):602–612.
47. Hassoun J, Soylemezoglu F, Gambarelli D, et al. Central neurocytoma: a synopsis of clinical and histological features. *Brain Pathol.* 1993;3(3):297–306.
48. Soylemezoglu F, Scheithauer BW, Esteve J, et al. Atypical central neurocytoma. *J Neuropathol Exp Neurol.* 1997;56(5):551–556.
49. von Deimling A, Janzer R, Kleihues P, et al. Patterns of differentiation in central neurocytoma. An immunohistochemical study of eleven biopsies. *Acta Neuropathol.* 1990; 79(5):473–479.
50. Zhang D, Wen L, Henning TD, et al. Central neurocytoma: clinical, pathological and neuroradiological findings. *Clin Radiol.* 2006;61(4):348–357.
51. Donoho D, Zada G. Imaging of central neurocytomas. *Neurosurg Clin N Am.* 2015; 26(1):11–19.

52. Vasiljevic A, Francois P, Loundou A, et al. Prognostic factors in central neurocytomas: a multicenter study of 71 cases. *Am J Surg Pathol.* 2012;36(2):220–227.
53. Rades D, Schild SE. Treatment recommendations for the various subgroups of neurocytomas. *J Neurooncol.* 2006;77(3):305–309.
54. Sweiss FB, Lee M, Sherman JH. Extraventricular neurocytomas. *Neurosurg Clin N Am.* 2015;26(1):99–104.
55. Vyberg M, Ulhoi BP, Teglbjaerg PS. Neuronal features of oligodendrogliomas–an ultrastructural and immunohistochemical study. *Histopathology.* 2007;50(7):887–896.
56. Preusser M, Laggner U, Haberler C, et al. Comparative analysis of NeuN immunoreactivity in primary brain tumours: conclusions for rational use in diagnostic histopathology. *Histopathology.* 2006;48(4):438–444.
57. Ishiuchi S, Tamura M. Central neurocytoma: an immunohistochemical, ultrastructural and cell culture study. *Acta Neuropathol (Berl).* 1997;94(5):425–435.
58. Perry A, Scheithauer BW, Macaulay RJ, et al. Oligodendrogliomas with neurocytic differentiation. A report of 4 cases with diagnostic and histogenetic implications. *J Neuropathol Exp Neurol.* 2002;61(11):947–955.
59. Rodriguez FJ, Mota RA, Scheithauer BW, et al. Interphase cytogenetics for 1p19q and t(1;19)(q10;p10) may distinguish prognostically relevant subgroups in extraventricular neurocytoma. *Brain Pathol.* 2009;19(4):623–629.
60. Imber BS, Braunstein SE, Wu FY, et al. Clinical outcome and prognostic factors for central neurocytoma: twenty year institutional experience. *J Neurooncol.* 2016;126(1): 193–200.
61. Brat DJ, Scheithauer BW, Eberhart CG, et al. Extraventricular neurocytomas: pathologic features and clinical outcome. *Am J Surg Pathol.* 2001;25(10):1252–1260.
62. Zhou XP, Marsh DJ, Morrison CD, et al. Germline inactivation of PTEN and dysregulation of the phosphoinositol-3-kinase/Akt pathway cause human Lhermitte-Duclos disease in adults. *Am J Hum Genet.* 2003;73(5):1191–1198.
63. Colby S, Yehia L, Niazi F, et al. Exome sequencing reveals germline gain-of-function EGFR mutation in an adult with Lhermitte-Duclos disease. *Cold Spring Harb Mol Case Stud.* 2016;2(6):a001230.
64. Abel TW, Baker SJ, Fraser MM, et al. Lhermitte-Duclos disease: a report of 31 cases with immunohistochemical analysis of the PTEN/AKT/mTOR pathway. *J Neuropathol Exp Neurol.* 2005;64(4):341–349.
65. Klisch J, Juengling F, Spreer J, et al. Lhermitte-Duclos disease: assessment with MR imaging, positron emission tomography, single-photon emission CT, and MR spectroscopy. *AJNR Am J Neuroradiol.* 2001;22(5):824–830.
66. Douglas-Akinwande AC, Payner TD, Hattab EM. Medulloblastoma mimicking Lhermitte-Duclos disease on MRI and CT. *Clin Neurol Neurosurg.* 2009;111(6):536–539.
67. Lok C, Viseux V, Avril MF, et al. Brain magnetic resonance imaging in patients with Cowden syndrome. *Medicine (Baltimore).* 2005;84(2):129–136.
68. Hair LS, Symmans F, Powers JM, et al. Immunohistochemistry and proliferative activity in Lhermitte-Duclos disease. *Acta Neuropathol (Berl).* 1992;84(5):570–573.
69. Hashimoto H, Iida J, Masui K, et al. Recurrent Lhermitte-Duclos disease–case report. *Neurol Med Chir (Tokyo).* 1997;37(9):692–696.
70. Inoue T, Nishimura S, Hayashi N, et al. Ectopic recurrence of dysplastic gangliocytoma of the cerebellum (Lhermitte-Duclos disease): a case report. *Brain Tumor Pathol.* 2007;24(1):25–29.
71. VandenBerg SR. Desmoplastic infantile ganglioglioma and desmoplastic cerebral astrocytoma of infancy. *Brain Pathol.* 1993;3(3):275–281.
72. VandenBerg SR, May EE, Rubinstein LJ, et al. Desmoplastic supratentorial neuroepithelial tumors of infancy with divergent differentiation potential ("desmoplastic infantile

gangliogliomas"). Report on 11 cases of a distinctive embryonal tumor with favorable prognosis. *J Neurosurg.* 1987;66(1):58–71.

73. Per H, Kontas O, Kumandas S, et al. A report of a desmoplastic non-infantile ganglioglioma in a 6-year-old boy with review of the literature. *Neurosurg Rev.* 2009;32(3): 369–374; discussion 374.
74. Qaddoumi I, Ceppa EP, Mansour A, et al. Desmoplastic noninfantile ganglioglioma: report of a case. *Pediatr Develop Pathol.* 2006;9(6):462–467.
75. Pommepuy I, Delage-Corre M, Moreau JJ, et al. A report of a desmoplastic ganglioglioma in a 12-year-old girl with review of the literature. *J Neurooncol.* 2006;76(3):271–275.
76. Trehan G, Bruge H, Vinchon M, et al. MR imaging in the diagnosis of desmoplastic infantile tumor: retrospective study of six cases. *AJNR Am J Neuroradiol.* 2004;25(6): 1028–1033.
77. Bachli H, Avoledo P, Gratzl O, et al. Therapeutic strategies and management of desmoplastic infantile ganglioglioma: two case reports and literature overview. *Childs Nerv Syst.* 2003;19(5–6):359–366.
78. Hoving EW, Kros JM, Groninger E, et al. Desmoplastic infantile ganglioglioma with a malignant course. *J Neurosurg Pediatr.* 2008;1(1):95–98.
79. Bianchi F, Tamburrini G, Massimi L, et al. Supratentorial tumors typical of the infantile age: desmoplastic infantile ganglioglioma (DIG) and astrocytoma (DIA). A review. *Childs Nerv Syst.* 2016;32(10):1833–1838.
80. Kros JM, Delwel EJ, de Jong TH, et al. Desmoplastic infantile astrocytoma and ganglioglioma: a search for genomic characteristics. *Acta Neuropathol (Berl).* 2002;104(2): 144–148.
81. Rout P, Santosh V, Mahadevan A, et al. Desmoplastic infantile ganglioglioma–clinicopathological and immunohistochemical study of four cases. *Childs Nerv Syst.* 2002; 18(9–10):463–467.
82. Brat DJ, Shehata BM, Castellano-Sanchez AA, et al. Congenital glioblastoma: a clinicopathologic and genetic analysis. *Brain Pathol.* 2007;17(3):276–281.
83. Suri V, Das P, Pathak P, et al. Pediatric glioblastomas: a histopathological and molecular genetic study. *Neurooncol.* 2009;11(3):274–280.
84. Schniederjan MJ, Alghamdi S, Castellano-Sanchez A, et al. Diffuse leptomeningeal neuroepithelial tumor: 9 pediatric cases with chromosome 1p/19q deletion status and IDH1 (R132H) immunohistochemistry. *Am J Surg Pathol.* 2013;37(5):763–771.
85. Rodriguez FJ, Schniederjan MJ, Nicolaides T, et al. High rate of concurrent BRAF-KIAA1549 gene fusion and 1p deletion in disseminated oligodendroglioma-like leptomeningeal neoplasms (DOLN). *Acta Neuropathol (Berl).* 2015;129(4):609–610.
86. Dodgshun AJ, SantaCruz N, Hwang J, et al. Disseminated glioneuronal tumors occurring in childhood: treatment outcomes and BRAF alterations including V600E mutation. *J Neurooncol.* 2016;128(2):293–302.
87. Rodriguez FJ, Perry A, Rosenblum MK, et al. Disseminated oligodendroglial-like leptomeningeal tumor of childhood: a distinctive clinicopathologic entity. *Acta Neuropathol (Berl).* 2012;124(5):627–641.
88. Rossi S, Rodriguez FJ, Mota RA, et al. Primary leptomeningeal oligodendroglioma with documented progression to anaplasia and t(1;19)(q10;p10) in a child. *Acta Neuropathol (Berl).* 2009;118(4):575–577.
89. Barnes NP, Pollock JR, Harding B, et al. Papillary glioneuronal tumour in a 4-year-old. *Pediatr Neurosurg.* 2002;36(5):266–270.
90. Tsukayama C, Arakawa Y. A papillary glioneuronal tumor arising in an elderly woman: a case report. *Brain Tumor Pathol.* 2002;19(1):35–39.
91. Dim DC, Lingamfelter DC, Taboada EM, et al. Papillary glioneuronal tumor: a case report and review of the literature. *Hum Pathol.* 2006;37(7):914–918.

92. Komori T, Scheithauer BW, Anthony DC, et al. Papillary glioneuronal tumor: a new variant of mixed neuronal-glial neoplasm. *Am J Surg Pathol*. 1998;22(10):1171–1183.
93. Javahery RJ, Davidson L, Fangusaro J, et al. Aggressive variant of a papillary glioneuronal tumor. Report of 2 cases. *J Neurosurg Pediatr.* 2009;3(1):46–52.
94. Newton HB, Dalton J, Ray-Chaudhury A, et al. Aggressive papillary glioneuronal tumor: case report and literature review. *Clin Neuropathol*. 2008;27(5):317–324.
95. Bridge JA, Liu XQ, Sumegi J, et al. Identification of a novel, recurrent SLC44A1-PRKCA fusion in papillary glioneuronal tumor. *Brain Pathol*. 2013;23(2):121–128.
96. Pages M, Lacroix L, Tauziede-Espariat A, et al. Papillary glioneuronal tumors: histological and molecular characteristics and diagnostic value of SLC44A1-PRKCA fusion. *Acta Neuropathol Communicat*. 2015;3:85.
97. Nagaishi M, Nobusawa S, Matsumura N, et al. SLC44A1-PRKCA fusion in papillary and rosette-forming glioneuronal tumors. *J Clin Neurosci*. 2016;23:73–75.
98. Anan M, Inoue R, Ishii K, et al. A rosette-forming glioneuronal tumor of the spinal cord: the first case of a rosette-forming glioneuronal tumor originating from the spinal cord. *Hum Pathol*. 2009;40(6):898–901.
99. Scheithauer BW, Silva AI, Ketterling RP, et al. Rosette-forming glioneuronal tumor: report of a chiasmal-optic nerve example in neurofibromatosis type 1: special pathology report. *Neurosurgery*. 2009;64(4):E771–E772; discussion E772.
100. Shah MN, Leonard JR, Perry A. Rosette-forming glioneuronal tumors of the posterior fossa. *J Neurosurg Pediatr*. 2010;5(1):98–103.
101. Komori T, Scheithauer BW, Hirose T. A rosette-forming glioneuronal tumor of the fourth ventricle: infratentorial form of dysembryoplastic neuroepithelial tumor? *Am J Surg Pathol*. 2002;26(5):582–591.
102. Marhold F, Preusser M, Dietrich W, et al. Clinicoradiological features of rosette-forming glioneuronal tumor (RGNT) of the fourth ventricle: report of four cases and literature review. *J Neurooncol*. 2008;90(3):301–308.
103. Zhang J, Babu R, McLendon RE, et al. A comprehensive analysis of 41 patients with rosette-forming glioneuronal tumors of the fourth ventricle. *J Clin Neurosci*. 2013;20(3): 335–341.
104. Ellezam B, Theeler BJ, Luthra R, et al. Recurrent PIK3CA mutations in rosette-forming glioneuronal tumor. *Acta Neuropathol (Berl)*. 2012;123(2):285–287.
105. Gessi M, Moneim YA, Hammes J, et al. FGFR1 mutations in Rosette-forming glioneuronal tumors of the fourth ventricle. *J Neuropathol Exp Neurol*. 2014;73(6):580–584.
106. Gessi M, Lambert SR, Lauriola L, et al. Absence of KIAA1549-BRAF fusion in rosette-forming glioneuronal tumors of the fourth ventricle (RGNT). *J Neurooncol*. 2012;110(1):21–25.
107. Aker FV, Ozkara S, Eren P, et al. Cerebellar liponeurocytoma/lipidized medulloblastoma. *J Neurooncol*. 2005;71(1):53–59.
108. Hortobagyi T, Bodi I, Lantos PL. Adult cerebellar liponeurocytoma with predominant pilocytic pattern and myoid differentiation. *Neuropathol Appl Neurobiol*. 2007;33(1): 121–125.
109. Pasquale G, Maria BA, Vania P, et al. Cerebellar liponeurocytoma: an updated follow-up of a case presenting histopathological and clinically aggressive features. *Neurol India*. 2009;57(2):194–196.
110. Patel N, Fallah A, Provias J, et al. Cerebellar liponeurocytoma. *Can J Surg*. 2009;52(4): E117–E119.
111. Tatke M, Singh AK. Cerebellar liponeurocytoma–a case report. *Indian J Pathol Microbiol*. 2005;48(1):29–31.
112. Nishimoto T, Kaya B. Cerebellar liponeurocytoma. *Arch Pathol Lab Med*. 2012;136(8): 965–969.

113. Kuchelmeister K, Nestler U, Siekmann R, et al. Liponeurocytoma of the left lateral ventricle–case report and review of the literature. *Clin Neuropathol.* 2006;25(2):86–94.
114. Alkadhi H, Keller M, Brandner S, et al. Neuroimaging of cerebellar liponeurocytoma. Case report. *J Neurosurg.* 2001;95(2):324–331.
115. Horstmann S, Perry A, Reifenberger G, et al. Genetic and expression profiles of cerebellar liponeurocytomas. *Brain Pathol.* 2004;14(3):281–289.
116. Giordana MT, Schiffer P, Boghi A, et al. Medulloblastoma with lipidized cells versus lipomatous medulloblastoma. *Clin Neuropathol.* 2000;19(6):273–277.
117. Gelabert-Gonzalez M. Paragangliomas of the lumbar region. Report of two cases and review of the literature. *J Neurosurg Spine.* 2005;2(3):354–365.

8

SELLAR AND SUPRASELLAR LESIONS

NORMAL PITUITARY

The pituitary resides in the *sella turcica* on the roof of sphenoid sinus, bounded superiorly by an encasing flap of dura (*diaphragma sellae*), over which rest the optic chiasm and the pituitary stalk. The cavernous sinuses, through which run the internal carotid arteries and a third of the cranial nerves, form a sheath of venous blood around the bony walls of the sella.

The main pituitary blood supply originates from the internal carotid arteries and flows first via the superior hypophyseal arteries to the median eminence of the hypothalamus, after which it forms a complex system of vascular channels, the hypophyseal portal system, that flow to the adenohypophysis. These vessels both convey the hypothalamic regulatory hormones to the adenohypophysis and distribute the pituitary hormones to the systemic circulation. Because these channels are under relatively low pressure under normotensive conditions, the anterior pituitary is prone to hypoperfusion and infarction at higher systemic pressures than other organs. The posterior lobe, or neurohypophysis, is perfused by the inferior hypophyseal arteries.

The anterior lobe, or adenohypophysis, develops from an ectodermal invagination (the *Rathke pouch*) of the palate during embryogenesis. The mature gland comprises three major epithelial cell populations (by hematoxylin and eosin [H&E] staining): acidophils, basophils, and chromophobes (Figure 8-1). These color classifications roughly correspond to the hormone produced by the cell, with acidophils producing growth hormone (GH), chromophobes producing prolactin, and basophils producing adrenocorticotropic hormone (ACTH), thyroid-stimulating hormone (TSH) or follicle-stimulating hormone (FSH), and luteinizing hormone (LH). Each cell produces one hormone type, except the gonadotrophs and occasional GH- and prolactin-producing "mammosomatotrophs." Morphologically, the only cells to show a specific identifying feature are the ACTH-secreting corticotrophs, which have a clear, spheroid, cytoplasmic vacuole called an *enigmatic body* (Figure 8-2) (1). Folliculostellate cells form the supporting structure for the epithelial cells and are similar to glia in that they extend numerous thin cytoplasmic processes and are positive

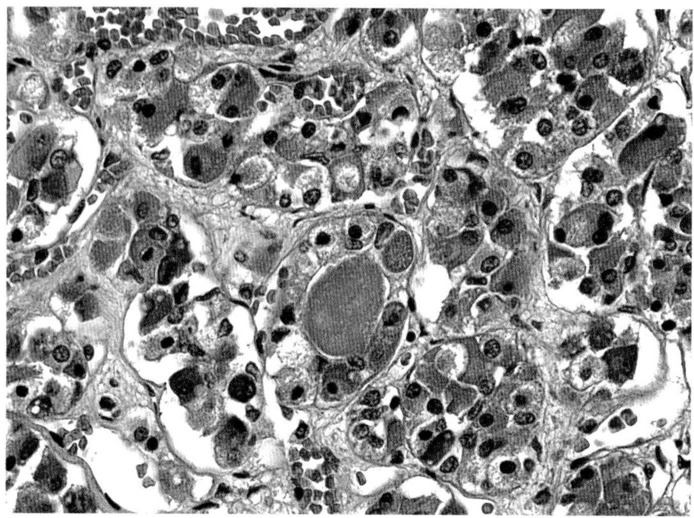

FIGURE 8-1 The normal adenohypophysis contains multiple cell types arranged in small nests, some of which contain hyaline globules.

for S100 and GFAP (2). Some have suggested that folliculostellate cells are fundamentally similar to dendritic cells and may play a role in antigen presentation (3).

The architecture of the adenohypophysis is similar to that of other endocrine organs, with nests of secretory epithelial cells trimmed with

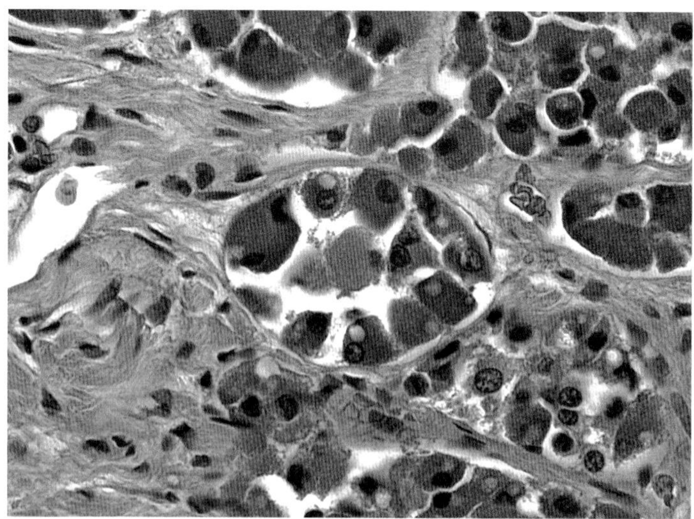

FIGURE 8-2 Basophilic, adrenocorticotropic hormone–secreting cells usually contain an "enigmatic body," a single clear perinuclear vacuole that is not present in adenoma cells.

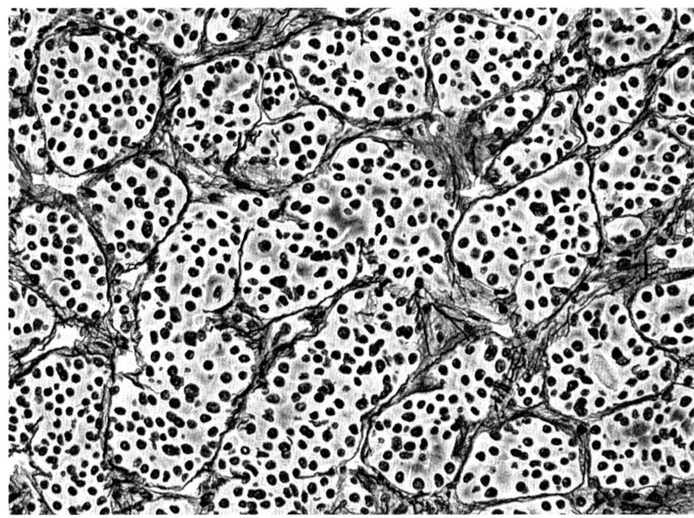

FIGURE 8-3 Reticulin staining accentuates the regular nested architecture of normal adenohypophysis, which is not a characteristic of adenomas.

permeable, thin-walled vascular channels, creating the "organoid" appearance of acinar architecture. Silver staining for reticulin emphasizes the borders of these nests (Figure 8-3), and can be useful in telling normal gland from adenoma, which would lack such a reticulin pattern. Many of the epithelial clusters contain a mixture of cell types, although this can be subtle in areas where one cell type makes up the majority. The cells in compressed adenohypophysis usually lose their distinctive cytoplasmic hues and become much more monotonous, making them appear more similar to adenoma cells.

The anterior lobe is further compartmentalized into areas where specific epithelial cell types predominate, although a mixture of cells is seen in all areas. This concept is important to remember in certain situations, discussed later. The lateral wings of the gland contain mostly acidophils and chromophobes, whereas the central portion, the "mucoid wedge," contains mostly basophils. At the frontier between the mucoid wedge and the neurohypophysis, basophils are normally seen wandering as groups and individuals into the posterior lobe in a phenomenon called "basophilic invasion," an alarming behavior for cells in other organs but innocent in the pituitary (Figure 8-4).

The posterior lobe of the pituitary, or neurohypophysis, is a native resident of the central nervous system, being essentially the swollen terminus for an extension of axons from hypothalamic nuclei. The histologic appearance of the neurohypophysis confirms its neuroepithelial origin and shows several features that distinguish it from other CNS tissues and neuroepithelial neoplasms. Although fibrillar, the overall texture is loose with a degree of condensation around small blood vessels,

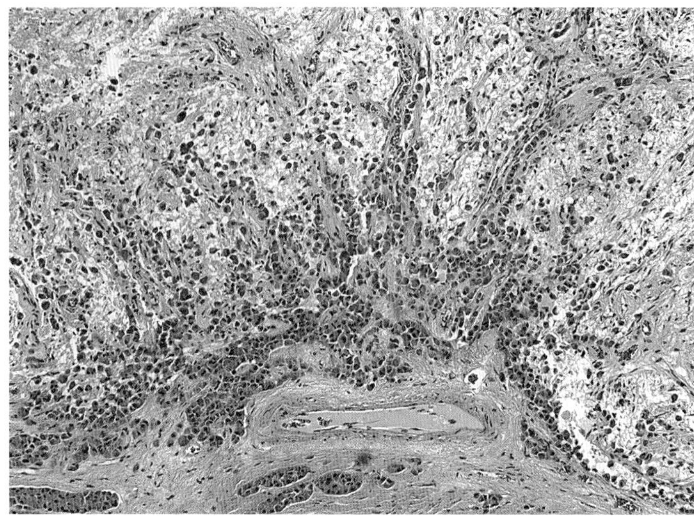

FIGURE 8-4 Basophilic invasion of normal, nonneoplastic corticotrophs into the neurohypophysis, a physiologic finding.

making the vessels appear prominent (Figure 8-5). The ends of the axons form eosinophilic, globose, granular structures called Herring bodies, which contain stores of vasopressin (ADH) and oxytocin. The supporting glial cells, or pituicytes, are conceptually similar to astrocytes and express GFAP and S100.

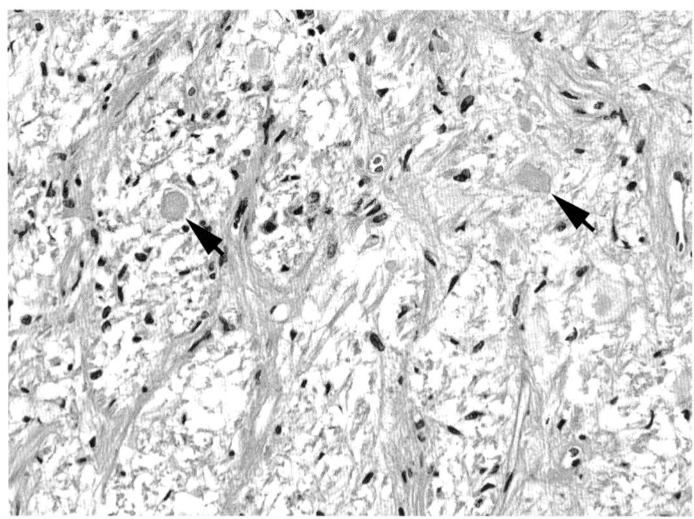

FIGURE 8-5 The neurohypophysis is fibrillar neuroglial tissue with round granular anucleate storage structures called Herring bodies (arrows) and subtle condensation of cellular processes around capillaries.

NONNEOPLASTIC CONDITIONS OF THE PITUITARY AND PARASELLAR AREA

Pituitary Hyperplasia

This condition is a numerical increase in anterior lobe epithelial cells of one or more types. The vast majority of pituitary hyperplasias are secondary, with vanishingly rare examples of primary hyperplasias reported (4). Biopsy of hyperplastic pituitary gland is rare and typically the result of mass effects.

The most common hyperplasia is that of lactotrophs during pregnancy and lactation, where these cells can make up almost three-quarters of the cells in the adenohypophysis and increase the mass of the gland. A mild hyperplasia also occurs due to "stalk effect" in situations where portal blood flow to the adenohypophysis is decreased due to compression of the infundibulum, releasing the lactotrophs from the inhibitory effects of dopamine from the hypothalamus. Dopamine antagonist medications, usually antipsychotics, also elicit this effect.

Hyperplasias of several other cell types are due to lack of feedback inhibition by the products of their target organs. The most common of these is thyrotroph hyperplasia, which occurs in the setting of primary hypothyroidism due to low thyroxine levels and is reversed after institution of hormone replacement therapy (5). Similar phenomena can be seen in corticotrophs among patients with adrenal insufficiency due to Addison disease or adrenalectomy, and in gonadotrophs among patients with primary hypogonadism. Somatotroph hyperplasia is extremely rare and has occurred in cases of ectopic growth-hormone–releasing hormone (GHRH) production by peripheral neuroendocrine neoplasms (6).

HISTOPATHOLOGY. Hyperplasias retain the nested, cytologically and immunohistochemically heterogeneous appearance of normal adenohypophysis, making the distinction from normal gland difficult. Reticulin staining may show expanded acini, but this finding is subjective and should be interpreted in the context of clinical and laboratory data.

Lymphocytic Hypophysitis

CLINICAL CONTEXT. This uncommon autoimmune illness occurs most often in women, although male cases are now thought to account for about 20% to 30% of cases (7). Although the third trimester and postpartum period were initially strongly associated with lymphocytic hypophysitis, a recent large series showed only about 10% of cases were associated with pregnancy (8). Children are rarely affected, and the disease is most common in the fourth decade. Patients present with symptoms similar to those of nonfunctioning pituitary macroadenomas, including headache, visual disturbances, and hypopituitarism. In a majority of cases, the hypopituitarism is hormone restricted, most often affecting ACTH, but reductions in other hormones occur with disease progression. Diabetes insipidus accompanies cases with posterior lobe damage. The inflammation extends into the posterior lobe in about 25% of cases but is limited to the neurohypophysis in only 10% (9).

Because of swelling and mass effects, this lesion is sometimes clinically mistaken for pituitary adenoma, especially when the gland bulges from the sella like a mass. Even when adenoma is not suspected, biopsy and/or decompressive surgery is attempted to confirm the diagnosis and to relieve pressure and prevent infarction, ameliorating headache and visual symptoms but not affecting the endocrine deficits. High-dose glucocorticoids have a dual role in relieving cortisol insufficiency and reducing inflammation. Almost three-quarters of reported cases require long-term hormone replacement (10).

HISTOPATHOLOGY. The characteristic appearance is lymphocytic infiltration of the pituitary, often so floridly as to distort the architecture of the gland and obscure native cells (Figure 8-6). This is in striking contrast to the normal gland, where scattered lymphocytes can be seen in the pars intermedia but do not populate the anterior or posterior lobes. Lymphoid follicles are present in a minority of cases. The lymphocytes are predominantly T cells, evenly split between $CD4^+$ and $CD8^+$ (11). Plasma cells, macrophages, eosinophils, and neutrophils may all appear in smaller numbers. Necrosis is seen in only about 5% of cases (10).

Granulomatous Hypophysitis

Idiopathic granulomatous hypophysis is the other major pattern of primary autoimmune pituitary disease, although it is controversial as to whether it is immunologically similar to lymphocytic hypophysitis (12).

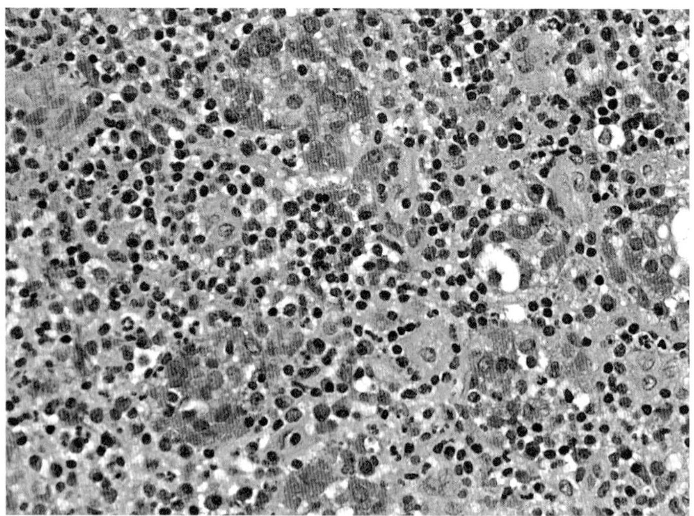

FIGURE 8-6 Lymphocytic hypophysitis can obscure native glandular structures with lymphocytes and plasma cells.

Granulomatous inflammation in the pituitary can also be secondary to a number of other processes, including tuberculosis, sarcoidosis, syphilis, or Rathke cyst rupture, so the idiopathic form is fundamentally a diagnosis of exclusion (13). Women are more affected than men. The patients tend to present with headache and visual disturbance and are treated with either partial excision to relieve mass effect, or excision plus corticosteroid replacement. Histologically, the process is characterized by lymphocytic inflammation with granulomas and usually giant cells. Necrosis, fibrosis, plasma cells and macrophages may also be seen in some cases.

Xanthomatous Hypophysitis

This form of hypophysitis is probably the least common and shares with lymphocytic and granulomatous hypophysitis similar age and sex distributions. At least one reported case evolved from lymphocytic hypophysitis (14). The salient histologic finding in this process is that of lipid-laden macrophages, typically in a milieu of chronic lymphoplasmacytic inflammation. As with granulomatous hypophysitis, there may be an association, possibly even in a majority of cases, with rupture of a Rathke cleft cyst and potential evolution to xanthogranuloma (15).

IgG4-Related Plasma Cell Hypophysitis

Sclerosis associated with IgG4 plasmacytosis, in addition to retroperitoneal fibrosis, autoimmune pancreatitis, and sclerosing sialadenitis, may involve the pituitary gland, where it tends to cause panhypopituitarism and/or central diabetes insipidus (16). Some cases of lymphocytic hypophysitis also have large complements of IgG4-expressing plasma cells, with or without sclerosis, so the boundary between those entities is somewhat amorphous and open to subjective judgment diagnostically. The relevance of the distinction may be insignificant clinically because both are treated with glucocorticoids.

Secondary Hypophysitis

The pituitary can suffer damage from systemic diseases such as sarcoidosis, granulomatosis with polyangiitis, syphilis, Langerhans cell histiocytosis, and tuberculosis. There is an iatrogenic secondary hypophysitis that is associated with administration of immunomodulatory therapy, typically as chemotherapy for malignancy. The strongest association is with the drug ipilimumab, a monoclonal antibody against cytotoxic T-lymphocyte–associated protein 4 (CTLA4), resulting in upregulation of immune response. It is thought the hypophysitis is related to expression of CTLA4 on the adenohypophyseal epithelial cells (17).

Hypothalamic Hamartoma

CLINICAL CONTEXT. The clinical and radiologic presentations of this lesion are so distinct that biopsy is frequently foregone due to the risk of damaging adjacent structures. There are two classic presenting syndromes associated with hypothalamic hamartomas: central precocious puberty and gelastic seizures, sometimes occurring in combination. Gelastic seizures, which are uncontrollable fits of "pressured" laughter, probably originate from activity of the neurons within the lesion (18). Surgical ablation or disconnection of the hamartoma from surrounding tissue can cure or greatly reduce seizure activity. Other successful treatment approaches include stereotactic radiosurgery, radiofrequency ablation, and thermal coagulation.

Hypothalamic hamartoma is a defining feature, along with cutaneous syndactyly of Pallister–Hall syndrome, which occurs in the setting of germline *GLI3* gene mutations (19). Sporadic hypothalamic hamartomas, which constitute the majority, have been shown to have somatic *GLI3* mutations (20) or other defects in the sonic hedgehog pathway (21).

HISTOPATHOLOGY. Small mature granule-type neurons are clustered in a background of granular, gray-matter type neuropil with individual neurons and astroglia at the periphery. The overall visual impression is that of gray matter but without organization or orientation of its elements like what is seen in cortex. Just as with normal gray matter, hypothalamic hamartomas show NeuN and synaptophysin staining in neurons and GFAP in scattered glial cells. Beyond recognizing the atypical appearance of the hamartomatous gray matter, one could potentially assess for sonic hedgehog pathway defects if necessary.

Rathke Cleft Cyst

GENERAL. The Rathke cleft is the plane of fusion between the adenohypophysis and the neurohypophysis created from the migration of the Rathke pouch from the palate and, in humans, contains the vestigial remnants of the intermediate lobe of the pituitary seen in lower animals. Small cystic spaces containing mucoid secretions normally inhabit the cleft, and the cuboidal to columnar cells do not have ciliated epithelium. Because they are lined with respiratory-type epithelium, Rathke cleft cysts fall within the rubric of benign *endodermal cysts*, along with colloid and "enterogenous" cysts (see Chapter 1).

CLINICAL CONTEXT. Most Rathke cleft cysts are asymptomatic and found incidentally on imaging or at autopsy. Women are overrepresented in reported cases, but the overall numbers are too small to draw firm conclusions. Symptomatic cases present with signs and symptoms similar to other sellar lesions, with headaches, visual deficits, and hypopituitarism, mostly in adults and occasionally in children (22,23). Most Rathke cleft cysts arise from the Rathke cleft, yet can be found along the infundibulum and be completely suprasellar (24). Magnetic resonance imaging (MRI) shows them to be T2/FLAIR hypointense relative to brain and of variable intensity on T1-weighted images with a characteristic indentation posteriorly in sagittal images ("ledge sign") (25). The cysts are noncontrast enhancing. Rathke cleft cysts are occasionally seen in collision with other lesions, mostly pituitary adenoma (26–28). A handful of reports have shown granulomatous hypophysitis after rupture of a Rathke cleft cyst (29–31). Hemorrhage into a Rathke cleft cyst can create "machinery oil" contents similar to that seen in adamantinomatous craniopharyngiomas (ACPs), giving the surgeon a strong suspicion for craniopharyngioma.

HISTOPATHOLOGY. A thin layer of epithelial cells surrounds the contents of a Rathke cleft cyst, ranging from one to several layers of columnar or cuboidal cells, often ciliated and showing interspersed goblet cells (Figure 8-7). The epithelium rests on a thin outer wall of paucicellular collagen and can become stretched to a single thin layer by the pressure of cyst contents. A potentially misleading finding is squamous metaplasia, which develops as a layer underneath the original epithelium and eventually can form dry, flaky keratin. The contents are inspissated mucous secretions that range from eosinophilic to amphophilic and are PAS positive with a gross appearance similar to thyroid cyst contents. Some Rathke cleft cysts show xanthogranulomatous degeneration that ranges from aggregates of macrophages to inflamed debris with cholesterol clefts, hemosiderin, and giant cells, similar to that seen in ACPs.

DIFFERENTIAL DIAGNOSIS. Cases with ciliated columnar cells require little consideration, but squamous metaplasia can cause a degree of overlap with epidermoid cysts. Epidermoid cysts, however, have a granular layer within the epithelium, but metaplastic cysts do not. In order to diagnose squamous metaplasia in a Rathke cleft cyst, one *must* observe dry keratin. Thin papillary craniopharyngiomas (PCPs), which do not produce any keratin, may develop inside of, or collide with, Rathke cleft cysts and have a higher potential for recurrence.

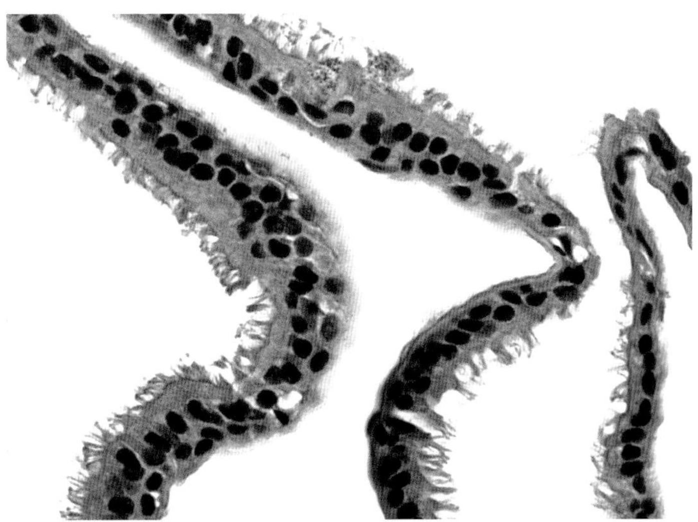

FIGURE 8-7 Rathke cleft cyst lining with ciliated columnar epithelium punctuated by mucin-bearing goblet cells.

Xanthogranuloma of the Sella

GENERAL. Xanthogranuloma, or cholesterol granuloma, of the sella remains a cryptic diagnosis. It is most often used to describe degenerating cellular debris found in and around the sella and occasionally elsewhere. The debris has no identifiable epithelium, yet many believe the findings are secondary to degeneration of other well-established epithelial lesions. Both ACPs and Rathke cleft cysts can develop similar xanthogranulomatous material, as can old hemorrhage or any other collection of degenerating cells. The term xanthogranuloma of the sella is essentially a stopgap used when a biopsy fails to yield a more specific diagnostic entity and indicates a short list of possible causes that should be considered. Whether sellar xanthogranulomas represent a common underlying process, or are a common endpoint for several processes, remains to be demonstrated.

CLINICAL CONTEXT. The defining series examining this lesion suggests that it is a unique and separate process from ACP, although some clinical features overlap. In that series, the peak age of incidence was in the second and third decades, coincident with the first peak of ACP occurrence. However, there was no second peak corresponding to that of ACP occurrence in middle age. Xanthogranulomas occurred around the sella but were more likely than ACP to have an intrasellar component. The most important differences between xanthogranuloma and ACP were that the former had a higher rate of gross total resection and better overall outcome, although the xanthogranuloma patients suffer higher rates of marked endocrine deficits (32). Additional investigation has strengthened the association between sellar xanthogranulomas and Rathke cleft cysts (15,33).

HISTOPATHOLOGY. By definition, all xanthogranulomas show cholesterol clefts with associated histiocytic inflammatory infiltrates (Figure 8-8). They also commonly show lymphoplasmacytic infiltrates, hemosiderin deposition, and granular necrotic debris (32). Minute fragments of squamous or cuboidal epithelium may be present but in such small quantities as to prohibit further classification. Scrupulous examination of deeper levels is warranted to search for potentially diagnostic epithelium.

TUMORS OF THE SELLAR REGION

Pituitary Adenoma (Pituitary Neuroendocrine Tumor)

CLASSIFICATION. If one were to fill two pails, one with pituitary "adenomas" and the other with pituitary "carcinomas," and then pour them into one pile on the floor, there would be no way, using any histopathologic, immunohistochemical, ultrastructural, or even genetic means, that one could confidently sort them back into their respective pails, the difference being a purely ex post facto designation based on demonstration of metastasis. Because pathologic examination cannot predict clinical behavior, and neuroendocrine tumors of other organs have undergone

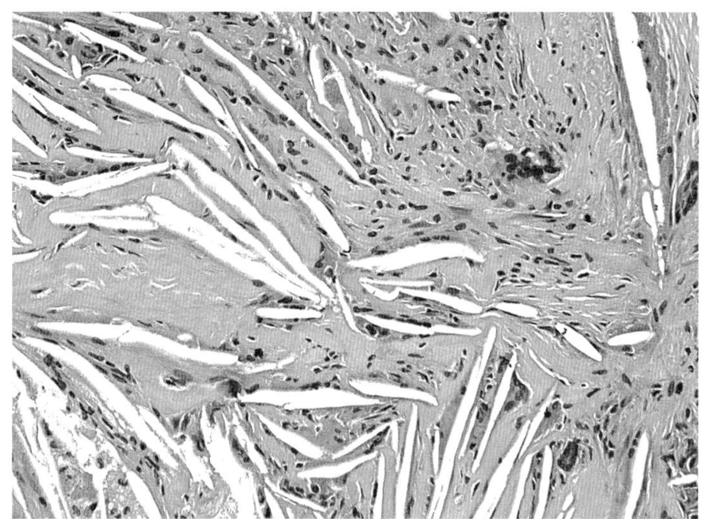

FIGURE 8-8 Xanthogranuloma of the sellar region usually results from degeneration and/or hemorrhage into a Rathke cleft cyst, yet can also result from several other precursor lesions.

similar renaming, the term *pituitary neuroendocrine tumor* (PitNET) has been proposed to represent all tumors arising from the anterior pituitary epithelium. This terminology is not a part of the 2017 WHO endocrine tumor update, but is preferred by the International Pituitary Pathology Club (34). Nevertheless, because the new PitNET terminology is not yet in wide use, the adenoma–carcinoma nomenclature is retained here for the sake of consistency.

Several tools are used to subdivide pituitary adenomas into meaningful groups: imaging, histology, immunohistochemistry, and electron microscopy. Grouping the adenomas by pure H&E morphology into acidophils, basophils, and chromophobes was common practice at one time but is unreliable and obsolete. The most common pathologic classification is based on hormones expressed immunohistochemically, described below. A further refinement is to immunostain for cell lineage groupings. Electron microscopy helps to further split adenoma types but is not practical for most community (and many academic) pathology practices and may be entirely supplanted by immunostaining for arguably its most important role, detecting the more aggressive "silent subtype III" (now *plurihormonal Pit-1 lineage*) adenomas.

DEMOGRAPHICS. Pituitary adenomas account for greater than 10% of all primary intracranial neoplasms in adults, putting them third in overall prevalence after meningeal and diffuse glial tumors. The incidence of adenomas in children is low, but increases with age, with those from 15 to 19 years constituting the majority (35). No clear sex predilection is evident for pituitary adenomas overall. Some variability in population characteristics is observed among the specific subtypes of pituitary adenoma, discussed later. Individuals with type I multiple endocrine neoplasia (MEN1) syndrome develop pituitary adenomas because of their disease, but syndromic tumor characteristics do not seem to substantially differ from those that are sporadic.

CLINICAL PRESENTATION. The clinical presentations of adenomas can be divided into two groups: endocrinologically apparent and anatomically apparent. Hormone-producing tumors typically present with syndromes attributable to excess of the secreted hormone: Cushing disease from ACTH, gigantism or acromegaly from GH, galactorrhea from prolactin (in women of reproductive age), and, rarely, hyperthyroidism from TSH. Adenomas that secrete FSH and LH, and prolactinomas in men and postmenopausal women, do not present with a specific hormonal syndrome, similar to nonsecreting tumors. Without a hormonal syndrome to herald their presence, these clinically silent tumors attain larger sizes and present with effects from anatomic disruption of neighboring structures. In this setting, headache, hypopituitarism, and loss of vision are the most common presentations.

NEUROIMAGING. MRI provides accurate preoperative diagnosis in most cases of pituitary adenoma. The main neuroimaging classification system assesses the extent to which the tumor expands and escapes the sella to invade adjacent structures, separating cases into invasive and noninvasive in five grades (36). A commonly used aspect of this system is that it categorizes by tumor size, those less than 1 cm being *microadenomas* and those greater being *macroadenomas*. "Giant" adenomas exceed 5 cm (37). With high-resolution techniques, microadenomas as small as 2 to 3 mm can be identified. On T1-weighted sequences, adenomas are slightly hypointense to adenohypophysis and do not enhance after-routine contrast administration. If T1-weighted images are taken quickly after contrast, adenomas can show early enhancement that is simultaneous with that of the posterior lobe (38). A small amount of delayed enhancement can also be seen (39).

INVASIVE ADENOMAS. Unlike adenomas occurring in other epithelial organs, pituitary adenomas have a tendency to invade adjacent tissue, specifically dura and bone. Most cases of macroadenoma show at least modest dural invasion if the dura is biopsied and inspected microscopically, with the presence of invasion increasing with tumor size and extension from the sella (40). The significance of this invasion is surprisingly little, with no evidence that it affects recurrence rates in one large series, although it may marginally increase mortality at 6 years (41). Invasion is also not correlated with the cytologic appearance of pituitary adenomas.

EXTRASELLAR ADENOMAS. Ectopic adenomas can occur anywhere from the third ventricle (42) to the nasopharynx (43) but very rarely appear farther abroad. They most likely arise from cellular rests stranded while migrating with Rathke pouch during development. Being immediately subjacent to the floor of the sella, the sphenoid sinus is the most common ectopic site for pituitary adenomas.

PITUITARY APOPLEXY. The term apoplexy (Greek: *apo*—away/from; *plexia*—to strike) originally referred to any precipitous, stroke-like onset of symptoms. In the context of the pituitary, the term is often used to refer to the lesion itself. Pituitary apoplexy is the sudden infarction and/or hemorrhage of a sellar tumor, usually a nonfunctioning pituitary adenoma, heralded by a syndrome of rapid-onset headache, vision problems, and hypopituitarism. Loss of consciousness, coma, and sudden death occur in a minority of cases (44). Emergent neurosurgery to preserve vision is necessary in cases where the lesion compresses the optic chiasm. Rarely, spontaneous infarction of an adenoma causes the lesion to vanish along with its symptoms (45). Incidental focal hemorrhage or necrosis within an adenoma is not unusual and, in the absence of the clinical syndrome, does not constitute apoplexy.

HISTOPATHOLOGY. The two core features that distinguish adenomas from normal pituitary tissue are loss of regular acinar architecture and cellular homogeneity. Most adenomas grow in a uniform sheetlike pattern punctuated by scattered blood vessels (Figure 8-9). Other patterns, including trabecular (Figure 8-10), papillary (Figure 8-11), oncocytic (not shown), fibrotic (Figure 8-12), nested (Figure 8-13), ribboned (Figure 8-14), and spindle cell/fascicular (Figure 8-15), are less common and have no practical significance other than to recognize that they are within the spectrum of morphologic appearance for pituitary adenomas. Papillary and trabecular patterns are associated with gonadotropin expression. The component epithelial cells vary

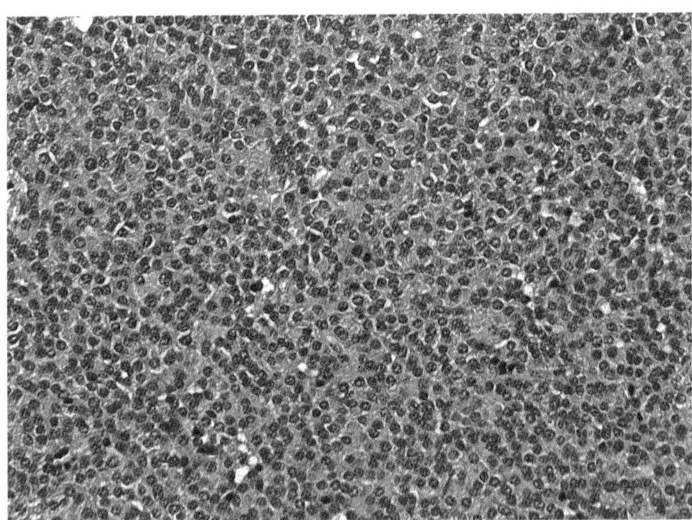

FIGURE 8-9 The typical sheetlike growth pattern of pituitary adenomas separates them from normal adenohypophysis.

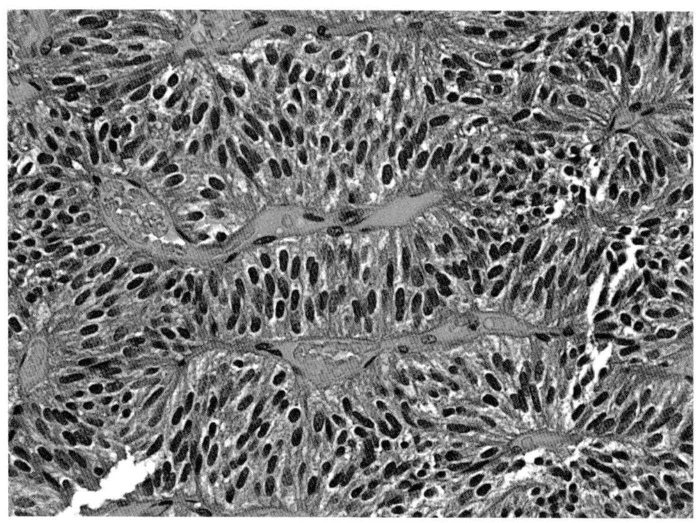

FIGURE 8-10 A distinct trabecular pattern formed by elongate epithelial cells is occasionally seen in gonadotroph adenomas.

from elongate to polygonal and may be organized along blood vessels or haphazard.

The cells of pituitary adenomas are typically small and monotonous with variably granular cytoplasm and mildly eccentric round nuclei that contain clumped, "salt and pepper" chromatin and a generally small nucleolus.

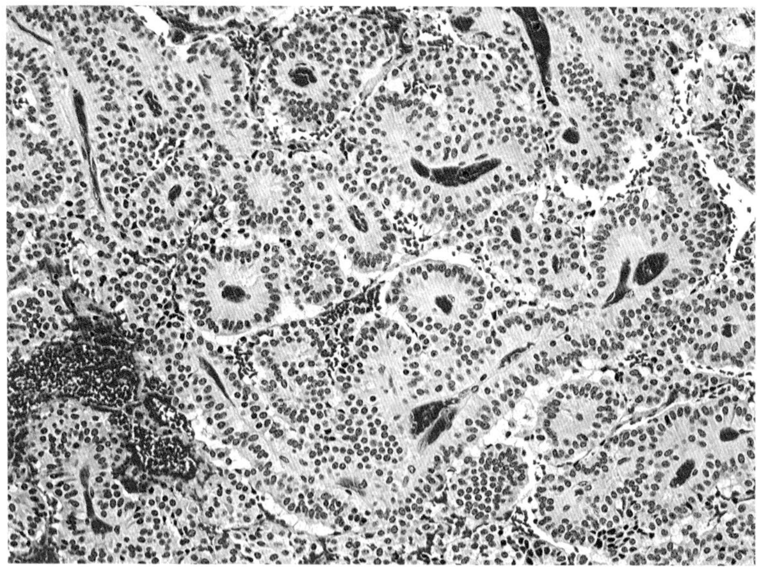

FIGURE 8-11 Papillary and pseudopapillary adenomas are also associated with gonadotropin expression.

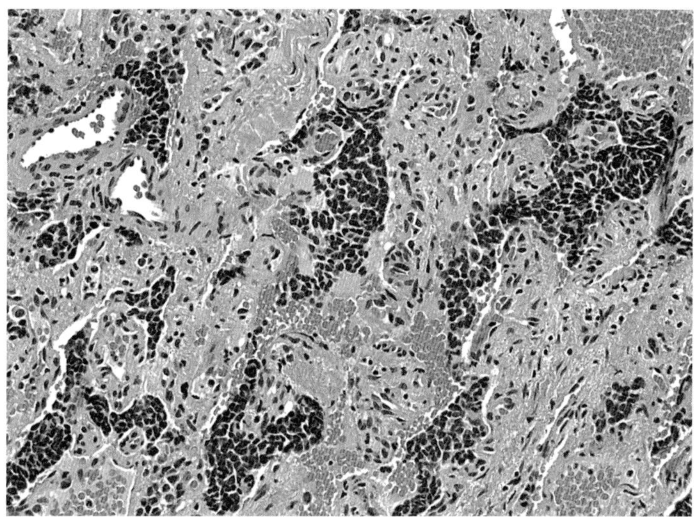

FIGURE 8-12 Dense fibrosis can be extensive and mimic the appearance of compressed peritumoral adenohypophyseal tissue.

Pleomorphism and tumor giant cells may be present but do not indicate tumor behavior necessarily, although plurihormonal Pit-1 lineage adenomas tend to display nuclear pleomorphism and are associated with higher recurrence rates.

INTRAOPERATIVE DIAGNOSIS. Macroadenomas generally present few challenges at the time of frozen section; the surgeon knows the biopsy contains

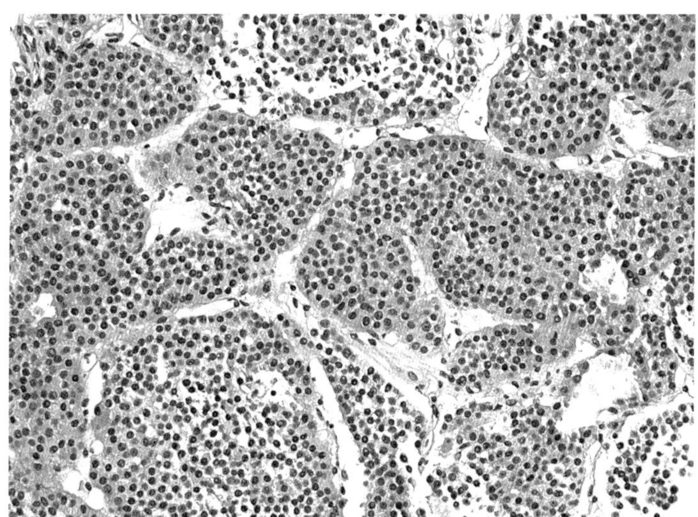

FIGURE 8-13 Nested adenomas can be similar to adenohypophysis but generally have larger and more heterogeneously sized cell clusters.

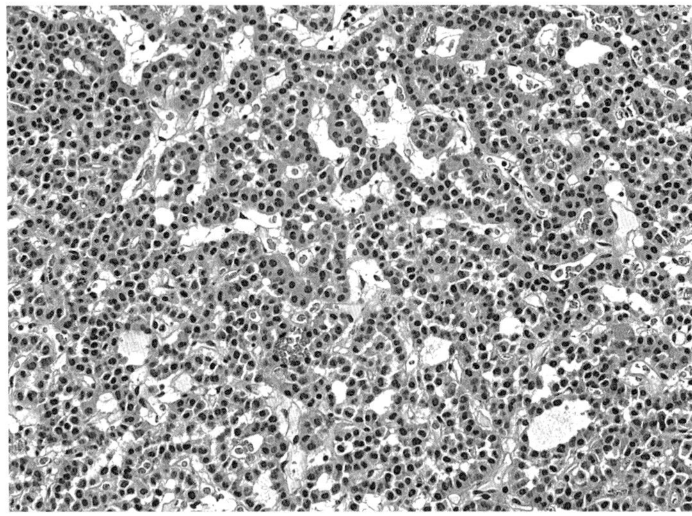

FIGURE 8-14 Ribbons and pseudoglands give a carcinoid-like pattern to some pituitary adenomas.

lesion and the radiologic and gross surgical appearances are almost diagnostic in themselves. Microadenomas, however, because of the often limited tissue and uncertainty of the exact location of the lesion, can produce a series of negative biopsies before the tumor is apprehended. Misidentifying normal pituitary as adenoma can lead to unnecessary repeat operations, while misidentifying adenoma as pituitary may result in oversampling, potentially resulting in permanent hypopituitarism. This situation occurs

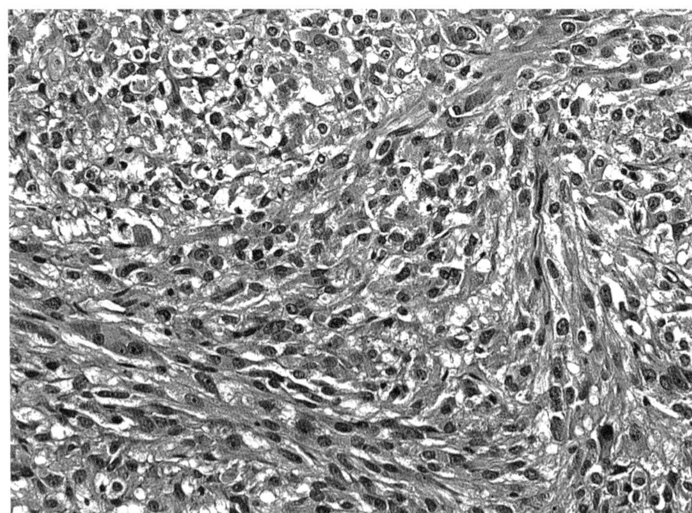

FIGURE 8-15 Rare spindle cell adenomas can form a fascicular architecture but retain the immunohistochemical characteristics of other adenomas.

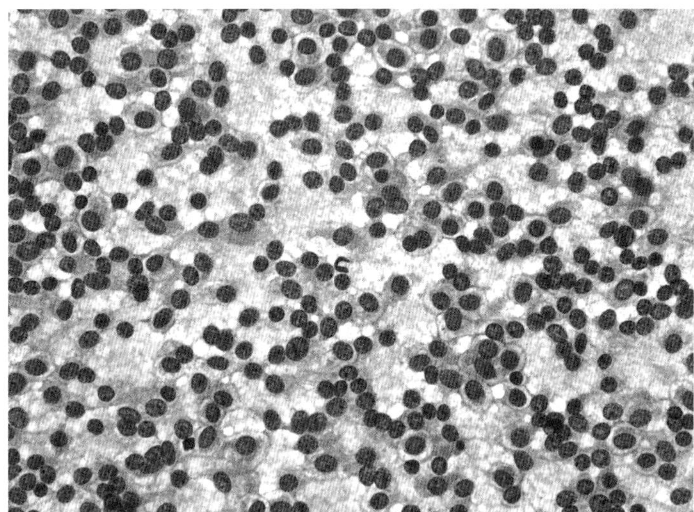

FIGURE 8-16 Gentle blotting of adenomas is sufficient to shed a thick layer of single cells onto a slide, a helpful diagnostic feature during intraoperative consultation.

most often in ACTH-secreting microadenomas, which can cause Cushing disease at only 2-mm diameter. Intraoperative ACTH levels afford an alternative method for determining whether the tumor has been excised.

Frozen sections and touch preparations both yield helpful information during intraoperative consultation. Frozen section is the most effective because it allows assessment of architecture and cellular homogeneity. Care must be taken, though, as nested architecture is seen occasionally in adenomas, and parts of the normal pituitary can have a nearly homogeneous dominance of one cell type. Touch preparations, especially with macroadenomas, can alone be sufficient for diagnosis. Because adenomas lose the cohesion of normal pituitary epithelium, gently blotting the specimen onto a slide spreads a thick coat of individual cells (Figure 8-16), while metastases and nonneoplastic adenohypophysis part with far fewer. Crush preparations, helpful for most other CNS tumor types, damage the fragile adenoma cells and help less.

CLASSIFICATION BY HORMONE IMMUNOSTAINING

NONIMMUNOREACTIVE (NULL CELL). Adenomas that lack secretion or immunohistochemical expression of hormones are one of the most commonly resected types, roughly as numerous as prolactinomas, although that number decreases when lineage markers are assessed (see section Classification by Lineage below). Like other silent adenomas, they attain larger size before diagnosis and are more likely to show invasion. In contrast to other subtypes, null cell adenomas occur more often in those older than 40 years (46).

Most hormonally inert adenomas grow in a sheetlike or sinusoidal pattern and are composed of uniform cells with a small amount of chromophobic cytoplasm. A minority show oncocytic change, with polygonal cells and abundant granular cytoplasm. No difference in behavior has been demonstrated between oncocytic adenomas and other null cell adenomas.

PROLACTIN. Prolactinomas are the most common subtype in autopsy series (47), but, because they can be treated medically, they are less common than gonadotropin-secreting adenomas among surgical specimens (48). The clinical presentation of prolactinomas is sexually dimorphic, with females presenting at younger ages with microadenomas (<1 cm) because they have prolactin-responsive breast and endometrial tissue, whereas males present at older ages with macroadenomas (>1 cm). The clinical syndrome in reproductive age women is galactorrhea and amenorrhea, while men generally present with headache and/or visual problems. Postmenopausal women present similarly to men.

Sheetlike growth of small chromophobic cells is typical in prolactinomas. The vast majority show sparse cytoplasmic granularity, but fewer than 5% of prolactinomas have dense acidophil granularity (48). Medical treatment with dopamine agonists (bromocriptine or cabergoline) alters the morphology by causing marked shrinkage of cytoplasm, condensation of nuclei, and fibrosis (49). The presence of psammoma bodies and amyloid (Figure 8-17) is relatively specific to prolactinomas but is not common.

GROWTH HORMONE. GH-producing adenomas present with gigantism in prepubertal patients, whose bones are still growing, and acromegaly in postpubertal patients. Most lesions are macroadenomas and present in the

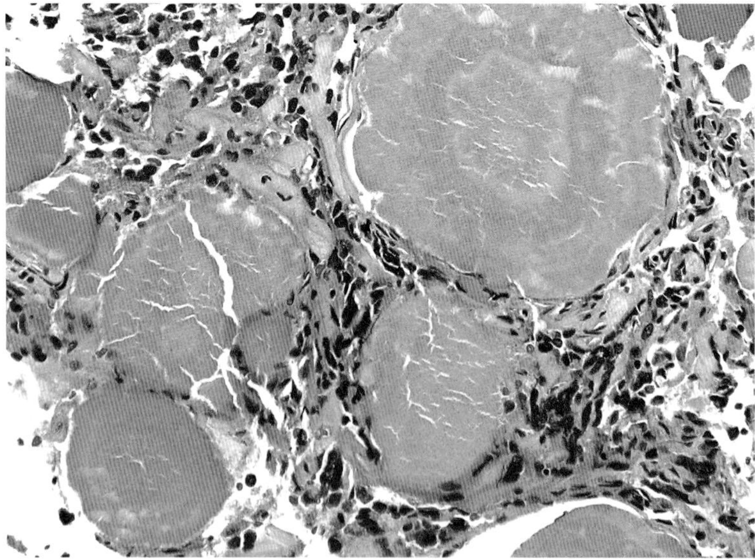

FIGURE 8-17 Amyloid spheroids generally occur in prolactinomas and can become so prominent as to overshadow the original tumor.

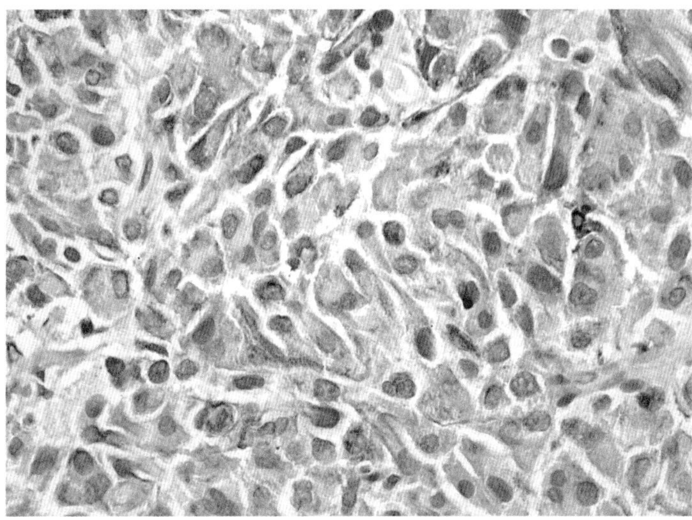

FIGURE 8-18 Densely granular GH-immunoreactive adenomas have a more diffuse cytoplasmic or perinuclear rim of cytokeratin staining.

third through fifth decades. In normal somatotroph cells, the hormone somatostatin causes feedback inhibition of GH production. As with prolactinomas, the inhibition mechanism is intact in GH-adenoma cells and allows some medical treatment of acromegaly with somatostatin analogs. Unlike prolactinomas, medical treatment does not significantly alter the GH adenoma's histologic appearance (50).

Many authors further subcategorize GH-producing lesions into pure somatotroph adenomas and mammosomatotrophs that also secrete prolactin. A third group has two distinct, separate populations of prolactin and GH-secreting cells and are called "acidophil stem cell" adenomas, after the putative progenitor. These categories, while immunohistochemically distinct, have not been shown to differ reliably in clinical behavior.

A distinction that has been shown to predict tumor behavior is that between sparsely granulated and densely granulated patterns. Densely granular GH adenomas resemble normal acidophils, with ample granular eosinophilic cytoplasm, and show diffuse cytoplasmic and perinuclear staining for cytokeratin (Figure 8-18). Sparsely granular adenomas, which have a higher rate of clinical recurrence, have plasmacytoid appearance created by their eccentric nucleus and pale pink "fibrous body." Cytokeratin staining shows dot-like spherical reactivity that highlights the fibrous body (Figure 8-19). Mixed lesions can be seen, and only those with a clear majority of densely granular cells qualify for the densely granular designation (51).

ADRENOCORTICOTROPIC HORMONE. ACTH-secreting adenomas cause Cushing disease by overstimulating the adrenals to produce cortisol, causing truncal obesity, moon facies, abdominal striae, diabetes mellitus, and

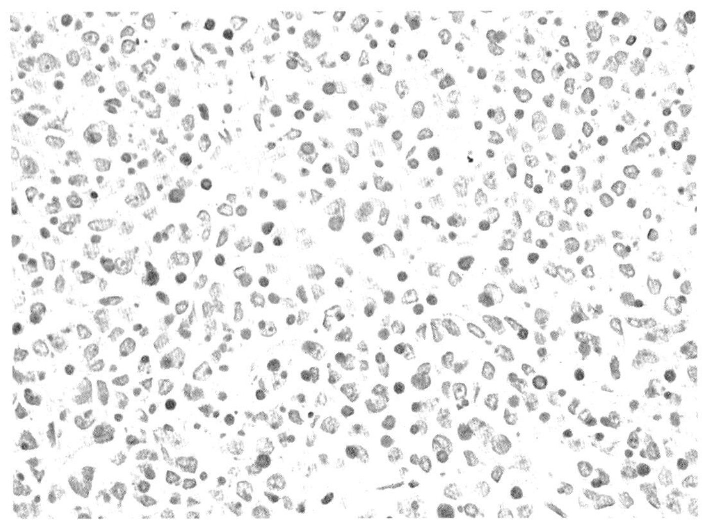

FIGURE 8-19 Sparsely granular GH-immunoreactive adenomas contain discrete perinuclear dots of cytokeratin immunoreactivity.

other effects. Most corticotroph adenomas occur in females between the ages of 30 and 40, with a female preponderance of about 8:1 (52). The vast majority of ACTH adenomas are microadenomas, measuring less than 1 cm. Some adenomas are ACTH positive by immunohistochemistry, yet are clinically silent. They are more often macroadenomas and present with mass effects. Some series have failed to show a difference in recurrence rates for silent corticotroph adenomas, but have suggested that recurrences are more aggressive when they happen, although this conclusion is based on a limited number of cases (53,54).

The cells of corticotroph adenomas are round with basophilic to amphophilic cytoplasmic granules that are intensely PAS positive. Granularity varies, though, and is less often seen in macroadenomas. Again, some authors separate the densely granular and sparsely granular types, but no difference has been demonstrated for this distinction in ACTH adenomas. The nonneoplastic adenohypophysis around ACTH-secreting adenomas often shows "Crooke hyaline change" in corticotroph cells. This appears as a circumferential band of hyaline around the cell edge that is composed of densely deposited cytokeratin filaments (Figure 8-20). Very rarely, the adenoma undergoes hyaline change and is called a Crooke cell adenoma.

GONADOTROPINS. Although they secrete active hormones, gonadotroph adenomas usually present with mass effect and are considered clinically nonfunctioning. The epidemiology of these tumors is incompletely understood, although, oddly, they are the most commonly resected adenoma subtype (48). They generally present as macroadenomas and more often affect men (55,56) than women.

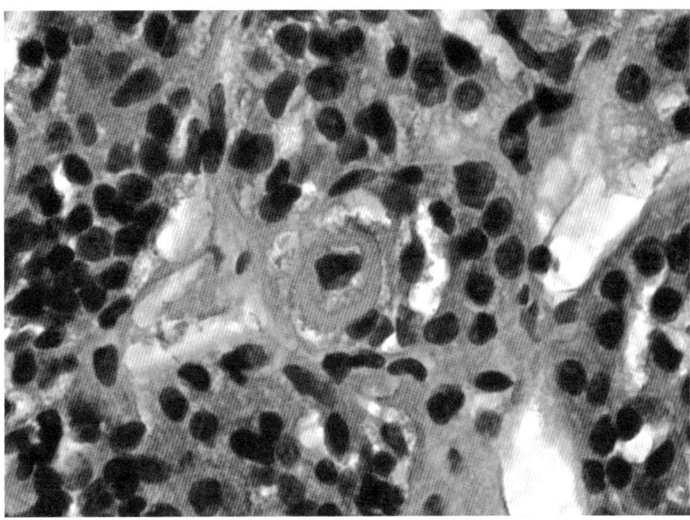

FIGURE 8-20 Crooke hyaline change: The high levels of cortisol in Cushing disease cause normal corticotroph cells to be banded with thick hyaline rims of cytokeratin.

Gonadotroph adenomas sometimes show distinctive architectural and cytologic patterns, either as papillary or trabecular arrangements of elongate cells. The appearance of these tumors can be surprisingly different from other pituitary adenomas but retain the same general immunostaining characteristics (synaptophysin and keratin).

THYROID-STIMULATING HORMONE. Pituitary adenomas rarely stain only for TSH, accounting for only about 1% (57). Patients may present with a Graves disease–like syndrome without ophthalmopathy and dermopathy. Some have clinically "silent" tumors. Most of the reported patients with this tumor are women, by a ratio of about 2:1, and have macroadenomas at diagnosis (57–59).

Histologically, TSH adenomas resemble other adenomas, displaying a solid or sinusoidal growth pattern. The cells are typically chromophobic. Some described cases meet criteria for "atypical adenoma," but this may not predict tumor behavior (58).

PLURIHORMONAL. A small percentage of adenomas express multiple hormones. They are grouped into "mammosomatotroph," acidophil stem cell, and mixed types. The acidophil stem cell type may be more aggressive than other adenomas and is characterized by fibrous bodies (see section Growth Hormone) and cytoplasmic vacuoles (50).

"Silent subtype III" adenomas were once considered to be a subcategory of silent corticotroph adenomas (after types I and II). They are now classified as plurihormonal Pit-1 lineage adenomas (PPLA) (see lineage below). This somewhat inaccurately named macroadenoma is frequently not plurihormonal and sometimes not hormonally silent. Some have suggested the term "poorly differentiated" replace the plurihormonal descriptor because the tumors are always poorly differentiated. PPLAs have the highest rate of recurrence of any adenoma and relatively aggressive course (60), but because diagnosis has been traditionally made by electron microscopy, the acceptance of this category has been limited in practice. More recently, immunostaining for GLG1, a Golgi apparatus protein, has shown promise in identifying PPLAs without electron microscopy (61). GLG-1 staining shows enlarged and irregular Golgi in PPLAs, and a small, round, compact Golgi in others.

CLASSIFICATION BY LINEAGE. Pituitary epithelial cells develop from stem cells in three basic lineages. Cells that produce prolactin, GH, or TSH form one lineage and all express the transcription factor Pit-1, which is thought to mediate their differentiation. Gonadotroph cells, those that produce LH and FSH, are under the control of steroidogenic factor-1 (SF1) and form another lineage. ACTH-producing cells form their own lineage and express T-box transcription factor (Tpit) (62). Incorporating these immunostains into the pathology workup in an algorithmic fashion may allow for more accurate subtyping and reduce the overall number of immunostains performed (62).

"ATYPICAL PITUITARY ADENOMA". A nebulous class of adenomas from the 2004 WHO classification of endocrine tumors based on immunostaining for p53 and MIB1 rates higher than 3%; this distinction has not shown any reliable difference in clinical behavior. Some have found MIB1 labeling indices to predict recurrence (63), but others have not shown this effect in nonfunctioning adenomas (64,65). Staining for p53 is even less consistent than MIB1 in predicting tumor recurrence (63,64). Among tumors with high (>3%) MIB1 staining, extent of surgical resection is the best predictor of recurrence (66). Using the WHO 2004 criteria for atypical adenoma, the results from several large series have been underwhelming with regard to association of atypia with recurrence (67–69). Mercifully, the WHO has not included the category of "atypical adenoma" in the 2017 classification.

IMMUNOHISTOCHEMISTRY. Beyond the expression of their specific hormone types, adenomas show immunostaining profiles similar to those of other neuroendocrine neoplasms, with cytoplasmic reactivity for cytokeratins and synaptophysin. Antibodies for neurofilaments and vimentin also label many adenomas (70).

DIFFERENTIAL DIAGNOSIS. Because pituitary adenomas have great variety in histologic appearance and are by far the most common tumors of the sella, they are best ruled out before considering other diagnostic options (Table 8-1). At the same time, overlap with other entities is enough that one should always stop and question whether another entity could be consistent with the histology under consideration. This is particularly true when pituitary hormone staining is negative. One is well advised to at least order a cytokeratin and synaptophysin and check the clinical history for possible sources of metastasis. Things that overlap the most with pituitary adenoma morphologically include metastatic carcinoma, plasmacytoma,

TABLE 8-1 Sellar and Parasellar Mass Lesions
Pituitary adenoma
Metastasis (usually carcinoma or melanoma)
Lymphoma (usually large B cell)
Plasmacytoma
Meningioma
Craniopharyngioma
Rathke cleft cyst
Pilocytic astrocytoma
Xanthogranuloma
Germinoma (or other germ cell tumor)
Chordoma
Granular cell tumor
Spindle cell oncocytoma
Pituicytoma
Hypophysitis

melanoma, and lymphoma. Immunostaining for the typical markers of those entities can help rule them in or out. Metastatic neuroendocrine tumors will have a similar immunoprofile, but are generally much more proliferative and anaplastic.

Pituitary Carcinoma (Pituitary Neuroendocrine Tumor)

Pituitary carcinomas are rare, with only 12 cases occurring in a series of 7,602 pituitary lesions (48). The term carcinoma can only be applied to adenohypophyseal neoplasms after they have produced metastases, either systemically or through the cerebrospinal fluid. Most cases express hormones, typically prolactin or ACTH, and progress from macroadenomas. Prognosis for these lesions is poor, with 66% mortality within 1 year of diagnosis in one series (71). No known histologic parameters can predict which cases of pituitary adenoma will metastasize, so diagnosis of this entity depends on neuroimaging studies.

Craniopharyngioma (WHO Grade I)

CLINICAL CONTEXT. Most cases of the adamantinomatous pattern occur in children and young adults with a small minority arising in middle-aged adults, whereas the much less common papillary variety is more common in adults. The distribution between the sexes varies by study, and there are no consistent differences. The vast majority of both types arise midline in the suprasellar/hypothalamic area, but some are intrasellar. Areas near the sella, for example, clivus, sphenoid bone, and nasopharynx, harbor an occasional case (72–74). Rare examples have been reported in the pineal region, distant from the parasellar bones and soft tissue (75,76).

Patients present with headache, visual disturbance, cognitive changes, nausea/vomiting, and hormonal changes, often in combination with one another (77). Imaging shows a heterogeneous, cystic, and solid mass with calcifications and contrast enhancement of the solid portions (78). Treatment consists of surgical excision and stereotactic radiosurgery.

Although most craniopharyngioma patients survive long term without recurrence, a large number (in some series, the vast majority) are left with lifelong endocrine, and/or visual abnormalities (79–81). The small fraction of patients who receive a gross total resection, with or without stereotactic radiosurgery, have much higher rates of long-term, recurrence-free survival than those with subtotal resection. Because of the difficulty in resecting these tumors without damaging the hypothalamus and other vital structures, conservative surgery is undertaken in many cases. Conflicting observations have been made as to whether the adamantinomatous ones are more aggressive than the papillary. BRAF mutations have been targeted successfully for treating PCPs (82).

HISTOPATHOLOGY

ADAMANTINOMATOUS. At low power, the appearance is multinodular, composed of irregular islands of squamoid epithelium separated by strips of fibrous tissue. These clusters may be thin walled and cystic. The periphery of each nodule is traced by a dark band of palisading basal cells, which apposes a layer of polygonal, epithelioid cells interiorly. The polygonal cells transition into a third cellular component of loosely arranged, star-shaped cells (the *stellate reticulum*). The interior of the cellular islands often contains fragments of "wet keratin," which are cohesive sheets of lightly eosinophilic, stratified squamous *ghost cells*, with visible outlines of what once were nuclei and cell borders (Figure 8-21). Calcification and ossification of

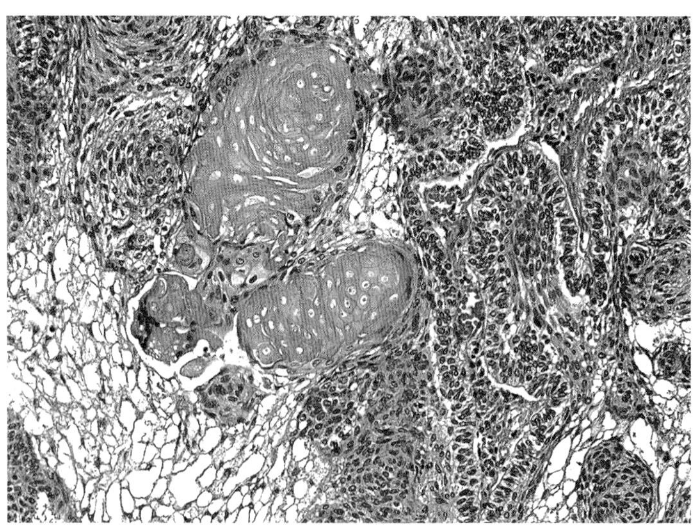

FIGURE 8-21 Adamantinomatous craniopharyngiomas contain nests of squamoid cells with peripheral palisading, "wet" keratin (center), calcifications, and stellate reticulum (lower left).

wet keratin are common. Small cystic spaces containing mucinous material can give an adenoid appearance. Cellular debris with granulomatous inflammation and cholesterol clefts is frequently seen microscopically and corresponds to the gross appearance of "machinery oil" fluid and grumous debris within cystic spaces. Occasionally, this xanthogranulomatous debris is the only element submitted, making diagnosis difficult because similar material can be found in other conditions in the suprasellar space (see below). The surrounding brain tissue can bear a surprising number of Rosenthal fibers that should not be mistaken for pilocytic astrocytoma on small biopsies that do not include the main lesion. The presence of entrapped, or invaded, brain appears to have no impact on rates of recurrence (83).

PAPILLARY. A solid proliferation of well-differentiated squamous cells arranged in a vaguely pseudopapillary architecture defines the papillary variant. The component squamous cells show very little, if any, maturation as they move away from the basal layer (Figure 8-22). Stellate reticulum, peripheral palisading, and keratin (wet or dry) are not seen. Calcification, xanthogranulomatous debris, and brain invasion are much less common in PCPs. Adenoid cysts of thick mucoid material are also seen in the papillary pattern and can be extensive (Figure 8-23). PCP can arise in the context of a Rathke cleft cyst, with ciliated, mucin-producing columnar epithelium overlying the tumor (Figure 8-24) (84).

IMMUNOHISTOCHEMISTRY. The squamous cells of craniopharyngioma stain for keratins and other epithelial markers, but these are rarely useful. Adamantinomatous cases (90%) have shown strong nuclear accumulation of beta catenin, a result of mutations in the gene for beta catenin, *CTNNB1*

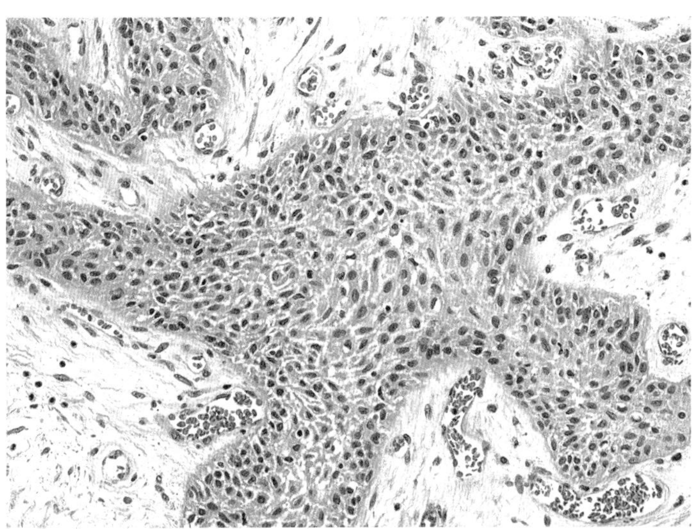

FIGURE 8-22 Papillary craniopharyngiomas contain well-differentiated squamous epithelium that lacks a granular layer, matures very little, and produces no keratin.

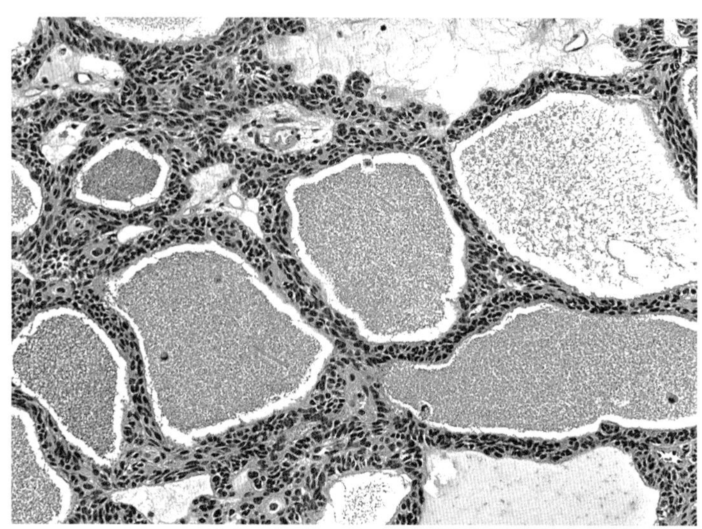

FIGURE 8-23 Some craniopharyngiomas, like this papillary example, contain numerous adenoid collections of mucinous substance.

(85). The VE1 immunostain can help screen for the BRAF V600E mutation in PCPs and assist in ruling out Rathke cleft cysts.

DIFFERENTIAL DIAGNOSIS. The xanthogranulomatous cellular debris seen in craniopharyngiomas can be seen in other sellar/suprasellar lesions,

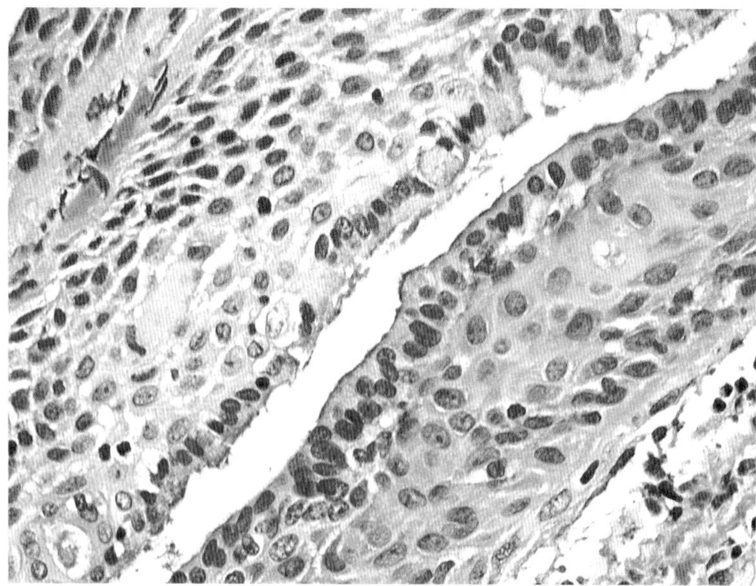

FIGURE 8-24 Papillary craniopharyngiomas may arise within Rathke cleft cysts as thin layers of nonkeratinizing squamous epithelium.

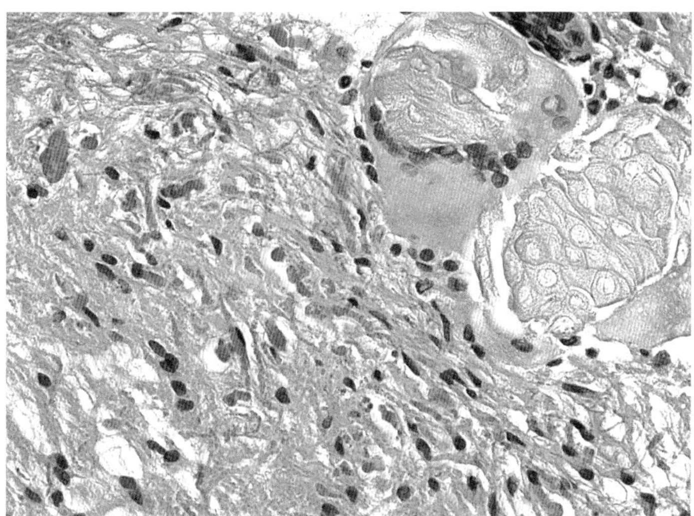

FIGURE 8-25 Brain tissue adjacent to craniopharyngiomas can show extensive piloid gliosis with numerous Rosenthal fibers and should not be mistaken for pilocytic astrocytoma.

especially Rathke cleft cyst, and should not be used to diagnose craniopharyngioma in the absence of an epithelial component. The term "xanthogranuloma of the sellar region" has been applied in this circumstance (see section Nonneoplastic Conditions of the Pituitary and Parasellar Area).

PCPs have more morphologic overlap with other entities than the ACPs. Epidermoid cysts are common in the sellar region and may appear similar to papillary craniopharyngioma but show maturation and "dry" keratinization of squamous cells. Rathke cleft cysts with extensive squamous metaplasia are also in the differential. Keratinization is the best morphologic confirmation of metaplasia in Rathke cleft cysts; it is never seen in PCP. DNA-based molecular testing can objectively confirm or refute the presence of PCP by demonstrating a BRAF V600E mutation, which is present in ~95% of cases (86).

The brain tissue surrounding a craniopharyngioma classically shows extensive piloid gliosis with numerous Rosenthal fibers that can simulate the densely fibrillar areas of pilocytic astrocytomas (Figure 8-25). Because of the overlap in age range and location, it could be easy to lunge at a diagnosis of pilocytic astrocytoma if biopsy material includes only the reactive tissue. Unlike a pilocytic astrocytoma, piloid gliosis is monophasic, lacks a myxoid background, and is nearly nonproliferative.

Granular Cell Tumor of the Sellar Region (WHO Grade I)

CLINICAL CONTEXT. Although granular cell "tumorlets" and asymptomatic granular cell tumors (GCTs) are common when assiduously sought at autopsy (87), symptomatic examples are rare, with fewer than 75 documented cases, most of which are case reports. Most patients are within the third through sixth decades of life, and women outnumber men by about 2:1. Although the most common presenting complaint is visual disturbance, endocrine abnormalities are frequent as well. Duration of symptoms before diagnosis varies from days to years (88).

GCTs, and their putative precursor tumorlets, arise in the pituitary stalk, possibly from the pituicytes that scaffold and support the neurohypophysis. Some GCTs may originate in the posterior pituitary itself. Imaging shows a circumscribed, homogeneous mass that is isointense to gray matter on T1-weighted MRI and isointense to white matter on T2. Edema of surrounding tissue is minimal or is not seen. Injection of IV contrast causes avid, uniform enhancement (89). Calcifications are rare.

Surgical excision is the treatment of choice for GCT. However, difficulty in developing a surgical plane around this firm and vascular tumor prevents complete excision in many cases, and can lead to collateral damage, especially to the pituitary stalk. Many patients will require postoperative hormone replacement, perhaps permanently. Although morbidity due to hormone disturbances is high, GCTs tend not to recur, even after subtotal resection. Radiation has been employed in some cases.

HISTOPATHOLOGY. GCT of the sellar region shows similar histologic findings to GCT elsewhere in the body, and identical findings to incidental tumorlets of the stalk. Large polygonal cells form large nests, vague fascicles, or sheets that contain abundant, granular, lightly eosinophilic cytoplasm and small monotonous nuclei (Figure 8-26). The nuclei may show some variation in size and shape, but overall are round to oval with open, granular chromatin and a prominent nucleolus. More fascicular examples display an elongate cytology. A meshwork of fine, thin-walled blood vessels

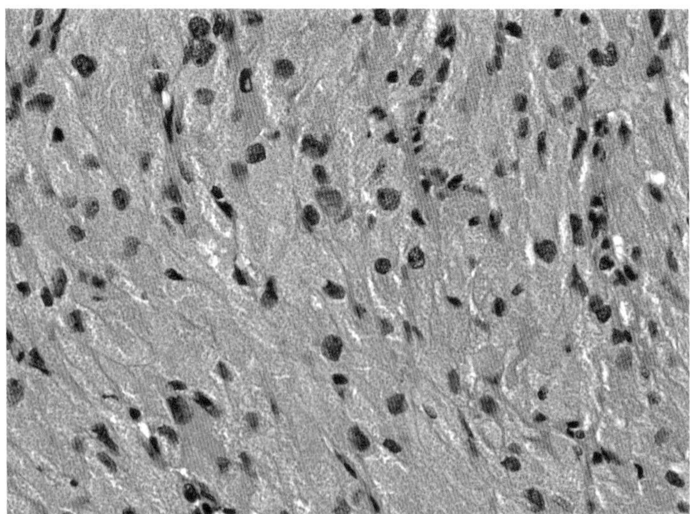

FIGURE 8-26 Granular cell tumor of the sellar region exhibits ample granular cytoplasm and bland uniform nuclei.

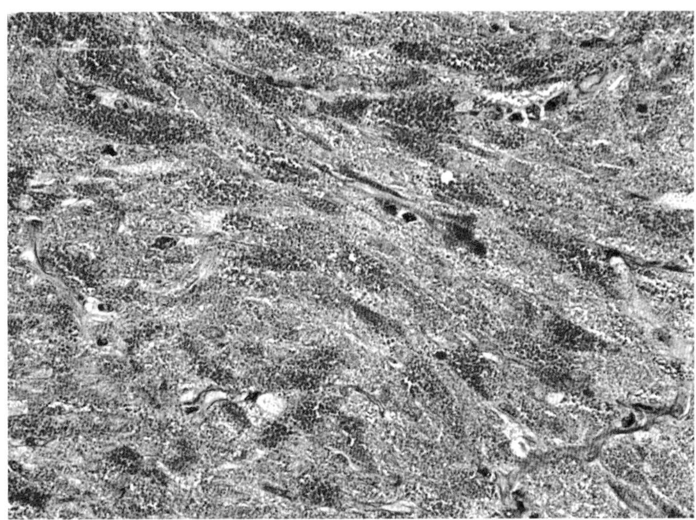

FIGURE 8-27 The lysosomes of granular cell tumors are PAS positive.

extends through the tumor, with occasional lymphocytic infiltrates. The cytoplasmic granules consist of lysosomes and are positive for PAS and CD68 (Figure 8-27). Antibodies against thyroid transcription factor 1 (TTF-1) mark the nucleus of GCT, pituicytoma, and spindle cell oncocytoma (SCO), adding some support to the notion that these three lesions are closely related and derive from pituicytes, which also express TTF-1 (90).

Pituicytoma (WHO Grade I)

GENERAL. This tumor is rare and, until the last decade, poorly defined in the literature, previously having been called "infundibuloma," "pituitary astrocytoma," as well as sharing the name pituicytoma with a few other lesions. Pituicytoma, as currently recognized, was added to the WHO classification in 2007 and still has fewer than 100 documented cases in the literature.

CLINICAL CONTEXT. Most reported pituicytomas become symptomatic in the fourth through sixth decades of life, causing hypopituitarism, visual defects, and headaches. Males make up about 50% more cases than females. The anatomic distribution follows the neurohypophysis, including the posterior lobe and pituitary stalk. MRI shows a solid, round, contrast-enhancing mass that arises in the suprasellar space or within the sella. No peritumoral edema should be seen. Most pituicytomas are effectively treated by simple excision and do not recur, even when subtotally resected. Radiation and chemotherapy are not typically used (91–95).

HISTOPATHOLOGY. The histologic appearance of pituicytoma is distinctive among tumors of the sellar region. The overall architecture shows small fascicles and storiform arrangements of elongate cells that are

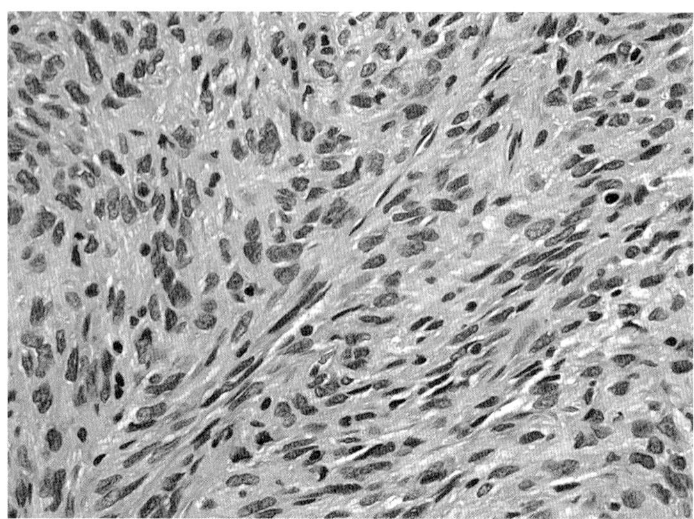

FIGURE 8-28 Pituicytoma composed of fibrillar cells in subtly flowing, vaguely fascicular architecture.

monomorphic and contain smooth, nongranular, nonvacuolated, lightly eosinophilic cytoplasm (Figure 8-28). The nuclei contain speckled, intermediate-density chromatin and a single small nucleolus. Mitoses are rare, with only a single mitotic figure appearing in a series of nine cases (91). Although the tumor may impinge on nearby vascular structures and appear to encase them, histologic evidence of invasion into surrounding tissue has not been demonstrated.

IMMUNOHISTOCHEMISTRY. Native pituicytes are the neurohypophyseal equivalent of astrocytes in that they are stellate cells that support and nourish the neuronal elements of the organ, thus pituicytomas express TTF-1, S100 protein, and GFAP (Figure 8-29). Epithelial membrane antigen staining is negative.

DIFFERENTIAL DIAGNOSIS. In the setting of a solid, contrast-enhancing, sellar/parasellar mass in an adult, the differential considerations can be limited to meningioma, pilocytic astrocytoma, pituitary adenoma, and the other rare sellar lesions such as GCT and SCO.

When examining sellar/parasellar biopsies containing spindle cell elements, the first decision is whether the sample could be neuroglial tissue from the posterior lobe of the pituitary. Round, granular, anucleate Herring bodies are only seen in neurohypophysis, as are neurofilament-positive axons descending from hypothalamic nuclei. Meningiomas are common lesions that can imitate pituicytoma, although they lack fibrillarity and GFAP or TTF-1 immunoreactivity. Sellar schwannomas, themselves rare, are also fascicular and can express S100 and sometimes GFAP, but have extensive pericellular reticulin and collagen IV staining.

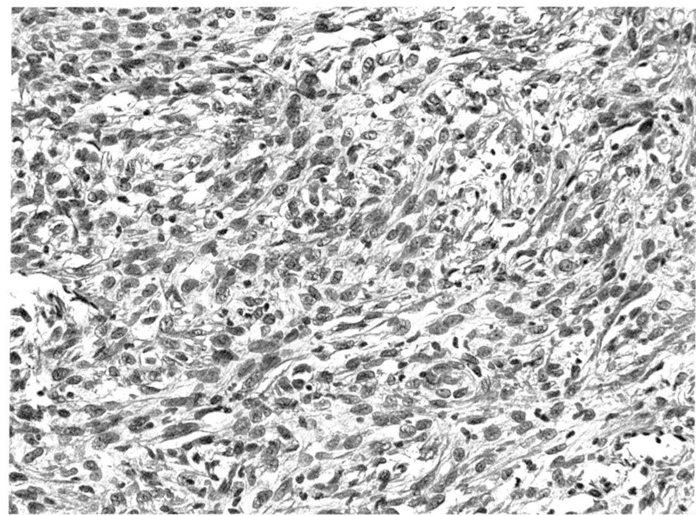

FIGURE 8-29 Pituicytomas show cytoplasmic reactivity for GFAP and S100.

The spindle cell pattern of pituitary adenoma almost equals pituicytoma in rarity and can appear histologically similar, but expresses cytokeratins, synaptophysin, and (with luck) one or more pituitary hormones.

The cytologic crush prep proves its worth in intraoperative examination of pituicytoma, where it elicits the fine glial fibrillar cytoplasmic processes and small cytoplasm that separate it from meningioma and other nonglial tumors (Figure 8-30).

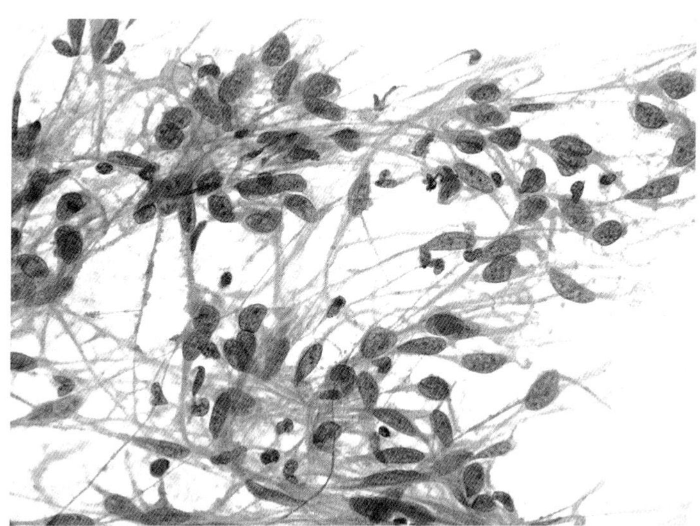

FIGURE 8-30 Crush preparations ease the difficulty of identifying the fibrillar glial processes of pituicytomas and facilitate intraoperative diagnoses.

Spindle Cell Oncocytoma (WHO Grade I)

CLINICAL CONTEXT. Of neoplasms peculiar to the sellar and parasellar space, SCO has the lowest number of reported cases, at fewer than 30. Formerly called SCO of the adenohypophysis, the finding of TTF-1 expression has linked these tumors with pituicytomas, GCTs, and neurohypophyseal pituicytes (90). SCO presents in middle-aged adults (mean age around 60 years, range 26 to 76) with signs and symptoms similar to nonsecreting pituitary adenomas, with loss of vision, headache, and hypopituitarism. Cases are distributed evenly between the sexes. Neuroimaging fails to show any differences between SCOs and pituitary adenomas (96). Although too few cases are described to accurately generalize about their behavior, SCOs are generally low-grade neoplasms that are effectively treated by surgery. Of 13 reported cases, 5 have recurred, ranging in latency from less than 1 year to more than 10 years, all following simple surgical excision (96–102).

HISTOPATHOLOGY. Similar in concept to oncocytic neoplasms from the kidney, salivary glands, thyroid, and elsewhere, SCO is a tumor characterized by cells with finely granular eosinophilic cytoplasm containing an abundance of mitochondria. Unlike other oncocytic neoplasms, SCO also shows a fascicular architecture with plump spindle-shaped cells (Figure 8-31). The nuclei are monotonous and round to elongate with coarse open chromatin and a single, prominent, eosinophilic nucleolus. Focal lymphocytic infiltrates and hemosiderin-laden macrophages have been noted (96). Mitotic rates are generally less than 1/10 high-power fields. Necrosis can be found occasionally but does not seem to indicate a more aggressive course.

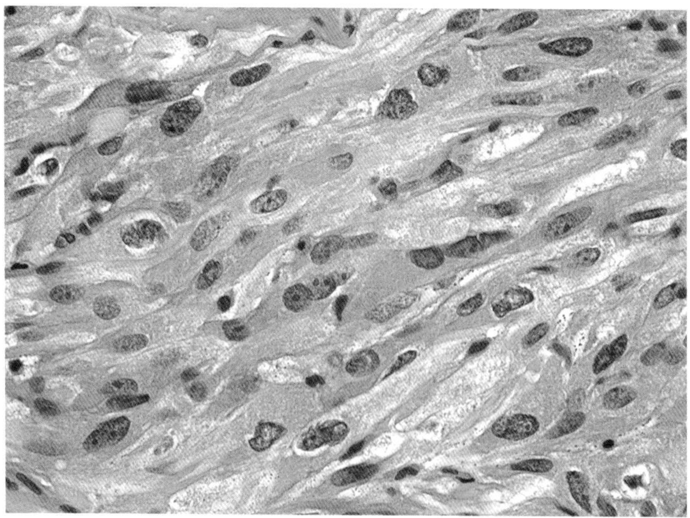

FIGURE 8-31 Spindle cell oncocytoma of the adenohypophysis has plump elongate cells with finely granular, oncocytic cytoplasm filled with mitochondria.

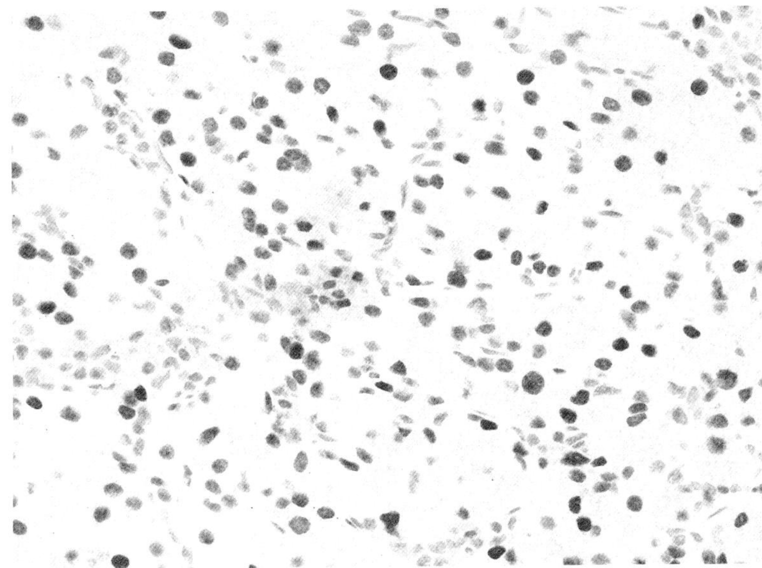

FIGURE 8-32 Thyroid transcription factor-1 (TTF-1) immunostaining labels the nuclei of spindle cell oncocytomas (seen here), pituicytomas, granular cell tumors of the sella, and normal pituicytes, suggesting a common lineage.

Immunohistochemistry shows reactivity for TTF-1 (Figure 8-32), S100 protein, vimentin, EMA, and galectin-3, whereas GFAP, synaptophysin, pituitary hormones, keratin, and CD68 are negative (96). MIB1 proliferation rates should be less than 5%, but figures up to 20% have been reported and associated with recurrence (100). However, the most aggressive case reported to date had a low MIB1 index of 2% to 3% (99).

DIFFERENTIAL DIAGNOSIS. Although the histology of SCO is unique, several other entities that occur in the sellar region can enter the differential diagnosis. Pituitary adenomas can have spindle-shaped cells with granular cytoplasm and can rarely form a fascicular architecture. In the setting of this morphology, immunoreactivity for synaptophysin and keratin firmly refutes any notion of SCO and supports a diagnosis of adenoma, as does reactivity for any of the anterior pituitary hormones. Pituicytoma shares architectural and some cytologic features with SCO, but it is not granular and fails to stain with EMA. GCT of the neurohypophysis comes the closest to SCO in appearance, being distinguished by staining for lysosomal markers like CD68.

Pilocytic Astrocytoma and Pilomyxoid Astrocytoma

Both of these low-grade astrocytomas commonly occur in the suprasellar region in children and are discussed in detail in Chapter 4 with other astrocytic neoplasms.

Germ Cell Tumors

In the pediatric and young adult populations, germ cell tumors are common in the suprasellar region. Females are more likely than males to have suprasellar involvement (103). These lesions are discussed in more detail in Chapter 15.

Salivary Gland Tumors

Microscopic nests of salivary gland tissue can be seen in the normal pituitary. These presumably give rise to rare cases of primary salivary gland neoplasms within the sella (104,105).

Metastases

Neoplastic disease from extrasellar sources can present as pituitary masses. Carcinomas occasionally metastasize to the pituitary, but only a fraction of them cause symptomatic disease (106). As with the rest of the CNS, lung and breast are the most common sources. Patients with metastatic disease are more likely to present with diabetes insipidus than those with pituitary adenomas (106,107). Hematopoietic lesions rarely manifest in the sella, with most cases consisting of large B-cell lymphoma (108,109) and plasmacytoma (110).

REFERENCES

1. Asa S. Tumors of the Pituitary Gland. Atlas of Tumor Pathology. Vol 22. Bethesda, MD: Armed Forces Institute of Pathology; 1998.
2. Marin F, Boya J, Lopez-Carbonell A, et al. Immunohistochemical localization of intermediate filament and S-100 proteins in several non-endocrine cells of the human pituitary gland. *Arch Histol Cytol.* 1989;52(3):241–248.
3. Allaerts W, Fluitsma DM, Hoefsmit EC, et al. Immunohistochemical, morphological and ultrastructural resemblance between dendritic cells and folliculo-stellate cells in normal human and rat anterior pituitaries. *J Neuroendocrinol.* 1996;8(1):17–29.
4. Horvath E, Kovacs K, Scheithauer BW. Pituitary hyperplasia. *Pituitary.* 1999;1(3–4): 169–179.
5. Khawaja NM, Taher BM, Barham ME, et al. Pituitary enlargement in patients with primary hypothyroidism. *Endocr Pract.* 2006;12(1):29–34.
6. Sano T, Asa SL, Kovacs K. Growth hormone-releasing hormone-producing tumors: clinical, biochemical, and morphological manifestations. *Endocr Rev.* 1988;9(3):357–373.
7. Bellastella G, Maiorino MI, Bizzarro A, et al. Revisitation of autoimmune hypophysitis: knowledge and uncertainties on pathophysiological and clinical aspects. *Pituitary.* 2016;19(6):625–642.
8. Honegger J, Schlaffer S, Menzel C, et al. Diagnosis of primary hypophysitis in Germany. *J Clin Endocrinol Metab.* 2015;100(10):3841–3849.
9. Caturegli P, Lupi I, Landek-Salgado M, et al. Pituitary autoimmunity: 30 years later. *Autoimmun Rev.* 2008;7(8):631–637.
10. Caturegli P, Newschaffer C, Olivi A, et al. Autoimmune hypophysitis. *Endocr Rev.* 2005;26(5):599–614.

11. Gutenberg A, Buslei R, Fahlbusch R, et al. Immunopathology of primary hypophysitis: implications for pathogenesis. *Am J Surg Pathol.* 2005;29(3):329–338.
12. Rao S, Mahadevan A, Maiti T, et al. Granulomatous and lymphocytic hypophysitis – are they immunologically distinct? *APMIS.* 2016;124(12):1072–1077.
13. Hunn BH, Martin WG, Simpson S, Jr, et al. Idiopathic granulomatous hypophysitis: a systematic review of 82 cases in the literature. *Pituitary.* 2014;17(4):357–365.
14. Hanna B, Li YM, Beutler T, et al. Xanthomatous hypophysitis. *J Clin Neurosci.* 2015; 22(7):1091–1097.
15. Kleinschmidt-DeMasters BK, Lillehei KO, et al. Review of xanthomatous lesions of the sella. *Brain Pathol.* 2017;27(3):377–395.
16. Bernreuther C, Illies C, Flitsch J, et al. IgG4-related hypophysitis is highly prevalent among cases of histologically confirmed hypophysitis. *Brain Pathol.* 2016.
17. Iwama S, De Remigis A, Callahan MK, et al. Pituitary expression of CTLA-4 mediates hypophysitis secondary to administration of CTLA-4 blocking antibody. *Sci Transl Med.* 2014;6(230):230ra45.
18. Munari C, Kahane P, Francione S, et al. Role of the hypothalamic hamartoma in the genesis of gelastic fits (a video-stereo-EEG study). *Electroencephalogr Clin Neurophysiol.* 1995;95(3):154–160.
19. Kang S, Graham JM, Jr, Olney AH, et al. GLI3 frameshift mutations cause autosomal dominant Pallister-Hall syndrome. *Nat Genet.* 1997;15(3):266–268.
20. Saitsu H, Sonoda M, Higashijima T, et al. Somatic mutations in GLI3 and OFD1 involved in sonic hedgehog signaling cause hypothalamic hamartoma. *Ann Clin Transl Neurol.* 2016;3(5):356–365.
21. Hildebrand MS, Griffin NG, Damiano JA, et al. Mutations of the sonic hedgehog pathway underlie hypothalamic hamartoma with gelastic epilepsy. *Am J Hum Genet.* 2016; 99(2):423–429.
22. Raper DM, Besser M. Clinical features, management and recurrence of symptomatic Rathke's cleft cyst. *J Clin Neurosci.* 2009;16(3):385–389.
23. Christophe C, Flamant-Durand J, Hanquinet S, et al. MRI in seven cases of Rathke's cleft cyst in infants and children. *Pediatr Radiol.* 1993;23(2):79–82.
24. Itoh J, Usui K. An entirely suprasellar symptomatic Rathke's cleft cyst: case report. *Neurosurgery.* 1992;30(4):581–584; discussion 584–585.
25. Kleinschmidt-DeMasters BK, Lillehei KO, Stears JC. The pathologic, surgical, and MR spectrum of Rathke cleft cysts. *Surg Neurol.* 1995;44(1):19–26; discussion 26–27.
26. Bader LJ, Carter KD, Latchaw RE, et al. Simultaneous symptomatic Rathke's cleft cyst and GH secreting pituitary adenoma: a case report. *Pituitary.* 2004;7(1):39–44.
27. Noh SJ, Ahn JY, Lee KS, et al. Pituitary adenoma and concomitant Rathke's cleft cyst. *Acta Neurochir (Wien).* 2007;149(12):1223–1228.
28. Sumida M, Migita K, Tominaga A, et al. Concomitant pituitary adenoma and Rathke's cleft cyst. *Neuroradiology.* 2001;43(9):755–759.
29. Albini CH, MacGillivray MH, Fisher JE, et al. Triad of hypopituitarism, granulomatous hypophysitis, and ruptured Rathke's cleft cyst. *Neurosurgery.* 1988;22(1 Pt 1):133–136.
30. Murakami M, Nishioka H, Izawa H, et al. Granulomatous hypophysitis associated with Rathke's cleft cyst: a case report. *Minim Invasive Neurosurg.* 2008;51(3):169–172.
31. Sonnet E, Roudaut N, Meriot P, et al. Hypophysitis associated with a ruptured Rathke's cleft cyst in a woman, during pregnancy. *J Endocrinol Invest.* 2006;29(4):353–357.
32. Paulus W, Honegger J, Keyvani K, et al. Xanthogranuloma of the sellar region: a clinicopathological entity different from adamantinomatous craniopharyngioma. *Acta Neuropathol (Berl).* 1999;97(4):377–382.

33. Amano K, Kubo O, Komori T, et al. Clinicopathological features of sellar region xanthogranuloma: correlation with Rathke's cleft cyst. *Brain Tumor Pathol.* 2013;30(4): 233–241.
34. Asa SL, Casar-Borota O, Chanson P, et al. From pituitary adenoma to pituitary neuroendocrine tumor (PitNET): an International Pituitary Pathology Club proposal. *Endocr Relat Cancer.* 2017;24(4):C5–C8.
35. Ostrom QT, Gittleman H, Xu J, et al. CBTRUS statistical report: primary brain and other central nervous system tumors diagnosed in the United States in 2009–2013. *Neurooncol.* 2016;18(suppl 5):v1–v75.
36. Hardy J, Vezina JL. Transsphenoidal neurosurgery of intracranial neoplasm. *Adv Neurol.* 1976;15:261–273.
37. Chacko G, Chacko AG, Lombardero M, et al. Clinicopathologic correlates of giant pituitary adenomas. *J Clin Neurosci.* 2009;16(5):660–665.
38. Yuh WT, Fisher DJ, Nguyen HD, et al. Sequential MR enhancement pattern in normal pituitary gland and in pituitary adenoma. *AJNR Am J Neuroradiol.* 1994;15(1):101–108.
39. Bartynski WS, Lin L. Dynamic and conventional spin-echo MR of pituitary microlesions. *AJNR Am J Neuroradiol.* 1997;18(5):965–972.
40. Selman WR, Laws ER, Jr, Scheithauer BW, et al. The occurrence of dural invasion in pituitary adenomas. *J Neurosurg.* 1986;64(3):402–407.
41. Meij BP, Lopes MB, Ellegala DB, et al. The long-term significance of microscopic dural invasion in 354 patients with pituitary adenomas treated with transsphenoidal surgery. *J Neurosurg.* 2002;96(2):195–208.
42. Kleinschmidt-DeMasters BK, Winston KR, Rubinstein D, et al. Ectopic pituitary adenoma of the third ventricle. Case report. *J Neurosurg.* 1990;72(1):139–142.
43. Alexander AA, Niktash N, Kardon DE, et al. Ectopic nasopharyngeal pituitary adenoma resected with endoscopic technique. *Ear Nose Throat J.* 2008;87(7):E8–E10.
44. Semple PL, Jane JA, Lopes MB, et al. Pituitary apoplexy: correlation between magnetic resonance imaging and histopathological results. *J Neurosurg.* 2008;108(5):909–915.
45. Yoshino A, Katayama Y, Watanabe T, et al. Vanishing pituitary mass revealed by timely magnetic resonance imaging: examples of spontaneous resolution of nonfunctioning pituitary adenoma. *Acta Neurochir (Wien).* 2005;147(3):253–257; discussion 257.
46. Martinez AJ. The pathology of nonfunctional pituitary adenomas. *Semin Diagn Pathol.* 1986;3(1):83–94.
47. Buurman H, Saeger W. Subclinical adenomas in postmortem pituitaries: classification and correlations to clinical data. *Eur J Endocrinol.* 2006;154(5):753–758.
48. Saeger W, Ludecke DK, Buchfelder M, et al. Pathohistological classification of pituitary tumors: 10 years of experience with the German Pituitary Tumor Registry. *Eur J Endocrinol.* 2007;156(2):203–216.
49. Mori H, Maeda T, Saitoh Y, et al. Changes in prolactinomas and somatotropinomas in humans treated with bromocriptine. *Pathol Res Pract.* 1988;183(5):580–583.
50. Ezzat S, Horvath E, Harris AG, et al. Morphological effects of octreotide on growth hormone-producing pituitary adenomas. *J Clin Endocrinol Metab.* 1994;79(1):113–118.
51. Obari A, Sano T, Ohyama K, et al. Clinicopathological features of growth hormone-producing pituitary adenomas: difference among various types defined by cytokeratin distribution pattern including a transitional form. *Endocr Pathol.* 2008;19(2):82–91.
52. Arafah BM, Nasrallah MP. Pituitary tumors: pathophysiology, clinical manifestations and management. *Endocr Relat Cancer.* 2001;8(4):287–305.
53. Bradley KJ, Wass JA, Turner HE. Non-functioning pituitary adenomas with positive immunoreactivity for ACTH behave more aggressively than ACTH immunonegative tumours but do not recur more frequently. *Clin Endocrinol (Oxf).* 2003;58(1):59–64.

54. Cho HY, Cho SW, Kim SW, et al. Silent corticotroph adenomas have unique recurrence characteristics compared with other nonfunctioning pituitary adenomas. *Clin Endocrinol (Oxf)*. 2010;72(5):648–653.
55. Snyder PJ. Gonadotroph cell adenomas of the pituitary. *Endocr Rev*. 1985;6(4):552–563.
56. Yamada S, Ohyama K, Taguchi M, et al. A study of the correlation between morphological findings and biological activities in clinically nonfunctioning pituitary adenomas. *Neurosurgery*. 2007;61(3):580–584; discussion 584–585.
57. Bertholon-Gregoire M, Trouillas J, Guigard MP, et al. Mono- and plurihormonal thyrotropic pituitary adenomas: pathological, hormonal and clinical studies in 12 patients. *Eur J Endocrinol*. 1999;140(6):519–527.
58. Marucci G, Faustini-Fustini M, Righi A, et al. Thyrotropin-secreting pituitary tumours: significance of "atypical adenomas" in a series of 10 patients and association with Hashimoto thyroiditis as a cause of delay in diagnosis. *J Clin Pathol*. 2009;62(5):455–459.
59. Sanno N, Teramoto A, Osamura RY. Long-term surgical outcome in 16 patients with thyrotropin pituitary adenoma. *J Neurosurg*. 2000;93(2):194–200.
60. Erickson D, Scheithauer B, Atkinson J, et al. Silent subtype 3 pituitary adenoma: a clinicopathologic analysis of the Mayo Clinic experience. *Clin Endocrinol (Oxf)*. 2009;71(1):92–99.
61. Richardson TE, Mathis DA, Mickey BE, et al. Clinical outcome of silent subtype III pituitary adenomas diagnosed by immunohistochemistry. *J Neuropathol Exp Neurol*. 2015;74(12):1170–1177.
62. McDonald WC, Banerji N, McDonald KN, et al. Steroidogenic factor 1, pit-1, and adrenocorticotropic hormone: a rational starting place for the immunohistochemical characterization of pituitary adenoma. *Arch Pathol Lab Med*. 2017;141(1):104–112.
63. Gejman R, Swearingen B, Hedley-Whyte ET. Role of Ki-67 proliferation index and p53 expression in predicting progression of pituitary adenomas. *Hum Pathol*. 2008;39(5):758–766.
64. Hentschel SJ, McCutcheon E, Moore W, et al. P53 and MIB-1 immunohistochemistry as predictors of the clinical behavior of nonfunctioning pituitary adenomas. *Can J Neurol Sci* 2003;30(3):215–219.
65. Mahta A, Haghpanah V, Lashkari A, et al. Non-functioning pituitary adenoma: immunohistochemical analysis of 85 cases. *Folia Neuropathol*. 2007;45(2):72–77.
66. Ogawa Y, Ikeda H, Tominaga T. Clinicopathological study of prognostic factors in patients with pituitary adenomas and ki-67 labeling index of more than 3%. *J Endocrinol Invest*. 2009;32(7):581–584.
67. Chiloiro S, Doglietto F, Trapasso B, et al. Typical and atypical pituitary adenomas: a single-center analysis of outcome and prognosis. *Neuroendocrinology*. 2015;101(2):143–150.
68. Del Basso De Caro M, Solari D, Pagliuca F, et al. Atypical pituitary adenomas: clinical characteristics and role of ki-67 and p53 in prognostic and therapeutic evaluation. A series of 50 patients. *Neurosurg Rev*. 2017;40(1):105–114.
69. Zada G, Woodmansee WW, Ramkissoon S, et al. Atypical pituitary adenomas: incidence, clinical characteristics, and implications. *J Neurosurg*. 2011;114(2):336–344.
70. Ogawa A, Sugihara S, Hasegawa M, et al. Intermediate filament expression in pituitary adenomas. *Virchows Arch B Cell Pathol Incl Mol Pathol*. 1990;58(5):341–349.
71. Pernicone PJ, Scheithauer BW, Sebo TJ, et al. Pituitary carcinoma: a clinicopathologic study of 15 cases. *Cancer*. 1997;79(4):804–812.
72. Cooper PR, Ransohoff J. Craniopharyngioma originating in the sphenoid bone. Case report. *J Neurosurg*. 1972;36(1):102–106.

73. Shuman AG, Heth JA, Marentette LJ, et al. Extracranial nasopharyngeal craniopharyngioma: case report. *Neurosurgery*. 2007;60(4):E780–E781; discussion E781.
74. Zhou L, Luo L, Xu J, et al. Craniopharyngiomas in the posterior fossa: a rare subgroup, diagnosis, management and outcomes. *J Neurol Neurosurg Psychiatry*. 2009;80(10): 1150–1154.
75. Solarski A, Panke ES, Panke TW. Craniopharyngioma in the pineal gland. *Arch Pathol Lab Med*. 1978;102(9):490–491.
76. Usanov EI, Hatomkin DM, Nikulina TA, et al. Craniopharyngioma of the pineal region. *Childs Nerv Syst*. 1999;15(1):4–7.
77. Petito CK, DeGirolami U, Earle KM. Craniopharyngiomas: a clinical and pathological review. *Cancer*. 1976;37(4):1944–1952.
78. Rennert J, Doerfler A. Imaging of sellar and parasellar lesions. *Clin Neurol Neurosurg*. 2007;109(2):111–124.
79. Karavitaki N, Brufani C, Warner JT, et al. Craniopharyngiomas in children and adults: systematic analysis of 121 cases with long-term follow-up. *Clin Endocrinol (Oxf)*. 2005;62(4):397–409.
80. Lin LL, El Naqa I, Leonard JR, et al. Long-term outcome in children treated for craniopharyngioma with and without radiotherapy. *J Neurosurg Pediatr*. 2008;1(2):126–130.
81. Yasargil MG, Curcic M, Kis M, et al. Total removal of craniopharyngiomas. Approaches and long-term results in 144 patients. *J Neurosurg*. 1990;73(1):3–11.
82. Aylwin SJ, Bodi I, Beaney R. Pronounced response of papillary craniopharyngioma to treatment with vemurafenib, a BRAF inhibitor. *Pituitary*. 2016;19(5):544–546.
83. Gupta DK, Ojha BK, Sarkar C, et al. Recurrence in pediatric craniopharyngiomas: analysis of clinical and histological features. *Childs Nerv Syst*. 2006;22(1):50–55.
84. Alomari AK, Kelley BJ, Damisah E, et al. Craniopharyngioma arising in a Rathke's cleft cyst: case report. *J Neurosurg Pediatr*. 2015;15(3):250–254.
85. Hofmann BM, Kreutzer J, Saeger W, et al. Nuclear beta-catenin accumulation as reliable marker for the differentiation between cystic craniopharyngiomas and rathke cleft cysts: a clinico-pathologic approach. *Am J Surg Pathol*. 2006;30(12):1595–1603.
86. Kim JH, Paulus W, Heim S. BRAF V600E mutation is a useful marker for differentiating Rathke's cleft cyst with squamous metaplasia from papillary craniopharyngioma. *J Neurooncol*. 2015;123(1):189–191.
87. Tomita T, Gates E. Pituitary adenomas and granular cell tumors. Incidence, cell type, and location of tumor in 100 pituitary glands at autopsy. *Am J Clin Pathol*. 1999;111(6): 817–825.
88. Cohen-Gadol AA, Pichelmann MA, Link MJ, et al. Granular cell tumor of the sellar and suprasellar region: clinicopathologic study of 11 cases and literature review. *Mayo Clin Proc*. 2003;78(5):567–573.
89. Aquilina K, Kamel M, Kalimuthu SG, et al. Granular cell tumour of the neurohypophysis: a rare sellar tumour with specific radiological and operative features. *Br J Neurosurg*. 2006;20(1):51–54.
90. Mete O, Lopes MB, Asa SL. Spindle cell oncocytomas and granular cell tumors of the pituitary are variants of pituicytoma. *Am J Surg Pathol*. 2013;37(11):1694–1699.
91. Brat DJ, Scheithauer BW, Staugaitis SM, et al. Pituicytoma: a distinctive low-grade glioma of the neurohypophysis. *Am J Surg Pathol*. 2000;24(3):362–368.
92. Figarella-Branger D, Dufour H, Fernandez C, et al. Pituicytomas, a mis-diagnosed benign tumor of the neurohypophysis: report of three cases. *Acta Neuropathol (Berl)*. 2002;104(3):313–319.
93. Nakasu Y, Nakasu S, Saito A, et al. Pituicytoma. Two case reports. *Neurol Med Chir (Tokyo)*. 2006;46(3):152–156.

94. Takei H, Goodman JC, Tanaka S, et al. Pituicytoma incidentally found at autopsy. *Pathol Int.* 2005;55(11):745–749.
95. Ulm AJ, Yachnis AT, Brat DJ, et al. Pituicytoma: report of two cases and clues regarding histogenesis. *Neurosurgery.* 2004;54(3):753–757; discussion 757–758.
96. Roncaroli F, Scheithauer BW, Cenacchi G, et al. 'Spindle cell oncocytoma' of the adenohypophysis: a tumor of folliculostellate cells? *Am J Surg Pathol.* 2002;26(8):1048–1055.
97. Borota OC, Scheithauer BW, Fougner SL, et al. Spindle cell oncocytoma of the adenohypophysis: report of a case with marked cellular atypia and recurrence despite adjuvant treatment. *Clin Neuropathol.* 2009;28(2):91–95.
98. Coire CI, Horvath E, Smyth HS, et al. Rapidly recurring folliculostellate cell tumor of the adenohypophysis with the morphology of a spindle cell oncocytoma: case report with electron microscopic studies. *Clin Neuropathol.* 2009;28(4):303–308.
99. Demssie YN, Joseph J, Dawson T, et al. Recurrent spindle cell oncocytoma of the pituitary, a case report and review of literature. *Pituitary.* 2011;14(4):367–370.
100. Kloub O, Perry A, Tu PH, et al. Spindle cell oncocytoma of the adenohypophysis: report of two recurrent cases. *Am J Surg Pathol.* 2005;29(2):247–253.
101. Dahiya S, Sarkar C, Hedley-Whyte ET, et al. Spindle cell oncocytoma of the adenohypophysis: report of two cases. *Acta Neuropathol (Berl).* 2005;110(1):97–99.
102. Vajtai I, Sahli R, Kappeler A. Spindle cell oncocytoma of the adenohypophysis: report of a case with a 16-year follow-up. *Pathol Res Pract.* 2006;202(10):745–750.
103. Jennings MT, Gelman R, Hochberg F. Intracranial germ-cell tumors: natural history and pathogenesis. *J Neurosurg.* 1985;63(2):155–167.
104. Chimelli L, Gadelha MR, Une K, et al. Intra-sellar salivary gland-like pleomorphic adenoma arising within the wall of a Rathke's cleft cyst. *Pituitary.* 2000;3(4):257–261.
105. Hampton TA, Scheithauer BW, Rojiani AM, et al. Salivary gland-like tumors of the sellar region. *Am J Surg Pathol.* 1997;21(4):424–434.
106. Teears RJ, Silverman EM. Clinicopathologic review of 88 cases of carcinoma metastatic to the pituitary gland. *Cancer.* 1975;36(1):216–220.
107. Morita A, Meyer FB, Laws ER, Jr, Symptomatic pituitary metastases. *J Neurosurg.* 1998; 89(1):69–73.
108. Kaufmann TJ, Lopes MB, Laws ER, Jr, et al. Primary sellar lymphoma: radiologic and pathologic findings in two patients. *AJNR Am J Neuroradiol.* 2002;23(3):364–367.
109. Rudnik A, Larysz D, Blamek S, et al. Primary pituitary lymphoma. *Folia Neuropathol.* 2007;45(3):144–148.
110. Yaman E, Benekli M, Coskun U, et al. Intrasellar plasmacytoma: an unusual presentation of multiple myeloma. *Acta Neurochir (Wien).* 2008;150(9):921–924; discussion 924.

9

MENINGEAL LESIONS

MENINGIOMA

General

Meningiomas arise from the *arachnoid cap cells* that inhabit the most superficial portion of the arachnoid membrane, just below the inner surface of the dura. These cells are most concentrated around the arachnoid villi where they form a cap over each villus, yet can be found wherever there are meninges, both as single cells and as small syncytial clusters that resemble minute meningiomas. Electron microscopy and immunohistochemistry support these histologic similarities, with intercellular tight junctions and epithelial membrane antigen (EMA) reactivity being seen in both. Rests of these cells created during development explain the appearance of meningiomas in extradural locations, such as the ventricles (Figure 9-1).

Although the great majority of meningiomas are benign and have a characteristic appearance, some can prove challenging both in appropriate grading and in identification. The 2016 World Health Organization (WHO) classification of central nervous system (CNS) tumors codifies a grading system for meningiomas that is among the most complicated of any tumor type, the application of which can be intimidating without experience or guidance. However, grading of meningiomas has become standard practice and has important prognostic implications and should never be omitted from the pathology report. In some cases, grading of meningiomas can be a secondary issue when a lesion presents with one of the more unusual patterns, and identification of the tumor as meningothelial takes precedence.

Clinical Context

Meningiomas constitute approximately 37% of all primary CNS-related neoplasms, making them the most common primary intracranial tumors (1). They are primarily a tumor of adults, and among those younger than 20 years, they are not even among the 10 most frequent tumor types (2). Meningiomas preferentially affect women at a ratio of approximately 3:2, although sex differences in meningioma incidence vary by location, with thoracic spinal meningiomas occurring at a 9:1 female to male ratio. Meningiomas present at a mean age of around 64 years, with no difference

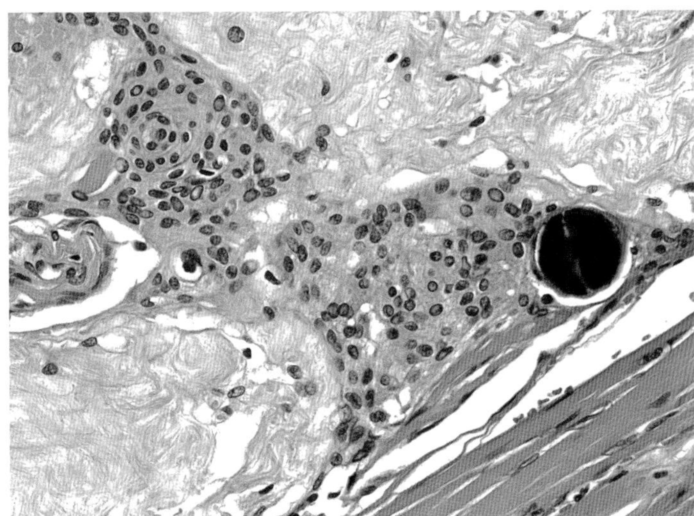

FIGURE 9-1 Meningothelial clusters such as these in the parasagittal dura (arachnoid villi) are physiologic, small, and nonproliferating.

in incidence among races. Groups who have lower incidences of meningiomas, specifically men and children, tend to have more aggressive tumors when they do occur. Most meningiomas present with symptoms and/or signs related to location and mass effect or to peritumoral edema, but lesions that invade the full thickness of the skull can present as fleshy scalp masses (3).

The familial tumor syndrome most consistently associated with the development of meningiomas is neurofibromatosis type 2 (NF2), in which patients harbor a germline mutation in the *NF2* gene at locus 22q12. Although meningiomas have been reported in patients with other tumor syndromes, the statistical relevance of such observations is unclear. In general, meningiomas in the context of NF2 occur earlier in life, are multiple, and are slightly more clinically aggressive than sporadic meningiomas (4,5). Dozens of meningiomas may pepper the dura of patients with NF2. NF2 also predisposes one to developing schwannomas and spinal ependymomas.

Germline mutations in the *SMARCB1* gene, which is also the gene responsible for the familial rhabdoid tumor predisposition syndrome, have been implicated in familial cases of multiple meningiomas (6,7). *SMARCE1* germline mutations are associated specifically with clear cell meningiomas (see below section Clear Cell Meningioma). Other germline mutations associated with meningiomas have included *SUFU* (8) and *BAP1* (9).

Prior exposure to ionizing radiation has been solidly linked to the development of meningiomas in the setting of low-dose x-ray treatment for tinea capitis (10), and in the setting of high-dose therapeutic radiation for malignancy (11,12).

Meningiomas may occur anywhere in the neuraxis, with a strong preference for the meninges overlying the cerebral convexities and parasagittal areas (lateral to the superior sagittal sinus). Other common sites for meningiomas include the falx, wing of the sphenoid bone ("sphenoid ridge" that is the anterior limit of the temporal fossa), cribriform plate (olfactory groove), tentorium, and supra- or parasellar region. Intraventricular meningiomas typically form in the trigone of the posterior-lateral ventricle, where the bulk of the choroid plexus lies, and may rarely arise in other parts of the lateral ventricles or even the third and fourth ventricles.

Radiology

Most meningiomas can be diagnosed clinically on the basis of their characteristic appearance on contrast-enhanced neuroimaging, where they cut a lens-shaped silhouette that tapers off into the surrounding dura. Meningiomas are best visualized radiologically with administration of contrast material because they are generally isointense to gray matter on computed tomography (CT) and T1-weighted magnetic resonance imaging (MRI), and can be difficult to distinguish from their surroundings. Fortunately, gadolinium contrast agent brilliantly illuminates meningiomas, such that lesions as small as a grain of rice can be detected. The "dural tail" sign, or the thin edge of surrounding contrast enhancement, provides the radiologist with a reasonably reliable means of identifying a meningioma (Figure 9-2). Although many other dura-based lesions also show a dural tail, the great majority of such cases will be meningiomas. T2-weighted MRI can often discriminate between meningiomas and their surroundings, although the intensity of the lesion's signal may vary, depending on the histologic pattern

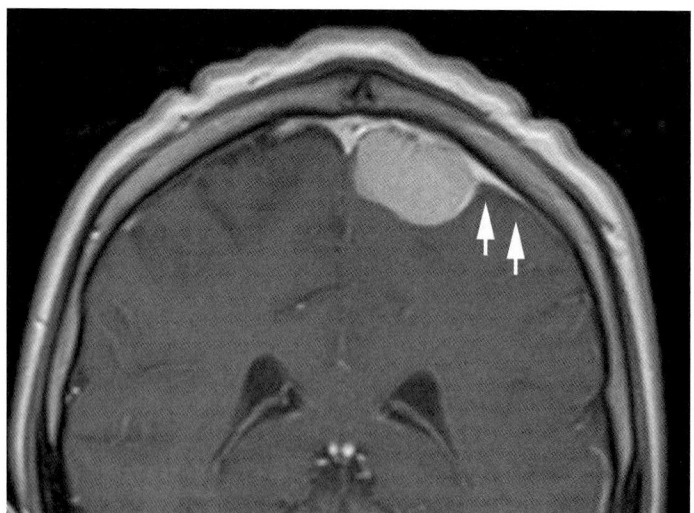

FIGURE 9-2 An enhancing dural lesion that tapers into a "dural tail" is the characteristic, though nonspecific, neuroimaging finding of meningioma.

(13). Peritumoral edema is highly variable, being associated with more aggressive meningiomas and either secretory or angiomatous histologic pattern. Other features that signal meningioma on imaging are hyperostosis and calcification (on CT).

Meningiomas may also present with unusual radiologic findings. Occasionally, a cystic space will form along the edge or in the middle of the lesion, giving it an overall cyst with nodule configuration. *En plaque* growth of meningiomas usually occurs along the base of the brain in the middle fossa and can give the impression of other processes. Osteolytic growth, bone invasion, and primary intradiploic occurrence are all seen in meningiomas but are much less common.

Prognosis/Treatment

Surgical removal is the treatment of choice for meningiomas, except in cases where the risks of surgery may outweigh the benefits. In cases with subtotal resection, or with a grade II or grade III diagnosis, adjuvant radiotherapy may be employed to effectively reduce the risk of recurrence and mortality (14); however, clear class I evidence for its efficacy is lacking, as are uniform guidelines for its application (15).

Most patients with meningiomas are cured of their disease by surgical excision, if the entire lesion can be removed. This is an important point because incomplete resection is the single best predictor of recurrence; around 90% of patients with a completely resected grade I meningioma will be free of recurrence at 5 years, but that percentage falls to 60% to 70% with incomplete removal (16). Whether a meningioma can be totally resected is mostly a function of location, with those in the skull base or involving major vascular structures being among the most difficult to excise. Grade II meningiomas have an increased rate of recurrence, around 40%, even when the tumor is completely resected, and grade III lesions have a recurrence rate of 60% or more (17,18). Survival is not adversely affected in cases of grade I meningioma, but the mortality rates for grade II and grade III meningiomas are approximately 20% and 70% at 5 years, respectively (17). Neuroimaging findings may also be used with extent of resection to predict risk of recurrence (19).

Invasion into bone may also be a factor in tumor recurrence and has been shown to negatively impact recurrence and overall survival in cases of atypical meningioma (20), but currently it has no clear place in the WHO grading scheme. Whether bone resection or radiation affects outcomes in these cases deserves to be explored.

Although the incidence of metastasis is only approximately 1 per 1,000 primary meningiomas, it is a well-documented phenomenon, even in cases with grade I histology (21–25). The most common metastatic site is the lung, with reports of vertebra and scattered other sites making up the remainder. Some of the suggested risk factors for metastasis in meningiomas are invasion of venous sinuses, aggressive histologic features, and craniotomy for primary tumor resection (25).

Histopathology

Where applicable, although this section mainly addresses the histologic patterns of meningioma, specific genetic findings that are characteristic for a given pattern are discussed along with the defining microscopic findings. The genetics of meningiomas as a general group are discussed in the following section.

WHO GRADE I MENINGIOMAS. Differentiating between the patterns of grade I meningiomas in the diagnostic line of the pathology report is generally not necessary, but an awareness of the many faces of meningioma will prevent diagnostic confusion when unusual patterns arise. All of these patterns below are generally WHO grade I but may be higher grade if they meet other histologic criteria or invade the brain.

MENINGOTHELIAL. This pattern is composed of whorls and small sheets of syncytial, polygonal cells with smooth eosinophilic cytoplasm, regularly contoured oval nuclei, minute nucleoli, and pale, finely granular chromatin (Figures 9-3 and 9-4). Scattered nuclei contain pseudoinclusions, or cytoplasmic intrusions, similar to those seen in papillary thyroid carcinoma. Present in most patterns of meningioma, pseudoinclusions are sharply circumscribed, devoid of contents, and compress the surrounding chromatin against the nuclear envelope. The whorls in this pattern are often vague and lobular, their edges blending with the surrounding tumor cells (Figure 9-5). Collagen deposition is minor, but fibrous septa and perivascular collagen can be present.

FIBROUS. Fibrous meningiomas share few of the morphologic characteristics of their meningothelial siblings and can be mistaken for other

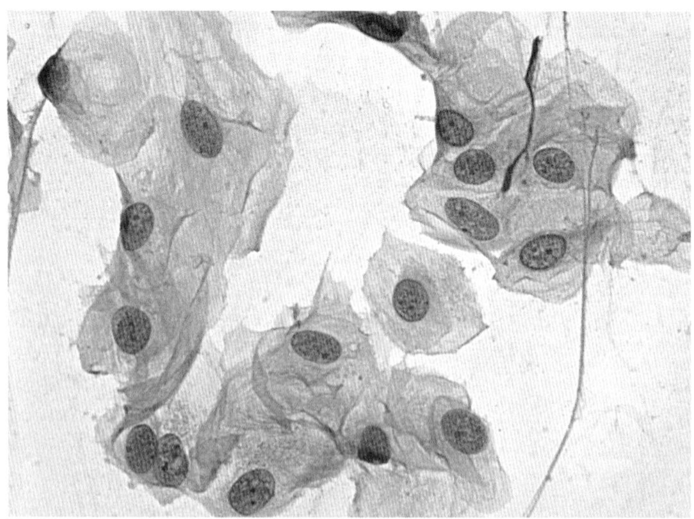

FIGURE 9-3 Cytologic crush preparations show the individual cells of meningioma: monotonous, pale, oval, regular nuclei, and vaguely tissue-paper–like cytoplasm.

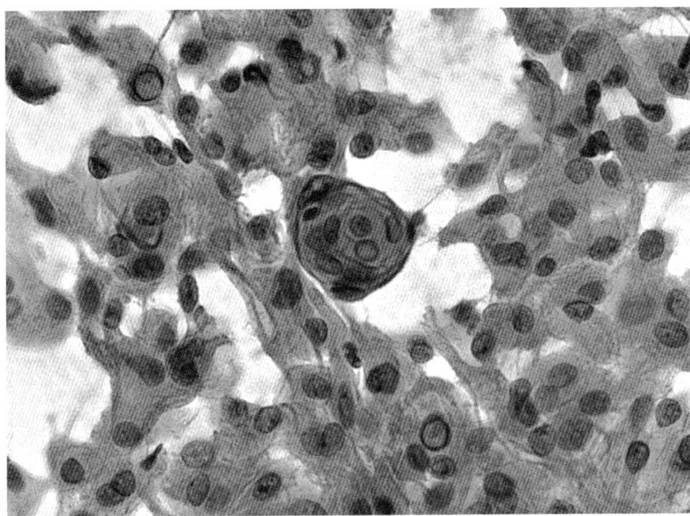

FIGURE 9-4 Most meningiomas are resistant to crushing. Tight cellular whorls and monotonous nuclei with pseudoinclusions are characteristic.

entities, specifically schwannoma (when in the cerebellopontine angle) and solitary fibrous tumor. The architecture ranges from fascicular to storiform (Figures 9-6 and 9-7), with few whorls or psammoma bodies and abundant collagen deposition. Collagen is deposited both in thick bands along blood vessels and as a dense, diffuse background matrix admixed with tumor cells. Dense bands of acellular collagen can replace the vast majority of the tumor, leaving only traces of the tumor's cells. These cases

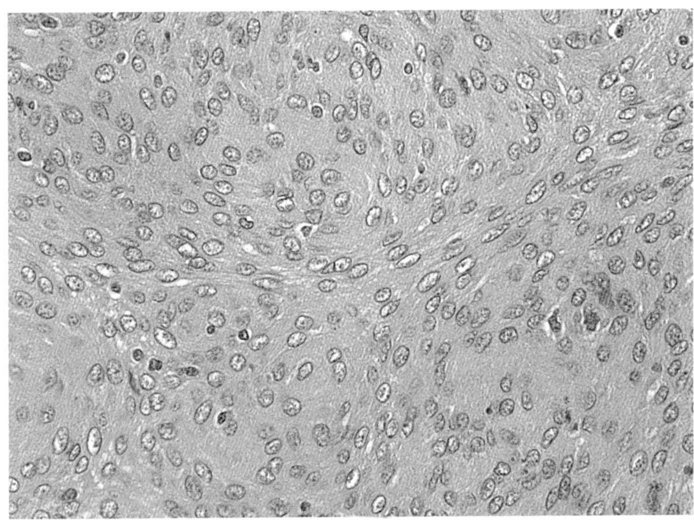

FIGURE 9-5 Meningothelial meningiomas are highly syncytial with subtle whorls and little background collagen.

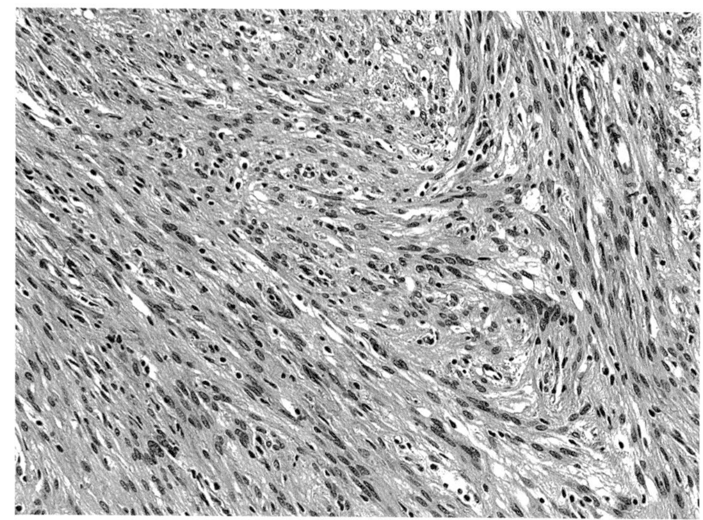

FIGURE 9-6 Fibrous meningiomas often grow in fascicles with irregular nuclei and lack whorls and psammoma bodies.

are sometimes called "sclerotic" meningiomas (Figure 9-8). The typical nuclear features of oval shape with regular outlines and pale chromatin are distorted into elongate nuclei with irregular outlines.

TRANSITIONAL. This pattern, transitional between meningothelial and fibrous, comprises the largest fraction of meningiomas and is the archetype of meningioma (Figure 9-9). The centers of the cellular whorls often hyalinize over time, leaving bubble-gum–colored spheres of protein, which,

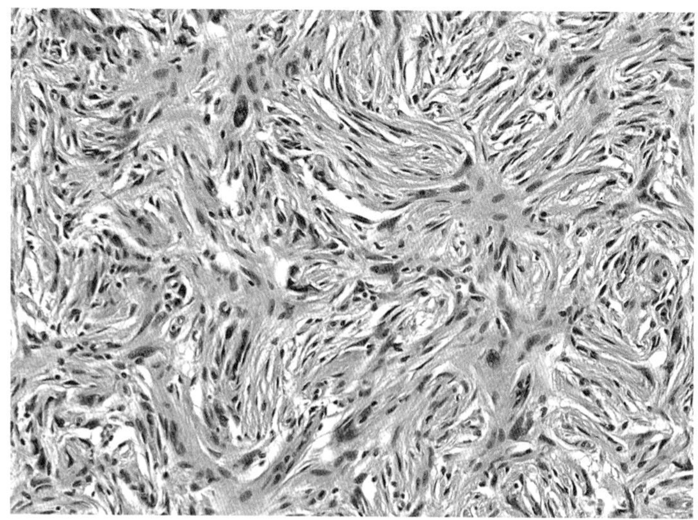

FIGURE 9-7 A storiform pattern manifests in some fibrous meningiomas.

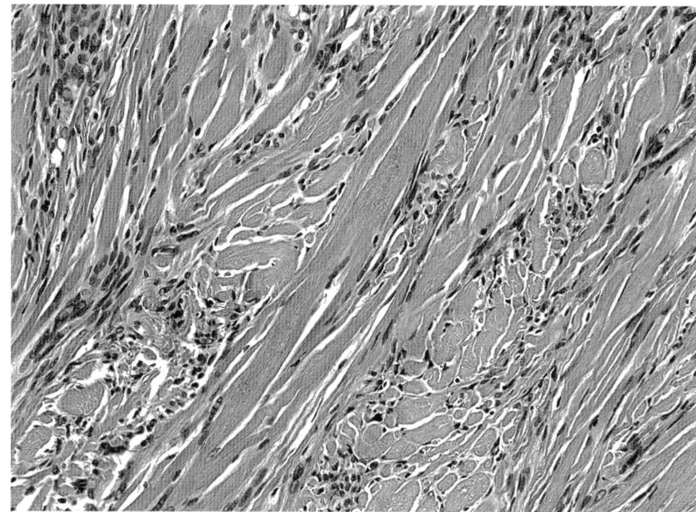

FIGURE 9-8 Dense acellular bands of collagen crowd the few remaining tumor cells in sclerotic fibrous meningiomas.

after more time, transform into psammoma bodies. Psammoma bodies are common in several patterns of meningioma and can provide a helpful diagnostic cue when other features are lacking.

PSAMMOMATOUS. This striking pattern is an ordinary meningioma that has numerous whorls that have mineralized and formed lamellated spheres of calcium, or psammoma bodies (Figure 9-10). As might be inferred from the heavy calcification, these lesions are generally slow-growing (if at all),

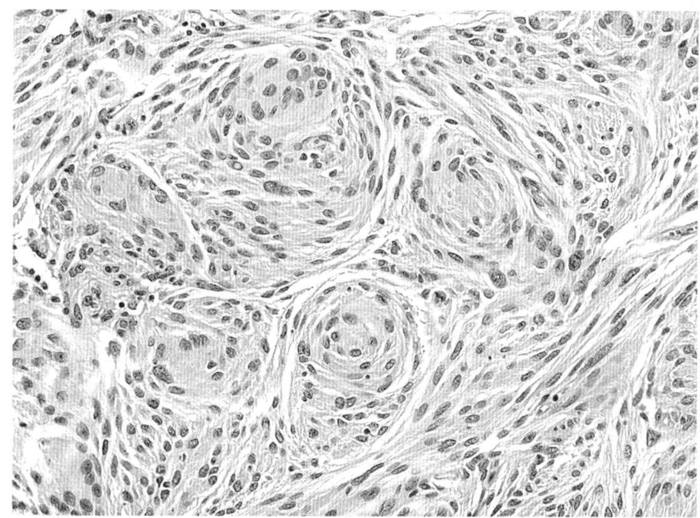

FIGURE 9-9 The transitional pattern of meningioma, with whorls and collagen deposition, spans the gap in appearance between meningothelial and fibrous patterns.

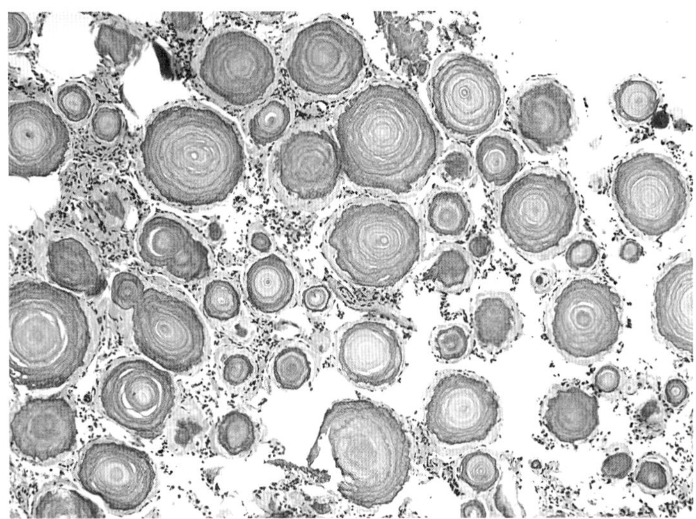

FIGURE 9-10 Psammomatous meningiomas result from extensive calcification of meningothelial whorls, sometimes with little of the original tumor left.

lack atypical features, and have a low MIB1 index. In extreme cases, it may be difficult to identify the residual meningioma cells among the extensive calcifications. Most psammomatous meningiomas occur in the spinal canal in women older than 40 years. Even among intracranial examples, there remains a strong predilection for women (26).

ANGIOMATOUS. This pattern overlaps with microcystic meningioma, with vacuolated cells and cobweb cytoplasm in many cases, but requires 50% or greater area of blood vessels to tumor tissue for inclusion, as put forward in one large series examining these lesions pathologically (27). The authors of this series recognized two patterns of angiomatous meningioma, macrovascular and microvascular, the macrovascular comprising a little more than half of the total cases. The macrovascular pattern displayed mostly large blood vessels with prominent hyalinization and intervening areas of usual meningioma, with syncytial whorls and short fascicles. The microvascular pattern was composed of small blood vessels with delicate walls in a background of microcystic meningioma in almost all cases, at least focally (27) (Figure 9-11). The vast majority of angiomatous meningiomas are grade I. Like secretory meningiomas, angiomatous ones are also associated with exaggerated peritumoral edema (28).

Theoretically, in the rare instance of an angiomatous meningioma in the posterior fossa, one could mistake a microvascular angiomatous meningioma with microcystic change for a hemangioblastoma. A dural-based location on imaging would heavily favor the former, as would positive immunostaining for somatostatin receptor 2A (SSTR2A), EMA, or progesterone receptors, and no inhibin immunostaining.

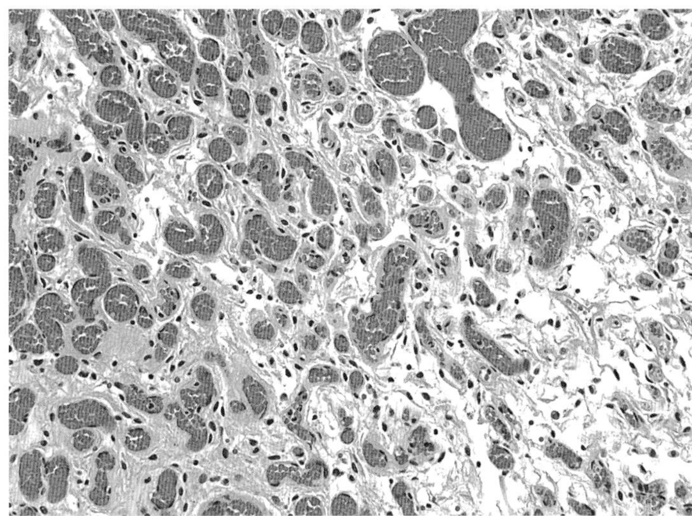

FIGURE 9-11 Angiomatous meningioma with striking vascularity and intervening microcystic cells (microvascular pattern).

MICROCYSTIC. Microcystic meningioma is most notable for not resembling the other members of the meningioma group. Although microcystic change is common focally in meningiomas of other patterns, some cases express it diffusely, creating diagnostic confusion for the pathologist expecting whorls and regular oval nuclei. In contrast to other subtypes, microcystic meningioma has large cells with clear cytoplasm formed from large vacuoles separated by cobweb-like strands (Figure 9-12). The cytoplasmic vacuoles in this lesion

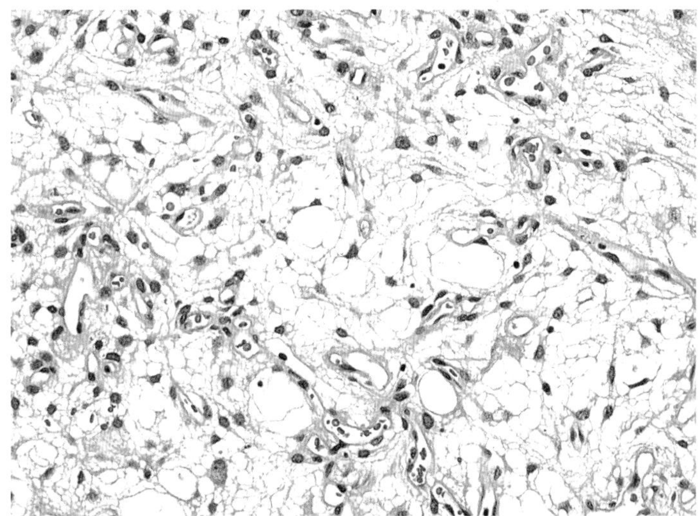

FIGURE 9-12 Microcystic meningiomas typically exhibit variably sized cells containing clear cytoplasm, "cobweb-like" vacuolization, and degenerative nuclear atypia.

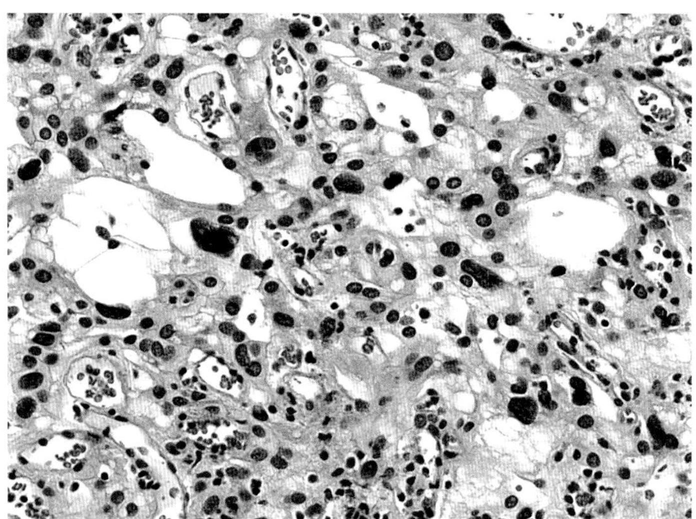

FIGURE 9-13 Degenerative nuclear atypia is common in microcystic and angiomatous meningiomas and is prognostically unimportant.

vary greatly in size, lacking the regularity of those usually seen in renal clear cell carcinoma or hemangioblastoma, with single large vacuoles sometimes occupying the entire cytoplasm. Nuclei in microcystic meningioma are prone to degenerative atypia, becoming hyperchromatic, irregular, and variable in size, ranging from small to gigantic (Figure 9-13). Some of the meningioma characteristics that microcystic lesions retain are hyalinized blood vessels and thick collagen bands, either of which can be diagnostically helpful. Nuclear pseudoinclusions are also retained. Although the cytoplasm of microcystic meningioma is clear, or nearly so, this generally indolent grade I pattern should not be mistaken for the grade II clear cell meningioma. Microcystic meningioma can occur as a purely intraosseous lesion and can be mistaken clinically for metastasis (29).

SECRETORY. The defining feature of this meningioma pattern is the "pseudopsammoma body," which is an intracellular, eosinophilic, spherical cytoplasmic inclusion that occurs in scattered cells within an otherwise usual meningioma (Figure 9-14). These structures are periodic acid-Schiff (PAS)-positive and immunoreactive for cytokeratins and carcinoembryonic antigen (CEA) (30). Secretory meningiomas usually also contain mast cell infiltrates. Although overwhelmingly benign, these lesions may have a higher rate of postoperative complication due to severe peritumoral edema. About 35% of patients with secretory meningiomas in one series had severe peritumoral edema that persisted after excision, and over a third of these patients required mechanical ventilation and intracranial pressure monitoring (31).

In a recent series, mutations in two genes, *KLF4* and *TRAF7*, were both present in nearly all tested cases of secretory meningioma and were not found together in a large group of meningiomas of other patterns,

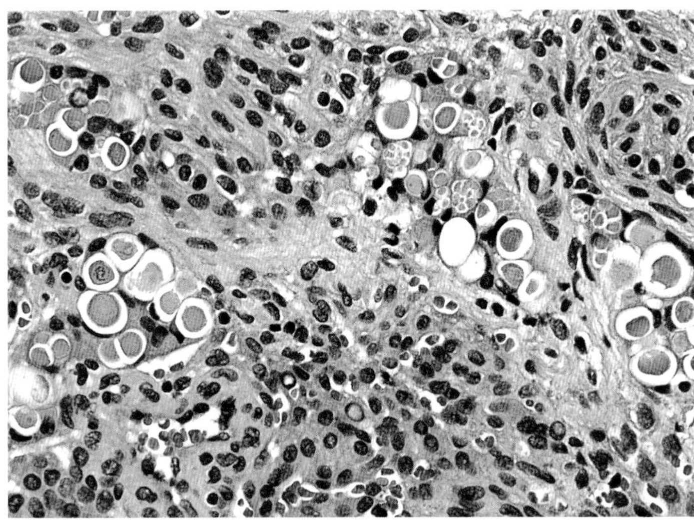

FIGURE 9-14 The distinctive secretory bodies of secretory meningioma are periodic acid-Schiff–positive and immunoreactive for cytokeratin and carcinoembryonic antigen, causing potential for confusion with carcinoma.

other brain tumors, metastatic tumors, or a small set of tumors from other organs, although isolated *TRAF7* mutations were found in a few other meningiomas. *KLF4* is more restricted to secretory meningiomas and has only shown one hotspot mutation in that context, K409Q. These mutations appear to be mutually exclusive with mutations in *NF2*, which are the most common genetic finding in meningiomas overall, suggesting that secretory meningiomas arise through a related but separate pathway from most others (32).

LYMPHOPLASMACYTE RICH. This rare class of meningiomas has not been studied in great numbers, the largest series being 19 cases, and remains controversial as a distinct pathologic entity (33). A dense, sometimes overwhelming, lymphoplasmacytic infiltrate crowds, and sometimes conceals, the native tumor cells (Figure 9-15). Plasma cells in these lesions frequently contain Russell bodies. Some patients with this lesion have had a polyclonal hypergammaglobulinemia (33–35). No evidence suggests that the lymphoplasmacytic infiltrate is neoplastic. An examination of 16 cases showed that plasma cells make up a minor component of the inflammation and generally don't express IgG4. That work also found that the predominant inflammatory cell type was macrophages and recommended the term "inflammation-rich meningioma" as a more accurate term (36). Immunostaining for SSTR2A might sometimes be useful to demonstrate the meningothelial component of this lesion. EMA immunostaining would label both tumor cells and plasma cells. Dural lesions that could possibly be confused with this entity include low-grade lymphoma, sarcoidosis, Rosai–Dorfman disease, Castleman disease, Langerhans histiocytosis, idiopathic pachymeningitis, and "plasma cell granuloma."

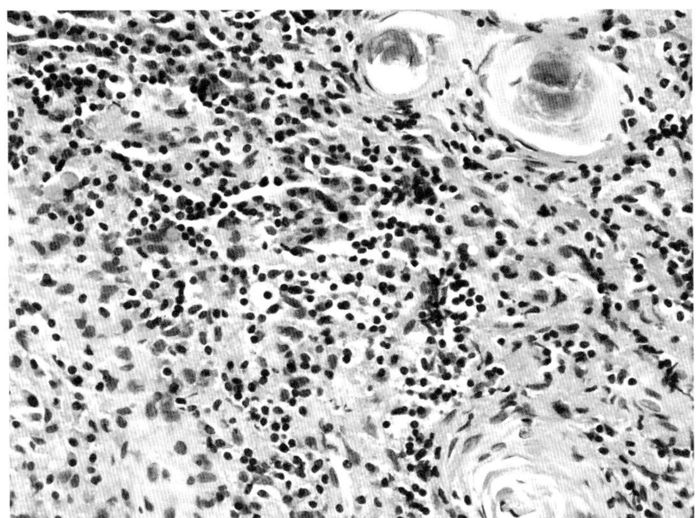

FIGURE 9-15 The rare lymphoplasmacyte-rich meningioma can be obscured by inflammatory cells and raise a long differential diagnosis of inflammatory lesions and lymphomas.

METAPLASTIC. Mesenchymal tissue including bone and cartilage can develop within otherwise regular meningiomas. Although still generally considered a part of metaplastic meningiomas, evidence suggests that those with apparent adipose metaplasia (Figure 9-16) may result from lipidization of tumor cells (37,38). The term metaplastic has been applied to meningiomas with a prominent myxoid background into which tumor cells are singly dispersed, a description that overlaps significantly with that

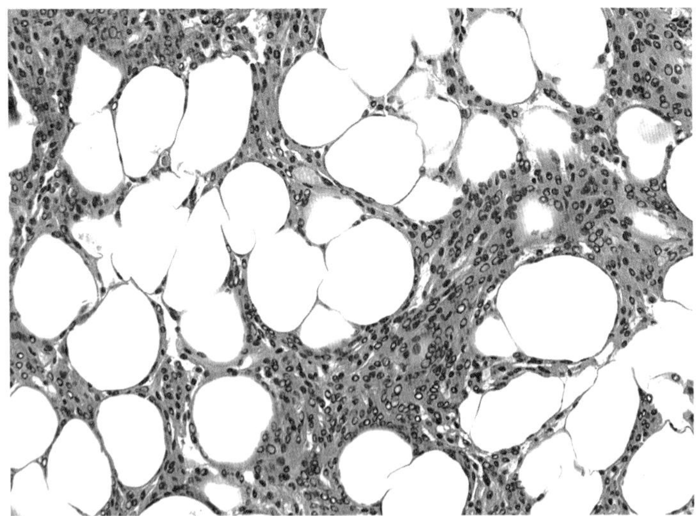

FIGURE 9-16 Lipidized tumor cells give the appearance of metaplastic adipose tissue in some meningiomas.

TABLE 9-1 Summary of World Health Organization 2016 Meningioma Grading Scheme

Grade I	Grade II	Grade III
0–3 mitoses/10 hpf Two or fewer atypical histologic features	4–19 mitoses/10 hpf OR Three or more of necrosis, macronucleoli, loss of architecture, small cell change, or hypercellularity OR Brain invasion OR Clear cell or chordoid pattern	≥20 mitoses/10 hpf OR Papillary or rhabdoid pattern OR Otherwise overtly sarcoma- or carcinoma-like

of chordoid meningioma. Although the vast majority of metaplastic meningiomas are grade I, metaplasia has also been described rarely in malignant meningiomas (39).

WHO GRADE II MENINGIOMAS. WHO grade II meningiomas have an increased rate of recurrence and tumor-associated mortality compared with WHO grade I meningiomas. In addition to the chordoid and clear cell patterns that automatically earn grade II status, there are three other avenues by which this grade can be achieved: increased mitotic count, a total of three or more atypical histologic features, or brain invasion (17,18) (Table 9-1). Atypia of mitotic figures, pleomorphism, and nuclear atypia do not predict the behavior of meningiomas and are not components of their grading. About 15% to 20% of all meningiomas are grade II.

ATYPICAL MENINGIOMA. Atypical meningiomas, WHO grade II, may be diagnosed by two sets of histologic criteria: (1) mitotic rate; or (2) a combination of three or more histologic features of atypia. In meningiomas, an elevated mitotic count is defined as a rate of 4 or more mitoses in 10 contiguous 400× fields, in the area of greatest mitotic activity in the examined tissue. Twenty or more mitoses elevate the neoplasm to grade III. Although not part of the meningioma grading scheme itself, a MIB1 immunostain is helpful in finding the area of maximal proliferation. Examining contiguous fields within the area of greatest proliferation is not specifically suggested in the WHO manual but recapitulates the methodology used in the articles that established these criteria (17,18).

There are five histologic features that indicate increased aggressiveness of meningiomas, even when the mitotic rate is lower than that required for atypical status: necrosis, loss of architecture, hypercellularity, macronucleoli,

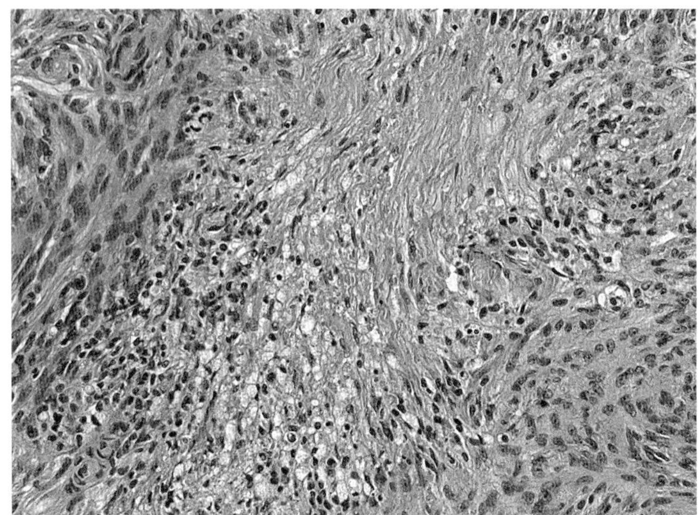

FIGURE 9-17 Necrosis and loss of architecture are two atypical features in this image of an atypical meningioma, World Health Organization grade II.

and high nucleus to cytoplasm ratio (small cell formation) (Figures 9-17 to 9-19). If three or more of these features are identified in a lesion, in any amount, the lesion meets criteria for "atypical meningioma, WHO grade II" according to the 2016 classification (40). Necrosis can be multifocal or geographic throughout a lesion and need not be in a particular pattern or amount. That is, any necrosis counts, as long as it is spontaneous. Widespread necrosis occasionally can be the result of presurgical embolization

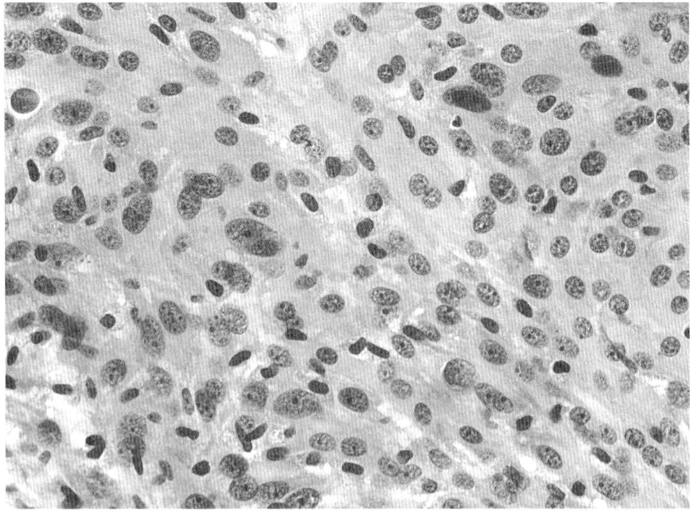

FIGURE 9-18 Macronucleoli indicate increased protein production and a feature of atypical meningiomas.

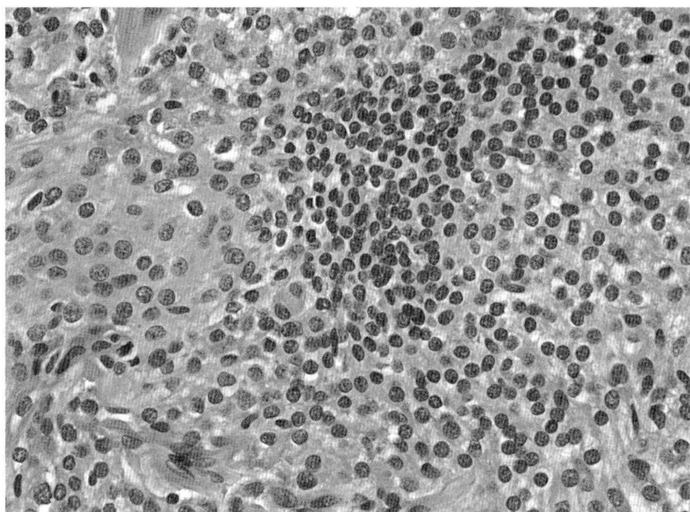

FIGURE 9-19 The atypical feature of small cell change can be mistaken for focal infiltrates of lymphocytes.

of a meningioma, in which case it does not count as an atypical feature (Figure 9-20). Loss of architecture, or "sheetlike" growth pattern, means that the tumor cells lose their whorling or fascicular arrangement and grow in a homogeneous, patternless fashion. Hypercellularity has been quantified as 53 or more nuclei per high-power field (hpf) diameter (18) but can be evaluated subjectively in most cases. Small cell formation typically

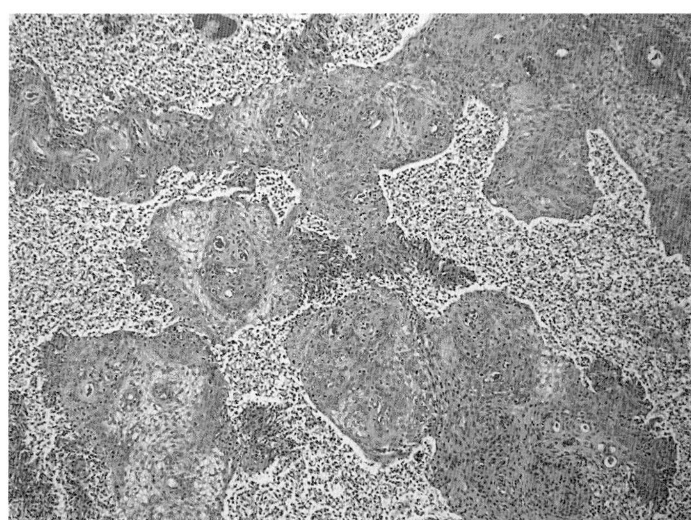

FIGURE 9-20 Preoperative embolization of meningiomas may result in extensive necrosis and prevent that from being used as a grading criterion.

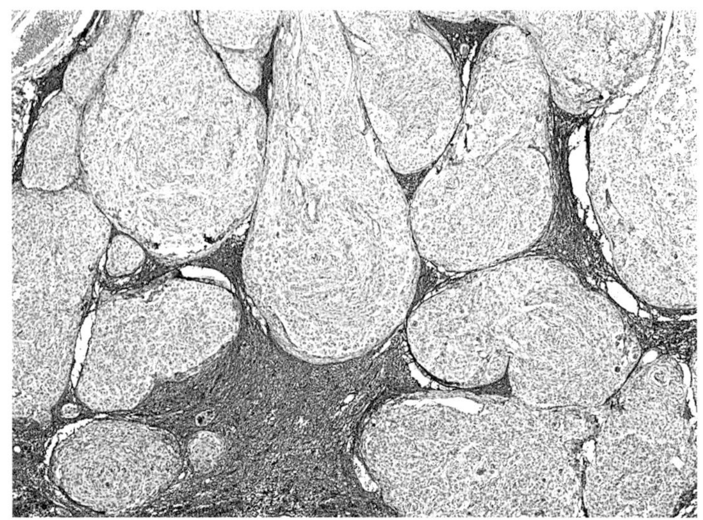

FIGURE 9-21 Glial fibrillary acidic protein immunohistochemistry highlights brain invasion that can be difficult to recognize on hematoxylin and eosin stain.

occurs as multifocal aggregates of very small tumor cells with round nuclei and scant cytoplasm that resemble lymphocytes.

Brain invasion is associated with increased recurrence and by itself justifies a diagnosis of atypical meningioma (18). Invasion usually manifests as tongue-like projections of tumor into the underlying cerebral cortex. Sometimes invasion can be subtle, but an immunostain for glial fibrillary acidic protein (GFAP) will highlight any areas of entrapped neural tissue (Figure 9-21). Any time adherent brain tissue or an irregular, scalloped edge is identified, it should trigger a closer look for invasion and possibly immunostaining for GFAP. Some meningiomas show fragments of brain adherent to the tumor surface, perhaps indicating early invasion into the pia mater, but show no invasion into the brain itself. The significance of this finding is not understood at present but may also increase the likelihood of recurrence.

CLEAR CELL MENINGIOMA. This pattern is characterized by polygonal cells with small round nuclei and abundant clear cytoplasm distributed in a background of dense stromal and perivascular hyalinization (Figure 9-22). This unusual pattern of meningioma has several tendencies that diverge from traditional meningiomas and can present diagnostic challenges. They usually lack typical meningothelial features (whorls, oval nuclei, psammoma bodies), or other patterns of meningioma, and occur in unusual locations (cerebellopontine angle and cauda equina) in younger patients (41,42). The clear cytoplasm in the tumor cells results from massive accumulation of glycogen, which is strongly PAS-positive and sensitive to diastase (Figure 9-23). As with other meningiomas, those with a clear cell

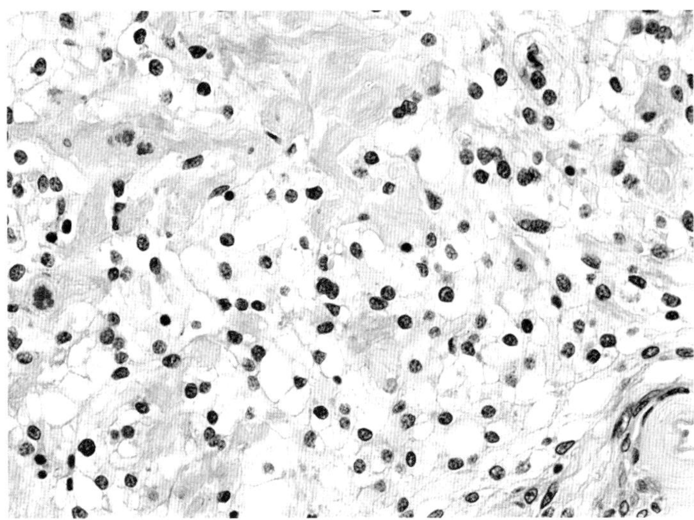

FIGURE 9-22 Clear cell meningiomas (World Health Organization grade II) have a monotonous population of clear cells with small round nuclei, with strands of collagen scattered throughout.

pattern show immunohistochemical reactivity for EMA and vimentin. Clear cell meningiomas are clinically more aggressive and can disseminate throughout the CNS, justifying their categorization as WHO grade II tumors (42). Fortunately, the radiologic appearance of clear cell meningiomas does not differ from those of other meningiomas, improving chances that this unusual pattern will not elude correct diagnosis.

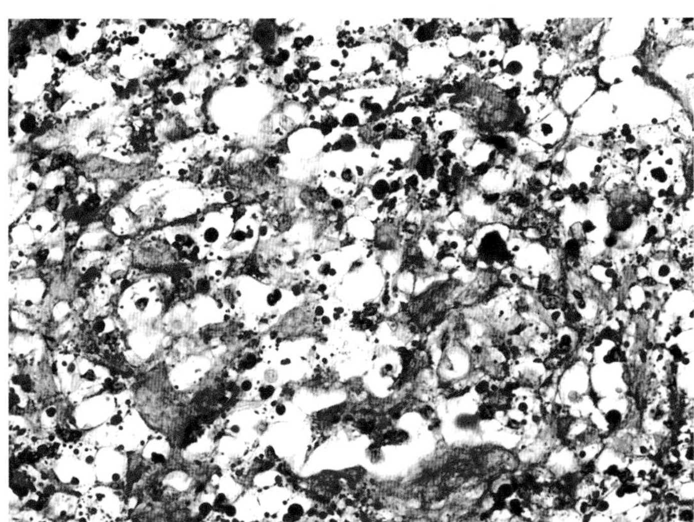

FIGURE 9-23 Periodic acid-Schiff–positive (diastase-labile) granules fill the cytoplasm in clear cell meningioma.

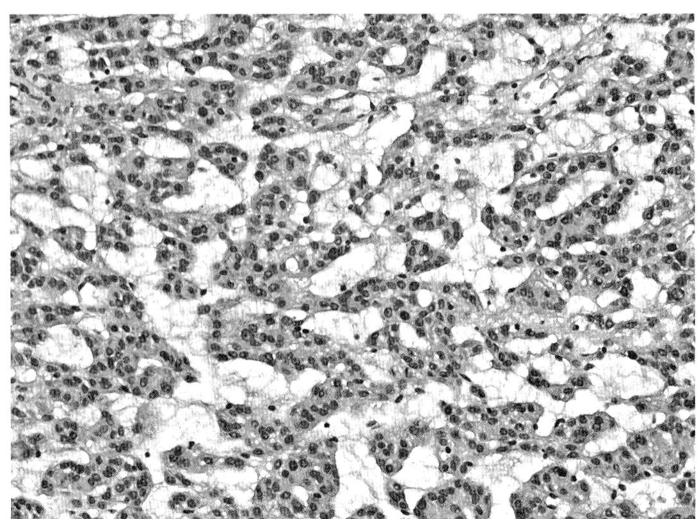

FIGURE 9-24 Chordoid meningiomas (World Health Organization grade II) are composed of cords, nests, and single cells in a basophilic matrix of myxoid material.

In addition to having a unique clinical context, arising in the cerebellopontine angle and cauda equina in younger patients, clear cell meningiomas also have a distinct genetic background, frequently developing in the context of germline *SMARCE1* mutations (43). Whether in the context of a known germline mutation or not, every case in a series of 15 exhibited loss of *SMARCE1* immunostaining, whereas other meningiomas and clear cell tumors did not, suggesting that loss of *SMARCE1* function is a critical event clear cell meningioma development (44). Because of the inherited nature of at least some of the *SMARCE1* mutations in these tumors, it is important to inform the treating clinician of this association for potential testing of the patient and family members, if indicated.

CHORDOID MENINGIOMA. The distinguishing features of chordoid meningiomas are nests and cords of meningothelial tumor cells in a background of baso- or amphophilic mucoid substance (Figure 9-24). This morphology is associated with a higher rate of recurrence than standard meningiomas and warrants its categorization as WHO grade II. As with other patterns, half of the tumor must have this appearance to be labeled "chordoid meningioma," an important concept because the pattern commonly occurs focally in nonchordoid meningiomas.

WHO GRADE III MENINGIOMAS

ANAPLASTIC MENINGIOMA. According to the 2016 WHO criteria, anaplastic meningioma, grade III, can be diagnosed by one or more of three criteria: (1) 20 or more mitotic figures in 10 contiguous 400× fields; (2) papillary or rhabdoid pattern; or (3) overt carcinomatous or sarcomatous cytology (Figure 9-25). Mitotic rates and histologic patterns represent somewhat

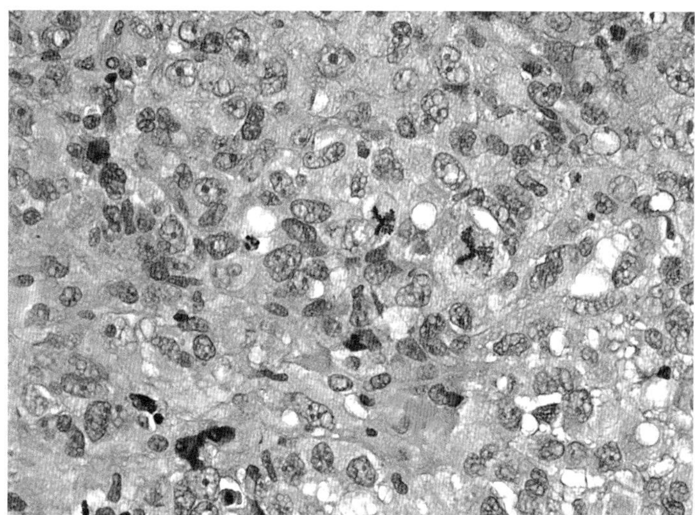

FIGURE 9-25 Anaplastic meningiomas like this tend to grow in a sheetlike pattern and are highly mitotically active, taking on the appearance of a poorly differentiated carcinoma.

objective and reproducible diagnostic criteria, but very rarely a meningioma may display a frankly malignant morphology that does not technically meet the other criteria for anaplasia. In that instance, some discretion is left to the pathologist to judge whether a meningioma is best categorized as anaplastic or atypical. Anaplastic or grade III status can be applied to only about 1% to 2% of all meningiomas. Anaplastic meningiomas are usually fatal and have a median overall survival of about 2.5 to 3 years (45,46).

PAPILLARY MENINGIOMA. This pattern of meningioma is composed of cells similar to other meningiomas; however, rather than being arranged in whorls and small sheets, the tumor cells radiate from blood vessels in a "peritheliomatous" architecture, giving them an appearance of free-floating perivascular pseudopapillae (Figure 9-26). This appearance is thought to result from dehiscence of the cells farther from the blood vessels in zones of incipient necrosis, similar to peritheliomatous metastatic lesions.

RHABDOID MENINGIOMA. This aggressive pattern of meningioma is characterized by its unique cytologic appearance, with eccentric, lightly eosinophilic, round, cytoplasmic inclusions that compress the nucleus against the plasma membrane, which is, unlike most meningiomas, distinct from that of its neighbors' (Figure 9-27). The inclusions, as in other rhabdoid tumors, are composed of whorled aggregates of intermediate filaments, sometimes containing organelles (47). Rhabdoid cells can be seen focally in meningiomas of lower grades; however, unless the rhabdoid cells constitute half or more of the lesion, it does not meet WHO 2016 criteria for the diagnosis of "rhabdoid meningioma." In many of the reported cases, a rhabdoid morphology occurs at the time of reresection of a more typical appearing meningioma (47).

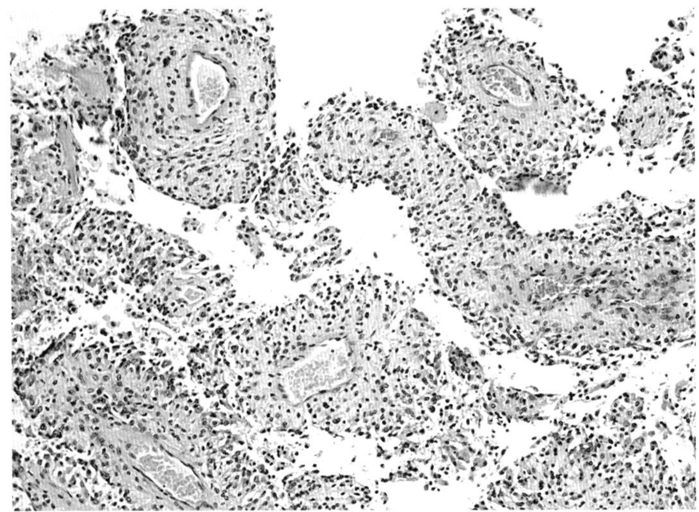

FIGURE 9-26 The fibrovascular cores of papillary meningioma (World Health Organization grade III) dehisce and create the appearance of floating freely.

Although rhabdoid pattern is, in itself, sufficient for a grade III designation, meningiomas with rhabdoid pattern often occur in a setting of other histologic parameters that can independently qualify a lesion as grade II or III.

Genetics

The most common genetic features in meningiomas are monosomy of chromosome 22 and mutations in NF2, frequently in combination, occurring in

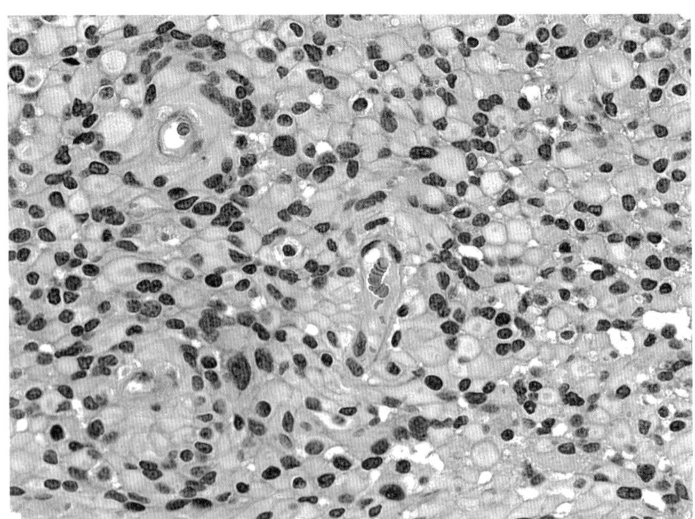

FIGURE 9-27 Rhabdoid meningioma (World Health Organization grade III) loses its syncytial appearance and develops eccentric eosinophilic cytoplasm.

a majority of cases. Other chromosomal abnormalities include losses of 1p, 6q, 9p, 10, 14q and 18q, all as elements of progression (48). In general, as meningiomas increase in grade, they have more chromosomal abnormalities, which form the basis of a proposed cytogenetic system for scoring risk based on the number of changes present (49). Similar to increasing grades of infiltrating gliomas, higher-grade meningiomas gain mutations in the promoter for the *hTERT* gene, causing overexpression and increased proliferation potential (50). Another proposed system for grading and classifying meningiomas is based on DNA methylation profiling and may take on more importance in the future (51).

Differential Diagnosis

The distinction between meningioma and other intracranial tumors is not usually an issue, given its vast majority among dural lesions and generally characteristic histology, but in some cases the location and/or unusual pattern may lead to incorrect diagnosis.

In the cerebellopontine angle and spinal cord, fibrous meningiomas, with their fascicular architecture, hyalinized vessels, and long fibroblast-like nuclei, can have considerable morphologic overlap with schwannomas. Review of the surgical and radiologic reports may help clarify the association between the lesion and the dura, or the eighth cranial nerve. The presence of psammoma bodies virtually rules out schwannoma, although they are frequently absent from meningiomas of the fibrous pattern. Meningiomas will display immunoreactivity for SSTR2A, EMA, and S100 protein (weak), whereas schwannomas lack SSTR2A and EMA staining and show strong and diffuse positivity for S100.

Differentiating anaplastic meningioma from a metastatic malignancy can sometimes be impossible by routine histology and immunohistochemistry. The most common diagnostic decision is between an anaplastic meningioma and a metastatic carcinoma, two lesions that can appear radiologically and microscopically similar, and, as the lesions become more poorly differentiated, express more confusing and overlapping antigen profiles. Strong vimentin positivity is seen in meningiomas, and its expression tends to be retained through tumor progression, whereas progesterone receptor and EMA staining are often lost. SSTR2A is expressed in nearly all meningiomas (Figure 9-28), even those of high grade, and is not expressed by most carcinomas (49), neuroendocrine ones being the exceptions (52), a possibility easily evaluated by staining for synaptophysin. Carcinomas should have strong and diffuse staining for a pancytokeratin, but many anaplastic meningiomas can also strongly express cytokeratins, though usually more focally. Myriad additional epithelial markers can be attempted, such as CEA, Ber-EP4, CD15, and B72.3, all of which should be positive in carcinoma and negative in meningioma, but not one of them is completely reliable (53).

Until the advent of clinical electron microscopy, meningeal solitary fibrous tumors (mSFTs), formerly hemangiopericytomas, were classified as

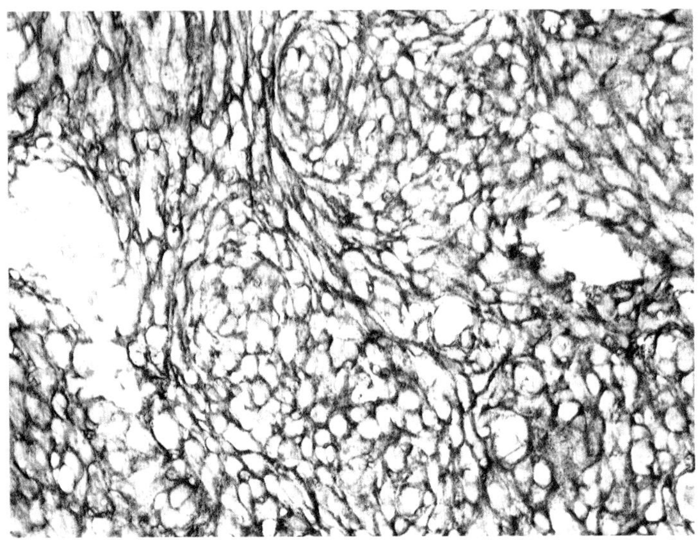

FIGURE 9-28 Immunostaining for somatostatin receptor 2A shows strong cytoplasmic reactivity in almost all meningiomas, even those of high grade.

"angioblastic meningiomas," reflecting the clinical and histologic overlap between them and meningiomas. Discriminating between SFTs and meningioma pathologically may seem trivial on the surface, but it is extremely important because of the more aggressive nature of SFTs. SFTs tend to be more hypercellular than even atypical meningiomas and are more cytologically uniform, with cells that show nuclear grooves and sometimes a degree of nuclear molding. A "staghorn" pattern of vascular channels, if present, is reasonably reliable for differentiating mSFT from meningioma, although ectatic vascular channels in meningiomas can sometimes give an appearance of staghorn shape. Fortunately, immunostaining for SSTR2A and STAT6 can reliably distinguish between meningioma and SFT. Meningiomas should immunostain for EMA, weakly for S100, and claudin-1, whereas mSFTs are negative for these markers and show some reactivity for CD34. Reticulin staining can be very helpful in demonstrating the fine network of intercellular reticulin that envelops individual SFT cells.

Not surprisingly, the tumors in the differential diagnosis with chordoid meningioma are those that also have a chordoid appearance. Although a single case of chordoid meningioma has been described within the third ventricle (54), chordoid glioma should generally take a low place on one's list of suspicions for a dura-based mass, because it almost always occurs in the anterior third ventricle. Chordomas can be differentiated by their immunoreactivity for keratins and for the notochord-specific transcription factor brachyury. Low-grade chondrosarcoma can take on a chordoid appearance but is distinguished by its individual cells separated by basophilic stroma and lack of nests and cords of tumor cells. Extraskeletal mesenchymal chondrosarcoma, long ago called "chordoid sarcoma," may simulate chordoid meningioma, but its occurrence within the CNS is rare. The diagnosis of extraskeletal myxoid chondrosarcoma is most appropriately confirmed with molecular studies for the characteristic t(9;22)(q22;q12) translocation. In difficult cases, radiologic data can provide helpful clues to the nature of the lesion. For a more complete review of the immunohistochemistry of chordoid meningiomas and similar appearing lesions, see Sangoi et al. (55).

Rhabdoid meningiomas display eccentric eosinophilic cytoplasm and sharply defined cell borders that could lead them to be confused with several other entities, including metastatic carcinoma, atypical teratoid rhabdoid tumor (AT/RT), and gemistocytic astrocytoma. Age and radiologic appearance will, in almost all cases, prevent confusion with the latter two, with AT/RT occurring largely in infants and gemistocytic astrocytomas being intra-axial and much less circumscribed. That most AT/RTs lack significant rhabdoid elements is also helpful. Metastatic carcinoma, which can be radiologically very similar to meningioma, is usually much less uniform than rhabdoid meningioma and usually can be ruled out with negative keratin staining.

The prominent collagenous background and singly dispersed cells of clear cell meningioma should distinguish it from metastatic renal clear cell carcinoma, which is not usually very collagenized and mostly grows in an "organoid" pattern of cell clusters separated by vascular channels (Figure 9-29). If the question arises, cytokeratin staining identifies the

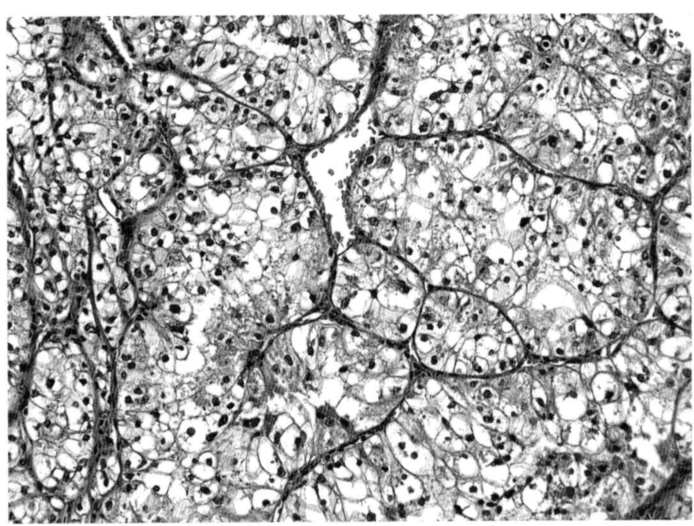

FIGURE 9-29 Metastatic renal clear cell carcinoma shows organoid architecture and a lack of hyalinized blood vessels.

metastatic renal cell carcinoma. Microcystic meningiomas also have clear cytoplasm, although the cells vary in size, have cobweb-like cytoplasmic vacuolization, and frequently have degenerative nuclear atypia. To support a diagnosis of clear cell meningioma, one may look for abundant coarse and variably sized cytoplasmic granules of diastase-labile PAS-positive material. Sequencing for *SMARCE1* mutations or staining for loss of expression can also reliably identify clear cell meningiomas.

Rarely, a reactive proliferation of meningothelial cells will grow large enough to warrant suspicion of neoplasm, classically around the edges of an optic nerve glioma. Knowledge of this phenomenon is the probably most effective way to prevent diagnosing it as meningioma. Corroborative testing might include looking for monosomy 22, as no immunostains are known to label only one and not the other. Even progesterone receptors, which are present in meningiomas and not seen in normal, quiescent meningothelial cells, are expressed in meningothelial hyperplasia (56).

MENINGIOANGIOMATOSIS

Clinical Context

This uncommon and enigmatic hamartomatous lesion is diagnosed mostly in children and young adults, with a mean age around 19 years at diagnosis. Men represent more cases in the literature than do women, surpassing them at a ratio of 2:1 in sporadic cases (57), although the ratio is even when occurring in the context of NF2. Although patients with NF2 are at a higher risk for this lesion, they make up less than 20% of the cases reported (57,58). Compared with sporadic cases, those with NF2 present earlier, are more likely to have multiple lesions, and almost always present incidentally without seizures. A majority of sporadic cases present with complex or simple partial seizures.

On imaging, both classes of meningioangiomatosis show a cerebral cortical lesion in the temporal or frontal lobe, although cases have been described throughout the CNS. CT shows a calcified lesion with a corona of hypodensity, whereas MRI displays a T1- and T2-hypointense lesion with surrounding T2 brightness (59). The lesions are plaque-like, firm, white, and circumscribed and characteristically widen the affected gyrus and, when resected, are found not to attach to the dura. Meningiomas, vascular anomalies, and other lesions have occurred in conjunction with meningioangiomatosis but represent a minority of cases. Simple excision permanently cures most cases and usually mitigates or eliminates associated seizures.

Histopathology

Cortical neuropil is perforated by uniform hyalinized small-caliber blood vessels coated with thin proliferations of meningothelial and fibroblastic

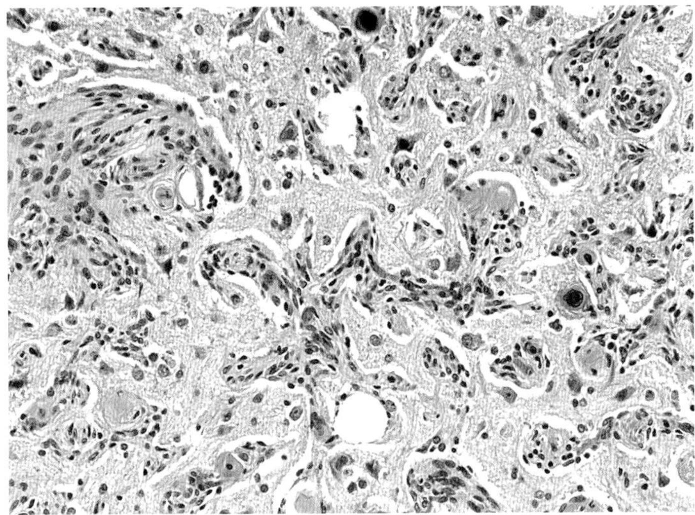

FIGURE 9-30 Meningioangiomatosis showing penetration of cortex by numerous vascular channels and nests of meningothelial cells.

spindle-shaped cells that occasionally contain psammoma bodies and whorls (Figure 9-30). The cellular component may not be prominent, leaving only the hyalinized vessels (Figure 9-31). Neurons and glia are entrapped among the vessels and can show reactive changes, commonly including tau-positive neurofibrillary tangles within neurons (60). Immunohistochemistry is not helpful in the identification of this lesion because

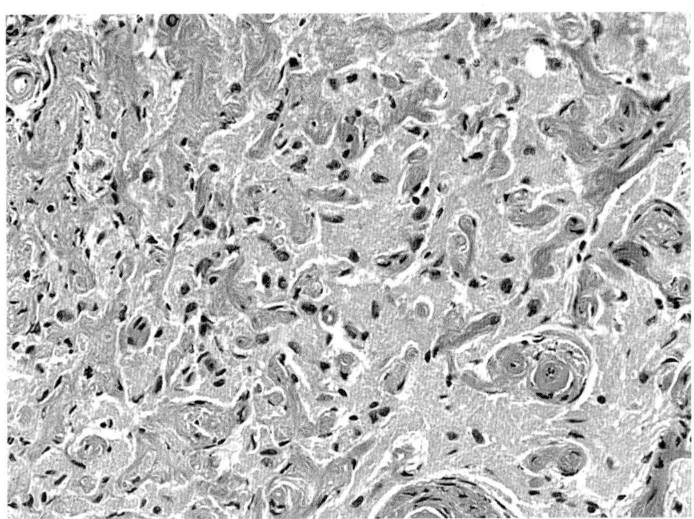

FIGURE 9-31 Some cases of meningioangiomatosis are paucicellular and show few meningothelial-like cells.

the component cells do not typically express EMA as meningiomas do. MIB-1 positivity should be less than 1%.

INTRACRANIAL SOLITARY FIBROUS TUMOR (FORMERLY HEMANGIOPERICYTOMA) (WHO GRADES I TO III)

Now recognized to be a single tumor entity with a spectrum of histologic findings and clinical aggressiveness, SFT encompasses what was formerly known as hemangiopericytoma. Instead of giving the different histologic patterns different names, we now give them different grades. WHO grade I cases correspond to what were always called SFT, and WHO grades II and III correspond to what were formerly called hemangiopericytoma and anaplastic hemangiopericytoma, respectively. Most intracranial cases are grade II.

Clinical Context

This uncommon tumor, when it occurs in the CNS, usually arises from the meninges, although intracerebral and intraventricular cases have been reported. Patients develop meningeal SFT (mSFT) at a mean age of around 40 to 50 years, which is somewhat younger than the average for meningiomas (61–67).

Most mSFTs are thought to be meningiomas prior to resection because of their similar radiologic appearance, characterized by a broad dural base, T1-isointensity to cortex, variable T2 intensity, avid uniform contrast enhancement, and peritumoral edema (68,69). Unlike meningiomas, mSFTs typically lack calcification on CT and tend to show osteolysis rather than hyperostosis (68,69). Angiography, which is not frequently attempted because a meningioma is suspected, can help to raise the suspicion for mSFT preoperatively (70).

In contrast to meningiomas, mSFTs are more likely to be WHO grade II or grade III, with grade I cases being relatively uncommon. Although the grades for mSFT compare with those of meningiomas, their rates of recurrence and mortality are, grade for grade, higher (62). Unlike most other CNS tumors, grades II and III mSFTs have a tendency to metastasize out of the CNS to other organs, mostly lung, liver, and bone, which commonly leads to death within 2 years (62). Treatment of grades II and III mSFTs with postoperative radiotherapy may reduce recurrence and mortality, but these findings have yet to be confirmed by larger prospective series (61,62). A series of 38 patients showed a 93% 5-year survival rate with postoperative radiotherapy, suggesting that prognosis for higher-grade mSFTs is improving with more aggressive therapy (71–74).

Histopathology

SFTs outside of the CNS are classed into benign and malignant based on the presence of mitotic activity (≥5/10 hpf), hypercellularity, and necrosis. However, it has been demonstrated the mSFTs with a “hemangiopericytoma”

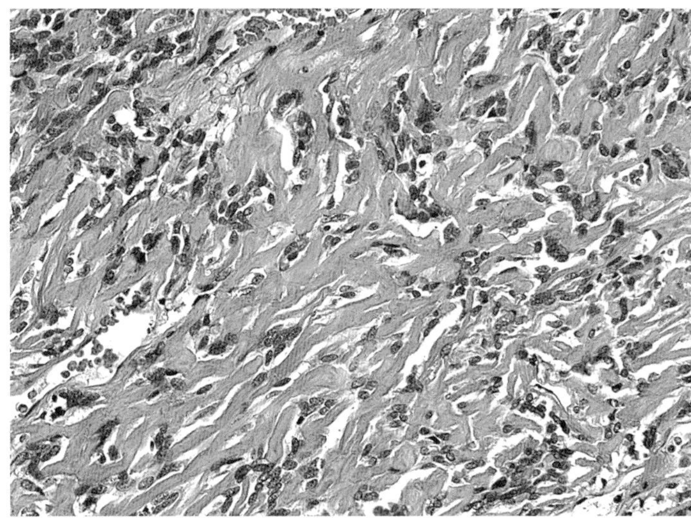

FIGURE 9-32 Solitary fibrous tumor is a generally patternless growth of elongate cells in a dense fibrous stroma.

histologic pattern and fewer mitotic figures than 5/10 hpf (WHO grade II) have a higher rate of recurrence and metastasis and benefit from radiotherapy, so it would be a disservice to the patients to discontinue grading mSFTs on three tiers (40,72–74).

Grade I mSFTs are densely collagenized lesions composed of thick paucicellular fascicles with elongate spindle-shaped cells (Figure 9-32). "Staghorn" vascular channels are common. The nuclei range from thin and wavy to oval and regular. SFT contains no whorls or psammoma bodies but can have focal areas of increased cellularity. Distinction from fibrous meningioma can be difficult on purely morphologic grounds, but applying immunohistochemistry for STAT6 will reveal nuclear staining in only SFT, not meningioma. SFTs also exhibit diffuse CD34 staining, with no immunoreactivity for SSTR1A, EMA, or S100 (65). Grade I mSFTs also have stronger and more diffuse CD34 and Bcl-2 immunostaining than higher-grade cases (66).

Grade II mSFT corresponds to what was formerly "hemangiopericytoma" which is characterized by dense cellularity with haphazardly oriented, monotonous, oval to elongate cells and "staghorn" vascular channels (Figures 9-33 and 9-34). The vascular channels are sometimes surrounded by a thin rim of collagen, or may create small intervening clusters out of tumor cells, giving at least a vague impression of meningothelial whorls. The lining of the vascular spaces is generally flattened, nonproliferating endothelial cells. The cytoplasm is minimal and is not bounded by obvious cell borders, giving a syncytial appearance. The nuclei are oval to elongate with more compact chromatin and less apparent nucleoli than meningiomas and do not show intranuclear pseudoinclusions. The grooves or folds in the

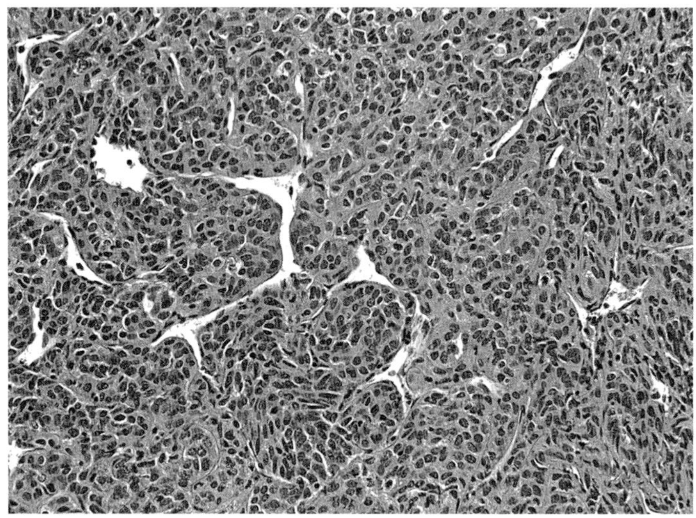

FIGURE 9-33 The hemangiopericytoma pattern of meningeal solitary fibrous tumor (WHO grade II) is densely cellular with "staghorn" vascular channels and a vaguely lobulated arrangement of cells.

nuclear membrane noted in some grade II mSFTs are less common in meningiomas. Avascular band of collagen, psammoma bodies, and tight concentric whorls is not present, helping to winnow meningioma from the differential diagnosis. A dense network of fine collagen fibrils invests the individual cells of mSFTs and is readily apparent on reticulin staining, a feature lacking in meningioma (Figure 9-35).

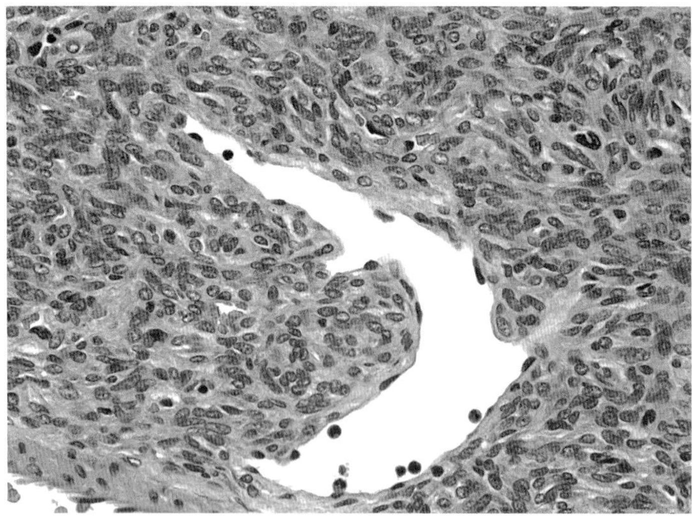

FIGURE 9-34 Like meningiomas, the cells of the hemangiopericytoma pattern of meningeal solitary fibrous tumor (WHO grade II) are syncytial and monomorphic.

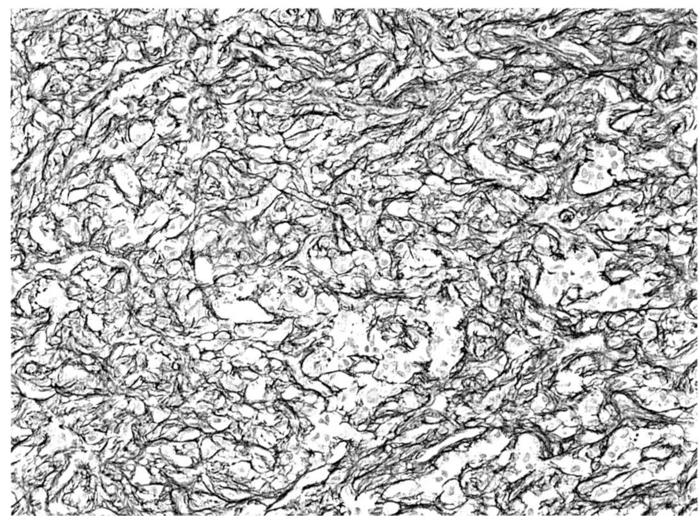

FIGURE 9-35 The dense network of intercellular reticulin in hemangiopericytomas is not seen in meningiomas.

WHO grade III is achieved when the mSFT shows 5 or more mitoses per 10 hpf, often, but not necessarily, in the context of moderate to high cellularity and necrosis. This grading scheme is based on that proposed by Mena et al. (63). Immunohistochemical markers of proliferation have not proven useful for predicting the behavior of meningeal hemangiopericytomas (64). Another grading scheme has been proposed that uses mitotic count ≥6/10 hpf as a criterion along with hypercellularity and necrosis (75).

Genetics

Nearly 100% of SFTs have a translocation involving the genes *NAB2* and *STAT6* regardless of histologic findings, resulting in an overexpression of a number of growth-related genes that induce proliferation (76). Although the points of fusion vary from tumor to tumor, the end result from the pathologist's perspective is the same: nuclear overexpression of STAT6 protein (Figure 9-36) that can be detected immunohistochemically as a sensitive and specific marker for SFT (77). Along with mutations in *TP53* and *PDGFRA*, different fusion variants may be associated with more aggressive clinical behavior (78).

MELANOCYTIC NEOPLASMS

General

Melanocytic lesions in the CNS occur in various patterns, from benign to malignant and focal to diffuse, and fundamentally arise in the meninges from meningeal melanocytes. As a category, primary melanocytic neoplasms of the CNS are unusual and account for a fraction of 1% of all

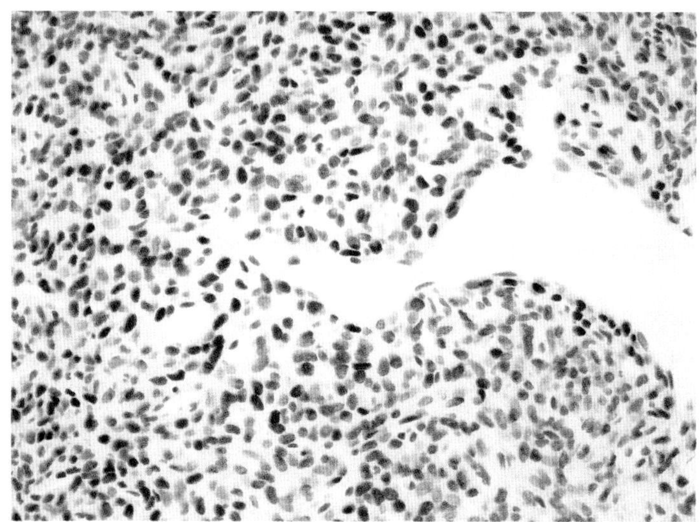

FIGURE 9-36 Strong nuclear immunostaining for STAT6 protein is present in all but a few meningeal solitary fibrous tumors, regardless of grade.

primary intracranial tumors. For practical purposes, these tumors can be grouped into three general categories: melanocytosis, melanocytoma, and primary CNS melanoma.

Clinical Context

MELANOCYTOSIS/MELANOMATOSIS. Melanocytosis almost always occurs in the context of an inherited phakomatosis, neurocutaneous melanosis, which is a syndrome composed of giant or multiple large, hairy, congenital nevi with diffuse meningeal melanocytosis or melanomatosis (79). This condition is usually diagnosed within the first 2 years of life and presents, aside from the nevi, with hydrocephalus, seizures, ataxia, and cranial nerve deficits. No gender or racial predilection exists (79,80). Even in patients with benign CNS melanocytosis, the outlook is grim, with a median survival of less than 3 years from presentation (79). Chemotherapy and radiation fail to significantly alter the course of disease. Most patients with this syndrome have somatic mutations, usually Q61R, in the *NRAS* gene (81), and a few have been noted to have *BRAF* V600E mutations (82). Radiographically, melanocytosis presents with meningeal thickening with bright homogeneous contrast enhancement, T1 hyperintensity due to melanin deposition, and adjacent T2 hyperintensity, probably due to edema (83).

MELANOCYTOMA (AND MELANOCYTIC TUMOR OF INTERMEDIATE GRADE). Middle-aged adults produce most of the reported melanocytomas and melanocytic tumors of intermediate grade (MTIG), with a median age of about 56 years in one review, although the range of ages is wide (84). Women account for slightly more cases than do men, with a female–male ratio similar to that for meningiomas. Melanocytomas present with symptoms similar to those of meningioma. Pigmented examples are identifiable on MRI by their singularly bright intrinsic T1 hyperintensity and T2 hypointensity due to the paramagnetic qualities of melanin (85). The anatomic distribution of these lesions favors the posterior fossa, brainstem, and spinal cord, presumably because the majority of meningeal melanocytes are in these places. Although few cases exist in the literature, survival without recurrence for melanocytomas is typical, even following incomplete resection (84). Too few cases of intermediate-grade melanocytic lesions have been described to accurately assess their prognosis, but they are probably more prone to recurrence. Extent of resection, as with many brain tumors, appears to play a large role in rates of recurrence (86).

MELANOMA. The age and anatomic distribution of CNS melanomas mirrors that of melanocytomas. As with melanomas elsewhere, those primary to the CNS tend to be aggressive and frequently fatal, regardless of their clinical management (84).

Histopathology and Genetics

Melanocytosis is characterized by a monotonous population of cells that can be spindled, oval, or polygonal (79). Tumor cells fill and expand the subarachnoid space and track down the cortical perivascular (Virchow–Robin) spaces, a feature that should not be misidentified as true parenchymal invasion. Nuclear atypia, mitosis, necrosis, large or multiple nucleoli, and invasion of neuropil all signal malignant transformation (Figure 9-37).

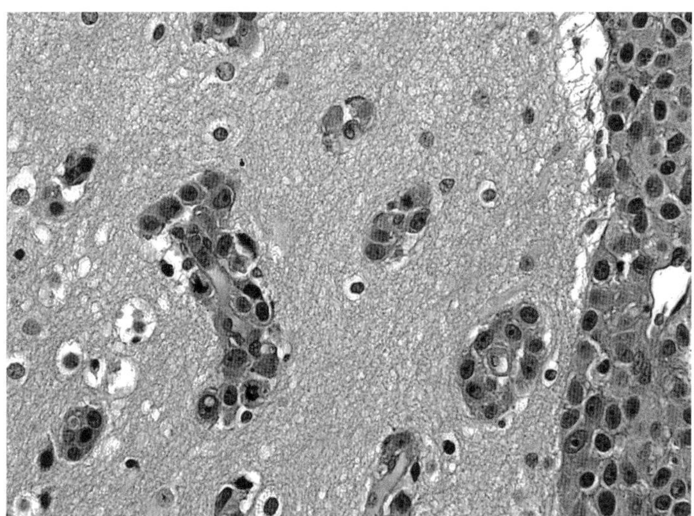

FIGURE 9-37 Mitoses and prominent nucleoli are worrisome in all central nervous system melanocytic tumors and indicate that this case of congenital melanocytosis has progressed to melanoma.

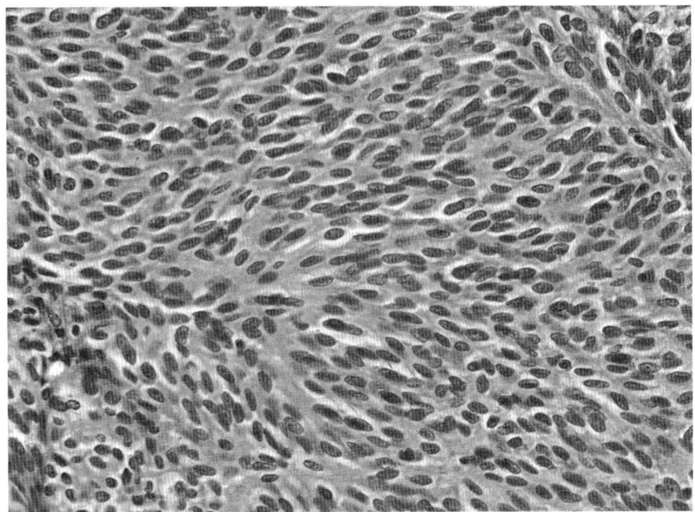

FIGURE 9-38 Melanocytoma with mildly elongate cells in small fascicles and sheets.

Pigment deposition is variable from scant to extremely heavy with numerous melanophages.

Melanocytomas generally contain mildly spindled cells with oval to elongate grooved nuclei that are arranged into small sheets and variably dense clusters (Figure 9-38), although a minority have an epithelioid component (84). Nucleoli should be single and small. Lobular clusters of cells can vaguely mimic the appearance of meningothelial whorls (Figure 9-39). The same histologic features that signify malignancy in melanocytosis

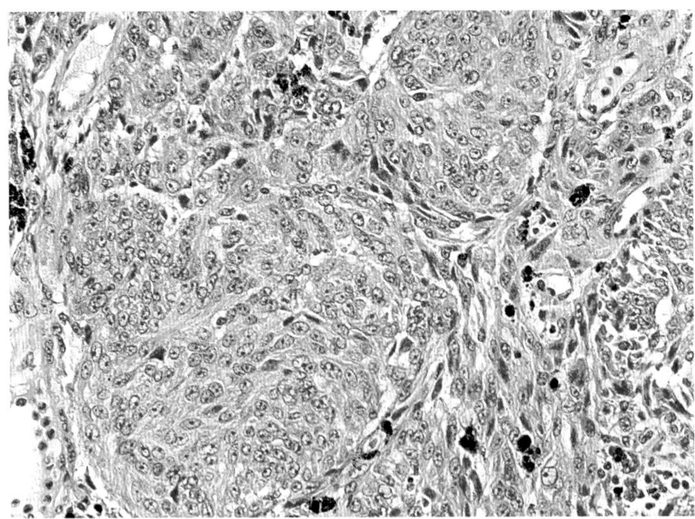

FIGURE 9-39 Vague lobules in melanocytoma may give the impression of meningothelial whorls.

apply to melanocytomas, with occasional (≤1/10 hpf) mitotic figures allowed (84). Because of the relative rarity of CNS melanocytic lesions, no clear boundaries exist between melanocytoma and MTIG, although cases described as such have lacked tight clusters of tumor cells and have shown brain invasion (84).

Genetically, melanocytomas are more similar to melanocytic tumors of the uvea than those of the skin, harboring *GNAQ* and *GNA11* activating mutations rather than mutations in *BRAF*, *HRAS*, and *NRAS* (87,88). Markers of poor prognosis in uveal melanoma have also been found in meningeal melanocytoma, including loss of chromosome 3 and inactivation of BAP1, although the significance of those findings in the CNS is unknown (89).

Primary CNS melanoma resembles its dermal counterpart histopathologically, featuring varying combinations of the above-mentioned traits. With potential occult primary sights, it can be difficult to prove histopathologically that a CNS lesion is not metastatic; however, DNA-based testing can frequently find changes that are more typical of one or the other. Similar to melanocytomas, melanomas of the CNS more resemble uveal examples, harboring activating mutations in the genes *GNAQ* and *GNA11*. Immunohistochemistry in primary CNS melanocytic lesions follows that of extracranial cases, with immunoreactivity for S100, HMB-45, tyrosinase (MART-1), and microphthalmia transcription factor (MITF).

IDIOPATHIC HYPERTROPHIC PACHYMENINGITIS

Hypertrophic pachymeningitis is a thickening of the dura that may be secondary to a number of processes, autoimmune and infectious, and may present as a mass lesion. A few rare cases have presented in absence of any known primary cause and been called "idiopathic hypertrophic pachymeningitis (IHP)," a subset of which has more recently been reported to result from IgG4-related sclerosing disease (90), which should be kept among diagnostic considerations when faced with a sclerotic dural lesion with lymphoplasmacytic infiltrates. This diagnosis remains otherwise one of exclusion.

HEMATOLYMPHOID AND OTHER INFLAMMATORY LESIONS

The meninges occasionally harbor hematologic neoplasms and inflammatory processes that clinically and radiographically mimic meningiomas. These entities usually do not overlap histologically with meningiomas, but they may present a challenge in differentiating them from one another. The following lesions are mentioned here for the sake of differential diagnosis and are discussed in more depth elsewhere: marginal zone B-cell lymphoma ("MALT-oma"), follicular lymphoma, plasmacytoma, Castleman disease, Rosai–Dorfman disease, "plasma cell granuloma," sarcoidosis, tuberculoma, and systemic granulomatous vasculitis.

OTHER MESENCHYMAL LESIONS

Virtually every grade and type of tumor of vascular, fibroblastic, myofibroblastic, skeletal muscle, smooth muscle, adipocytic, nerve sheath, cartilaginous, and osseous differentiation has made at least a cameo appearance in the dura and meninges, but cumulatively they account for far less than 1% of all meningeal tumors. A detailed discussion of each of these entities is beyond the scope of this text.

REFERENCES

1. Ostrom QT, Gittleman H, Xu J, et al. CBTRUS statistical report: primary brain and other central nervous system tumors diagnosed in the United States in 2009–2013. *Neurooncol.* 2016;18(Suppl 5):v1–v75.
2. Ostrom QT, de Blank PM, Kruchko C, et al. Alex's Lemonade Stand Foundation infant and childhood primary brain and central nervous system tumors diagnosed in the United States in 2007–2011. *Neurooncol.* 2015;16(Suppl 10):x1–x36.
3. Ghosal N, Kapila K, Sharma MC, et al. Fine needle aspiration cytology of a meningioma with extracranial extension after irradiation for medulloblastoma. *Acta Cytol.* 2001;45(6):1092–1093.
4. Antinheimo J, Haapasalo H, Haltia M, et al. Proliferation potential and histological features in neurofibromatosis 2-associated and sporadic meningiomas. *J Neurosurg.* 1997;87(4):610–614.
5. Perry A, Giannini C, Raghavan R, et al. Aggressive phenotypic and genotypic features in pediatric and NF2-associated meningiomas: a clinicopathologic study of 53 cases. *J Neuropathol Exp Neurol.* 2001;60(10):994–1003.
6. van den Munckhof P, Christiaans I, Kenter SB, et al. Germline SMARCB1 mutation predisposes to multiple meningiomas and schwannomas with preferential location of cranial meningiomas at the falx cerebri. *Neurogenetics.* 2012;13(1):1–7.
7. Christiaans I, Kenter SB, Brink HC, et al. Germline SMARCB1 mutation and somatic NF2 mutations in familial multiple meningiomas. *J Med Genet.* 2011;48(2):93–97.
8. Aavikko M, Li SP, Saarinen S, et al. Loss of SUFU function in familial multiple meningioma. *Am J Hum Genet.* 2012;91(3):520–526.
9. Pilarski R, Rai K, Cebulla C, et al. BAP1 tumor predisposition syndrome. In: Pagon RA, Adam MP, Ardinger HH, et al., eds. Seattle, WA: University of Washington. GeneReviews®; 1993.
10. Ron E, Modan B, Boice JD, Jr, et al. Tumors of the brain and nervous system after radiotherapy in childhood. *N Engl J Med.* 1988;319(16):1033–1039.
11. Banerjee J, Paakko E, Harila M, et al. Radiation-induced meningiomas: a shadow in the success story of childhood leukemia. *Neurooncol.* 2009;11(5):543–549.
12. Neglia JP, Robison LL, Stovall M, et al. New primary neoplasms of the central nervous system in survivors of childhood cancer: a report from the childhood cancer survivor study. *J Natl Cancer Inst.* 2006;98(21):1528–1537.
13. Engelhard HH. Progress in the diagnosis and treatment of patients with meningiomas. Part I: diagnostic imaging, preoperative embolization. *Surg Neurol.* 2001;55(2):89–101.
14. Aghi MK, Carter BS, Cosgrove GR, et al. Long-term recurrence rates of atypical meningiomas after gross total resection with or without postoperative adjuvant radiation. *Neurosurgery.* 2009;64(1):56–60.
15. Marcus HJ, Price SJ, Wilby M, et al. Radiotherapy as an adjuvant in the management of intracranial meningiomas: are we practising evidence-based medicine? *Br J Neurosurg.* 2008;22(4):520–528.

16. Nanda A, Bir SC, Maiti TK, et al. Relevance of Simpson grading system and recurrence-free survival after surgery for World Health Organization grade I meningioma. *J Neurosurg.* 2017;126(1):201–211.
17. Perry A, Scheithauer BW, Stafford SL, et al. "Malignancy" in meningiomas: a clinicopathologic study of 116 patients, with grading implications. *Cancer.* 1999;85(9):2046–2056.
18. Perry A, Stafford SL, Scheithauer BW, et al. Meningioma grading: an analysis of histologic parameters. *Am J Surg Pathol.* 1997;21(12):1455–1465.
19. Hwang WL, Marciscano AE, Niemierko A, et al. Imaging and extent of surgical resection predict risk of meningioma recurrence better than WHO histopathological grade. *Neurooncol.* 2016;18(6):863–872.
20. Gabeau-Lacet D, Aghi M, Betensky RA, et al. Bone involvement predicts poor outcome in atypical meningioma. *J Neurosurg.* 2009;111(3):464–471.
21. Abboud M, Haddad G, Kattar M, et al. Extraneural metastases from cranial meningioma: a case report. *Radiat Oncol.* 2009;4:20.
22. Adlakha A, Rao K, Adlakha H, et al. Meningioma metastatic to the lung. *Mayo Clin Proc.* 1999;74(11):1129–1133.
23. Fulkerson DH, Horner TG, Hattab EM. Histologically benign intraventricular meningioma with concurrent pulmonary metastasis: case report and review of the literature. *Clin Neurol Neurosurg.* 2008;110(4):416–419.
24. Gladin CR, Salsano E, Menghi F, et al. Loss of heterozygosity studies in extracranial metastatic meningiomas. *J Neurooncol.* 2007;85(1):81–85.
25. Sujit Kumar GS, Chacko G, Chacko AG, et al. Multiple extracranial metastases from intradiploic meningioma. *Neurol India.* 2009;57(1):96–97.
26. Lin Z, Zhao M, Ren X, et al. Clinical features, radiologic findings, and surgical outcomes of 65 intracranial psammomatous meningiomas. *World Neurosurg.* 2017;100:395–406.
27. Hasselblatt M, Nolte KW, Paulus W. Angiomatous meningioma: a clinicopathologic study of 38 cases. *Am J Surg Pathol.* 2004;28(3):390–393.
28. Ben Nsir A, Chabaane M, Krifa H, et al. Intracranial angiomatous meningiomas: a 15-year, multicenter study. *Clin Neurol Neurosurg.* 2016;149:111–117.
29. Velazquez Vega JE, Rosenberg AE. Microcystic meningioma of the calvarium: a series of 9 cases and review of the literature. *Am J Surg Pathol.* 2015;39(4):505–511.
30. Probst-Cousin S, Villagran-Lillo R, Lahl R, et al. Secretory meningioma: clinical, histologic, and immunohistochemical findings in 31 cases. *Cancer.* 1997;79(10):2003–2015.
31. Regelsberger J, Hagel C, Emami P, et al. Secretory meningiomas: a benign subgroup causing life-threatening complications. *Neurooncol.* 2009;11(6):819–824.
32. Reuss DE, Piro RM, Jones DT, et al. Secretory meningiomas are defined by combined KLF4 K409Q and TRAF7 mutations. *Acta Neuropathol (Berl).* 2013;125(3):351–358.
33. Zhu HD, Xie Q, Gong Y, et al. Lymphoplasmacyte-rich meningioma: our experience with 19 cases and a systematic literature review. *Int J Clin Exp Med.* 2013;6(7):504–515.
34. Gi H, Nagao S, Yoshizumi H, et al. Meningioma with hypergammaglobulinemia. Case report. *J Neurosurg.* 1990;73(4):628–629.
35. Horten BC, Urich H, Stefoski D. Meningiomas with conspicuous plasma cell-lymphocytic components: a report of five cases. *Cancer.* 1979;43(1):258–264.
36. Lal A, Dahiya S, Gonzales M, et al. IgG4 overexpression is rare in meningiomas with a prominent inflammatory component: a review of 16 cases. *Brain Pathol.* 2014;24(4):352–359.
37. Colnat-Coulbois S, Kremer S, Weinbreck N, et al. Lipomatous meningioma: report of 2 cases and review of the literature. *Surg Neurol.* 2008;69(4):398–402; discussion 402.
38. Ohba S, Yoshida K, Akiyama T, et al. Lipomatous meningioma. *J Clin Neurosci.* 2007;14(10):1003–1006.

39. Takayama Y, Nobusawa S, Ochiai I, et al. Malignant meningioma with adenocarcinoma-like metaplasia: demonstration of intestinal phenotype. *Neuropathology*. 2015;35(2): 158–164.
40. Louis DN, Ohgaki H, Wiestler OD, et al., eds. WHO Classification of Tumours of the Central Nervous System. 4th, revised ed. Lyon, France: IARC Press; 2016.
41. Jain D, Sharma MC, Sarkar C, et al. Clear cell meningioma, an uncommon variant of meningioma: a clinicopathologic study of nine cases. *J Neurooncol*. 2007;81(3):315–321.
42. Zorludemir S, Scheithauer BW, Hirose T, et al. Clear cell meningioma. A clinicopathologic study of a potentially aggressive variant of meningioma. *Am J Surg Pathol*. 1995; 19(5):493–505.
43. Smith MJ, Wallace AJ, Bennett C, et al. Germline SMARCE1 mutations predispose to both spinal and cranial clear cell meningiomas. *J Pathol*. 2014;234(4):436–440.
44. Tauziede-Espariat A, Parfait B, Besnard A, et al. Loss of SMARCE1 expression is a specific diagnostic marker of clear cell meningioma: a comprehensive immunophenotypical and molecular analysis. *Brain Pathol*. 2017. doi: 10.1111/bpa.12524. [Epub ahead of print]
45. Moliterno J, Cope WP, Vartanian ED, et al. Survival in patients treated for anaplastic meningioma. *J Neurosurg*. 2015;123(1):23–30.
46. Ferraro DJ, Funk RK, Blackett JW, et al. A retrospective analysis of survival and prognostic factors after stereotactic radiosurgery for aggressive meningiomas. *Radiat Oncol*. 2014;9:38.
47. Perry A, Scheithauer BW, Stafford SL, et al. "Rhabdoid" meningioma: an aggressive variant. *Am J Surg Pathol*. 1998;22(12):1482–1490.
48. Zang KD. Meningioma: a cytogenetic model of a complex benign human tumor, including data on 394 karyotyped cases. *Cytogenet Cell Genet*. 2001;93(3–4):207–220.
49. Menke JR, Raleigh DR, Gown AM, et al. Somatostatin receptor 2a is a more sensitive diagnostic marker of meningioma than epithelial membrane antigen. *Acta Neuropathol (Berl)*. 2015;130(3):441–443.
50. Sahm F, Schrimpf D, Olar A, et al. TERT promoter mutations and risk of recurrence in meningioma. *J Natl Cancer Inst*. 2015;108(5).
51. Sahm F, Schrimpf D, Stichel D, et al. DNA methylation-based classification and grading system for meningioma: a multicentre, retrospective analysis. *Lancet Oncol*. 2017;18(5): 682–694.
52. Kimura N, Pilichowska M, Date F, et al. Immunohistochemical expression of somatostatin type 2A receptor in neuroendocrine tumors. *Clin Cancer Res*. 1999;5(11):3483–3487.
53. Liu Y, Sturgis CD, Bunker M, et al. Expression of cytokeratin by malignant meningiomas: diagnostic pitfall of cytokeratin to separate malignant meningiomas from metastatic carcinoma. *Mod Pathol*. 2004;17(9):1129–1133.
54. Song KS, Park SH, Cho BK, et al. Third ventricular chordoid meningioma in a child. *J Neurosurg Pediatr*. 2008;2(4):269–272.
55. Sangoi AR, Dulai MS, Beck AH, et al. Distinguishing chordoid meningiomas from their histologic mimics: an immunohistochemical evaluation. *Am J Surg Pathol*. 2009;33(5): 669–681.
56. Perry A, Lusis EA, Gutmann DH. Meningothelial hyperplasia: a detailed clinicopathologic, immunohistochemical and genetic study of 11 cases. *Brain Pathol*. 2005;15(2): 109–115.
57. Jallo GI, Kothbauer K, Mehta V, et al. Meningioangiomatosis without neurofibromatosis: a clinical analysis. *J Neurosurg*. 2005;103(Suppl 4):319–324.
58. Omeis I, Hillard VH, Braun A, et al. Meningioangiomatosis associated with neurofibromatosis: report of 2 cases in a single family and review of the literature. *Surg Neurol*. 2006;65(6):595–603.

59. Wiebe S, Munoz DG, Smith S, et al. Meningioangiomatosis. A comprehensive analysis of clinical and laboratory features. *Brain.* 1999;122 (Pt 4):709–726.
60. Halper J, Scheithauer BW, Okazaki H, et al. Meningio-angiomatosis: a report of six cases with special reference to the occurrence of neurofibrillary tangles. *J Neuropathol Exp Neurol.* 1986;45(4):426–446.
61. Dufour H, Metellus P, Fuentes S, et al. Meningeal hemangiopericytoma: a retrospective study of 21 patients with special review of postoperative external radiotherapy. *Neurosurgery.* 2001;48(4):756–762.
62. Guthrie BL, Ebersold MJ, Scheithauer BW, et al. Meningeal hemangiopericytoma: histopathological features, treatment, and long-term follow-up of 44 cases. *Neurosurgery.* 1989;25(4):514–522.
63. Mena H, Ribas JL, Pezeshkpour GH, et al. Hemangiopericytoma of the central nervous system: a review of 94 cases. *Hum Pathol.* 1991;22(1):84–91.
64. Vuorinen V, Sallinen P, Haapasalo H, et al. Outcome of 31 intracranial haemangiopericytomas: poor predictive value of cell proliferation indices. *Acta Neurochir (Wien).* 1996;138(12):1399–1408.
65. Carneiro SS, Scheithauer BW, Nascimento AG, et al. Solitary fibrous tumor of the meninges: a lesion distinct from fibrous meningioma. A clinicopathologic and immunohistochemical study. *Am J Clin Pathol.* 1996;106(2):217–224.
66. Tihan T, Viglione M, Rosenblum MK, et al. Solitary fibrous tumors in the central nervous system. A clinicopathologic review of 18 cases and comparison to meningeal hemangiopericytomas. *Arch Pathol Lab Med.* 2003;127(4):432–439.
67. Weon YC, Kim EY, Kim HJ, et al. Intracranial solitary fibrous tumors: imaging findings in 6 consecutive patients. *AJNR Am J Neuroradiol.* 2007;28(8):1466–1469.
68. Akiyama M, Sakai H, Onoue H, et al. Imaging intracranial haemangiopericytomas: study of seven cases. *Neuroradiology.* 2004;46(3):194–197.
69. Sibtain NA, Butt S, Connor SE. Imaging features of central nervous system haemangiopericytomas. *Eur Radiol.* 2007;17(7):1685–1693.
70. Servo A, Jaaskelainen J, Wahlstrom T, et al. Diagnosis of intracranial haemangiopericytomas with angiography and CT scanning. *Neuroradiology.* 1985;27(1):38–43.
71. Ecker RD, Marsh WR, Pollock BE, et al. Hemangiopericytoma in the central nervous system: treatment, pathological features, and long-term follow-up in 38 patients. *J Neurosurg.* 2003;98(6):1182–1187.
72. Ghia AJ, Allen PK, Mahajan A, et al. Intracranial hemangiopericytoma and the role of radiation therapy: a population based analysis. *Neurosurgery.* 2013;72(2):203–209.
73. Ghia AJ, Chang EL, Allen PK, et al. Intracranial hemangiopericytoma: patterns of failure and the role of radiation therapy. *Neurosurgery.* 2013;73(4):624–630.
74. Stessin AM, Sison C, Nieto J, et al. The role of postoperative radiation therapy in the treatment of meningeal hemangiopericytoma-experience from the SEER database. *Int J Radiat Oncol Biol Phys.* 2013;85(3):784–790.
75. Bouvier C, Metellus P, de Paula AM, et al. Solitary fibrous tumors and hemangiopericytomas of the meninges: overlapping pathological features and common prognostic factors suggest the same spectrum of tumors. *Brain Pathol.* 2012;22(4):511–521.
76. Robinson DR, Wu YM, Kalyana-Sundaram S, et al. Identification of recurrent NAB2-STAT6 gene fusions in solitary fibrous tumor by integrative sequencing. *Nat Genet.* 2013;45(2):180–185.
77. Schweizer L, Koelsche C, Sahm F, et al. Meningeal hemangiopericytoma and solitary fibrous tumors carry the NAB2-STAT6 fusion and can be diagnosed by nuclear expression of STAT6 protein. *Acta Neuropathol (Berl).* 2013;125(5):651–658.

78. Akaike K, Kurisaki-Arakawa A, Hara K, et al. Distinct clinicopathological features of NAB2-STAT6 fusion gene variants in solitary fibrous tumor with emphasis on the acquisition of highly malignant potential. *Hum Pathol.* 2015;46(3):347–356.
79. Kadonaga JN, Frieden IJ. Neurocutaneous melanosis: definition and review of the literature. *J Am Acad Dermatol.* 1991;24(5 Pt 1):747–755.
80. Pavlidou E, Hagel C, Papavasilliou A, et al. Neurocutaneous melanosis: report of three cases and up-to-date review. *J Child Neurol.* 2008;23(12):1382–1391.
81. Kinsler VA, Thomas AC, Ishida M, et al. Multiple congenital melanocytic nevi and neurocutaneous melanosis are caused by postzygotic mutations in codon 61 of NRAS. *J Invest Dermatol.* 2013;133(9):2229–2236.
82. Salgado CM, Basu D, Nikiforova M, et al. BRAF mutations are also associated with neurocutaneous melanocytosis and large/giant congenital melanocytic nevi. *Pediatr Dev Pathol.* 2015;18(1):1–9.
83. Byrd SE, Darling CF, Tomita T, et al. MR imaging of symptomatic neurocutaneous melanosis in children. *Pediatr Radiol.* 1997;27(1):39–44.
84. Brat DJ, Giannini C, Scheithauer BW, et al. Primary melanocytic neoplasms of the central nervous systems. *Am J Surg Pathol.* 1999;23(7):745–754.
85. Offiah CJ, Laitt RD. Case report: intracranial meningeal melanocytoma: a cause of high signal on T1- and low signal on T2-weighted MRI. *Clin Radiol.* 2006;61(3):294–298.
86. Wang H, Zhang S, Wu C, et al. Melanocytomas of the central nervous system: a clinicopathological and molecular study. *Eur J Clin Invest.* 2013;43(8):809–815.
87. Kusters-Vandevelde HV, Klaasen A, Kusters B, et al. Activating mutations of the GNAQ gene: a frequent event in primary melanocytic neoplasms of the central nervous system. *Acta Neuropathol (Berl).* 2010;119(3):317–323.
88. Gessi M, Hammes J, Lauriola L, et al. GNA11 and N-RAS mutations: alternatives for MAPK pathway activating GNAQ mutations in primary melanocytic tumours of the central nervous system. *Neuropathol Appl Neurobiol.* 2013;39(4):417–425.
89. van de Nes J, Gessi M, Sucker A, et al. Targeted next generation sequencing reveals unique mutation profile of primary melanocytic tumors of the central nervous system. *J Neurooncol.* 2016;127(3):435–444.
90. Chan SK, Cheuk W, Chan KT, et al. IgG4-related sclerosing pachymeningitis: a previously unrecognized form of central nervous system involvement in IgG4-related sclerosing disease. *Am J Surg Pathol.* 2009;33(8):1249–1252.

10

EMBRYONAL NEOPLASMS

INTRODUCTION

Embryonal tumors of the CNS are poorly differentiated malignant neoplasms that preferentially affect children. Categories of embryonal CNS neoplasms recognized by the World Health Organization (WHO) include medulloblastoma; CNS neuroblastoma; CNS ganglioneuroblastoma; embryonal tumor with multilayered rosettes (ETMR), C19C-altered; medulloepithelioma; CNS-embryonal tumor, NOS; and atypical teratoid/rhabdoid tumor (AT/RT) (1). Additional NOS categories are present when confirmatory diagnostic testing is unavailable or cannot be performed for technical reasons. Notably missing from the classification is the term primitive neuroectodermal tumor (PNET), which has been abandoned in the 2016 WHO update. Pineoblastomas are also malignant tumors that may have an embryonal phenotype, yet are usually addressed with other pineal parenchymal tumors (see Chapter 12). As a group, these lesions are treated aggressively, with both craniospinal radiation and multiagent chemotherapy. Although response to therapy and survival varies among the different entities, all embryonal tumors of the CNS are malignant and considered WHO grade IV.

MEDULLOBLASTOMA (WHO GRADE IV)

General

The concept of medulloblastoma has undergone a foundational shift since the 2007 WHO classification in which the entire disease spectrum was described and categorized by three histopathologic patterns. Since then, a number of large-scale genetic investigations have elucidated the biology of medulloblastoma and provided an objective genetic framework with which to classify them, separating them into four major separate tumor types with further subtyping of one of those groups (2,3). The result has been a hybrid medulloblastoma classification that provides criteria for both the genetic and histomorphologic categories, with the latter having been more or less subsumed as patterns within the larger genetic context, allowing for an "integrated" approach that improves prognostic and therapeutic precision.

Demographics and Clinical Context

Medulloblastomas tend to occur in children, in whom they are the most common primary CNS malignancy. Most cases occur in the first 4 years of life, with incidence becoming progressively lower through young adulthood (4). Although rare, medulloblastomas may occur in older patients, up to the seventh decade, so patient age alone cannot rule it out as a diagnostic consideration. The male to female ratio is about 1.5:1 (5).

Medulloblastomas present with histories similar to those of other posterior fossa masses, particularly ependymoma. Infants may present with an enlarging head due to increased intracranial pressure with incompletely fused cranial sutures, whereas slightly older children will often experience increased intracranial pressure and hydrocephalus with headaches, nausea/vomiting, dizziness, and ataxia.

By definition, medulloblastomas occur in the posterior fossa. Most cases are centered in the midline cerebellum, or vermis, and extend into the fourth ventricle, sometimes causing obstruction of cerebrospinal fluid flow (Figure 10-1). The older the age at presentation, the more likely the tumor will arise in the lateral cerebellum, where it may display a "grape-like" pattern of nodularity that corresponds to the extent of nodularity in the histologic pattern, discussed later (6,7). Nodular/desmoplastic medulloblastoma in early childhood suggests the presence of Gorlin syndrome. On imaging, medulloblastomas are usually ring-enhancing or have a heterogeneous pattern with contrast and tend to be solid with discrete circumscription. Distant seeding of the subarachnoid space may

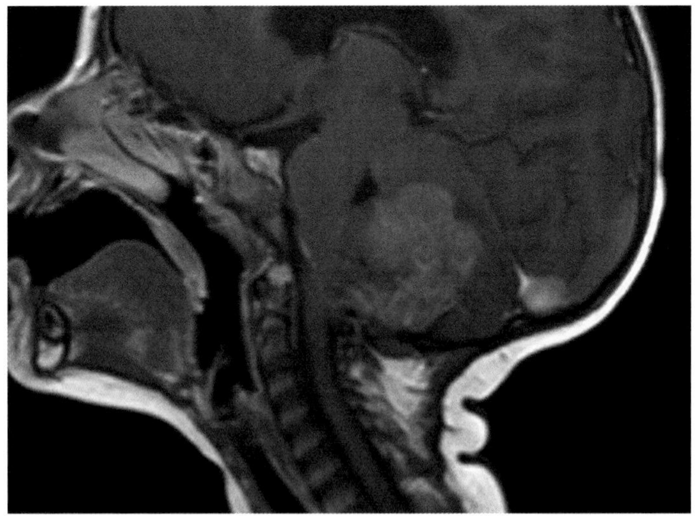

FIGURE 10-1 T1-weighted magnetic resonance imaging showing a midline cerebellar vermis mass extending into the fourth ventricle, the classic imaging appearance of medulloblastoma.

be identified on neuroimaging and is associated with decreased rates of survival. Extensive or geographic necrosis is uncommon on radiographic examination.

Prognosis by Clinical Factors

The outlook for patients with medulloblastoma can be stratified by clinical and radiologic factors into two groups, poor (high) risk and average, or standard, risk (8). The single most predictive clinical factor is the presence of leptomeningeal dissemination or "drop" metastases at the time of diagnosis. This is evaluated both by magnetic resonance imaging (MRI) of the brain and spinal cord and lumbar puncture for cytologic evidence of metastasis. In one series, given combination of radio- and chemotherapy, patients with evidence of tumor dissemination at diagnosis have around a 67% 5-year survival rate, in contrast to a 90% 5-year survival in patients with no evidence of spread (9). Patient age is the other major risk factor, with those younger than 3 years being at higher risk. Not surprisingly, extent of surgical resection plays a role in patient survival. Compared with other embryonal CNS malignancies, survival in cases of medulloblastoma is high overall, up to almost 80% at 5 years, when treated with radiation and multiagent chemotherapy (9). Occasionally, medulloblastomas will metastasize outside of the CNS, usually to bone but also occasionally to solid organs and soft tissue (10).

Histopathology

CLASSIC MEDULLOBLASTOMA. Most medulloblastomas fit the "classic" pattern, composed of sheets of monotonous, embryonal cells with minimal cytoplasm. In addition to sheet-like growth, other patterns such as palisading, prominent rosettes, and perivascular clearing can be seen. Fibrillar, or neuroblastic, rosettes (Homer Wright) (Figure 10-2) are present in fewer than half of cases and are not specific to medulloblastoma, thus are not a necessary diagnostic criterion; however, their presence heavily favors a lesion of immature neuronal differentiation. Foci of necrosis are common, although they usually make up only a small fraction of the tumor bulk. The nuclei are typically hyperchromatic with smooth chromatin and range from round and regular to angular with some nuclear molding. Nucleoli are usually inconspicuous, if identifiable at all. These cells often extend along the surface of the cerebellum underneath the leptomeninges and into the parenchyma along the perivascular spaces of penetrating arteries (Figure 10-3). Occasionally, tumor cells may encircle and arrange themselves around blood vessels, creating structures similar to the perivascular pseudorosettes seen in ependymomas.

Occasionally, one will receive a biopsy from a previously treated medulloblastoma patient that shows almost complete transition from small blue cells to large, mature ganglion cells (Figure 10-4) (11–13). These could represent maturation of residual medulloblastoma cells induced by radiation and chemotherapy or dysplasia of native cerebellar granular neurons.

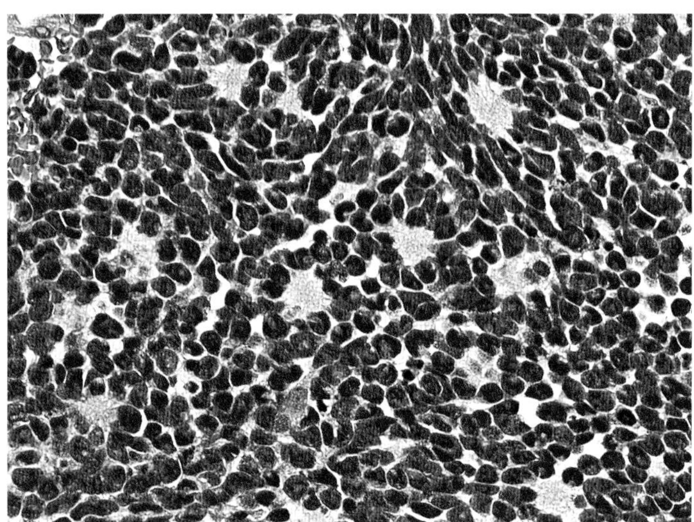

FIGURE 10-2 Homer Wright rosettes often dot the sheets of poorly differentiated cells in classic medulloblastoma, but they are not necessary for the diagnosis.

DESMOPLASTIC/NODULAR PATTERN. Conceptually, this pattern represents a medulloblastoma with foci of increased neuronal differentiation. The prototype consists of circumscribed, round, reticulin-poor nodules composed of well-spaced tumor cells in a neuropil-like background, separated by more cellular strands of tumor with a reticulin-rich background (Figures 10-5 and 10-6). The pale nodules show increased synaptophysin and neurofilament expression, more uniform nuclear features, and decreased proliferation.

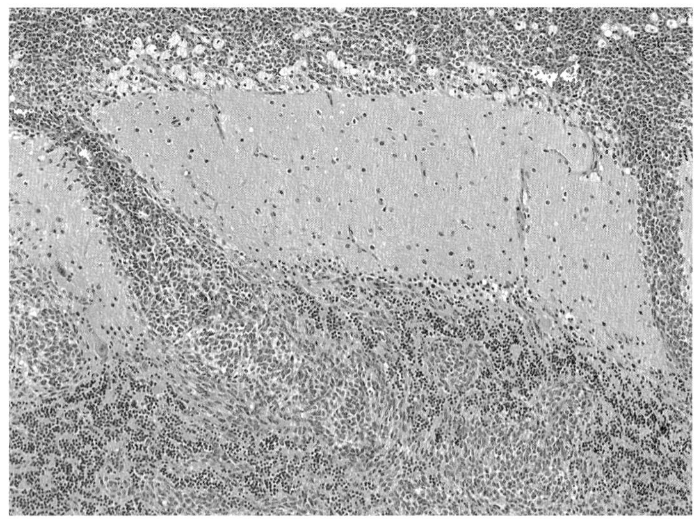

FIGURE 10-3 Medulloblastoma extending through the subarachnoid space and along perivascular spaces.

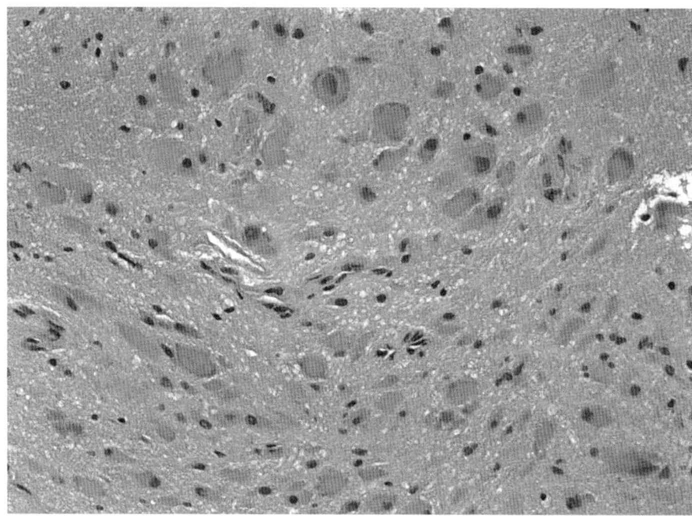

FIGURE 10-4 Posttreatment biopsies of medulloblastoma occasionally show mature ganglion cells in places suspected to be recurrence.

Maturing or mature ganglion cells may reside within nodules. In contrast, the internodular tissue is less differentiated, more pleomorphic, and more proliferative. Occasionally, nodules are so prominent that they abut each other with virtually no intervening tissue. When this pattern forms the entirety of the lesion, it can be categorized as ***medulloblastoma with extensive nodularity*** (MBEN) (Figures 10-7 and 10-8) according to WHO 2016 classification. MBEN is associated with infant patients and Gorlin syndrome.

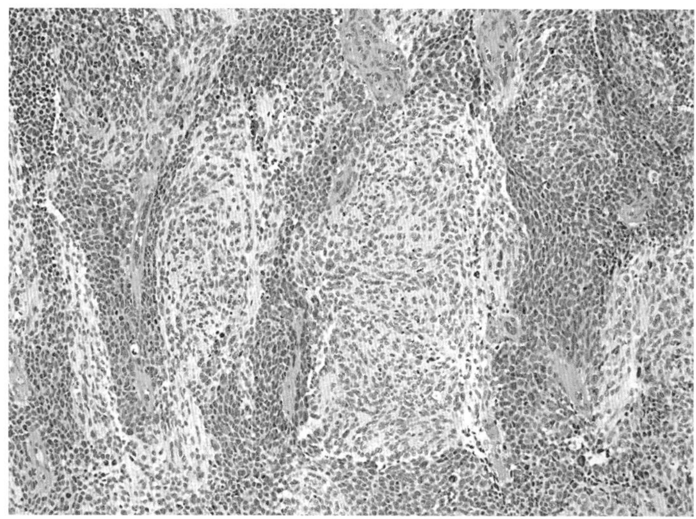

FIGURE 10-5 The "pale islands" of nodular/desmoplastic medulloblastoma give an impression of lymph node tissue at low magnification.

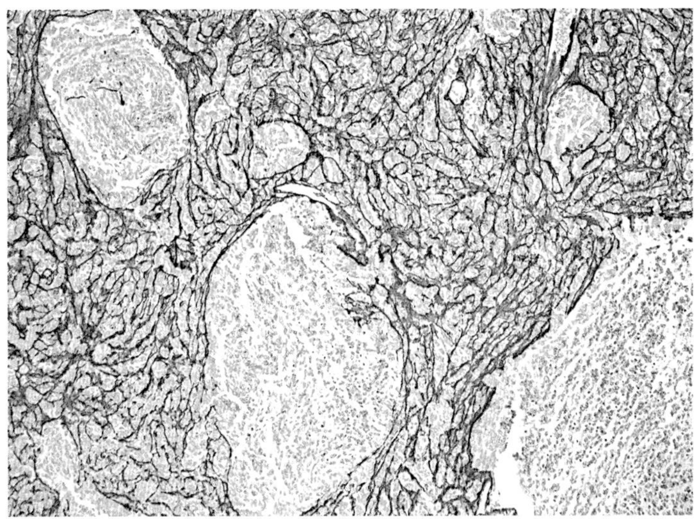

FIGURE 10-6 Reticulin staining marks the internodular tissue in nodular/desmoplastic medulloblastoma and spares the nodule contents.

In some cases, desmoplasia presents as a solid background of dense collagen impregnated with small files of tumor cells (Figure 10-9). Although technically desmoplastic, this feature does not constitute a desmoplastic/nodular pattern by itself and is most likely a reactive fibrosis due to activation of leptomeningeal fibroblasts (14). Similarly, one may see pale nodules

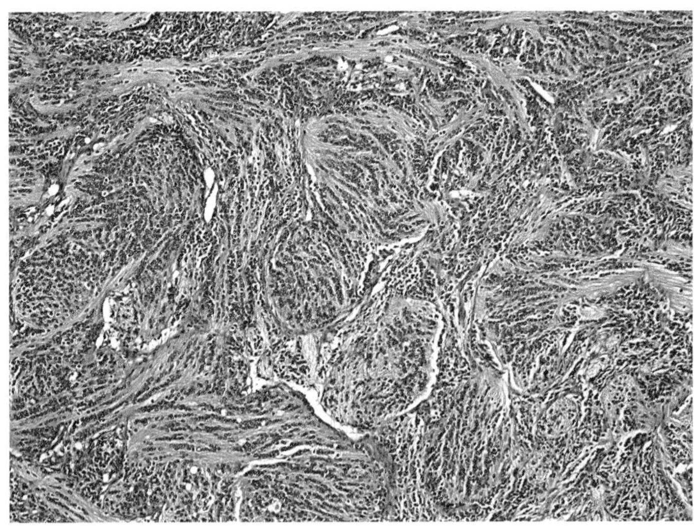

FIGURE 10-7 When the nodules constitute the vast majority of the tissue and there is only a scant internodular element, it is a medulloblastoma with extensive nodularity.

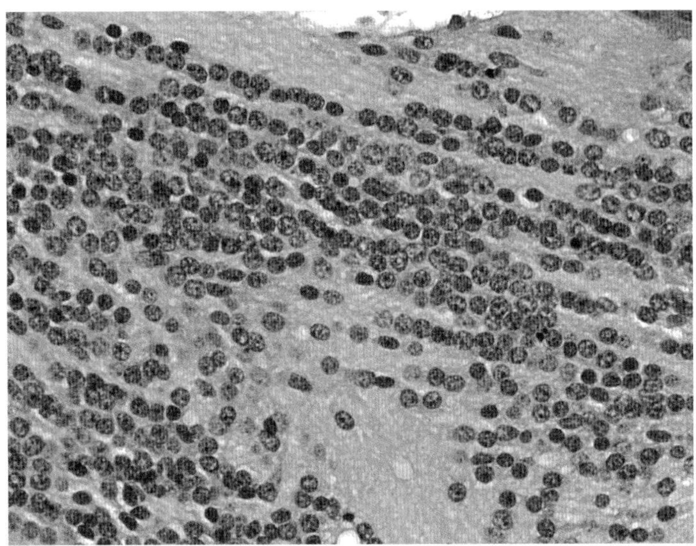

FIGURE 10-8 Linear streaming of neurocytic tumor cells within nodules is common on medulloblastoma with extensive nodularity.

without reticular, internodular reticular desmoplasia that also do not qualify a tumor as desmoplastic/nodular; both elements must be present. Absence of evidence for SHH-activation (sonic hedgehog) can be taken as evidence that a medulloblastoma is not desmoplastic/nodular (see below). Cases with nodules but no internodular desmoplasia (Figure 10-10) have

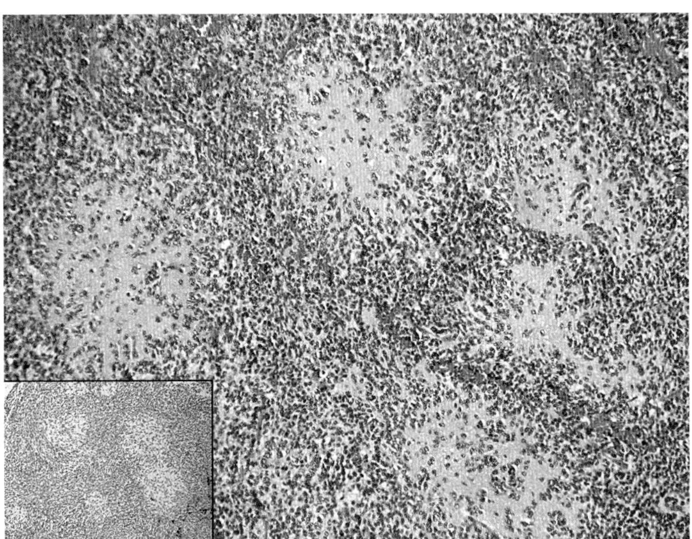

FIGURE 10-9 Pale nodules appear in classic and large cell/anaplastic histologies without internodular reticular desmoplasia (inset). Such lesions do not qualify as desmoplastic/nodular.

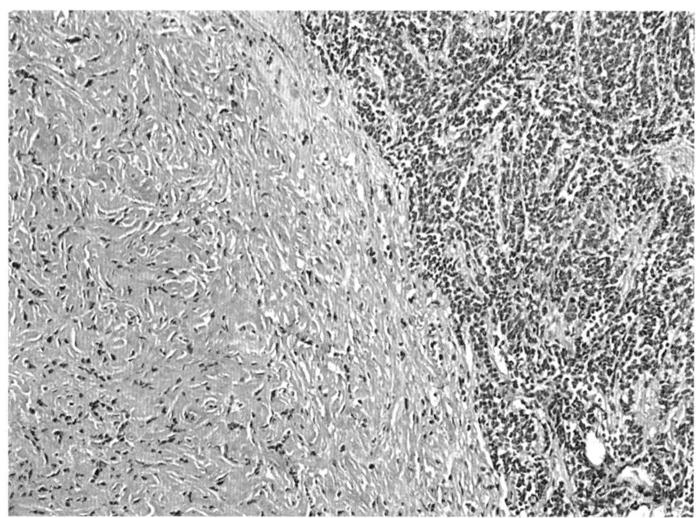

FIGURE 10-10 Dense, sclerotic collagen containing scant tumor cells is a reactive phenomenon and is not relevant to the desmoplastic/nodular histologic pattern.

been termed "biphasic" and shown to behave clinically more like classic medulloblastomas (15). Such biphasic cases are not of the SHH-activated group and should be considered histologically classic.

LARGE CELL/ANAPLASTIC PATTERN. These tumors have a higher degree of cytologic atypia and larger cell size, and retain a sheetlike growth pattern. The term anaplastic is applied where large, pleomorphic, and hyperchromatic nuclei mold to each other in a pattern similar to mosaic tiles (Figure 10-11). In contrast, the "large cell" nucleus is more round with open or vesicular chromatin, a prominent nucleolus, and a thin rim of eosinophilic cytoplasm (Figure 10-12). Both patterns show increased mitoses, frequent apoptotic debris, and cell–cell wrapping. Although originally described as separate entities, large cell and anaplastic medulloblastoma are thought to represent similarly aggressive phenotypes, more prone to metastasis, and less amenable to treatment (16).

HETEROLOGOUS ELEMENTS. Several heterologous elements have been reported in otherwise classic or anaplastic medulloblastomas, including cartilage (17), muscle, fat (18), and melanocytes (19–21). Myogenic and melanocytic are the two most common types and cases with them were formerly classified as separate entities. However, now such examples are merely considered rare morphologic variants with nondistinctive clinical behavior. It is unclear as to whether medulloblastomas with heterologous elements tend to fall into any specific molecular category; they have been reported in WNT-activated (22) and non-WNT/non-SHH (23,24). In the case of medulloblastoma with adipocytic differentiation, one should proceed with caution to prevent confusion with a less aggressive

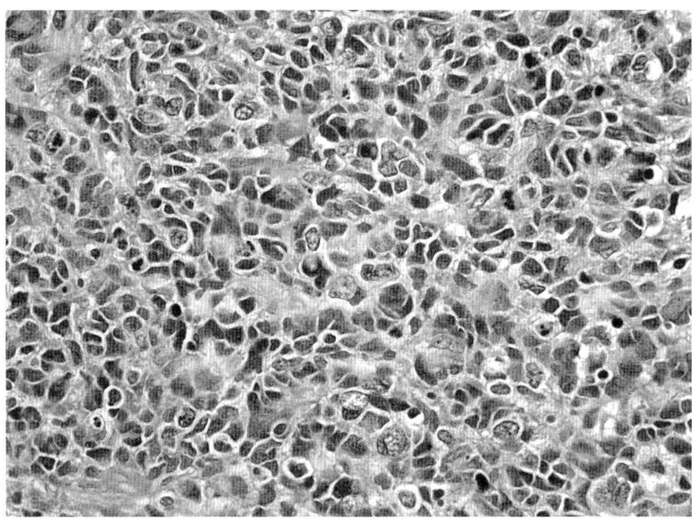

FIGURE 10-11 Angular large nuclei mold to form mosaic tile patterns in anaplastic medulloblastoma.

tumor, cerebellar liponeurocytoma, discussed in Chapter 6 with neuronal and glioneuronal tumors.

Medulloblastoma Genetic Groups

MEDULLOBLASTOMA, WNT-ACTIVATED

CLINICAL CONTEXT. This group accounts for the fewest of any medulloblastoma molecular group, around 10% (Table 10-1). Patients with

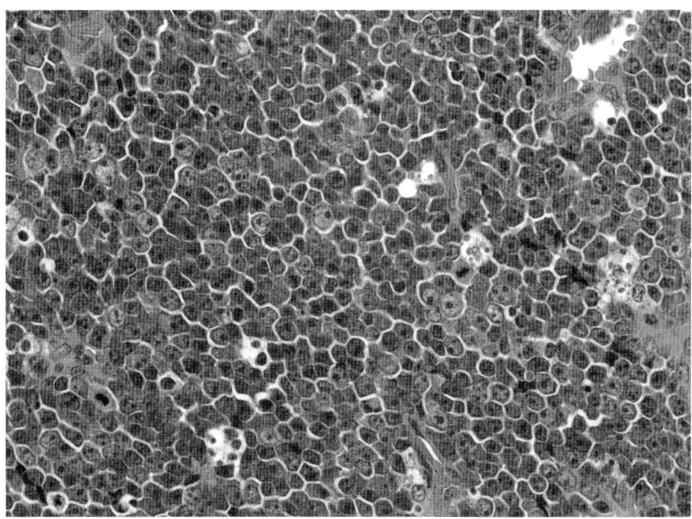

FIGURE 10-12 Large round nuclei with open chromatin and prominent nucleoli are the signature features of purely large cell medulloblastoma.

TABLE 10-1 Clinically Relevant Medulloblastoma Molecular Groups (WHO 2016)

		SHH-activated		Non-WNT/non-SHH	
	WNT-activated	TP53 Wild Type	TP53 Mutant	Group 3	Group 4
Ages	Mostly children, some adults	Bimodal: infants and adults	Children	Children, some infants	Mostly children, few infants and adults
Histology	Classic, rare LCA	Desmoplastic, MBEN, classic, LCA	Classic, LCA	Classic or LCA	Classic > LCA
Chromosomal Abnormalities	Monosomy 6 (~85–90%)	del9q (~50%), occasional *MYCN amp*	*MYCN amp., GLI2 amp.* del17p	i17q, *MYC* amp, 1q+	i17q (>50%), occasional *MYCN* amp
Gene Mutations	*CTNNB1(95%), DDX3X, SMARCA4, TP53*	*PTCH, SUFU, SMO*	*TP53*	None consistent	None consistent
Immunohistochemistry	Nuclear β-catenin, YAP1+; GAB1 neg	GAB1, YAP1 +	p53, GAB1, YAP1+	GAB1, YAP1 neg	GAB1, YAP1 neg
Prognosis	Very good	Infants good, others intermediate	Poor	Poor	Intermediate
Percent of total (approx.)	15%	20%	5%	20%	40%

Modified from (25) and (2).

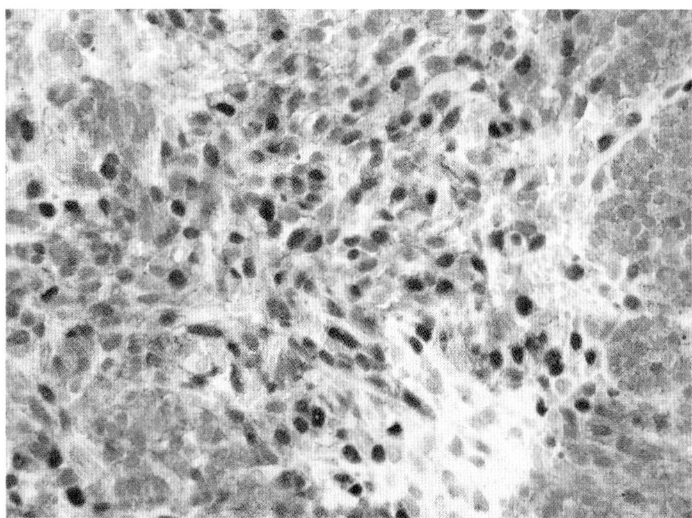

FIGURE 10-13 Nuclear accumulation of beta-catenin, which can be focal and subtle, identifies WNT-activated medulloblastomas.

WNT-activated medulloblastomas are typically children or young adults, infant cases being rare, and are equally likely to be male or female. Although rare, medulloblastomas that arise within the context of familial adenomatous polyposis (germline *APC* mutation; Turcot syndrome, type 2) are presumably in the WNT-activated group by virtue of gene's involvement in the same pathway (26). WNT-activated medulloblastomas rarely present with metastases and have an excellent prognosis overall, with greater than 95% 5-year survival, although adult patients may not fare as well (27).

HISTOPATHOLOGY. Almost all cases from the WNT-activated group have the classic histology and very rarely will have a LC/A histology. Immunostaining for beta-catenin is an important surrogate marker for WNT-activated tumors, it showing nuclear accumulation that is usually focal (Figure 10-13) in a majority of cases (28). Like SHH-activated cases, WNT group tumors also express YAP1 in most cases, but not GAB1. One recent series suggests that ALK immunostaining may be useful in identifying WNT-activated medulloblastomas (29).

GENETICS. Around 90% of tumors from this group have inactivating point mutations in *CTNNB1*, the gene for beta-catenin (30), making it the most common genetic feature. Almost as many also have monosomy 6, which has long been known to be a marker of WNT-driven biology and good prognosis in medulloblastomas (31). Other mutations are common in WNT-driven medulloblastomas, such as in *DDX3X* or *SMARCA4*, yet their exact roles are unknown (32). TP53 mutations are seen, but do not convey the poor prognosis that they do in the SHH group. Occasional WNT-driven medulloblastomas may have *MYC* amplification (33).

MEDULLOBLASTOMA, SHH-ACTIVATED (*TP53*-WILD TYPE AND *TP53*-MUTANT)

CLINICAL CONTEXT. SHH-activated medulloblastomas may occur at any age and form a bimodal distribution, with the younger peak from birth to about 4 years and the older peak rising from adolescence to adulthood. Whereas tumors from the other genetic groups tend to occur in the midline, SHH-driven ones are more likely to be laterally situated. Given a medulloblastoma in a lateral cerebellar hemisphere, the likelihood of it being SHH-group is high. Several tumor syndromes are associated with SHH medulloblastomas, including Gorlin syndrome (34), Li-Fraumeni syndrome (35), and Fanconi anemia (36). Gorlin-associated cases tend to present before the age of 3 years, be extensively nodular, and have an excellent prognosis (34,37).

As a group, SHH-driven medulloblastomas have an age-dependent prognosis, with those in younger children having better outcomes and those in adults having intermediate outcomes. The main dichotomy in prognosis is between cases that are *TP53*-wild type and *TP53*-mutant, the latter associated so strongly with poor survival that *TP53* mutation constitutes a separate subcategory of SHH medulloblastoma in the 2016 WHO (1). *MYCN* and *GLI2* amplification are thought to be associated with poor survival.

HISTOPATHOLOGY. All desmoplastic/nodular and extensively nodular medulloblastomas are SHH-driven, but the converse is not true. Given an SHH tumor, only half of the time will it be D/N, with the remaining cases being mostly classic and a few anaplastic (28). Immunohistochemistry is a convenient method to classify a medulloblastoma as SHH-driven and can involve any of a number of markers, including GAB1, YAP1, and SFRP1 (28,38). Immunostaining for p53 provides useful surrogate for *TP53* mutation testing, showing strong nuclear accumulation in the vast majority of cases where mutations are present (39).

GENETICS. TP53-wild type, SHH-driven medulloblastomas tend to have mutations in SHH pathway genes, particularly *PTCH1*, *SUFU*, and *SMO*. Cytogenetically, these cases are more likely to have deletions of 9q (PTCH1) and 10q, yet generally have an overall intact chromosomal profile with few gains and losses.

TP53-wild type, SHH-driven medulloblastomas tend to have amplifications of *GLI2* and/or *MYCN* in the setting of a complex profile of chromosomal gains and losses. The finding of *chromothripsis*, or a hypercomplex chromosomal rearrangement affecting one chromosome or even just one segment, in the setting of SHH-driven medulloblastoma is strongly associated with TP53 mutation (35). TP53-mutant tumors in this group also have losses of 17p, but without gain of 17q as seen in non-SHH/non-WNT cases. Most of the SHH-activated tumors with LC/A histology fall into the TP53-mutant group (40).

MEDULLOBLASTOMA, NON-WNT/NON-SHH

CLINICAL CONTEXT. This WHO 2016 category of medulloblastoma combines the groups 3 and 4 of the consensus molecular grouping from 2012 and together account for around 60% of all medulloblastomas (2). There is as of yet no great clinical utility in distinguishing between the two somewhat overlapping molecular categories, nor any method to do so that is readily available to the pathologist on a clinically relevant timescale. The patients of this group range in age from infancy to early adulthood and are almost twice as likely to be male than female (41). Rubinstein–Taybi syndrome (broad thumb-hallux) has been described in the setting of a group 3 medulloblastoma (42).

Non-WNT/non-SHH medulloblastomas have the worst overall prognosis, having the highest rates of metastasis, *MYC* or *MYCN* amplification, and LC/A histology. Most of the risk in this WHO category comes from the molecular group 3, which is particularly enriched for most of the risk factors in medulloblastoma.

HISTOPATHOLOGY. Although most LC/A medulloblastomas fall into this category, most of the cases in the category are still classic histology. Reactive leptomeningeal desmoplasia and nondesmoplastic nodularity may both be seen among the non-WNT/non-SHH tumors and should be worked up appropriately to exclude the possibility of an SHH-activated tumor.

GENETICS. Isochromosome 17q (typically with loss of 17p) is the most common genetic abnormality overall in medulloblastoma, occurring in about 30% to 60% of cases (43,44) and has been reported to convey a worse prognosis (43–46). Isochromosome 17q is present in the majority of non-WNT/non-SHH tumors, almost 70%, and essentially does not occur in other molecular groups.

MYC and *MYCN* amplifications are more likely in this group and restricted respectively to groups 3 and 4. Although the significance of *MYCN* amplification in group 4 tumors is less certain, MYC amplification conveys a poor prognosis in group 3 (47).

Medulloblastoma, NOS

When a medulloblastoma cannot be characterized with certainty into a histomorphologic or molecular genetic category, the term medulloblastoma, NOS may be applied. This may be due to insufficient sampling or other issues of tissue quality. In the event that such a diagnosis is rendered, additional tissue collection should be encouraged if possible. If the tissue is such that even histologic categorization is not possible, one may want to avoid specifying it as a medulloblastoma altogether, given that other CNS malignancies can have similar histology focally and express overlapping immunohistochemical markers.

Ancillary Testing

A workup for medulloblastoma should place the tumor into both a histologic and molecular genetic group. Providing both is not quite yet universal, but is already the standard of care in many places and many clinical trials now require such information for enrollment. The only thing needed beyond routine H&Es for histologic classification is reticulin staining to assess for internodular desmoplasia in the desmoplastic/nodular variety, assuming other diagnoses have been ruled out.

For molecular categorization, a panel of three immunostains will be able to place most cases into one of the three WHO groups: beta-catenin, GAB1, and YAP1. WNT-activated cases show nuclear accumulation of beta-catenin at least focally on immunostaining and YAP1 in the cytoplasm and some nuclei. GAB1 should not be expressed by WNT-activated medulloblastomas. SHH-activated cases will express both YAP1 and GAB1, but not have nuclear beta-catenin. In desmoplastic/nodular cases, both are more likely to label the internodular tissue (Figure 10-14), whereas the staining is diffuse in SHH cases with classic or LC/A histology. The non-WNT/non-SHH tumors will not exhibit any of those immunohistochemical features (28). Other immunostains can be used, although these are probably the most common.

Testing for chromosomal abnormalities can be helpful for molecular categorization when immunostaining is inconclusive. Monosomy 6, frequently as the sole chromosomal defect, is present in the vast majority of WNT-group cases and is highly unlikely in other groups. Deletions of 9q at

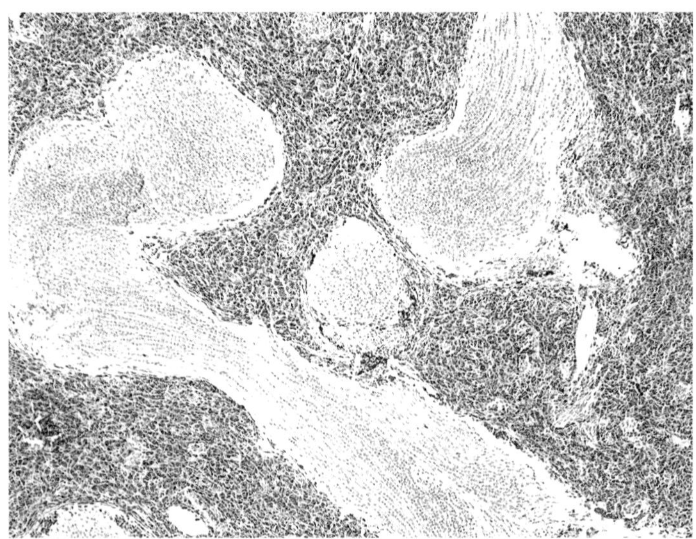

FIGURE 10-14 YAP1 (seen here) and GAB1 are immunohistochemical markers of SHH-activated medulloblastomas and tend to label the internodular areas of nodular desmoplastic cases.

the *PTCH1* locus are present in a little less than half of SHH-activated medulloblastomas and rare in other groups (38,41). Isochromosome 17q (gain of 17q with loss of 17p) identifies a medulloblastoma as non-WNT/ non-SHH. Amplifications of *MYC* are typically restricted to the WNT-activated group and group 3, while *MYCN* amplifications are restricted to SHH-activated and group 4. Fluorescence in situ hybridization (FISH) is commonly used for a number of these, although one may also use copy-number changes on DNA microarrays or other DNA-based methods.

Differential Diagnosis

The differential diagnosis for medulloblastoma is that of posterior fossa tumors in children, including ependymoma, AT/RT, and ETMR. Because of its hypercellular, small blue cell appearance, the cerebellar granular layer must also remain on the pathologist's mind during intraoperative consultation, where freezing artefact can distort histologic features (Figure 10-15). This normal structure occasionally provokes a mistaken diagnosis of medulloblastoma. In young adults who are immunosuppressed, primary CNS lymphoma can also appear in a sheetlike pattern reminiscent of medulloblastoma.

AT/RTs overlap histologically with medulloblastomas, especially the LC/A pattern. Both have large nuclei with vesicular, "open," chromatin with prominent nucleoli, although AT/RT can be composed of small cells that give an appearance more of classic medulloblastoma. While there can be a large amount of morphologic similarity, medulloblastoma tends to be more uniform and lacks the round eosinophilic cytoplasmic inclusions often seen in AT/RT. However, rhabdoid cytoplasmic inclusions are usually

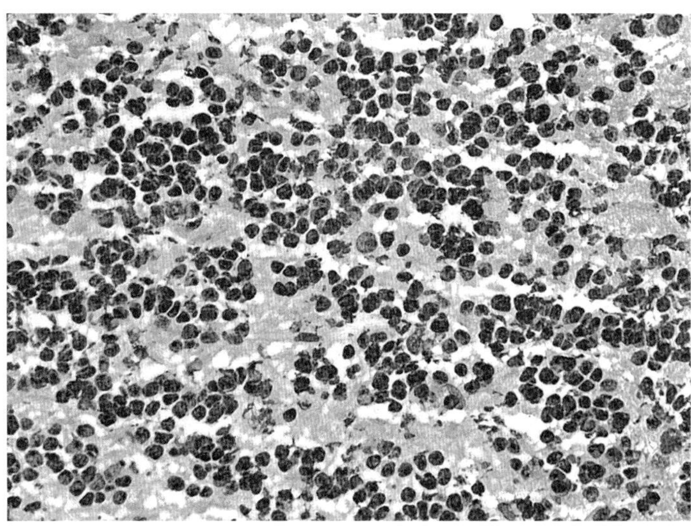

FIGURE 10-15 Freezing distorts and lends a suspicious look to cerebellar granule neurons, which should not be mistaken intraoperatively for medulloblastoma or any other malignancy.

subtle and focal. As a soft sign, medulloblastoma is also frequently peppered with apoptotic debris and pyknotic nuclei that are not as apparent in AT/RT. The distinction between medulloblastoma and AT/RT on H&E staining can be difficult, so additional evidence should always accompany the morphologic impression. Medulloblastoma should display diffuse nuclear immunostaining for SMARCB1/INI1within tumor cells, whereas AT/RT nuclei should be negative. Vascular endothelial cells provide a ready internal positive control and prevent misdiagnosis of AT/RT when absent staining results from technical failure (see Atypical Teratoid/Rhabdoid Tumor section). Negative INI1 staining with a positive internal control essentially confirms the diagnosis of AT/RT in the CNS, in the setting of a malignant intracranial neoplasm (48,49).

Clinically, because of the large overlap in age and anatomic distribution, ependymomas sometimes appear like medulloblastoma, especially in small specimens. Highly cellular (usually anaplastic) ependymomas may occasionally appear embryonal, yet can usually be separated from medulloblastomas on morphologic grounds by the presence of prominently fibrillar perivascular pseudorosettes and an overall more prominent vasculature. The perivascular pseudorosettes in medulloblastoma are more finely fibrillar and granular but can appear very similar to those of ependymoma (Figure 10-16). Instances with ambiguous features can usually be solved by immunohistochemistry; the fibrillar areas of ependymomas show strong positivity for GFAP, whereas the fibrillar areas of medulloblastoma express synaptophysin. Although not highly sensitive, EMA staining produces a cytoplasmic "dot-and-ring" pattern and traces the luminal surface of true ependymal rosettes in ependymoma.

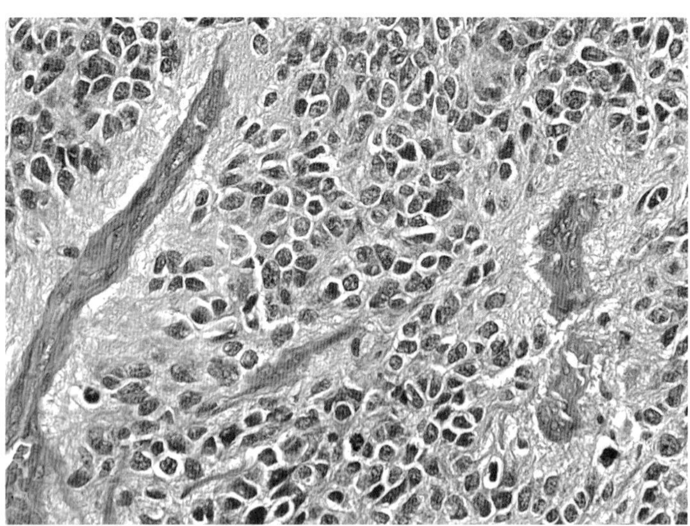

FIGURE 10-16 Ependymoma-like perivascular pseudorosettes are a focal feature of some medulloblastomas.

CENTRAL NERVOUS SYSTEM NEUROBLASTOMA AND GANGLIONEUROBLASTOMA (WHO GRADE IV)

Clinical Context

Because the term "PNET" covered such a heterogeneous group of entities for so long, including cerebral neuroblastoma, it is difficult to draw any firm conclusions about cerebral neuroblastomas based on literature before 2016, when the WHO made it once more a discrete entity (1). Histopathologically defined cerebral neuroblastomas are rare, and true cerebral neuroblastomas are vanishingly rare when genetic features are taken into account. Of a series of 323 archival tumors diagnosed as CNS-PNET from a number of institutions, only 44 fell into a neuroblastoma category, with all of the remaining going to other known tumor entities, such as AT/RT and glioblastoma, and novel new categories of embryonal tumor (50).

Histopathology

CNS neuroblastoma is a malignant tumor composed of embryonal, neuroblastic cells that may grow in sheets or have nodules and small amounts of fibrillar neuropil, similar to a peripheral neuroblastoma. Those cells may be arranged in fibrillar, Homer Wright rosettes, similar to what one might see in medulloblastoma (Figure 10-17). Maturation into fully differentiated ganglion cells may be seen, and, depending on the prominence of that population, one may further refine the diagnosis to CNS ganglioneuroblastoma (Figure 10-18), similar to the nomenclature of related lesions in peripheral ganglia, except there is no schwannian stroma in the vast majority of CNS cases.

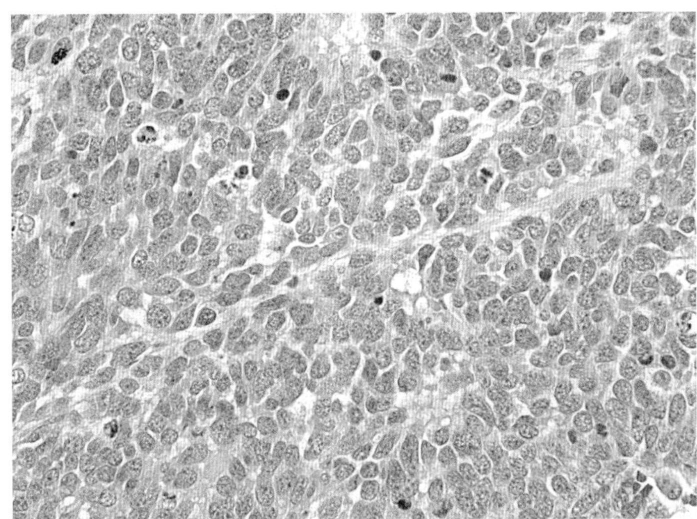

FIGURE 10-17 CNS neuroblastoma recapitulates the appearance of medulloblastoma, with sheets of neuroblastic embryonal cells and fibrillar Homer Wright rosettes.

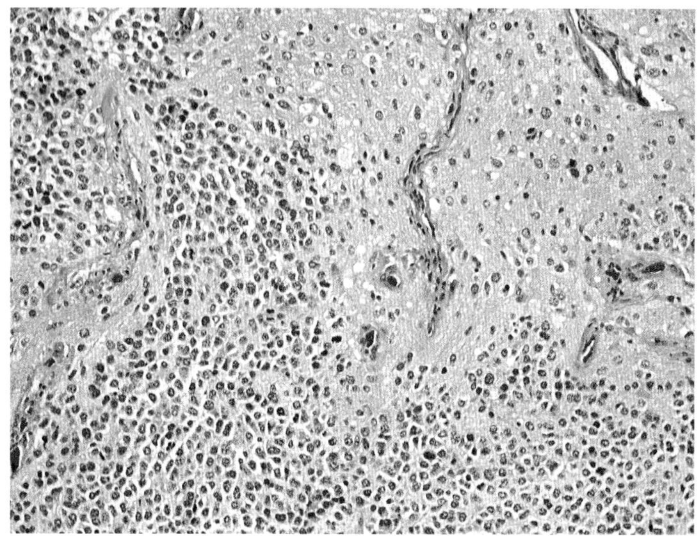

FIGURE 10-18 CNS ganglioneuroblastoma has mature ganglionic elements (upper right) and malignant neuroblastic elements (lower left).

Immunohistochemistry

CNS neuroblastoma displays an immunophenotype similar to medulloblastoma, with widespread synaptophysin staining and GFAP possibly occurring focally within tumor cells. Neurofilament is not widely expressed and is mostly limited to the mature neuronal elements. NeuN positivity is also not frequently seen, except in mature neuronal elements.

Differential Diagnosis

Glioblastoma must be considered when faced with a poorly differentiated supratentorial embryonal tumor, because glioblastomas treated with a more limited field of radiation and receive a vastly different chemotherapy regimen than CNS neuroblastomas. Radiographic findings can favor one of these two diagnoses; CNS neuroblastoma is typically more circumscribed with pushing borders and occasionally has a cystic component, whereas glioblastoma has an irregular and less-defined silhouette. Infiltration along white matter tracts, such as the corpus callosum, on MRI heavily favors a diagnosis of glioblastoma. Leptomeningeal metastasis on MRI heavily favors CNS neuroblastoma. Histologically, glioblastomas can exactly mimic the morphology and immunophenotype of CNS neuroblastoma, usually as a separate component that arises from the glial population, so it is advisable to examine genetic testing and other specific markers of glioblastoma, which are covered in Chapter 3.

Another tumor commonly confused with CNS neuroblastoma is AT/RT. As with medulloblastoma, AT/RT may be distinguished from

CNS-neuroblastoma by the extent of its morphologic and immunophenotypic heterogeneity. The distinction between these two tumors is vitally important to the clinicians because both the treatment regimen and survival rates are markedly different.

Small blue cell malignancies, metastatic or primary, such as Ewing sarcoma, neuroblastoma, rhabdomyosarcoma, NUT midline carcinoma, and others, must remain in consideration among embryonal CNS neoplasms.

EMBRYONAL TUMOR WITH MULTILAYERED ROSETTES, C19MC-ALTERED

General

ETMR was formerly classified by the WHO (2007) under three separate headings as subcategories of CNS-PNET: embryonal tumor with abundant neuropil and true rosettes (ETANTR), ependymoblastoma, and medulloepithelioma. The genetic basis for ETMR as a novel category of embryonal CNS-neoplasm is an amplification, or sometimes fusion, of a small segment of DNA on 19q13.42 that contains the largest cluster of miRNAs in humans (51,52). This area is referred to as C19MC, which abbreviates "chromosome 19 microRNA cluster."

Clinical Context

Most EMTRs present before the age of 2 years and all but the rarest cases before five (53–55). Most of them arise in the cerebral hemispheres, yet they can also appear in the ventricles, cerebellum, and pineal gland. The most common MRI appearance is a non- to inhomogeneously enhancing, well-circumscribed, solid mass that arises within the supratentorial and infratentorial compartments with frequencies roughly according to the volumes of nervous tissue contained in each (54). Overall survival in patients with ETMR is typically less than 1 year from diagnosis.

Histopathology

ETANTR AND EPENDYMOBLASTOMA PATTERNS. Histologically, this pattern of ETMR is composed of islands of embryonal tumor cells in a sea of less cellular, finely fibrillar, neuropil-like matrix, forming luminal, or "ependymoblastic," multilayered rosettes (Figure 10-19). The ependymoblastic rosettes appear in both the hypo- and hypercellular areas and are formed of pseudostratified, elongate tumor cells arranged radially around a well-defined, round to slit-like lumen. Sometimes, the lumen is rudimentary and contains small amounts of granular material. Although luminal rosettes define ETANTR, perivascular and fibrillar rosettes may also be seen. Similar to nodular medulloblastomas, ETANTR tumor cells show varying levels of differentiation, from embryonal within the areas of cellularity to neurocytic, and even occasionally ganglionic, within the hypocellular areas. The "ependymoblastoma" pattern is essentially the same as

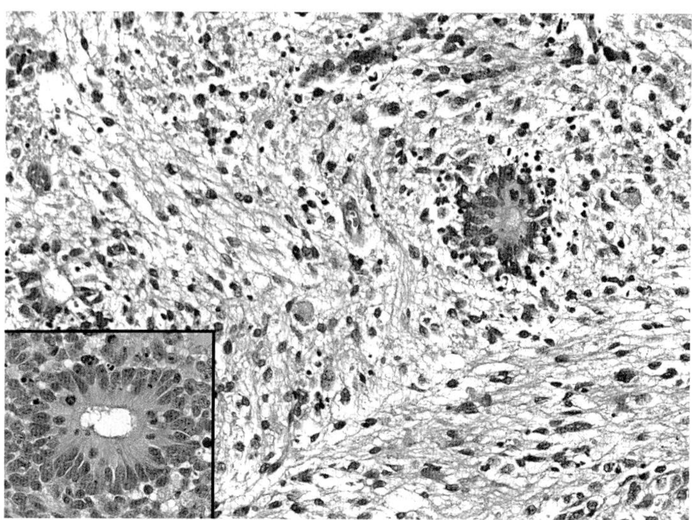

FIGURE 10-19 Embryonal tumor multilayered rosettes is characterized by cellular islands of embryonal cells and true rosettes (inset) in a background of loose neuropil-rich tumor (ETANTR pattern).

ETANTR, except that most or all of the tissue is the densely cellular element (Figure 10-20).

Although the undifferentiated cells within the clusters generally fail to stain for neuronal or glial markers, NeuN, synaptophysin, and neurofilament staining can be strong within the more differentiated cells of the

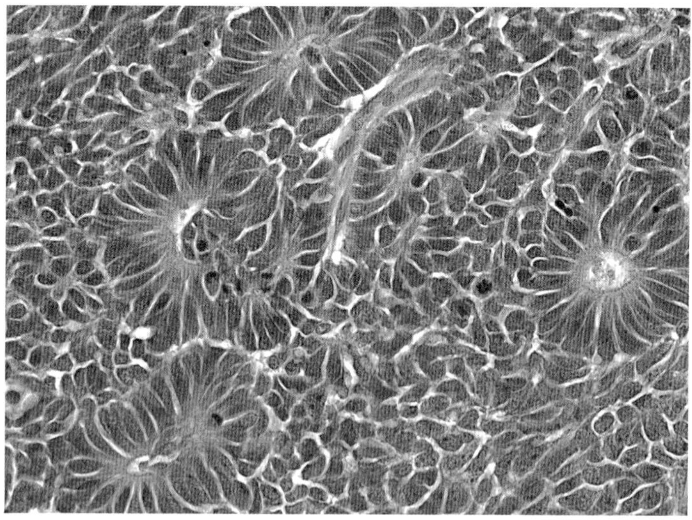

FIGURE 10-20 "Ependymoblastomatous" rosettes are pseudostratified with sharply defined lumens within sheets of embryonal tumor cells.

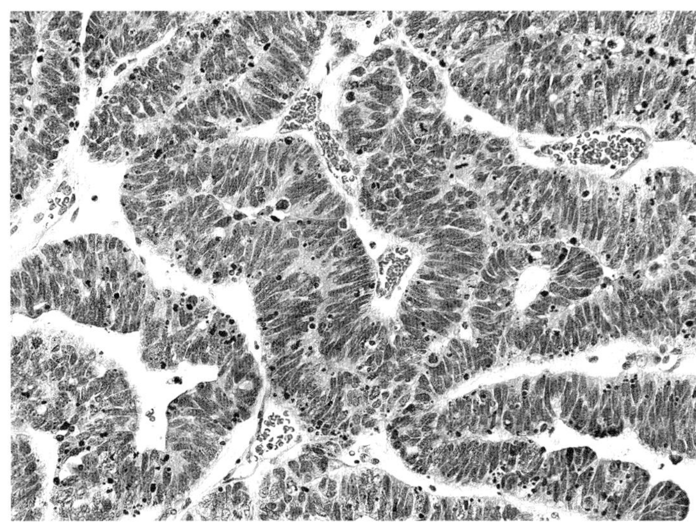

FIGURE 10-21 The medulloepithelioma pattern exhibits gland-like epithelioid structures that resemble primitive neural tube.

neuropil-like areas. GFAP stains scattered, entrapped astrocytes and the occasional tumor cell.

Medulloepithelioma Pattern

HISTOPATHOLOGY. The medulloepithelioma pattern is characterized by a "back-to-back" proliferation of tubular structures that resemble the primitive/embryonic neural tube composed of pseudostratified columnar cells (Figure 10-21). Similar to the malignant glands of well-differentiated adenocarcinoma the columnar cells of medulloepithelioma rest on a shared basement membrane. Although tubules and papillary structures dominate the histologic picture of this lesion, areas of undifferentiated proliferation are also seen. Tumor cells often lack significant pleomorphism, and have a high nucleus to cytoplasm ratio, with large, regular, elliptical nuclei that contain coarse, open chromatin. Mitosis is abundant. As with other embryonal CNS tumors, medulloepitheliomas may show divergent differentiation into glial, neural, and mesenchymal lineages (56–59). Care must be taken in the face of non-neuroepithelial differentiation that the lesion in question is not actually an immature teratoma.

Rare medulloepitheliomas may not show alterations of C19MC, yet they still strongly express LIN28A protein and should be considered as ETMRs (60).

Immunohistochemistry

Reticulin staining and immunostaining for type IV collagen emphasize the shared basement membrane of tumor epithelium, as does PAS staining. Typical neuroepithelial markers, such as S100, synaptophysin, and GFAP, are not expressed in the epithelial cells of medulloepithelioma, although they may be seen in nonepithelial areas. LIN28A, a protein that binds miRNAs and is thought to regulate the pluripotency of stem cells, is highly expressed in ETMR and not in other pediatric CNS tumors, providing a useful immunohistochemical surrogate to C19MC amplification testing. The staining pattern is cytoplasmic, strong, and diffuse (60). AT/RTs can also demonstrate small foci of LIN28A immunostaining, yet these consist of only a few cells and are unlikely to be mistaken for the pattern seen in ETMRs.

Genetics

The unifying feature of ETMRs is amplification or, much less commonly, fusion of the C19MC locus at 19q13.42 (51). The micro-RNAs coded in that area are thought to be the drivers of ETMRs malignancy. Amplification of C19MC is usually detected via FISH; the relative small size of the amplification makes it difficult to detect with some array-based copy-number platforms. LIN28 immunostaining is a strong surrogate for the DNA-based testing (60).

Other common features in ETMRs include whole gains of chromosome 2 (~75%), gain of 1q (25%), and loss of 6q (~20%) (52).

Differential Diagnosis

The main diagnostic pitfall with ETMRs is placing them in a less aggressive diagnostic category. In the posterior fossa, one may focus on the areas of cellular embryonal tissue or have a, "ependymoblastoma" pattern and mistakenly diagnose medulloblastoma, which is much more common there and has a much better prognosis. Large multilayered rosettes should not be seen in medulloblastoma. This can also happen in the pineal gland, where pineoblastomas may have rosette structures. These are less of a concern with the medulloepithelioma pattern, which is so distinctive that it is unlikely to be mistaken as another tumor.

CNS EMBRYONAL TUMOR, NOS

Inevitably there are idiosyncratic malignant tumors, particularly in children, that defy discrete categorization. This diagnosis of exclusion is available for such circumstances once one has ruled out all of the known CNS embryonal tumors and embryonal-appearing cases from other categories, such as glioblastoma, AT/RT, anaplastic ependymoma, choroid plexus carcinoma, and Ewing sarcoma.

ATYPICAL TERATOID/RHABDOID TUMOR (WHO GRADE IV)

Clinical Context

AT/RT is an aggressive malignant tumor of the CNS that is pathogenetically related and morphologically similar to the malignant rhabdoid tumors of the kidney and soft tissue that occur both sporadically and in the setting of the "familial rhabdoid tumor predisposition syndrome" (61). Rhabdoid tumor predisposition syndrome is due to a germline mutation in the *SMARCB1* chromatin modeling (SWI/SNF complex) gene on chromosome 22q11.2, causing a nonfunctioning allele and subsequent tumors when a somatic "second hit" occurs. Sporadic AT/RTs also show mutations or deletions of the *SMARCB1* gene, providing a pathogenetically relevant target for molecular and immunohistochemical interrogation. SMARCA4 mutations have been associated with AT/RTs in the setting of wild type SMARCB1, sometimes as a germline allele (62).

Most cases of AT/RT occur sporadically and before 3 years of age, with less than a quarter occurring in ages greater than 3 years (63–65). Rarely, AT/RT may affect adults (66). As with medulloblastoma, AT/RTs show a modest male predominance, with male:female ratios around 1.5:1 (65). Up to a third of patients with rhabdoid tumors may have germline mutations and genetic counseling should be suggested to all patients diagnosed with AT/RT and their families (67).

AT/RTs may occur anywhere in the brain, with somewhat more coming from the supratentorial compartment (63,64,68). Infants tend to get AT/RTs in the posterior fossa. Cases rarely arise within the spinal cord, probably at a rate lower than the relative volume of the cord to the brain (65,69). On MRI, AT/RT is generally circumscribed, with heterogeneous contrast enhancement and signal intensity, usually secondary to areas of hemorrhage and necrosis. Leptomeningeal spread is a common radiologic finding, being present in approximately a fifth to a quarter of cases at diagnosis (68). Some AT/RTs show a characteristic "band-like wavy pattern" of enhancement, although this finding is not diagnostic and often not present (69).

Histopathology

Microscopically, AT/RT is usually mildly heterogeneous in tissue pattern. Most cases have areas composed of sheets of poorly differentiated embryonal cells with monotonous nuclei with variably open chromatin and prominent nucleoli and a small to moderate amount of lightly eosinophilic cytoplasm (Figures 10-22 and 10-23). Some areas may have a streaming appearance and more elliptical nuclei. Other areas may contain foci of cells with prominent cytoplasmic vacuoles (Figure 10-24). Occasionally, the cells in AT/RT will form cords and clusters in a myxoid background (Figure 10-25). Epithelial structures can be seen rarely. Although the variability of the cells and tissue patterns in AT/RT is high, the nuclear features tend to be consistent, with pale chromatin and prominent nucleoli.

Most cases of AT/RT have focal and relatively subtle rhabdoid morphology. Relatively few cases have overtly rhabdoid morphology with large, eccentric, smooth, pink cytoplasmic inclusions that may indent the nucleus (Figure 10-26) (70,71). These cytoplasmic inclusions, as with other rhabdoid tumors, are composed ultrastructurally of whorled aggregates of

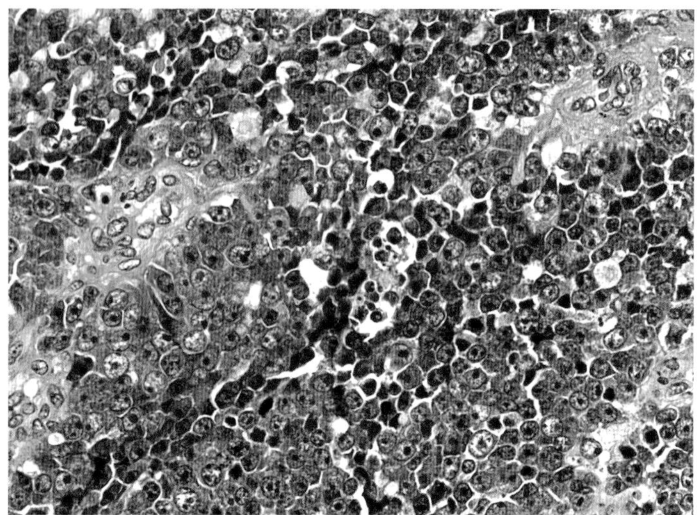

FIGURE 10-22 Large round nuclei with prominent nucleoli in AT/RT (seen here) may closely replicate those of large cell/anaplastic medulloblastoma.

intermediate filaments (72). Rhabdoid inclusions are not a necessary criterion for the diagnosis of AT/RT and can be completely absent.

Histologic heterogeneity is characteristic of AT/RT, with neuroectodermal, mesenchymal, and, rarely, epithelial differentiation being evident. The neuroectodermal component can closely mimic medulloblastoma or CNS neuroblastoma, even with neuroblastic-like rosette structures (Figure 10-27). Necrosis, hemorrhage, and numerous mitoses are often present. Establishing a diagnosis of AT/RT on a purely morphologic basis can be

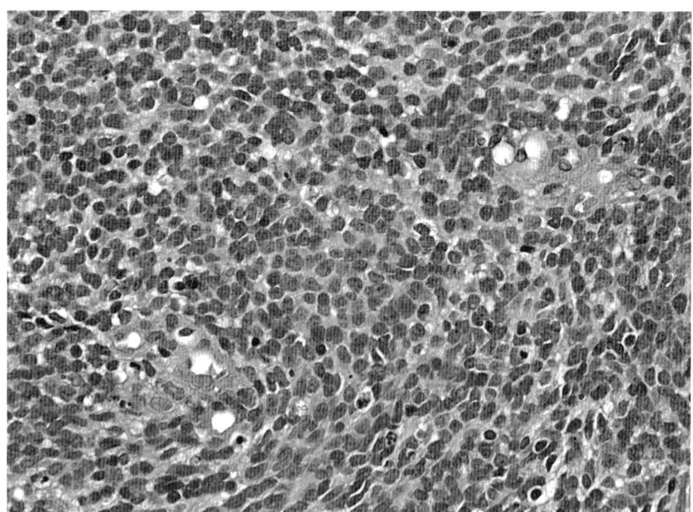

FIGURE 10-23 Atypical teratoid/rhabdoid tumors often contain fields of monotonous undifferentiated cells similar to medulloblastoma.

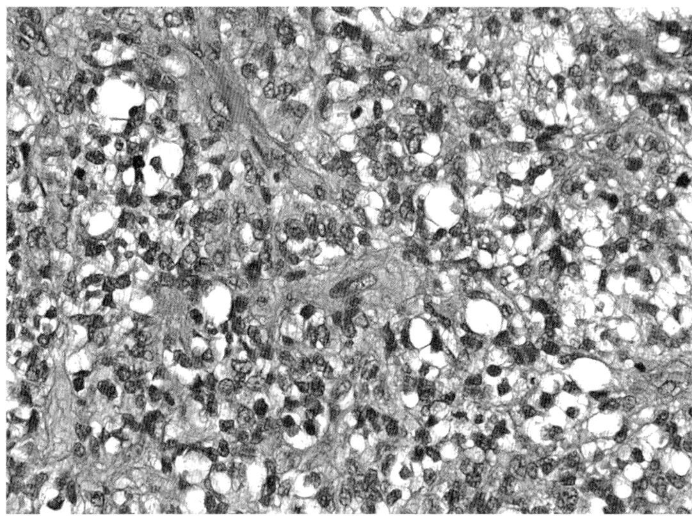

FIGURE 10-24 Patches of prominent cytoplasmic vacuolation are a common and distinctive histologic feature of atypical teratoid/rhabdoid tumor.

extremely difficult and risky, so its diagnosis should always be augmented with confirmatory ancillary testing.

Immunohistochemistry

AT/RT, in accordance with its heterogeneous histologic appearance, has a characteristically heterogeneous immunophenotype (Figure 10-28). Focal membranous and cytoplasmic staining for EMA is one of the most consistent

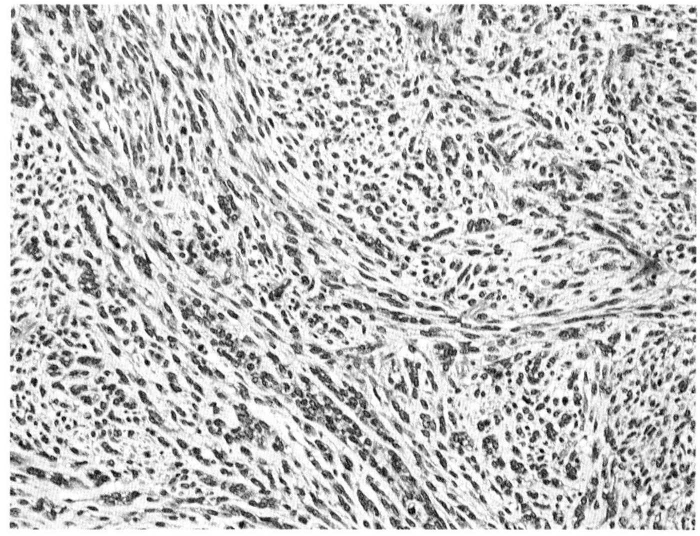

FIGURE 10-25 AT/RTs occasionally have cords and nests of cells, some of which are elongate, in a myxoid background.

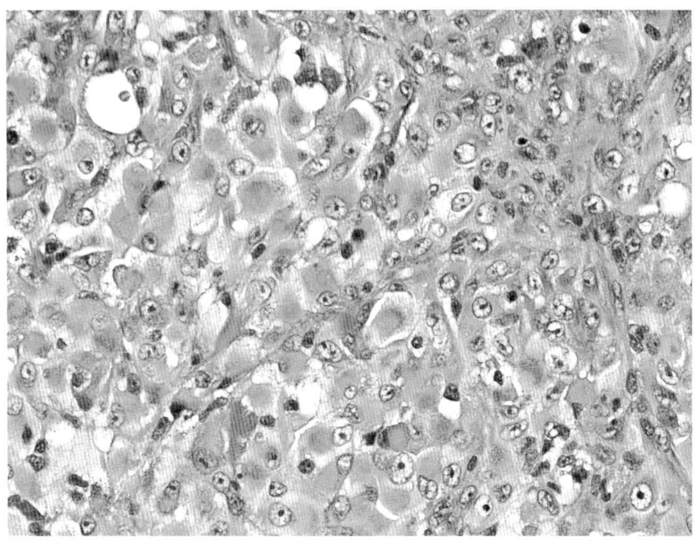

FIGURE 10-26 Overtly rhabdoid cells such as these are absent from many AT/RTs and are not required for the diagnosis.

features, with foci of smooth muscle actin (SMA), vimentin, cytokeratin, GFAP, synaptophysin, and neurofilament reactivity also common.

The most important immunohistochemical feature of AT/RT is the absence of nuclear staining for the tumor suppressor INI1 (Figure 10-29). Because loss of INI1 function is thought to be a necessary proximal event in the formation of AT/RT, demonstration of its loss by immunohistochemistry,

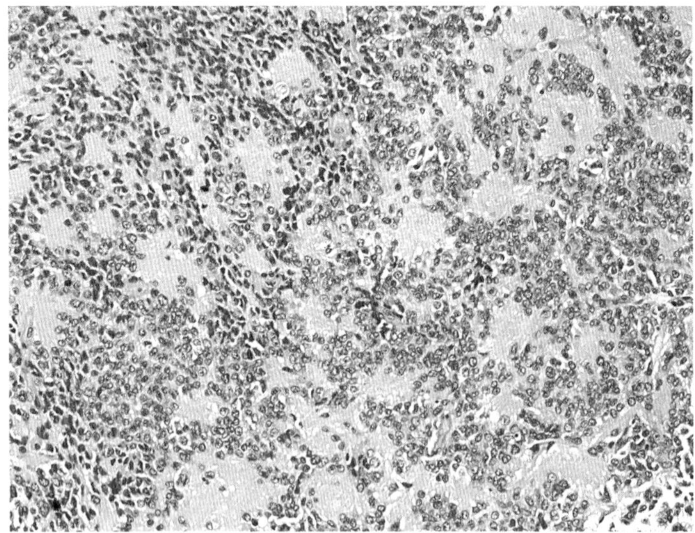

FIGURE 10-27 A small number of AT/RTs will express apparent neuroblastic differentiation, replete with neuroblastic-like rosettes.

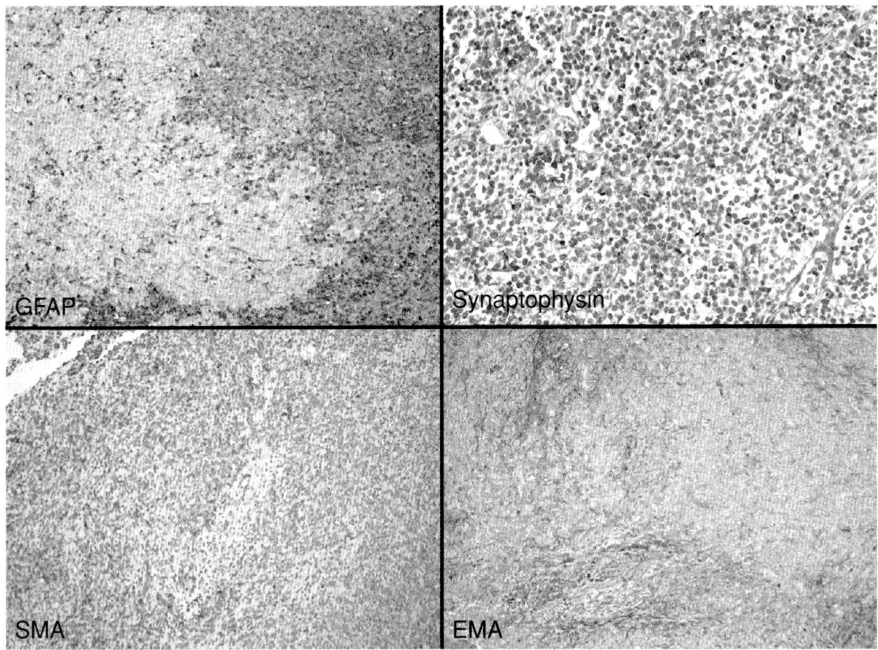

FIGURE 10-28 Immunohistochemistry shows heterogeneous mesenchymal, epithelial, and neuroepithelial expression in atypical teratoid/rhabdoid tumor.

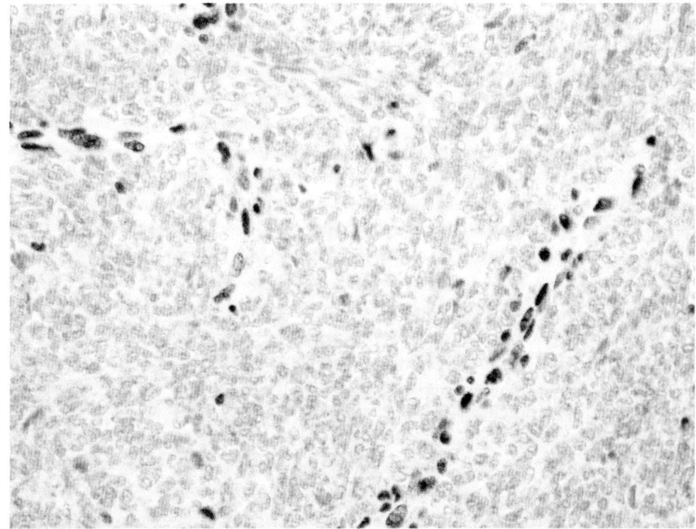

FIGURE 10-29 Nuclear INI1 immunoreactivity in atypical teratoid/rhabdoid tumor is limited to the nonneoplastic endothelial cells and is absent from tumor cells.

FISH, another method is a reliable way to diagnose AT/RT in the setting of an embryonal brain tumor. The epitopes recognized by some antibodies to SMARCB1/INI1, including BAF47, are thermally labile, causing loss of immunoreactivity in areas of cautery artefact, even when the morphologic features of cautery are missing.

Genetics

Loss of SMARCB1 protein expression is the primary genetic feature of AT/RT with essentially no other consistent findings. The loss is either by a combination of inactivating mutation and deletion of the other allele, which is more common, or simply homozygous deletion (67). No other chromosomal abnormalities or mutations have a consistent role in AT/RT development.

DNA methylation profiling has identified three subgroups that overlap in age and anatomic distributions, except for the ATRT-TYR group which tends to be in the posterior fossa and in younger patients (73). The significance of this grouping is not yet clear.

Differential Diagnosis

AT/RT should always be ruled out when one encounters a malignant intracranial neoplasm in a child, especially when younger than 3 years. Pale, monotonous nuclei and prominent nucleoli should even prompt suspicion in adult brain tumor patients.

Given the reliable and specific SMARCB1/INI1 immunostain for AT/RT and its necessity for confirming the diagnosis, it is unlikely that one would mistakenly diagnose another malignant brain tumor as AT/RT; however, the converse is frequently true. The tumors most likely to be mimicked by AT/RT include medulloblastoma (particularly LC/A), choroid plexus carcinoma, CNS neuroblastoma, and occasionally high-grade glioma (epithelioid glioblastoma). Assessment if SMARCB1/INI1 status is appropriate in any malignant brain tumor in a child and with even the slightest suspicion in older patients.

On the other hand, in the rare event that one has a tumor that is strongly suspicious for AT/RT but has retained SMARCB1/INI1 expression, consideration should be given to testing for the loss of SMARCA4/BRG1 expression.

SMARCB1 loss has been reported in at least two other CNS tumor entities that have lower-grade morphology and good prognosis: cribriform neuroepithelial tumor (CRINET) (74) and papillary glial tumor of the spinal cord (75). Neither of these resembles AT/RT histologically, so it is unlikely that one would mistake them, but it important to remember that INI1 loss in the context of histologic malignancy constitutes AT/RT.

Prognosis

In the recent past, the prognosis for patients with AT/RT was grim, with median event-free survival of about 10 months (63). Newer regimens have led to a long-term cure in a minority of patients (76). In tumor registry data from the United States from 2001 to 2009, age at diagnosis was related to survival: patients 0 to 3 years had 22% survival at 2 years, versus around 50% for patients 4 to 19 years (65).

REFERENCES

1. Louis DN, Ohgaki H, Wiestler OD, et al., eds. WHO Classification of Tumours of the Central Nervous System. 4th ed. Lyon, France: IARC Press; 2016.
2. Taylor MD, Northcott PA, Korshunov A, et al. Molecular subgroups of medulloblastoma: the current consensus. *Acta Neuropathol.* 2012;123(4):465–472.
3. Zhukova N, Ramaswamy V, Remke M, et al. Subgroup-specific prognostic implications of TP53 mutation in medulloblastoma. *J Clinical Oncol.* 2013;31(23):2927–2935.
4. Ostrom QT, Gittleman H, Xu J, et al. CBTRUS statistical report: Primary brain and other central nervous system tumors diagnosed in the United States in 2009-2013. *Neuro Oncol.* 2016;18(suppl 5):v1–v75.
5. Roberts RO, Lynch CF, Jones MP, et al. Medulloblastoma: a population-based study of 532 cases. *J Neuropathol Exp Neurol.* 1991;50(2):134–144.
6. Buhren J, Christoph AH, Buslei R, et al. Expression of the neurotrophin receptor p75NTR in medulloblastomas is correlated with distinct histological and clinical features: evidence for a medulloblastoma subtype derived from the external granule cell layer. *J Neuropathol Exp Neurol.* 2000;59(3):229–240.
7. Giangaspero F, Perilongo G, Fondelli MP, et al. Medulloblastoma with extensive nodularity: a variant with favorable prognosis. *J Neurosurg.* 1999;91(6):971–977.
8. Packer RJ, Cogen P, Vezina G, et al. Medulloblastoma: clinical and biologic aspects. *Neuro Oncol.* 1999;1(3):232–250.
9. Packer RJ, Sutton LN, Elterman R, et al. Outcome for children with medulloblastoma treated with radiation and cisplatin, CCNU, and vincristine chemotherapy. *J Neurosurg.* 1994;81(5):690–698.
10. Eberhart CG, Cohen KJ, Tihan T, et al. Medulloblastomas with systemic metastases: evaluation of tumor histopathology and clinical behavior in 23 patients. *J Pediatr Hematol Oncol.* 2003;25(3):198–203.
11. Cai DX, Mafra M, Schmidt RE, et al. Medulloblastomas with extensive posttherapy neuronal maturation. Report of two cases. *J Neurosurg.* 2000;93(2):330–334.
12. Geyer JR, Schofield D, Berger M, et al. Differentiation of a primitive neuroectodermal tumor into a benign ganglioglioma. *J Neurooncol.* 1992;14(3):237–241.
13. Kane W, Aronson SM. Gangliogliomatous maturation in cerebellar medulloblastoma. *Acta Neuropathol.* 1967;9(3):273–279.
14. Rubinstein LJ, Northfield DW. The medulloblastoma and the so-called "arachnoidal cerebellar sarcoma". *Brain.* 1964;87:379–412.
15. McManamy CS, Pears J, Weston CL, et al. Nodule formation and desmoplasia in medulloblastomas-defining the nodular/desmoplastic variant and its biological behavior. *Brain Pathol.* 2007;17(2):151–164.
16. Verma S, Tavare CJ, Gilles FH. Histologic features and prognosis in pediatric medulloblastoma. *Pediatr Dev Pathol.* 2008;11(5):337–343.
17. Anwer UE, Smith TW, DeGirolami U, et al. Medulloblastoma with cartilaginous differentiation. *Arch Pathol Lab Med.* 1989;113(1):84–88.
18. Giordana MT, Schiffer P, Boghi A, et al. Medulloblastoma with lipidized cells versus lipomatous medulloblastoma. *Clin Neuropathol.* 2000;19(6):273–277.
19. Kubota KC, Itoh T, Yamada Y, et al. Melanocytic medulloblastoma with ganglioneurocytomatous differentiation: a case report. *Neuropathology.* 2009;29(1):72–77.

20. Polydorides AD, Perry A, Edgar MA. Large cell medulloblastoma with myogenic and melanotic differentiation: a case report with molecular analysis. *J Neurooncol.* 2008; 88(2):193–197.
21. Zanini C, Mandili G, Pulera F, et al. Immunohistochemical and proteomic profile of melanotic medulloblastoma. *Pediatr Blood Cancer.* 2009;52(7):875–877.
22. Rajeshwari M, Kakkar A, Nalwa A, et al. WNT-activated medulloblastoma with melanotic and myogenic differentiation: report of a rare case. *Neuropathology.* 2016;36(4):372–375.
23. Stefanits H, Ebetsberger-Dachs G, Weis S, et al. Medulloblastoma with multi-lineage differentiation including myogenic and melanotic elements: a case report with molecular data. *Clin Neuropathol.* 2014;33(2):122–127.
24. Wright KD, von der Embse K, Coleman J, et al. Isochromosome 17q, MYC amplification and large cell/anaplastic phenotype in a case of medullomyoblastoma with extracranial metastases. *Pediatr Blood Cancer.* 2012;59(3):561–564.
25. Ellison DW, Eberhart C, Pietsch T, et al. Medulloblastoma. In: Louis DN, Ohgaki H, Wiestler OD, et al., eds. WHO Classification of Tumours of the Central Nervous System. 4th ed. Lyon, France: IARC Press; 2016:184–188.
26. Huang H, Mahler-Araujo BM, Sankila A, et al. APC mutations in sporadic medulloblastomas. *Am J Pathol.* 2000;156(2):433–437.
27. Clifford SC, Lannering B, Schwalbe EC, et al. Biomarker-driven stratification of disease-risk in non-metastatic medulloblastoma: results from the multi-center HIT-SIOP-PNET4 clinical trial. *Oncotarget.* 2015;6(36):38827–38839.
28. Ellison DW, Dalton J, Kocak M, et al. Medulloblastoma: clinicopathological correlates of SHH, WNT, and non-SHH/WNT molecular subgroups. *Acta Neuropathol.* 2011;121(3): 381–396.
29. Lastowska M, Trubicka J, Niemira M, et al. ALK expression is a novel marker for the WNT-activated type of pediatric medulloblastoma and an indicator of good prognosis for patients. *Am J Surg Pathol.* 2017;41(6):781–787.
30. Northcott PA, Shih DJ, Peacock J, et al. Subgroup-specific structural variation across 1,000 medulloblastoma genomes. *Nature.* 2012;488(7409):49–56.
31. Clifford SC, Lusher ME, Lindsey JC, et al. Wnt/Wingless pathway activation and chromosome 6 loss characterize a distinct molecular sub-group of medulloblastomas associated with a favorable prognosis. *Cell Cycle.* 2006;5(22):2666–2670.
32. Robinson G, Parker M, Kranenburg TA, et al. Novel mutations target distinct subgroups of medulloblastoma. *Nature.* 2012;488(7409):43–48.
33. Pfaff E, Remke M, Sturm D, et al. TP53 mutation is frequently associated with CTNNB1 mutation or MYCN amplification and is compatible with long-term survival in medulloblastoma. *J Clin Oncol.* 2010;28(35):5188–5196.
34. Brugieres L, Remenieras A, Pierron G, et al. High frequency of germline SUFU mutations in children with desmoplastic/nodular medulloblastoma younger than 3 years of age. *J Clin Oncol.* 2012;30(17):2087–2093.
35. Rausch T, Jones DT, Zapatka M, et al. Genome sequencing of pediatric medulloblastoma links catastrophic DNA rearrangements with TP53 mutations. *Cell.* 2012;148(1-2):59–71.
36. Miele E, Mastronuzzi A, Po A, et al. Characterization of medulloblastoma in Fanconi anemia: a novel mutation in the BRCA2 gene and SHH molecular subgroup. *Biomark Res.* 2015;3:13.
37. Garre ML, Cama A, Bagnasco F, et al. Medulloblastoma variants: age-dependent occurrence and relation to Gorlin syndrome–a new clinical perspective. *Clinical Cancer Res.* 2009;15(7):2463–2471.
38. Northcott PA, Korshunov A, Witt H, et al. Medulloblastoma comprises four distinct molecular variants. *J Clin Oncol.* 2011;29(11):1408–1414.

39. Tabori U, Baskin B, Shago M, et al. Universal poor survival in children with medulloblastoma harboring somatic TP53 mutations. *J Clin Oncol.* 2010;28(8):1345–1350.
40. Kool M, Jones DT, Jager N, et al. Genome sequencing of SHH medulloblastoma predicts genotype-related response to smoothened inhibition. *Cancer Cell.* 2014;25(3):393-405.
41. Kool M, Korshunov A, Remke M, et al. Molecular subgroups of medulloblastoma: an international meta-analysis of transcriptome, genetic aberrations, and clinical data of WNT, SHH, Group 3, and Group 4 medulloblastomas. *Acta Neuropathol.* 2012;123(4): 473–484.
42. Bourdeaut F, Miquel C, Richer W, et al. Rubinstein-Taybi syndrome predisposing to non-WNT, non-SHH, group 3 medulloblastoma. *Pediatr Blood Cancer.* 2014;61(2):383–386.
43. Cogen PH, Daneshvar L, Metzger AK, et al. Deletion mapping of the medulloblastoma locus on chromosome 17p. *Genomics.* 1990;8(2):279–285.
44. Giordana MT, Migheli A, Pavanelli E. Isochromosome 17q is a constant finding in medulloblastoma. An interphase cytogenetic study on tissue sections. *Neuropathol Appl Neurobiol.* 1998;24(3):233–238.
45. Pan E, Pellarin M, Holmes E, et al. Isochromosome 17q is a negative prognostic factor in poor-risk childhood medulloblastoma patients. *Clin Cancer Res* 2005;11(13):4733–4740.
46. Pfister S, Remke M, Benner A, et al. Outcome prediction in pediatric medulloblastoma based on DNA copy-number aberrations of chromosomes 6q and 17q and the MYC and MYCN loci. *J Clin Oncol.* 2009;27(10):1627–1636.
47. Ramaswamy V, Remke M, Bouffet E, et al. Risk stratification of childhood medulloblastoma in the molecular era: the current consensus. *Acta Neuropathol.* 2016;131(6):821–831.
48. Judkins AR, Mauger J, Ht A, et al. Immunohistochemical analysis of hSNF5/INI1 in pediatric CNS neoplasms. *Am J Surg Pathol.* 2004;28(5):644–650.
49. Sigauke E, Rakheja D, Maddox DL, et al. Absence of expression of SMARCB1/INI1 in malignant rhabdoid tumors of the central nervous system, kidneys and soft tissue: an immunohistochemical study with implications for diagnosis. *Mod Pathol.* 2006;19(5): 717–725.
50. Sturm D, Orr BA, Toprak UH, et al. New brain tumor entities emerge from molecular classification of CNS-PNETs. *Cell.* 2016;164(5):1060–1072.
51. Korshunov A, Remke M, Gessi M, et al. Focal genomic amplification at 19q13.42 comprises a powerful diagnostic marker for embryonal tumors with ependymoblastic rosettes. *Acta Neuropathol.* 2010;120(2):253–260.
52. Korshunov A, Sturm D, Ryzhova M, et al. Embryonal tumor with abundant neuropil and true rosettes (ETANTR), ependymoblastoma, and medulloepithelioma share molecular similarity and comprise a single clinicopathological entity. *Acta Neuropathol.* 2014; 128(2):279–289.
53. Eberhart CG, Brat DJ, Cohen KJ, et al. Pediatric neuroblastic brain tumors containing abundant neuropil and true rosettes. *Pediatr Dev Pathol.* 2000;3(4):346–352.
54. Gessi M, Giangaspero F, Lauriola L, et al. Embryonal tumors with abundant neuropil and true rosettes: a distinctive CNS primitive neuroectodermal tumor. *Am J Surg Pathol.* 2009;33(2):211–217.
55. Pfister S, Remke M, Castoldi M, et al. Novel genomic amplification targeting the microRNA cluster at 19q13.42 in a pediatric embryonal tumor with abundant neuropil and true rosettes. *Acta Neuropathol.* 2009;117(4):457–464.
56. Molloy PT, Yachnis AT, Rorke LB, et al. Central nervous system medulloepithelioma: a series of eight cases including two arising in the pons. *J Neurosurg.* 1996;84(3):430–436.
57. Auer RN, Becker LE. Cerebral medulloepithelioma with bone, cartilage, and striated muscle. Light microscopic and immunohistochemical study. *J Neuropathol Exp Neurol.* 1983;42(3):256–267.

58. Deck JH. Cerebral medulloepithelioma with maturation into ependymal cells and ganglion cells. *J Neuropathol Exp Neurol.* 1969;28(3):442–454.
59. Scheithauer BW, Rubinstein LJ. Cerebral medulloepithelioma. Report of a case with multiple divergent neuroepithelial differentiation. *Child's Brain.* 1979;5(1):62–71.
60. Spence T, Sin-Chan P, Picard D, et al. CNS-PNETs with C19MC amplification and/or LIN28 expression comprise a distinct histogenetic diagnostic and therapeutic entity. *Acta Neuropathol.* 2014;128(2):291–303.
61. Sevenet N, Sheridan E, Amram D, et al. Constitutional mutations of the hSNF5/INI1 gene predispose to a variety of cancers. *Am J Hum Genet.* 1999;65(5):1342–1348.
62. Hasselblatt M, Nagel I, Oyen F, et al. SMARCA4-mutated atypical teratoid/rhabdoid tumors are associated with inherited germline alterations and poor prognosis. *Acta Neuropathol.* 2014;128(3):453–456.
63. Hilden JM, Meerbaum S, Burger P, et al. Central nervous system atypical teratoid/rhabdoid tumor: results of therapy in children enrolled in a registry. *J Clin Oncol.* 2004;22(14): 2877–2884.
64. Tekautz TM, Fuller CE, Blaney S, et al. Atypical teratoid/rhabdoid tumors (ATRT): improved survival in children 3 years of age and older with radiation therapy and high-dose alkylator-based chemotherapy. *J Clin Oncol.* 2005;23(7):1491–1499.
65. Ostrom QT, Chen Y, M de Blank P, et al. The descriptive epidemiology of atypical teratoid/rhabdoid tumors in the United States, 2001-2010. *Neuro Oncol.* 2014;16(10):1392–1399.
66. Raisanen J, Biegel JA, Hatanpaa KJ, et al. Chromosome 22q deletions in atypical teratoid/rhabdoid tumors in adults. *Brain Pathol.* 2005;15(1):23–28.
67. Biegel JA. Molecular genetics of atypical teratoid/rhabdoid tumor. *Neurosurg Focus.* 2006;20(1):E11.
68. Meyers SP, Khademian ZP, Biegel JA, et al. Primary intracranial atypical teratoid/rhabdoid tumors of infancy and childhood: MRI features and patient outcomes. *AJNR Am J Neuroradiol.* 2006;27(5):962–971.
69. Warmuth-Metz M, Bison B, Dannemann-Stern E, et al. CT and MR imaging in atypical teratoid/rhabdoid tumors of the central nervous system. *Neuroradiology.* 2008;50(5):447–452.
70. Rorke LB, Packer R, Biegel J. Central nervous system atypical teratoid/rhabdoid tumors of infancy and childhood. *J Neurooncol.* 1995;24(1):21–28.
71. Rorke LB, Packer RJ, Biegel JA. Central nervous system atypical teratoid/rhabdoid tumors of infancy and childhood: definition of an entity. *J Neurosurg.* 1996;85(1):56–65.
72. Inenaga C, Toyoshima Y, Mori H, et al. A fourth ventricle atypical teratoid/rhabdoid tumor in an infant. *Brain Tumor Pathol.* 2003;20(2):47–52.
73. Johann PD, Erkek S, Zapatka M, et al. Atypical teratoid/rhabdoid tumors are comprised of three epigenetic subgroups with distinct enhancer landscapes. *Cancer Cell.* 2016;29(3): 379–393.
74. Hasselblatt M, Oyen F, Gesk S, et al. Cribriform neuroepithelial tumor (CRINET): a nonrhabdoid ventricular tumor with INI1 loss and relatively favorable prognosis. *J Neuropathol Exp Neurol.* 2009;68(12):1249–1255.
75. Hasselblatt M, Kurniawan AD, Rozsnoki S, et al. Glial papillary tumour of the spinal cord with SMARCB1/INI1-loss and favourable long-term outcome. *Neuropathol Appl Neurobiol.* 2017. doi: 10.1111/nan.12395.
76. Chi SN, Zimmerman MA, Yao X, et al. Intensive multimodality treatment for children with newly diagnosed CNS atypical teratoid rhabdoid tumor. *J Clin Oncol.* 2009;27(3): 385–389.

11

CHOROID PLEXUS TUMORS

CHOROID PLEXUS PAPILLOMA (WHO GRADE I), ATYPICAL CHOROID PLEXUS PAPILLOMA (WHO GRADE II), AND CHOROID PLEXUS CARCINOMA (WHO GRADE III)

Clinical Context

Altogether, tumors of the choroid plexus epithelium represent a very small fraction of all primary central nervous system (CNS) tumors, making up less than 0.5% (1). Papillomas are more common than carcinomas by a margin of at least 2:1 (2–4). The age range for reported choroid plexus neoplasms is broad, extending from 0 to 72 years, yet the distribution is strongly skewed toward early childhood, with a median age for all cases of 3.5 years in one extensive review of the literature (5). One large tumor registry dataset showed choroid plexus tumors (CPTs) to account for 2.3% of childhood brain tumors, and about 10% of those in infancy (6). Although older patients tend to get choroid plexus papillomas (CPPs) rather than higher grade lesions, the median ages for all three histologic grades were below 3 years in a recent large clinical series (4). Older patients also tend to have more caudally located tumors than the young. Nonetheless, those patients in the first decade remain common at every anatomic location (5). Males and females are roughly equally represented among cases of CPTs. Patients most commonly present with obstructive hydrocephalus due to their intraventricular growth.

Patients with Aicardi syndrome may have an increased risk for developing CPPs, some developing multiple simultaneous lesions (7). Other features of this cryptogenic syndrome include agenesis of the corpus callosum, infantile spasms, and chorioretinal lacunae.

Choroid plexus carcinomas (CPCs) have been noted to occur in the context of Li–Fraumeni syndrome, frequently in the setting of confirmed germline *TP53* mutations (8,9). Although CPC is not particularly common among Li–Fraumeni-related cancers, it appears that Li–Fraumeni and Li–Fraumeni-like syndromes are more frequent in patients with CPC and even present in some children with CPP (10). Another series suggests that a significant number of CPT patients may have germline *TP53* mutations without any family history (11).

Neuroimaging of CPTs shows a solid, well-circumscribed, contrast-enhancing mass that is sometimes internally cystic. An identifying feature, when present, is a multinodular, bosselated profile. CPTs are typically unifocal but can be either truly multifocal (7) or disseminated via metastases (12).

The most common locations for CPTs include all four ventricles and the cerebellopontine (CP) angle, that is, places where normal choroid plexus is found, although they have been reported to occur in extraventricular locales. The lateral and fourth ventricles contain the vast majority of CPTs. Both location and histologic grade correlate with age; adults tend to get papillomas and these are common in the fourth ventricle, whereas children tend to have higher grade lesions that arise in the lateral ventricles (5).

The primary treatment approach for all CPTs is surgical resection, with the frequent addition of chemotherapy for carcinomas. Radiation therapy also seems to have benefit, but its role in the treatment of CPC and atypical choroid plexus papilloma (ACPP) is still being examined (12). Because of the rarity of these malignancies, treatment regimens are varied and standard approach has yet been determined. Grade I papillomas are essentially cured by gross total resection, with one series reporting 100% 5-year survival without recurrence, the rate dropping to 68% with subtotal resection (13). CPCs, in contrast, are aggressive and have 5-year overall survival rates around 60%, although long-term cures have been achieved after complete resection (14).

All grades of choroid plexus neoplasia have the potential to metastasize, and it is most common for carcinomas to disseminate in the cerebrospinal fluid. Abdominal dissemination via ventriculoperitoneal shunt has been described (15).

Besides histologic grade, completeness of resection is an important prognostic factor for all CPTs. In CPCs, the presence of TP53 mutations is associated with much worse outcomes, 0% survival at 5 years in one series (16).

Histopathology

Papillomas recapitulate many of the features of normal choroid plexus; a field of branching fibrovascular cores sporting a monolayer of bland epithelial cells (Figure 11-1). The regularity and organization of most papillomas is on the level of a normal anatomic structure; however, the epithelial component is not formed of the short and bump-like "hob-nail" cells of normal choroid plexus (Figure 11-2) but cuboidal to columnar cells with a more smooth and contiguous surface (Figure 11-3). This vertical exaggeration can pull the nuclei into oblong conformations, yet they remain orderly and nonoverlapping.

The cells of some papillomas are tethered to the fibrovascular stalk by a long strand of fibrillar eosinophilic cytoplasm, imparting an ependymal appearance; the distinction from ependymoma is discussed later in Differential Diagnosis section.

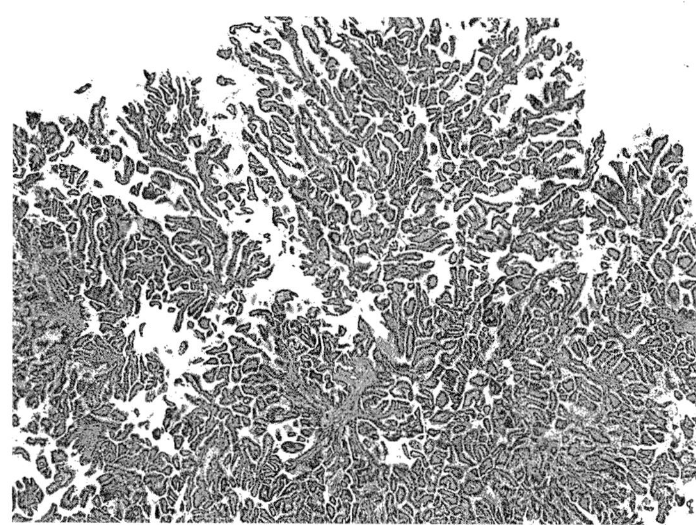

FIGURE 11-1 Choroid plexus papillomas are usually architecturally organized at low magnification.

ACPPs behave more aggressively then grade I CPPs and are more prone to recur (17,18). Although several histologic features have been investigated, proliferation rate as assessed by mitotic figures (Figure 11-4) is the most important prognostic indicator in otherwise standard papillomas. A rate of 2 mitoses per 10 HPF is the sole criterion for advancing a papilloma to atypical, or grade II, status (19). Overlapping and pseudostratified nuclei, nuclear pleomorphism, necrosis, and areas of solid

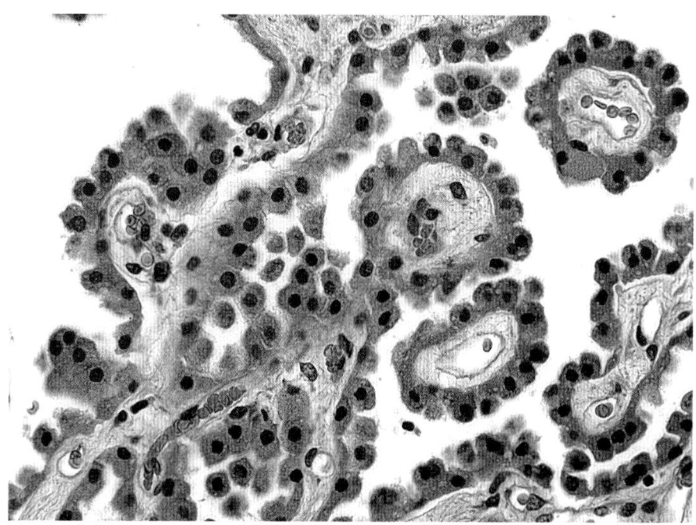

FIGURE 11-2 Normal choroid plexus displays robust fibrovascular cores covered with a cuboidal epithelium with a scalloped, or "hobnail," profile and hyperchromatic round nuclei.

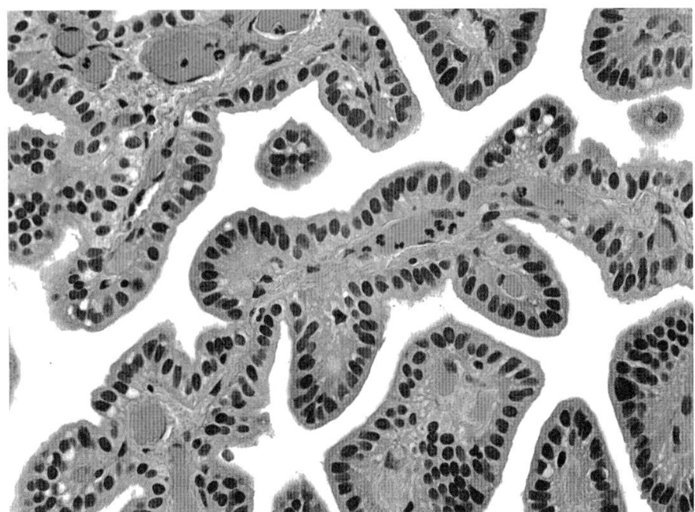

FIGURE 11-3 Well-differentiated papillomas resemble normal choroid plexus, except with more columnar epithelium and an even apical surface.

growth may also be seen in ACPPs, but only one or two of those and not together in constellation (17).

CPCs are proliferative, disorganized, and malignant (Figure 11-5). One study used four or more of the following criteria to diagnose carcinoma: mitotic count >5/10 HPF, hypercellularity, necrosis, loss of papillary architecture, and pleomorphism (17). CPC usually develops *de novo*, but occasionally develops from a preexisting papilloma (Figure 11-6).

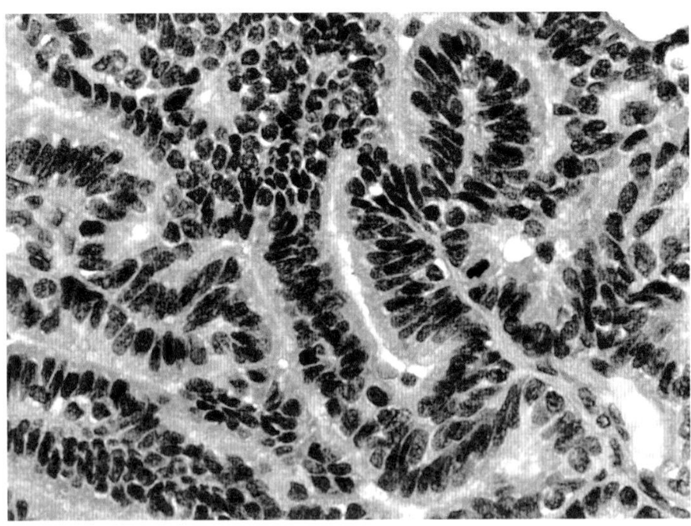

FIGURE 11-4 Atypical choroid plexus papillomas often have a crowded and tall columnar epithelium with less developed papillae, but mitoses (2/10 HPF) are required for inclusion into grade II.

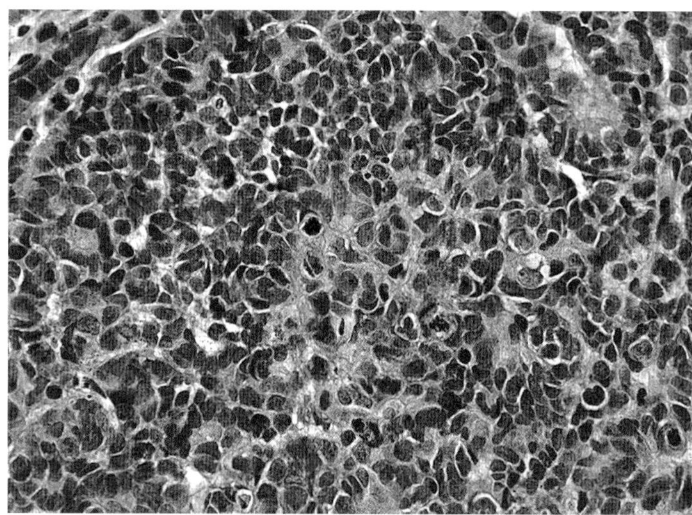

FIGURE 11-5 Choroid plexus carcinomas usually have areas of solid growth with necrosis, mitoses, and frankly malignant cytologic features.

Immunohistochemistry

Papillomas express similar immunohistochemical profiles as normal choroid plexus, including cytokeratin, vimentin, synaptophysin, and S100. Most papillomas are cytokeratin 7 positive and cytokeratin 20 negative, although this finding is not constant (20). Carcinomas usually retain expression of cytokeratins (Figure 11-7) but can be negative. GFAP reactivity is

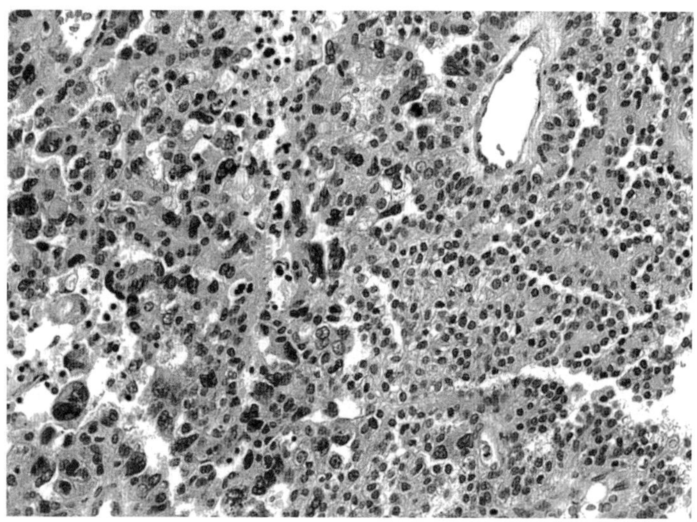

FIGURE 11-6 Choroid plexus carcinoma (left) can develop within a papilloma (right), but most cases arise de novo.

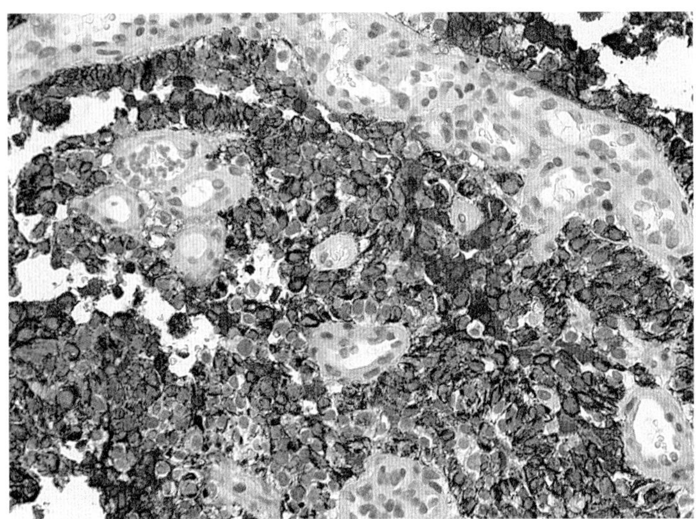

FIGURE 11-7 Choroid plexus carcinomas retain cytokeratin expression in most cases (AE1/3).

present in about 20%, especially where there is fibrillar, ependymoma-like basal cytoplasm (Figure 11-8). Papillomas usually express diffuse prealbumin (transthyretin) and S100, while CPCs more often do not (20,21). The potassium channel KIR7.1 has been suggested as a specific and sensitive marker for CPTs in which immunohistochemistry shows membranous staining (22). Although variable, mean MIB1 staining indices have been measured at 3% to 4% for papillomas and 14% for carcinomas (21).

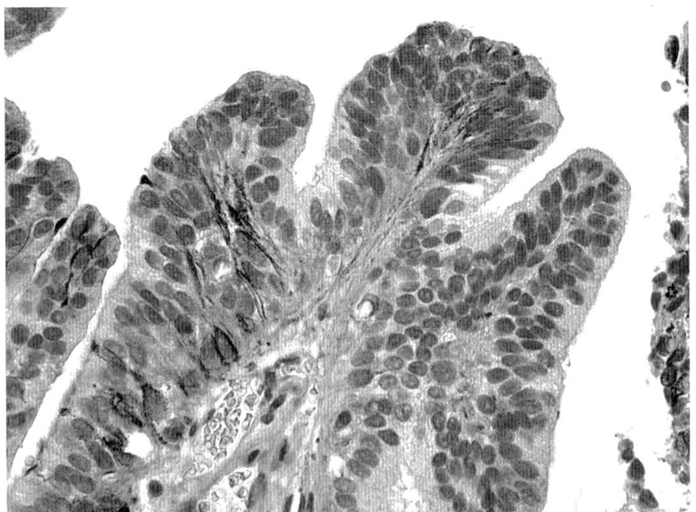

FIGURE 11-8 Glial fibrillary acidic protein reactivity is present in the basal cytoplasm of many choroid plexus papillomas.

Differential Diagnosis

In children, CPPs are difficult to confuse with other neoplasms; most of the other tumors that occur in the same age range are malignant and poorly differentiated. An occasional papilloma with fibrillary, GFAP-positive cytoplasm can have a vaguely ependymal appearance. However, papillary ependymomas lack a regular and continuous apical surface instead they bear a shaggy trim of unevenly situated nuclei. Although both can show GFAP reactivity, a papilloma will also generally have cytokeratin and synaptophysin staining and lack dot- and ring-like EMA positivity.

Although CPPs are usually morphologically innocent, the possibility of a metastatic, well-differentiated carcinoma could be entertained in an adult patient. For reassurance, staining for synaptophysin and S100 would confirm the identity of a papilloma and rule out a metastatic carcinoma. Transthyretin and KIR7.1 immunostaining can be used to confirm a diagnosis of CPT. Other markers of adenocarcinoma and their organs of origin, such as BerEP4, TTF-1, and CDX2, should be negative in CPTs.

Patients with von Hippel–Lindau syndrome develop papillary tumors of the endolymphatic sac that can protrude into the CP angle from the inner ear and be mistaken for CPP. Histologically, both have single layers of orderly cuboidal to columnar epithelium, but papillomas have finer papillary structure with more complex architecture and less collagen. The presence of fluid-filled cystic spaces, apically located nuclei, and multiple cytoplasmic vacuoles favors endolymphatic sac tumor (23). Preoperative imaging or intraoperative observations of a mass originating from the petrous ridge would strongly favor an endolymphatic sac tumor. Cytokeratin 5/6 is expressed by endolymphatic sac tumors and not CPP, whereas synaptophysin is only significantly expressed by CPPs (23).

CPCs can be difficult to distinguish from atypical teratoid/rhabdoid tumor (AT/RT) or primitive neuroectodermal tumor in children when no clear papillary architecture is found. Because CPCs are extremely rare in the posterior fossa, this distinction is mostly limited to cases in the lateral ventricles. INI1/BAF47 immunoreactivity is present in CPCs and absent in AT/RT (24).

A hypothetical prospect of having to differentiate metastatic carcinoma from CPC in adults exists, but the incidence of the latter in adults is extremely low (25). Any diagnosis of adult CPC should be accompanied by unambiguous evidence of a primary choroid plexus neoplasm and an absence of evidence for any other origin. Findings that support CPC include synaptophysin and S100 co-expression. The presence of BerEP4 reactivity strongly favors metastasis (26).

REFERENCES

1. Ostrom QT, Gittleman H, Xu J, et al. CBTRUS statistical report: primary brain and other central nervous system tumors diagnosed in the United States in 2009-2013. *Neuro Oncol.* 2016;18(suppl 5):v1–v75.

2. Ellenbogen RG, Winston KR, Kupsky WJ. Tumors of the choroid plexus in children. *Neurosurgery*. 1989;25(3):327–335.
3. Johnson DL. Management of choroid plexus tumors in children. *Pediatr Neurosci*. 1989; 15(4):195–206.
4. Wrede B, Hasselblatt M, Peters O, et al. Atypical choroid plexus papilloma: clinical experience in the CPT-SIOP-2000 study. *J Neurooncol*. 2009;95(3):383–392.
5. Wolff JE, Sajedi M, Brant R, et al. Choroid plexus tumours. *Br J Cancer*. 2002;87(10):1086–1091.
6. Ostrom QT, de Blank PM, Kruchko C, et al. Alex's Lemonade stand foundation infant and childhood primary brain and central nervous system tumors diagnosed in the United States in 2007-2011. *Neuro Oncol*. 2015;16(suppl 10):x1–x36.
7. Taggard DA, Menezes AH. Three choroid plexus papillomas in a patient with Aicardi syndrome. A case report. *Pediatr Neurosurg*. 2000;33(4):219–223.
8. Dickens DS, Dothage JA, Heideman RL, et al. Successful treatment of an unresectable choroid plexus carcinoma in a patient with Li-Fraumeni syndrome. *J Pediatr Hematol Oncol*. 2005;27(1):46–49.
9. Krutilkova V, Trkova M, Fleitz J, et al. Identification of five new families strengthens the link between childhood choroid plexus carcinoma and germline TP53 mutations. *Eur J Cancer*. 2005;41(11):1597–1603.
10. Gozali AE, Britt B, Shane L, et al. Choroid plexus tumors; management, outcome, and association with the Li-Fraumeni syndrome: The Children's Hospital Los Angeles (CHLA) experience, 1991-2010. *Pediatr Blood Cancer*. 2012;58(6):905–909.
11. Magnusson S, Gisselsson D, Wiebe T, et al. Prevalence of germline TP53 mutations and history of Li-Fraumeni syndrome in families with childhood adrenocortical tumors, choroid plexus tumors, and rhabdomyosarcoma: a population-based survey. *Pediatr Blood Cancer*. 2012;59(5):846–853.
12. Mazloom A, Wolff JE, Paulino AC. The impact of radiotherapy fields in the treatment of patients with choroid plexus carcinoma. *Int J Radiat Oncol Biol Phys*. 2010;78(1):79–84.
13. Krishnan S, Brown PD, Scheithauer BW, et al. Choroid plexus papillomas: a single institutional experience. *J Neurooncol*. 2004;68(1):49–55.
14. Packer RJ, Perilongo G, Johnson D, et al. Choroid plexus carcinoma of childhood. *Cancer*. 1992;69(2):580–585.
15. Donovan DJ, Prauner RD. Shunt-related abdominal metastases in a child with choroid plexus carcinoma: case report. *Neurosurgery*. 2005;56(2):E412.
16. Tabori U, Shlien A, Baskin B, et al. TP53 alterations determine clinical subgroups and survival of patients with choroid plexus tumors. *J Clin Oncol*. 2010;28(12):1995–2001.
17. Jeibmann A, Hasselblatt M, Gerss J, et al. Prognostic implications of atypical histologic features in choroid plexus papilloma. *J Neuropathol Exp Neurol*. 2006;65(11):1069–1073.
18. Cannon DM, Mohindra P, Gondi V, et al. Choroid plexus tumor epidemiology and outcomes: implications for surgical and radiotherapeutic management. *J Neurooncol*. 2015; 121(1):151–157.
19. Louis DN, Ohgaki H, Wiestler OD, et al., eds. WHO Classification of Tumours of the Central Nervous System. 4th ed. Lyon, France: IARC Press; 2016.
20. Gyure KA, Morrison AL. Cytokeratin 7 and 20 expression in choroid plexus tumors: utility in differentiating these neoplasms from metastatic carcinomas. *Mod Pathol*. 2000;13(6):638–643.
21. Vajtai I, Varga Z, Aguzzi A. MIB-1 immunoreactivity reveals different labelling in low-grade and in malignant epithelial neoplasms of the choroid plexus. *Histopathology*. 1996;29(2):147–151.

22. Hasselblatt M, Bohm C, Tatenhorst L, et al. Identification of novel diagnostic markers for choroid plexus tumors: a microarray-based approach. *Am J Surg Pathol.* 2006;30(1):66–74.
23. Du J, Wang J, Cui Y, et al. Clinicopathologic study of endolymphatic sac tumor (ELST) and differential diagnosis of papillary tumors located at the cerebellopontine angle. *Neuropathology.* 2015;35(5):410–420.
24. Judkins AR, Burger PC, Hamilton RL, et al. INI1 protein expression distinguishes atypical teratoid/rhabdoid tumor from choroid plexus carcinoma. *J Neuropathol Exp Neurol.* 2005;64(5):391–397.
25. Wyatt SS, Price RA, Holthouse D, et al. Choroid plexus carcinoma in an adult. *Australas Radiol.* 2001;45(3):369–371.
26. Gottschalk J, Jautzke G, Paulus W, et al. The use of immunomorphology to differentiate choroid plexus tumors from metastatic carcinomas. *Cancer.* 1993;72(4):1343–1349.

12

TUMORS OF THE PINEAL REGION

PINEOCYTOMA (WHO GRADE I), PINEAL PARENCHYMAL TUMOR OF INTERMEDIATE DIFFERENTIATION (WHO GRADE II TO III), AND PINEOBLASTOMA (WHO GRADE IV)

Pineal parenchymal tumors occupy a continuum of differentiation and clinical aggressiveness from the indolent pineocytoma to the overtly malignant pineoblastoma, with at least one category of intermediate differentiation. The criteria governing the boundaries within this spectrum remain undecided, complicating any effort to describe the component entities with accuracy. Nevertheless, enough of these rare cases have been amassed to establish a working approach to pathologic categorization that correlates with patient outcome. This approach was propounded by Jouvet et al. (1) and has been loosely adopted by the World Health Organization (WHO), as detailed later.

Clinical Context

Although mass lesions in and around the pineal gland are not uncommon, pineal parenchymal tumors are rather infrequent, constituting less than 1% of primary central nervous system (CNS) neoplasms and less than a third of pineal region tumors (1,2).

In general, both pineocytoma and pineal parenchymal tumor of intermediate differentiation (PPTID) are more likely to occur in young to middle-aged adults, but can also be seen in children. Pineoblastomas show the opposite distribution, with more cases occurring in childhood and early adulthood and fewer thereafter. No sex predilection exists for any category (1–4).

Pineal parenchymal tumors present with symptoms and signs similar to other pineal region tumors, the constellation of which may form Parinaud syndrome, an upward gaze paralysis with retraction nystagmus due to compression of the tectum. Acute obstructive hydrocephalus with signs of increased intracranial pressure is the most common presentation, which is likely due to the proximity of the cerebral aqueduct. Rarely, pineal parenchymal tumors present with spontaneous hemorrhage.

The most consistent association of pineal parenchymal tumors with a genetic syndrome is that of pineoblastoma with germline DICER1 mutations.

Certain inactivating *DICER1* mutations cause a tumor predisposition syndrome in which the rates of pleuropulmonary blastoma, cystic nephroma, Wilms tumor, Sertoli–Leydig cell tumors, differentiated thyroid carcinoma, and pineoblastoma, among others (5). In one series, about a third of children diagnosed with pineoblastoma who were tested showed a germline *DICER1* mutation, making the case that such patients and their families should be offered genetic counseling (6). Pineoblastomas are also occasionally seen in the context of retinoblastoma and/or germline *RB1* mutations (7). In such cases, the retinoblastomas are generally bilateral with a synchronous pineoblastoma, termed "trilateral retinoblastoma" (8). Children with this presentation have a much worse prognosis than those with retinoblastoma alone. Pineoblastoma has been reported in familial adenomatous polyposis but is rare among those patients (9).

Pineocytomas are round, homogeneous, and hypodense on computed tomography (CT), sometimes with calcifications. Signal intensities on magnetic resonance imaging (MRI) are variable (10). The mass is circumscribed and compresses the surrounding tissue, whereas germ cell tumors tend to invade the brain (11). Because any pineal tumor can grow anteriorly, they may present as a posterior third ventricle mass. Small internal cystic spaces can be seen in pineal parenchymal tumors of any grade. However, an overall cystic construction should be approached with skepticism and suspicion of a pineal cyst.

Treatment approaches for pineal parenchymal tumors are not standardized, but include surgical excision for pineocytomas, with radiation added for most PPTIDs. Pineoblastomas are often treated with both chemotherapy and radiation, the latter frequently being craniospinal. Well-differentiated pineocytomas have 80% to 100% 5-year survival following resection, commensurate with their WHO grade I status (1,3,12). Those same series show a poor survival rate for pineoblastoma, about 10% at 5 years, whereas more recent series indicate median survivals around 50% to 70% at 5 years (13–15). One recent review of the literature found a median overall survival rate for PPTID of 14 years and progression-free survival of about 5 years among 127 reported patients (16).

Histopathology

Pineocytomas are formed of expanses of monotonous cells interrupted by small anucleate areas of felt-like cortical neuropil, very similar to those seen in some neurocytomas (Figure 12-1). Better-differentiated tumors tend to have greater amounts of these "pineocytomatous rosettes." This classic architecture contrasts, with PPTIDs, which take on a lobular arrangement or diffuse, sheetlike growth.

The tumor cells are generally monotonous, with round regular nuclei that contain finely speckled chromatin and small, but easily found, nucleoli. A minority of pineocytoma and PPTID are pleomorphic with multinucleate, sometimes giant, tumor cells and irregular, hyperchromatic nuclei. Pleomorphism has not been shown to impact clinical outcomes, and

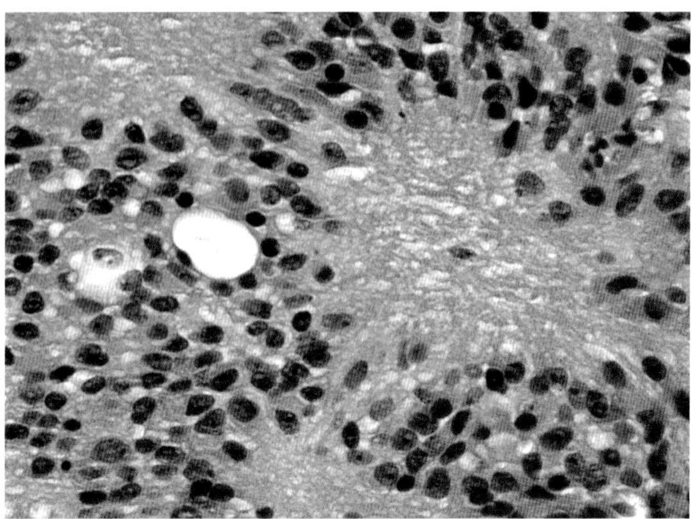

FIGURE 12-1 Pineocytomas usually contain areas of anucleate neuropil (pineocytomatous rosettes), similar to those seen in neurocytomas.

those cases behave according to the grade established by other criteria (17).

Mitosis (<1/10 HPF) and necrosis are not consistent with pineocytoma, WHO grade I (1). Ganglion cells are occasionally present, as in other tumors with neuronal or neurocytic differentiation. Lamellated calcifications with round or scalloped edges (*corpora arenacea*) are also seen and possibly represent overrun calcifications of the normal gland.

Pineoblastomas may closely resemble other malignant embryonal tumors and consist of sheets of small and poorly differentiated embryonal cells, frequently with necrosis, numerous mitoses, and vascular proliferation (Figure 12-2). Some cases may have large angular cells with prominent nucleoli and other features of anaplasia, the significance of which is unknown. Both lumen-forming (18) and fibrillary (Homer Wright) (19) rosettes sometimes appear. Pineoblastoma may also coexist with lower grade elements, in which case the tumor should still be classified pineoblastoma.

Some have observed heterologous elements within pineoblastoma, specifically skeletal muscle, cartilage, and melanotic epithelia. These cases resemble similar lesions of the retina and are called *pineal anlage tumors* (20,21). The significance of this exceptionally rare finding and how it relates to other pineoblastomas is unknown.

Grading

No formal WHO criteria exist by which to grade PPTs. One large series addressing the PPT grading suggests that they be divided into four categories based on mitotic figures and amount of neurofilament reactivity, with

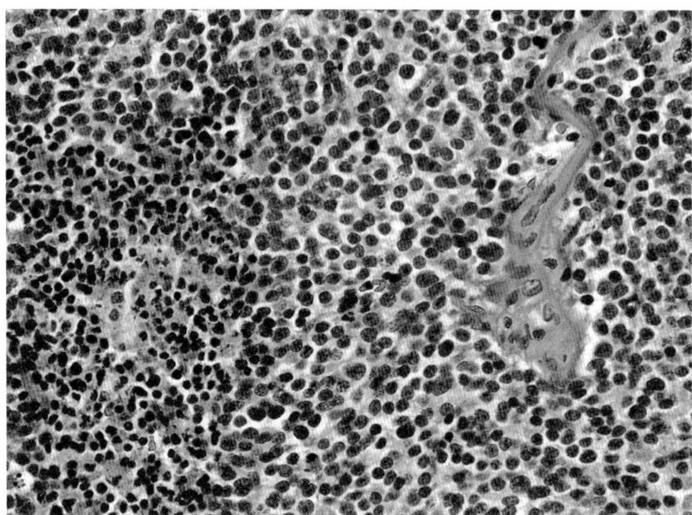

FIGURE 12-2 Pineoblastomas usually grow in sheetlike fashion and contain necrosis and multiple mitotic figures.

PPTID occupying grades II and III. Pineocytomas should not contain mitosis or necrosis and should display strong and widespread neurofilament staining by immunohistochemistry. Grade II PPTIDs have pineocytomatous rosettes and 1 to 5 mitoses per 10 random 400× fields. Grade III is achieved with mitosis >6/10 HPF, or with loss of neurofilament expression. Pineoblastoma is patently malignant with sheets of small embryonal cells. Although not a formal criterion, the authors of this grading system did not observe necrosis in any grade I or grade II lesions, suggesting its utility as an adjunct criterion (1).

Another series evaluating Ki-67 labeling and mitotic count suggests stratifying into high and low risk categories, defining high-risk cases as those that have three or more mitotic figures or 5% or greater Ki-67 immunolabeling (22).

Immunohistochemistry

PPTs are essentially neuronal in differentiation and express similar immunohistochemical profiles to the modified neuronal cells composing the pineal gland. Pineocytomas and PPTIDs usually show diffuse reactivity for synaptophysin, chromogranin, and neuron-specific enolase (NSE). Synaptophysin highlights subtle pineocytomatous rosettes (Figure 12-3). The extent of neurofilament staining is inversely correlated to tumor grade and has been included as a grading criterion in pineal parenchymal tumors by Jouvet et al. (1). GFAP and S100 do not label most pineocytoma cells but identify nonneoplastic astrocytes interspersed throughout. MIB1/Ki-67 proliferation indices are low in pineocytomas, usually less than 2%, and are negatively correlated with neurofilament reactivity (23,24).

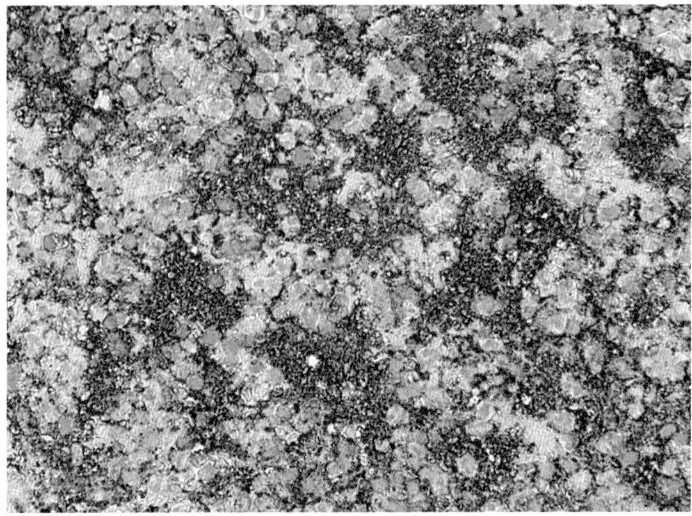

FIGURE 12-3 Pineocytomas are positive for synaptophysin, particularly within rosettes.

Genetics

Beyond germline and somatic defects in DICER1 and RB1 in pineoblastomas, there are no consistent known genetic findings in PPTs of any grade. One small series using comparative genomic hybridization suggests that chromosomal gains of 12q and 22 may be associated with higher grade PPTs, although that finding awaits corroboration (25). That series found no copy number defects in three grade I pineocytomas.

Differential Diagnosis

One of the most common diagnostic dilemmas in pineal parenchymal tumors is distinguishing between normal pineal gland and pineocytoma which, in minute biopsies, may be difficult. The pineal gland architecture comprises cellular lobules separated by thin fibrovascular septa (Figure 12-4), similar to other neuroendocrine organs, but a pseudopapillary nonnested configuration can also be seen (Figure 12-5). The component pinealocytes are uniform and fibrillar, the outermost of which are oriented perpendicularly to the fibrovascular septum in a single layer. Small pineocytic rosettes may be seen (18). A distinguishing feature of native pinealocytes in adults is the presence of cytoplasmic lipofuscin fragments (Figure 12-6), which are absent in neoplastic pinealocytes. Lipofuscin granules are larger and more numerous as age increases; thus, they are less helpful in younger patients. Pineocytomas also lack the lobulation and perivascular orientation of normal pineal gland and are more densely cellular. Lobular architecture is common in PPTID, but these higher-grade tumors can usually be distinguished from normal gland by proliferation markers.

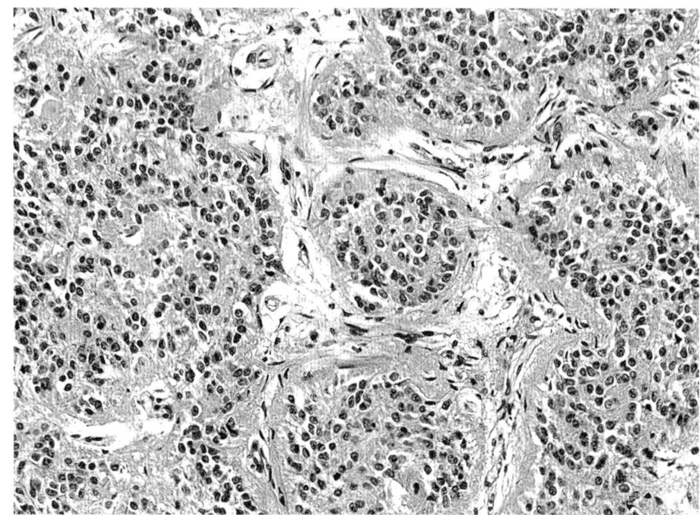

FIGURE 12-4 Normal pineal gland can grow in lobules containing small fibrillar pinealocytes.

Pineoblastoma is distinguished from other embryonal tumors more by its location than any morphologic or immunohistochemical findings. Metastatic neuroendocrine carcinoma could theoretically pose as pineoblastoma; however, the two overlap little in age distributions and the former would express cytokeratins.

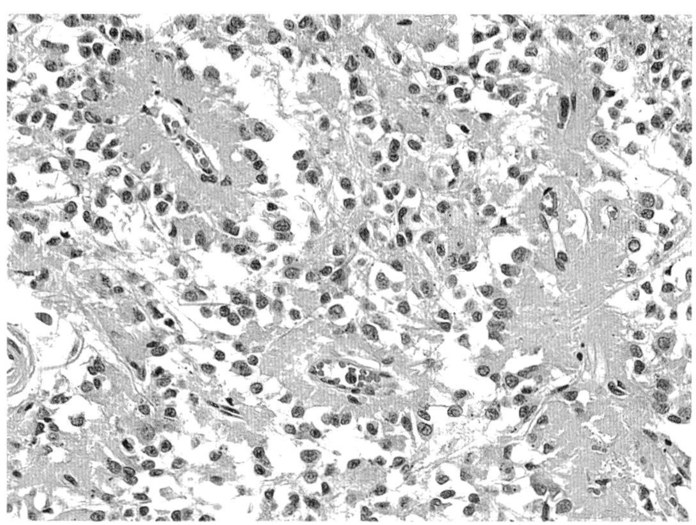

FIGURE 12-5 Normal pineal gland, a pseudopapillary arrangement of pinealocytes around blood vessels.

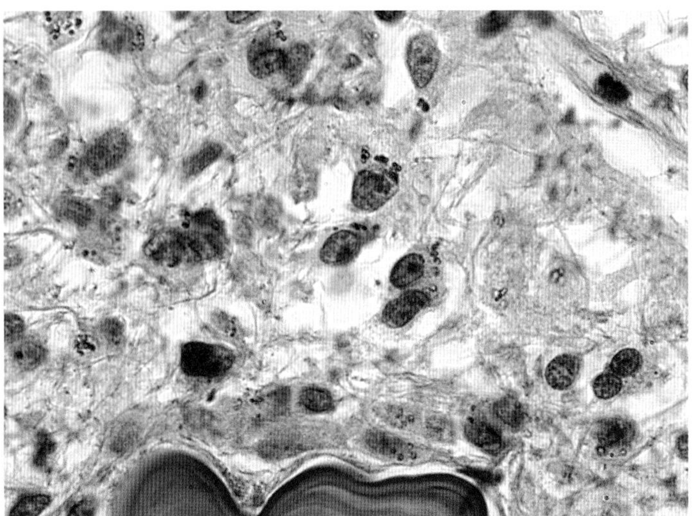

FIGURE 12-6 Although usually not as prominent as in this 60-year-old pineal gland, normal adult pinealocytes contain lipofuscin granules that are not seen in neoplastic cells.

PINEAL CYST

Clinical Context

Small cysts are very common in normal pineal glands and are most often identified incidentally on neuroimaging or at autopsy. Rare cases become symptomatic when the cyst compresses the neighboring structures, causing similar clinical syndromes to pineal region neoplasms.

T2/FLAIR MRI shows a hyperintense, unilocular, round intrapineal cavity with smooth and well-defined margins. Layering of hemorrhage and cyst fluid has been described. Calcifications are common in older patients on CT (26).

Most symptomatic cases are cured by surgical disruption of the cyst wall with few recurrences. Occasionally, the cyst will spontaneously rupture or even hemorrhage (pineal apoplexy).

Histopathology

The cyst wall is composed of an inner layer of fibrillar glial tissue that is unlined by ependymal cells and contains scattered hemosiderin deposits. Compressed pineal gland generally abuts the cyst wall. The glial element bears variable amounts of Rosenthal fibers as a testament to the constant pressure of the cyst contents (Figure 12-7).

The dense piloid gliosis, Rosenthal fibers, and normal pineal gland in pineal cysts have led some to be misdiagnosed as pilocytic astrocytomas or pineocytomas (27). Compared with pilocytic astrocytoma, the glial cyst wall tissue is not biphasic in appearance and does not have myxoid microcysts.

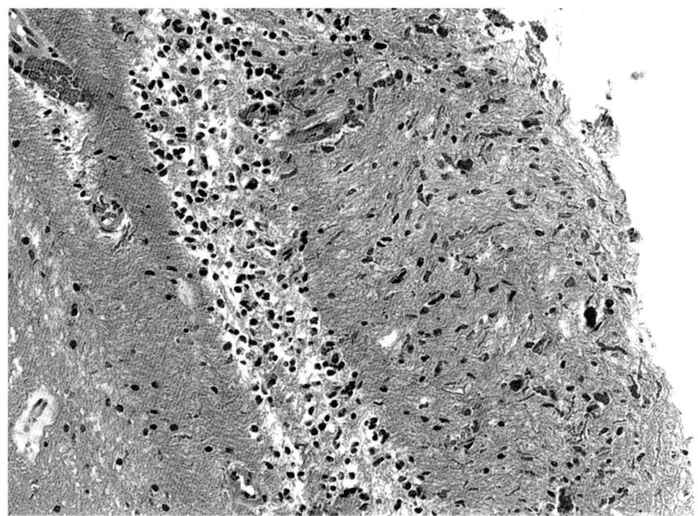

FIGURE 12-7 Pineal cyst wall composed of compressed glial tissue with Rosenthal fibers and a layer of compressed pineal gland.

A pineal cyst's well-delineated layer of piloid gliosis is not a feature of pineal parenchymal tumors and helps to rule them out.

PAPILLARY TUMOR OF THE PINEAL REGION (WHO GRADE II TO III)

Clinical Context

The rarest of primary pineal tumors, the papillary tumor of the pineal region (PTPR), suggested to be a distinct entity in 2003 (28), although the tumor had been described under different names at least back to 1982 (29). The median age of patients is around 32 years, with a range from 15 months to 71 years and no significant sex predilection (28,30–32). Patients present with similar complaints as other pineal region tumors.

Neuroimaging descriptions of PTPR in the literature are limited, but those available describe a generally circumscribed neoplasm with a mildly lobulated outline, heterogeneous contrast enhancement, small internal cysts, and variable T1 and T2 intensities (30).

Treatment of PTPR has been variable. It usually includes surgical resection followed by radiation therapy either immediately or at the time of recurrence. Local recurrence is common, greater than 90% at 7 years in one study, but mortality stabilized after 5 years, giving about 60% overall survival at 10 years (33).

Histopathology

The overall effect is one of a hybrid tumor of both choroid plexus and ependymal cells. Pseudopapillae of varying sizes are the dominant

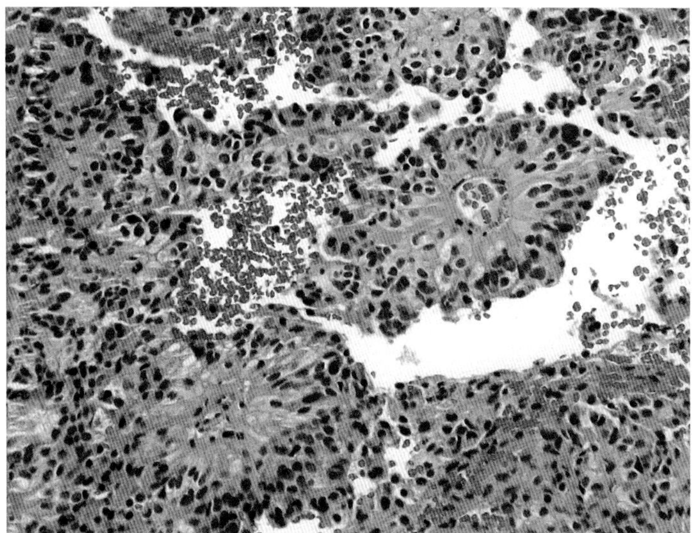

FIGURE 12-8 The papillae and pseudopapillae of papillary tumor of the pineal region can be poorly formed and irregular.

architecture and often coexist with more solid areas (Figure 12-8). Discreet epithelioid columnar and cuboidal cells extend radially from the vascular core with their nuclei tethered at different levels, giving a pseudostratified appearance. In addition to perivascular pseudorosettes, lumen-forming rosettes and tubes are common (Figure 12-9). Mitosis

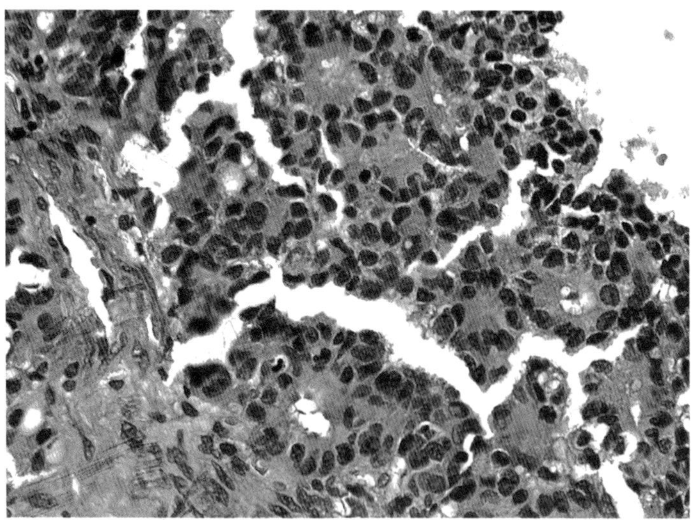

FIGURE 12-9 Papillary tumor of the pineal may exhibit more solid-appearing areas, which sometimes have lumen-forming rosettes and tubes, similar in concept to those seen in ependymomas.

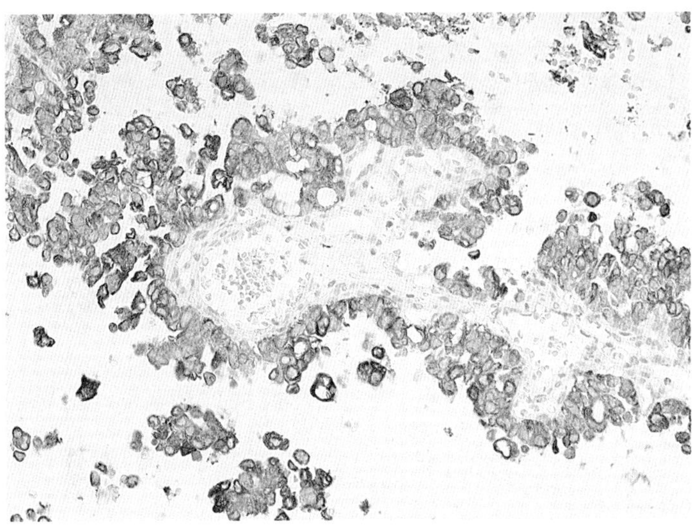

FIGURE 12-10 Cytokeratin (CAM 5.2) immunostaining highlights the cells of papillary tumor of the pineal region.

and focal necrosis can both be seen. It has been proposed that PTPR arises from the subcommissural organ, which is a modified ependymal structure and circumventricular organ (21).

Immunohistochemistry

PTPR consistently expresses cytokeratins (Figure 12-10) and NSE. Most will also react with S100 protein, vimentin, and microtubule-associated protein-2 (MAP2) antisera (33). EMA is most often negative but occasionally decorates cell surfaces and may form the intracytoplasmic dot- and ring-like structures seen in ependymomas (31). Weak and/or focal synaptophysin and chromogranin positivity is present in a minority, while GFAP and neurofilament are negative (33).

Genetics

The most consistent finding in PTPRs is whole loss of a copy of chromosome 10, a feature present in almost all cases (31,34–36). Loss of chromosome 10, thus one allele of *PTEN*, may be in concert with deletion or mutation of the other allele of *PTEN*, causing a disinhibition of the PI3K/AKT/mTOR pathway (36).

Although germ cell neoplasms in the CNS frequently occur in the pineal region, they are also found in other locations and are discussed separately in Chapter 15.

REFERENCES

1. Jouvet A, Saint-Pierre G, Fauchon F, et al. Pineal parenchymal tumors: A correlation of histological features with prognosis in 66 cases. *Brain Pathol.* 2000;10(1):49–60.

2. Cho BK, Wang KC, Nam DH, et al. Pineal tumors: Experience with 48 cases over 10 years. *Child's Nerv Syst.* 1998;14(1-2):53–58.
3. Mena H, Rushing EJ, Ribas JL, et al. Tumors of pineal parenchymal cells: A correlation of histological features, including nucleolar organizer regions, with survival in 35 cases. *Human Pathol.* 1995;26(1):20–30.
4. Schild SE, Scheithauer BW, Schomberg PJ, et al. Pineal parenchymal tumors. Clinical, pathologic, and therapeutic aspects. *Cancer.* 1993;72(3):870–880.
5. Doros L, Schultz KA, Stewart DR, et al. DICER1-related disorders. In: Pagon RA, Adam MP, Ardinger HH, et al., eds. GeneReviews(R). Seattle, WA: University of Washington; 1993.
6. de Kock L, Sabbaghian N, Druker H, et al. Germ-line and somatic DICER1 mutations in pineoblastoma. *Acta Neuropathol.* 2014;128(4):583–595.
7. Plowman PN, Pizer B, Kingston JE. Pineal parenchymal tumours: II. On the aggressive behaviour of pineoblastoma in patients with an inherited mutation of the RB1 gene. *Clin Oncol.* 2004;16(4):244–247.
8. Bader JL, Meadows AT, Zimmerman LE, et al. Bilateral retinoblastoma with ectopic intracranial retinoblastoma: Trilateral retinoblastoma. *Cancer Genet Cytogenet.* 1982; 5(3):203–213.
9. Ikeda J, Sawamura Y, van Meir EG. Pineoblastoma presenting in familial adenomatous polyposis (FAP): Random association, FAP variant or Turcot syndrome? *Br J Neurosurg.* 1998;12(6):576–578.
10. Chiechi MV, Smirniotopoulos JG, Mena H. Pineal parenchymal tumors: CT and MR features. *J Comput Assist Tomogr.* 1995;19(4):509–517.
11. Satoh H, Uozumi T, Kiya K, et al. MRI of pineal region tumours: Relationship between tumours and adjacent structures. *Neuroradiology.* 1995;37(8):624–630.
12. Fauchon F, Jouvet A, Paquis P, et al. Parenchymal pineal tumors: A clinicopathological study of 76 cases. *Int J Radiat Oncol Biol Phys.* 2000;46(4):959–968.
13. Farnia B, Allen PK, Brown PD, et al. Clinical outcomes and patterns of failure in pineoblastoma: A 30-year, single-institution retrospective review. *World Neurosurg.* 2014; 82(6):1232–1241.
14. Jakacki RI, Burger PC, Kocak M, et al. Outcome and prognostic factors for children with supratentorial primitive neuroectodermal tumors treated with carboplatin during radiotherapy: A report from the children's oncology group. *Pediatr Blood Cancer.* 2015;62(5): 776–783.
15. Raleigh DR, Solomon DA, Lloyd SA, et al. Histopathologic review of pineal parenchymal tumors identifies novel morphologic subtypes and prognostic factors for outcome. *Neuro Oncol.* 2017;19(1):78–88.
16. Mallick S, Benson R, Rath GK. Patterns of care and survival outcomes in patients with pineal parenchymal tumor of intermediate differentiation: An individual patient data analysis. *Radiother Oncol.* 2016;121(2):204–208.
17. Fevre-Montange M, Szathmari A, Champier J, et al. Pineocytoma and pineal parenchymal tumors of intermediate differentiation presenting cytologic pleomorphism: A multicenter study. *Brain Pathol.* 2008;18(3):354–359.
18. Hirato J, Nakazato Y. Pathology of pineal region tumors. *J Neuro Oncol.* 2001;54(3):239–249.
19. Borit A, Blackwood W, Mair WG. The separation of pineocytoma from pineoblastoma. *Cancer.* 1980;45(6):1408–1418.
20. McGrogan G, Rivel J, Vital C, Guerin J. A pineal tumour with features of "pineal anlage tumour". *Acta Neurochir.* 1992;117(1-2):73–77.
21. Schmidbauer M, Budka H, Pilz P. Neuroepithelial and ectomesenchymal differentiation in a primitive pineal tumor (pineal anlage tumor). *Clin Neuropathol.* 1989;8(1):7–10.

22. Yu T, Sun X, Wang J, et al. Twenty-seven cases of pineal parenchymal tumours of intermediate differentiation: Mitotic count, Ki-67 labelling index and extent of resection predict prognosis. *J Neurol Neurosurg Psychiatry*. 2016;87(4):386–395.
23. Numoto RT. Pineal parenchymal tumors: Cell differentiation and prognosis. *J Cancer Res Clin Oncol*. 1994;120(11):683–690.
24. Tsumanuma I, Tanaka R, Washiyama K. Clinicopathological study of pineal parenchymal tumors: Correlation between histopathological features, proliferative potential, and prognosis. *Brain Tumor Pathol*. 1999;16(2):61–68.
25. Rickert CH, Simon R, Bergmann M, et al. Comparative genomic hybridization in pineal parenchymal tumors. *Genes Chromosomes Cancer*. 2001;30(1):99–104.
26. Mena H, Armonda RA, Ribas JL, et al. Nonneoplastic pineal cysts: A clinicopathologic study of twenty-one cases. *Ann Diagn Pathol*. 1997;1(1):11–18.
27. Fain JS, Tomlinson FH, Scheithauer BW, et al. Symptomatic glial cysts of the pineal gland. *J Neurosurg*. 1994;80(3):454–460.
28. Jouvet A, Fauchon F, Liberski P, et al. Papillary tumor of the pineal region. *Am J Surg Pathol*. 2003;27(4):505–512.
29. Trojanowski JQ, Tascos NA, Rorke LB. Malignant pineocytoma with prominent papillary features. *Cancer*. 1982;50(9):1789–1793.
30. Amemiya S, Shibahara J, Aoki S, et al. Recently established entities of central nervous system tumors: Review of radiological findings. *J Comput Assist Tomogr*. 2008;32(2):279–285.
31. Hasselblatt M, Blumcke I, Jeibmann A, et al. Immunohistochemical profile and chromosomal imbalances in papillary tumours of the pineal region. *Neuropathol Appl Neurobiol*. 2006;32(3):278–283.
32. Fevre Montange M, Vasiljevic A, Bergemer Fouquet AM, et al. Histopathologic and ultrastructural features and claudin expression in papillary tumors of the pineal region: A multicenter analysis. *Am J Surg Pathol*. 2012;36(6):916–928.
33. Fevre-Montange M, Hasselblatt M, Figarella-Branger D, et al. Prognosis and histopathologic features in papillary tumors of the pineal region: A retrospective multicenter study of 31 cases. *J Neuropathol Exp Neurol*. 2006;65(10):1004–1011.
34. Heim S, Sill M, Jones DT, et al. Papillary tumor of the pineal region: A distinct molecular entity. *Brain Pathol*. 2016;26(2):199–205.
35. Gutenberg A, Brandis A, Hong B, et al. Common molecular cytogenetic pathway in papillary tumors of the pineal region (PTPR). *Brain Pathol*. 2011;21(6):672–677.
36. Goschzik T, Gessi M, Denkhaus D, et al. PTEN mutations and activation of the PI3K/Akt/mTOR signaling pathway in papillary tumors of the pineal region. *J Neuropathol Exp Neurol*. 2014;73(8):747–751.

13

CRANIAL AND SPINAL NERVE SHEATH TUMORS

SCHWANNOMA

Clinical Context

A large number of neurosurgical specimens originate outside of the central nervous system (CNS) proper from the perineural cells of the cranial and spinal nerve roots, the vast majority of which are schwannomas. In one large series including patients of all ages, schwannomas were the third most common tumor of the spinal cord area, following meningiomas and ependymomas and constituting more than 20% of all spinal tumors (1). Most patients are middle-aged adults, with no predilection for either sex. Vestibular schwannomas typically present with progressive sensorineural hearing loss (2), and spinal nerve root schwannomas present with local or radicular pain and/or sensory loss (3).

Type 2 neurofibromatosis (NF2), an autosomal dominant tumor predisposition syndrome caused by mutations in the *NF2* gene on chromosome 22q, is strongly associated with schwannomas both in and out of the CNS. In addition to bilateral vestibular nerve schwannomas, NF2 patients develop meningiomas and spinal ependymomas. The severity of disease phenotype varies greatly between affected families, but it is more consistent within families and correlates with the type of germline mutation, with deletions and frameshift mutations being more severe than point mutations (4). Most schwannomas are sporadic. Multiplicity, young age, or history of meningioma or spinal ependymoma should raise suspicion for NF2. Schwannomatosis is another inherited condition predisposing to schwannomas, but the patients lack germline *NF2* mutations. Some families with isolated schwannomatosis (without meningiomas or spinal ependymomas) have had wild type NF2 and germline mutations in either *SMARCB1* (5) or *LZTR1* (6), although most cases of schwannomatosis remain unexplained (7).

In spite of the patois moniker "acoustic neuroma," the vast majority of cerebellopontine angle schwannomas arise from the vestibular component of CN VIII. The dorsal sensory spinal nerve roots are thought to generate most other intradural schwannomas, yet schwannomas can arise anywhere there are peripheral nerves. Intracerebral examples, which are exceedingly rare, probably develop from minute nerves that travel along blood vessels (8).

Neuroimaging of schwannomas reveals a circumscribed extra-axial tumor with smooth contours compressing its surroundings. When arising within an intervertebral foramen, the tumor bulges from either end, forming a "dumbbell" configuration that is a radiologic signature of schwannoma. Most vestibular schwannomas grow at least partially within the internal auditory canal and protrude into the cerebellopontine angle (9). Gadolinium contrast causes heterogeneous enhancement that is peripheral or ring-shaped in some cases (9,10).

Most vestibular schwannomas grow slowly (0 to 3 mm/year) and can be monitored conservatively for long periods of time (2). When they progress, surgery results in long-term cures for most patients. Unfortunately, surgery incurs a risk of further irreversible hearing loss due to iatrogenic disruption of axons. Stereotactic radiosurgery is a less invasive approach that, although it may be slightly less effective at controlling tumor growth, may be better for preserving hearing (11,12). One large series suggests that observation results in higher quality of life measures than active treatment measures (13). Spinal nerve root schwannomas are similarly indolent and amenable to resection, with generally less serious sensory and motor impairment afterward. Malignant progression of schwannomas is exceedingly rare (14).

Histopathology

Although the vast majority of cases offer little challenge, schwannomas periodically test a pathologist's vigilance with unfamiliar patterns. Fortunately, schwannomas with unusual histologic patterns are still schwannomas and present with clinical scenarios similar to those with a conventional microscopic appearance. Several schwannoma patterns and variants with unique features are presented separately later.

Several features are consistent among schwannomas regardless of the other elements of histologic pattern; hyalinized blood vessels, collagenous encapsulation, and regionally variable cellularity are present in the vast majority of cases and are excellent adjunct features in recognizing schwannomas with unusual histology. Other elements seen in schwannomas that are less diagnostically helpful include hemosiderin-laden macrophages, "ancient change," and cystic degeneration. Pseudoepithelialized cystic spaces occasionally form. Recognition of the most common features is the key to diagnosing those few schwannomas with both subtle histology and unusual location or presentation.

CONVENTIONAL SCHWANNOMA. At low magnification, dense areas (Antoni A) contain cells with irregular elongate nuclei that are arranged in tight fascicles with no clear cell–cell borders, alternating with less cellular areas (Antoni B) composed of loosely arranged cells with hyperchromatic round to oval nuclei (Figure 13-1). The relative amount of Antoni A and B patterns

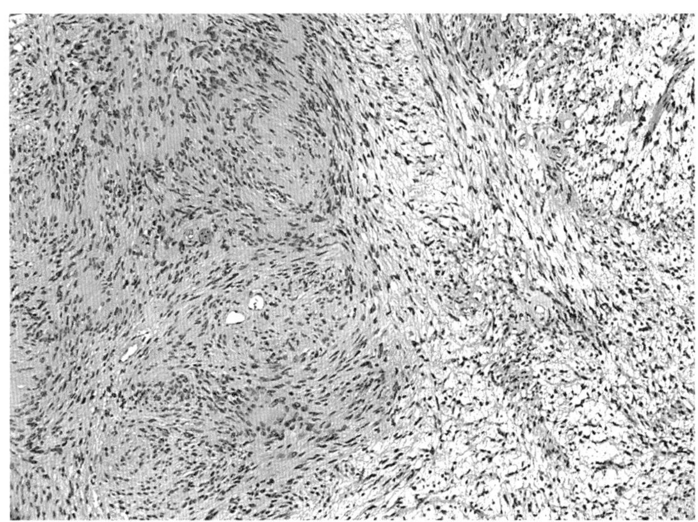

FIGURE 13-1 Most schwannomas contain cellular Antoni A and less cellular Antoni B areas.

is variable, and sometimes the two subtly blend and mute the biphasic effect. Periodically, nuclei within Antoni A areas align in ranks, creating stripes of nuclear palisades between belts of fibrillar pink cytoplasm (Figure 13-2). Many vestibular schwannomas are predominantly Antoni A tissue, are relatively hypocellular compared to other locations, and lack nuclear palisading (Figure 13-3). Cells with the characteristic irregular, elongate, club-shaped nuclei also form vague fascicles or whorls in Antoni A areas; their counterparts in Antoni B are far less organized.

CELLULAR SCHWANNOMA. This pattern is probably the most likely to be mistaken for a sarcoma because of its spindle-cell morphology, dense cellularity, and lack of Antoni B tissue or Verocay bodies (Figure 13-4). Additional unusual features such as hyperchromasia, mitosis, necrosis, and pleomorphism led to a malignant initial diagnosis in over a quarter of cases in one large series (15). Only a small number of reported cellular schwannomas have occurred in the intracranial and intraspinal compartments (16–18). Cellular schwannomas behave clinically like conventional schwannomas. Distinguishing between cellular schwannoma and malignant peripheral nerve sheath tumor (MPNST) is discussed with the latter entity. Cellular schwannomas express strong and diffuse S100 protein and diffuse SOX10 on immunostaining (19).

PLEXIFORM SCHWANNOMA. Occasionally, schwannomas grow in a complex or multinodular pattern that simulates the configuration of a plexiform neurofibroma. Most cases arise in the skin and subcutis of the trunk. Unlike the strong association between plexiform neurofibroma and NF1, this lesion is not a pathognomonic indicator of NF2 and occurs sporadically in many cases (20,21).

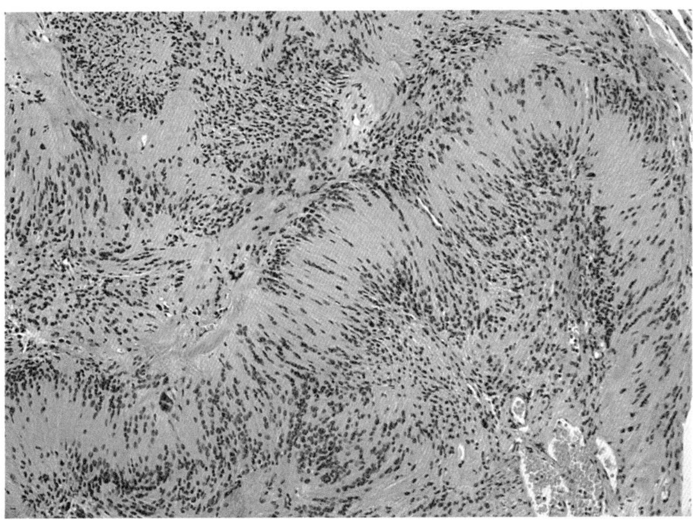

FIGURE 13-2 Nuclei align in palisades to form Verocay bodies in classic schwannomas.

EPITHELIOID AND "NEUROBLASTOMA-LIKE" SCHWANNOMA. Rarely, schwannomas lose their spindle-cell morphology and grow as sheets of small cells (Figure 13-5), which even more rarely arrange in rosette-like structures reminiscent of neuroblastoma. Some cases have shown malignant behavior, although most follow a benign course (22,23). Epithelioid morphology can also be seen focally in otherwise unremarkable schwannomas. In the spine, another cellular epithelioid neoplasm that also stains strongly for

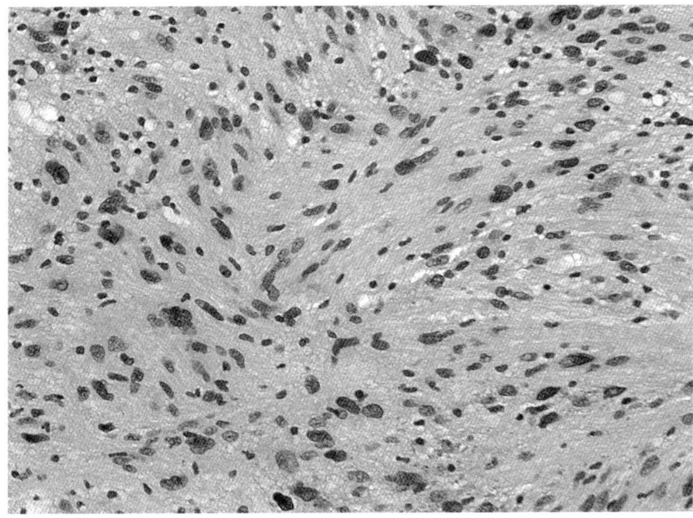

FIGURE 13-3 Many vestibular schwannomas are Antoni A predominant and relatively hypocellular with increased degenerative nuclear pleomorphism.

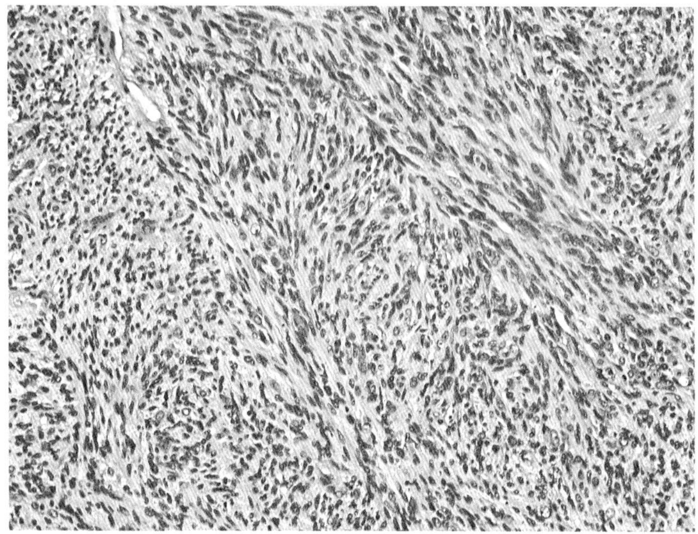

FIGURE 13-4 Cellular schwannomas resemble malignant peripheral nerve sheath tumor, with long fascicles of spindled cells and no Verocay bodies or Antoni B tissue.

S100 protein is ependymoma, which would be distinguished from schwannoma by strong and diffuse immunostaining for glial fibrillary acidic protein (GFAP). One large series of epithelioid schwannomas showed a majority to have loss of SMARCB1/INI1 immunostaining, which is usually noted in malignant tumors, although they had excellent outcomes, with no metastasis and only one recurrence (24).

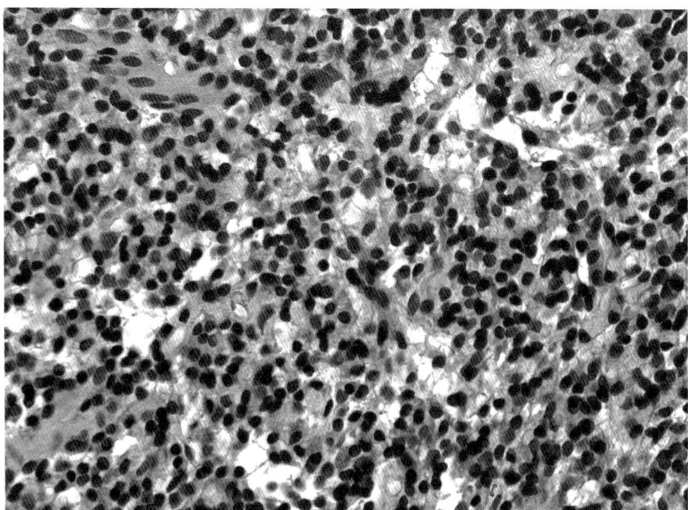

FIGURE 13-5 Epithelioid, neuroblastoma-like schwannomas are densely cellular with round cells but may contain residual areas of more classic schwannoma.

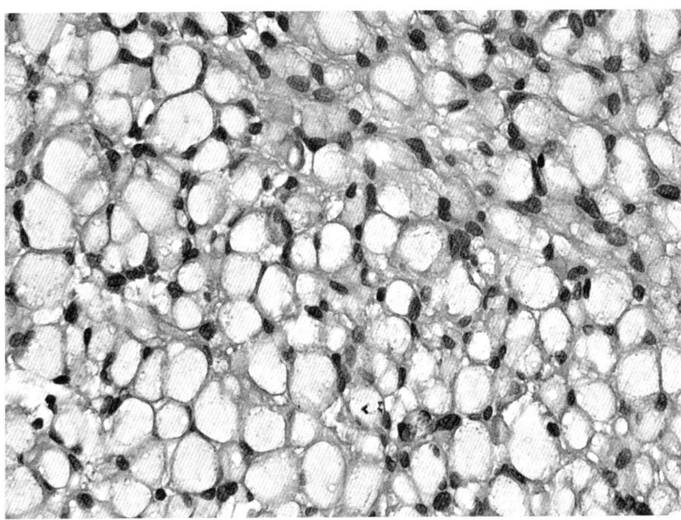

FIGURE 13-6 Myxoid, signet-ring-like change can be seen focally in schwannomas, but rarely involves the entire lesion, as in this case.

MYXOID SCHWANNOMA. This pattern is distinctly uncommon and has an appearance almost unrecognizable as schwannoma (Figure 13-6). Basophilic pools of mucin compress the nuclei to one side, causing a "signet-ring" appearance that may cause concern for more aggressive neoplasms (25). Unlike adenocarcinomas with similar cytomorphology, these myxoid-schwannomas are tightly coherent and well circumscribed. Immunohistochemically, these lesions retain the characteristic of strong and diffuse S100 immunostainingand meshwork of laminin and collagen IV staining of other schwannomas.

Immunohistochemistry

Schwannomas virtually always react strongly and diffusely with S100 protein immunostaining and in an intercellular latticework pattern for type IV collagen and laminin. Although not entirely specific, strong S100 protein staining is important supporting evidence of schwannoma, without which the diagnosis is tenuous. Type IV collagen and laminin can be useful in differentiating schwannomas from fibroblastic and myofibroblastic tumors. The strength and wide distribution of S100 protein and collagen IV staining in schwannomas is rarely seen in other tumor types. The transcription factor SOX10 is sensitive for identifying schwannomas, being expressed in almost all cases, but is also expressed in melanomas and myoepithelial tumors, among others (26). Ki-67/MIB1 proliferation indices are highly variable and do not predict the behavior of schwannomas. Many schwannomas also express GFAP to varying degrees (27).

Differential Diagnosis

Considerable overlap between neurofibromas and schwannomas can be seen histologically; indeed, hybrid schwannoma/neurofibromas are well documented (28). In the classic view, neurofibromas grow within nerves and incorporate axons to expand the nerve in a fusiform, concentric fashion, whereas schwannomas grow from the surface of nerves and do not incorporate axons, forming an eccentric, circumscribed mass. Immunohistochemistry for neurofilament is a good method for highlighting entrapped axons, but this method has recently been challenged (29). Neurofibromas also generally lack the distinct fascicles and hyalinized blood vessels of schwannomas. In any event, it is entirely acceptable to call a tumor with features of both tumors a "hybridschwannoma/neurofibroma," particularly in the setting of a patient with neurofibromatosis of either type, in which context such lesions are more common (28).

Especially in the cerebellopontine angle, where schwannomas often contain little Antoni B tissue, fibrous meningiomas should always be included in the differential diagnosis. Intraoperatively, crush preparations clearly differentiate the two, with schwannomas breaking into mesh-like fragments with punched-out "windows" between intact fascicles and minimal single-cell dispersion in the background (Figure 13-7). The free ends of the fascicles also appear cleanly snapped off, with few or no shaggy ends. Elongate fascicles within tissue fragments display the signature irregular, club-shaped nuclei (Figure 13-8). Fibrous meningiomas fragment into smaller pieces on crush preparations with greater shedding of individual tumor cells and more ragged edges and ends of fragments. Psammoma

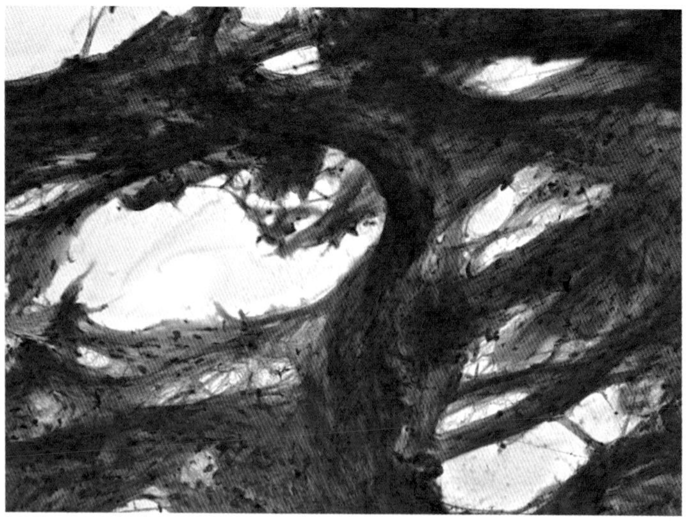

FIGURE 13-7 Schwannomas break into mesh-like fragments of fascicles that form "windows" in crush preparations, a feature that distinguishes them from meningiomas.

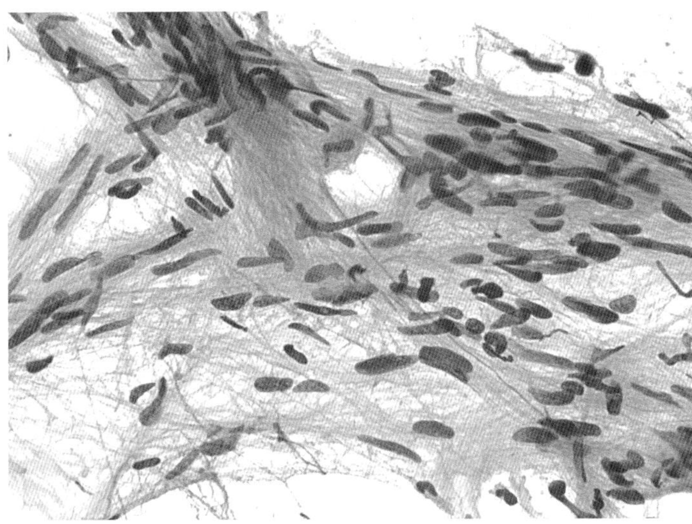

FIGURE 13-8 A forceful crush preparation reveals the typical nuclei of schwannoma, with asymmetrical tapering and irregular contours that reliably differentiate them from the nuclei of meningiomas.

bodies should not generally be seen in schwannomas. Immunohistochemistry for epithelial membrane antigen (EMA) will show membranous staining in meningiomas and only occasional focal or faint staining in schwannomas. S100 protein staining is often present in meningiomas but rarely to the degree seen in schwannomas.

The uncommon "tanycytic" spinal ependymoma, with vague fascicles, poorly formed perivascular pseudorosettes, and strong S100 protein positivity, can appear similar to schwannoma but shows diffuse GFAP staining and cytoplasmic "dot-and-ring" EMA immunoreactivity. They also grow, with only the rarest exceptions, within the substance of the spinal cord, an extremely unlikely location for schwannoma. Hyper cellular spinal ependymomas may occasionally be mistaken for epithelioid schwannomas.

NEUROFIBROMA

Clinical Context

Unlike schwannomas, neurofibromas are uncommon in the cranial and spinal nerves, at least within the confines of the dura. Of a recent series of 430 spinal tumors, neurofibromas accounted for no more than six cases, less than a tenth of the number of schwannomas (1). Patients present with pain and sensory loss in a dermatomal distribution.

As with neurofibromas peripherally, those of spinal and cranial nerves are mostly sporadic but can be associated with NF1. Those with a complex configuration involving multiple nerves, *plexiform neurofibromas*, are almost exclusive to NF1, with only a handful of reports in patients without the syndrome and no family history (30). The *NF1* gene, however, is large and therefore prone to *de novo* mutations, so around half of NF1 patients have no family history. Other features of NF1 include iris hamartomas (Lisch nodules), *café-au-lait* spots, axillary freckling, and optic pathway gliomas. NF1 patients are also at increased risk for developing infiltrating astrocytomas, although this is not a frequent occurrence (31).

Simple sporadic neurofibromas are curable by surgical excision alone but require complete transection of the involved nerve because of their typical diffuse growth that incorporates the native axons. Large plexiform neurofibromas are at risk for transformation into MPNSTs, which is discussed later.

Histopathology

At low magnification, neurofibromas are usually uniformly hypocellular with no clear architectural organization. At higher magnification, the tumor is composed of dispersed Schwann cells with wavy nuclei in a lightly basophilic background with unoriented irregular bundles of dense collagen (Figure 13-9), often compared with "shredded carrots." Alternatively, the collagen may form loose and undulating wisps of narrow fibers. The Schwann cells usually show a degree of orientation, being roughly parallel to the entrapped nerve axons. Mast cells frequently dot the background. The blood vessels in neurofibromas are small and lack hyalinization but stand out against their hypocellular surroundings. Neurofibromas occasionally contain lamellated round-to-oblong structures called Wagner–Meissner bodies that resemble normal Meissner corpuscles (Figure 13-10).

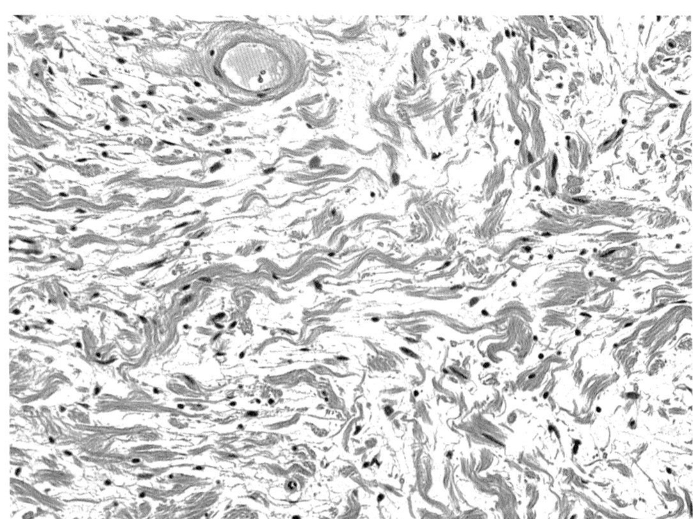

FIGURE 13-9 Neurofibromas are uniformly hypocellular with scattered collagen bundles in a myxoid background.

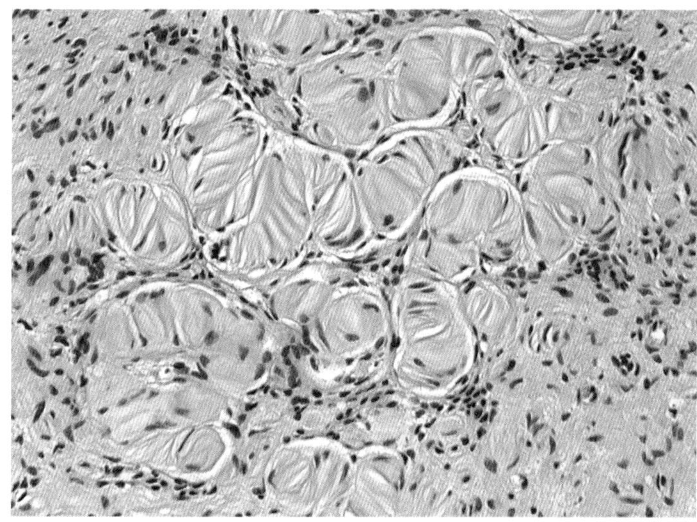

FIGURE 13-10 Wagner–Meissner bodies are characteristic of neurofibromas, though frequently not present.

Isolated nuclear atypia or hypercellularity may be present in some cases and are not by themselves cause for alarm or independently associated with aggressive behavior (Figure 13-11). According to a recent consensus recommendation by experts in peripheral nerve sheath tumors, such examples can be termed *neurofibroma with atypia* or *cellular neurofibroma*, respectively. However, atypia, hypercellularity, loss of architecture,

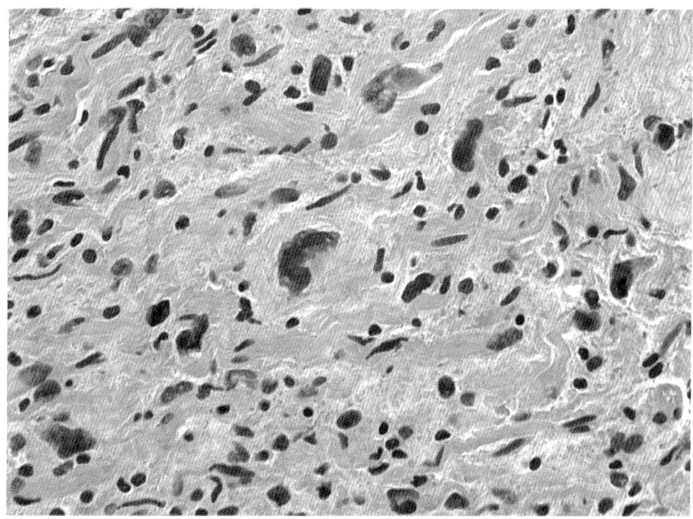

FIGURE 13-11 Although degenerative nuclear atypia is more common in schwannomas, it is also present in some neurofibromas without consequence.

TABLE 13-1 Proposed Diagnostic Spectrum of Malignancy From Neurofibroma to MPNST

Diagnosis	Proposed Features
Neurofibroma	Schwannian cells with thin, wavy nuclei in myxoid and collagenous stroma; diffuse S100 & SOX10; CD34+ lattice pattern (plexiform when involves multiple nerve trunks)
Neurofibroma With Atypia	Neurofibroma with scattered enlarged, irregular, and hyperchromatic nuclei
Cellular Neurofibroma	Neurofibroma with hypercellularity, retained architecture and mitosis <1/50 HPF
Atypical Neurofibromatous Neoplasm of Undetermined Biological Potential (ANNUBP)	Two or more of: nuclear atypia, hypercellularity, loss of architecture, or mitosis >1/50 HPF but <3/10HPF
MPNST, Low-grade	ANNUBP with 3–9 mitotic figures/10 HPF but no necrosis
MPNST, High-grade	Mitosis ≥10/10 HPF, or 3–9/10 HPF and necrosis

Modified from Miettinen MM, Antonescu CR, Fletcher CDM, et al. *Histopathologic evaluation of atypical neurofibromatous tumors and their transformation into malignant peripheral nerve sheath tumor in neurofibromatosis 1 patient—a consensus overview.* Hum Pathol. 2017;pii: S0046-8177(17)30167-3.

and mitotic activity (>1/50 HPF and <3/10 HPF) are features that in combination suggest an increased risk of progression to MPNST(32). The term "*atypical neurofibromatous neoplasm of uncertain biologic potential* (ANNUBP)" has been proposed for neurofibromas with at least two of those features (Table 13-1). Cases with those features and mitotic index of 3–9/10 HPF in the absence of necrosis may be called *low-grade MPNST* (32). High-grade MPNST is discussed below.

Plexiform neurofibromas are lesions that involve multiple nerve fascicles and have a gross appearance of a "bag of worms." Histologically, the tumor tissue is identical to conventional neurofibroma, the only difference being the presence of multiple involved nerve trunks. Large plexiform neurofibromas may contain areas of sarcomatous transformation and should therefore be sampled thoroughly. Except in rare cases, plexiform neurofibromas are pathognomonic for NF1, though not technically sufficient alone to meet syndrome criteria.

The differential diagnosis of spinal and cranial nerve neurofibromas, schwannomas, and MPNSTs is discussed below.

MALIGNANT MELANOTIC SCHWANNIAN TUMOR

Clinical Context

Formerly known as melanotic schwannoma, this rare tumor has recently been shown to cause death in a subset of patients and commonly have recurrences and metastasis, in stark contrast to typical schwannomas (33). The patients are adults with a wide range of ages and tend to have paraspinal tumors, sometimes involving the sympathetic ganglia, although they can occur anywhere. There seems to be no bias in the distribution of cases between men and women (33,34).

Histopathology and Genetics

Microscopic examination reveals an encapsulated, vaguely lobulated arrangement of predominantly spindled cells with lightly eosinophilic, somewhat fibrillar-appearing cytoplasm growing in short fascicles and sheets, and variably abundant melanin (Figure 13-12). Nucleoli are variable and may be prominent. Varying amounts of epithelioid and "adipocyte-like" vacuolated cells may be present. Psammomatous calcifications are present in a little less than half of cases. Mitotic figures are usually inconspicuous ≤1/10 HPF and have been associated with metastasis when ≥2/10 HPF (33).

Although the frequent presence of epithelioid tumor cells and immunoreactivity for S100 protein, HMB-45, tyrosinase, and melan-Acan cause concern for melanoma, paraspinal location, low proliferation, vacuolated cells, and psammoma bodies all favor MMST. Gene expression profiling does support the idea that MMSTs are genetically distinct from both melanoma

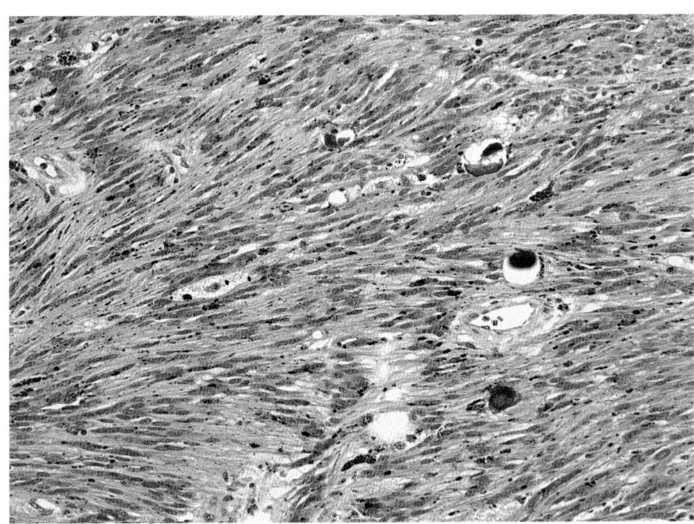

FIGURE 13-12 Malignant melanotic schwannian tumors show obvious melanin production and may contain psammoma bodies.

and schwannoma (33). In the original series by Carney, there was a high prevalence of MMSTs in Carney syndrome patients (34), yet the converse has not proven true: given an MMST, the likelihood of Carney syndrome is actually pretty low (33,35,36).

MALIGNANT PERIPHERAL NERVE SHEATH TUMOR

Clinical Context

The vast majority of MPNSTs arise either associated with a neurofibroma or spontaneously, presumably in relation to a peripheral nerve. MPNSTs are rather uncommon in the CNS, more often arising in larger peripheral nerve trunks in the buttocks, posterior thigh, brachial plexus, and paraspinal area. MPNST is uncommon in the general population, affecting only 0.001% of a reference center patient population in one series (37). Only slightly more patients are female than male. MPNSTs are generally tumors of adulthood, and most often present in the fourth through sixth decades. Children constitute about 10% to 15% of MPNST patients and are much more likely to have NF1 (38,39). The distribution of patient ages is bimodal, with NF1-associated cases occurring 4 to 8 years earlier than sporadic ones on average (37,38).

Although strongly associated with NF1, only half of MPNSTs occur in the setting of that syndrome, similar to several other syndrome-associated tumors (37,40). The lifetime risk for developing MPNST is estimated at approximately 10% for NF1 patients by one population-based study (41). However, another large population-based study found only 3% occurrence over a four-decade period (42). Radiation is another factor associated with MPNST, causing tumors after latencies of over 15 years on average (43,44). Incidence of MPNST is thought to be higher in patients with pre-existing large plexiform neurofibromas, but almost half occur *de novo* without a precursor lesion. Radiation is a risk factor for MPNST.

Imaging of MPNST typically shows fusiform expansion of a nerve or group of nerves with internal heterogeneity representing necrosis and hemorrhage, best seen on contrast-enhanced images (45,46).

Most of the data regarding treatment and outcome in MPNST are based on tumors occurring outside of the dural compartment, so they are not necessarily applicable to spinal and cranial nerve cases that are generally more difficult to resect than examples in the limbs. No standard protocol for treating MPNST exists, and many patients receive a combination of surgical resection and radiation therapy. The outcomes of these endeavors are highly variable and multifactorial. Overall, patients who have NF1, incomplete tumor resection, tumors larger than 5 cm, or axial tumor location have significantly shorter survival than those without (37,47,48). High (≥60 Gy) doses of radiation and brachytherapy are associated with improved local control (48). Histopathologic grading does not seem to predict tumor behavior in multivariate analysis (37,48).

Histopathology

Low-grade MPNSTs differ from high-grade ones in that they are generally less cellular, less proliferative, and do not exhibit necrosis. The vast majority of these arise within a pre-existing neurofibroma as a result of progression. A recent consensus statement suggested guidelines for low-grade MPNST as: features of ANNUBP (atypia, hypercellularity, loss of architecture; see above under neurofibroma) plus a mitotic rate of 3–9/10 HPF with no necrosis (Table 13-1). Loss of architecture can be demonstrated immunohistochemically by loss of the usual lattice-like pattern of CD34 reactivity (32).

At low magnification, high-grade MPNSTs usually have geographically variable cellularity that has been likened to marble, although the effect is usually subtle (Figure 13-13). Long, straight fascicles intersect and often form a herringbone pattern like that of fibrosarcoma (Figure 13-14). The nuclei are elongate to elliptical with irregular contours and generally tapered ends but should not have broad, rounded tips. The cytoplasm is indistinct. Necrosis is present in the majority of cases and can be widespread. Mitotic figures are frequently greater than 10/10 HPF, although a count of 3–9/10 HPF in the context of necrosis also may qualify as high-grade MPNST (32). The edges of many MPNSTs are invasive and infiltrate adjacent soft tissue structures or destroy neighboring bone. Although most cases have modest nuclear pleomorphism relative to their other malignant features, some display marked atypia similar to that seen in pleomorphic undifferentiated sarcoma with bizarre nuclei and tumor giant cells. Areas of residual neurofibroma are frequently seen in cases that develop from progression.

Rare MPNSTs contain foci of divergent differentiation, most famously rhabdomyosarcomatous elements that constitute a **"malignant Triton**

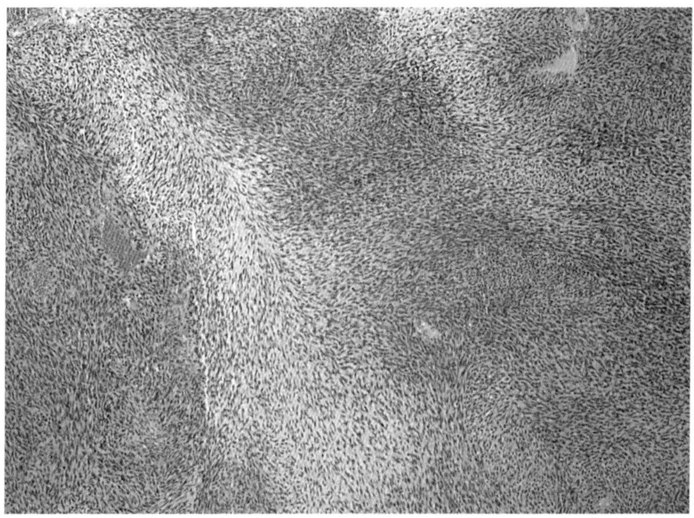

FIGURE 13-13 High-grade, malignant peripheral nerve sheath tumors usually have geographic variation in cellularity, although it is often more subtle than that seen here.

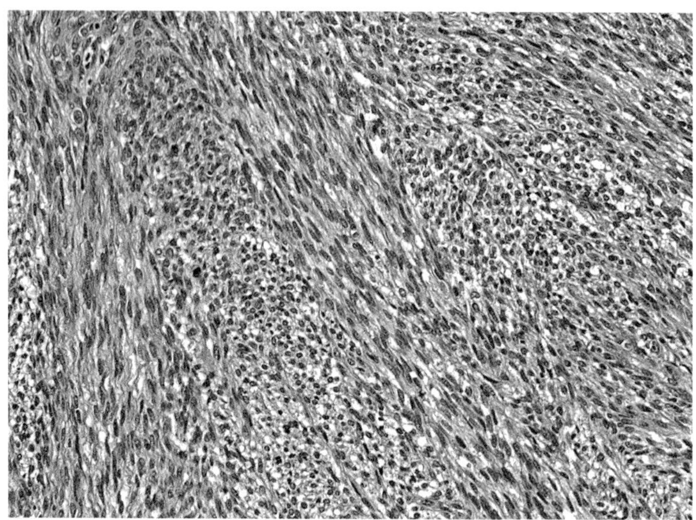

FIGURE 13-14 The classic picture of malignant peripheral nerve sheath tumor is of long intersecting fascicles, similar to fibrosarcoma and monophasic synovial sarcoma.

tumor" after an experimental lesion induced in the Triton salamander (49). Rhabdomyoblasts can be demonstrated by desmin immunohistochemistry and should be unevenly scattered and unoriented, whereas infiltrated skeletal muscle fibers will be evenly spaced and, at least subtly, parallel. Other heterologous elements may include epithelia, bone, and cartilage.

Immunohistochemistry

Many MPNSTs express S100 protein by immunohistochemistry, usually with a pattern differing from schwannoma by being weak and patchy or focal (50). The absence of S100 protein reactivity, however, is common and does not rule out the diagnosis of MPNST. SOX10 nuclear staining in MPNSTs tends to highlight entrapped cells and subsets of malignant cells in a mosaic fashion, rarely being and diffuse and strong (19,26). Other Schwann cell markers such as Leu-7 and myelin basic protein are also seen occasionally in MPNST but are neither specific nor sensitive for that diagnosis (50). Nuclear p53 reactivity is present at least focally in about two thirds of MPNST, with no differences in rates between sporadic and syndromic cases (51). Two independent series conclude that p53 staining of any amount strongly predicts a significantly shorter overall survival than in cases with no staining (51,52).

Differential Diagnosis

Cellular schwannoma should always be considered before diagnosing an MPNST because of their similarities in appearance and radically different clinical behavior; this is probably the most significant pitfall in diagnosing peripheral nerve sheath tumors. Occasional mitosis, hyaline necrosis, nuclear atypia, and striking hypercellularity can all be seen in schwannoma. In one series, only mitotic rate ≥10/10 HPF was seen almost exclusively in MPNST and not cellular schwannoma (19). Immunohistochemistry is helpful because S100 protein staining should only be weak and/or focal in MPNST and strong and diffuse in cellular schwannoma. SOX10 is frequently negative in MPNST or has a mosaic pattern of reactivity. Staining for p53 can be misleading in this situation, as it can be diffusely positive in both (19). Histone H3 K27 trimethylation (H3 K27me3) immunostaining is lost in around half of high-grade MPNSTs, but not in cellular schwannomas or other morphologically similar spindle cell tumors, making it a specific but not sensitive marker (53,54).

The remaining entities in the differential diagnosis with MPNST are sarcomas with similar architecture, specifically fibrosarcoma and monophasic synovial sarcoma. In contrast to MPNST, synovial sarcoma has more regular nuclei with blunt broad ends, binds keratin and EMA antibodies, and contains *SYT-SSX* gene fusions. Fibrosarcoma is histologically very similar to MPNST but should not show S100 reactivity, although many MPNSTs also lack appreciable staining. Fortunately, both monophasic synovial sarcoma and fibrosarcoma are rare metastatic visitors to the intradural compartment and their occurrence as CNS primaries could merit a case report.

Other Nerve Sheath Tumors

Several other nerve sheath neoplasms rarely involve the spinal and cranial nerves, such as perineurioma (55) and neurothekeoma (56), but are so infrequent that they are beyond the scope of this discussion.

REFERENCES

1. Engelhard HH, Villano JL, Porter KR, et al. Clinical presentation, histology, and treatment in 430 patients with primary tumors of the spinal cord, spinal meninges, or caudaequina. *J Neurosurg Spine*. 2010;13(1):67–77.
2. Bakkouri WE, Kania RE, Guichard JP, et al. Conservative management of 386 cases of unilateral vestibular schwannoma: tumor growth and consequences for treatment. *J Neurosurg*. 2009;110(4):662–669.
3. Safavi-Abbasi S, Senoglu M, Theodore N, et al. Microsurgical management of spinal schwannomas: evaluation of 128 cases. *J Neurosurg Spine*. 2008;9(1):40–47.
4. Ruttledge MH, Andermann AA, Phelan CM, et al. Type of mutation in the neurofibromatosis type 2 gene (NF2) frequently determines severity of disease. *Am J Hum Genet*. 1996;59(2):331–342.
5. Smith MJ, Wallace AJ, Bowers NL, et al. Frequency of SMARCB1 mutations in familial and sporadic schwannomatosis. *Neurogenetics*. 2012;13(2):141–145.
6. Piotrowski A, Xie J, Liu YF, et al. Germline loss-of-function mutations in LZTR1 predispose to an inherited disorder of multiple schwannomas. *Nat Genet*. 2014;46(2):182–187.
7. Hutter S, Piro RM, Reuss DE, et al. Whole exome sequencing reveals that the majority of schwannomatosis cases remain unexplained after excluding SMARCB1 and LZTR1 germline variants. *Acta Neuropathol*. 2014;128(3):449–452.

8. Sharma MC, Karak AK, Gaikwad SB, et al. Intracranial intraparenchymal schwannomas: a series of eight cases. *J Neurol Neurosurg Psychiatry*. 1996;60(2):200–203.
9. Duvoisin B, Fernandes J, Doyon D, et al. Magnetic resonance findings in 92 acoustic neuromas. *Eur J Radiol*.1991;13(2):96–102.
10. Friedman DP, Tartaglino LM, Flanders AE. Intradural schwannomas of the spine: MR findings with emphasis on contrast-enhancement characteristics. *AJR Am J Roentgenol*. 1992;158(6):1347–1350.
11. Karpinos M, Teh BS, Zeck O, et al. Treatment of acoustic neuroma: stereotactic radiosurgery vs. microsurgery. *Int J Radiat Oncol Biol Phys*. 2002;54(5):1410–1421.
12. Pollock BE, Driscoll CL, Foote RL, et al. Patient outcomes after vestibular schwannoma management: a prospective comparison of microsurgical resection and stereotactic radiosurgery. *Neurosurgery*. 2006;59(1):77–85; discussion77–85.
13. Soulier G, van Leeuwen BM, Putter H, et al. Quality of life in 807 patients with vestibular schwannoma: comparing treatment Modalities. *Otolaryngol Head Neck Surg*. 2017: 194599817695800.
14. Woodruff JM, Selig AM, Crowley K, et al. Schwannoma (neurilemoma) with malignant transformation. A rare, distinctive peripheral nerve tumor. *Am J Surg Pathol*. 1994;18(9): 882–895.
15. White W, Shiu MH, Rosenblum MK, et al. Cellular schwannoma. A clinicopathologic study of 57 patients and 58 tumors. *Cancer*. 1990;66(6):1266–1275.
16. Deruaz JP, Janzer RC, Costa J. Cellular schwannomas of the intracranial and intraspinal compartment: morphological and immunological characteristics compared with classical benign schwannomas. *J Neuropathol Exp Neurol*. 1993;52(2):114–118.
17. Koyye RT, Mahadevan A, Santosh V, et al. A rare case of cellular schwannoma involving the trigeminal ganglion. *Brain Tumor Pathol*. 2003;20(2):79–83.
18. Landeiro JA, Ribeiro CH, Galdino AC, et al. Cellular schwannoma: a rare spinal benign nerve-sheath tumor with a pseudosarcomatous appearance: case report. *Arquivos de neuro-psiquiatria*. 2003;61(4):1035–1038.
19. Pekmezci M, Reuss DE, Hirbe AC, et al. Morphologic and immunohistochemical features of malignant peripheral nerve sheath tumors and cellular schwannomas. *Mod Pathol*. 2015;28(2):187–200.
20. Iwashita T, Enjoji M. Plexiformneurilemmoma: a clinicopathological and immunohistochemical analysis of 23 tumours from 20 patients. *Virchows Arch A Pathol Anat Histopathol*. 1987;411(4):305–309.
21. Kao GF, Laskin WB, Olsen TG. Solitary cutaneous plexiformneurilemmoma (schwannoma): a clinicopathologic, immunohistochemical, and ultrastructural study of 11 cases. *Mod Pathol*. 1989;2(1):20–26.
22. Kroh H, Matyja E, Marchel A. Epithelioidschwannomas of the acoustic nerve. *Folia Neuropathol*. 2000;38(1):23–27.
23. Laskin WB, Weiss SW, Bratthauer GL. Epithelioid variant of malignant peripheral nerve sheath tumor (malignant epithelioidschwannoma). *Am J Surg Pathol*. 1991;15(12):1136–1145.
24. Jo VY, Fletcher CD. SMARCB1/INI1 loss in epithelioidschwannoma: aclinicopathologic and immunohistochemicalstudy of 65 cases. *Am J Surg Pathol*. 2017. doi: 10.1097/PAS.0000000000000849.
25. Tozbikian G, Shen R, Suster S. Signet ring cell gastric schwannoma: report of a new distinctive morphological variant. *Ann Diagn Pathol*. 2008;12(2):146–152.
26. Miettinen M, McCue PA, Sarlomo-Rikala M, et al. Sox10—a marker for not only schwannian and melanocytic neoplasms but also myoepithelial cell tumors of soft tissue: a systematic analysis of 5134 tumors. *Am J Surg Pathol*. 2015;39(6):826–835.

27. Memoli VA, Brown EF, Gould VE. Glial fibrillary acidic protein (GFAP) immunoreactivity in peripheral nerve sheath tumors. *Ultrastruct Pathol.* 1984;7(4):269–275.
28. Harder A, Wesemann M, Hagel C, et al. Hybrid neurofibroma/schwannoma is overrepresented among schwannomatosis and neurofibromatosis patients. *Am J Surg Pathol.* 2012;36(5):702–709.
29. Nascimento AF, Fletcher CD. The controversial nosology of benign nerve sheath tumors: neurofilament protein staining demonstrates intratumoral axons in many sporadic schwannomas. *Am J Surg Pathol.* 2007;31(9):1363–1370.
30. McCarron KF, Goldblum JR. Plexiformneurofibroma with and without associated malignant peripheral nerve sheath tumor: a clinicopathologic and immunohistochemical analysis of 54 cases. *Mod Pathol.* 1998;11(7):612–617.
31. Rodriguez FJ, Perry A, Gutmann DH, et al. Gliomas in neurofibromatosis type 1: a clinicopathologic study of 100 patients. *J Neuropathol Exp Neurol.* 2008;67(3):240–249.
32. Miettinen MM, Antonescu CR, Fletcher CDM, et al. Histopathologic evaluation of atypical neurofibromatous tumors and their transformation into malignant peripheral nerve sheath tumor in neurofibromatosis 1 patients—a consensus overview. *Hum Pathol.* 2017;pii: S0046-8177(17)30167-3.
33. Torres-Mora J, Dry S, Li X, et al. Malignant melanotic schwannian tumor: a clinicopathologic, immunohistochemical, and gene expression profiling study of 40 cases, with a proposal for the reclassification of "melanoticschwannoma". *Am J Surg Pathol.* 2014; 38(1):94–105.
34. Carney JA. Psammomatous melanotic schwannoma. A distinctive, heritable tumor with special associations, including cardiac myxoma and the Cushing syndrome. *Am J Surg Pathol.*1990;14(3):206–222.
35. Vallat-Decouvelaere AV, Wassef M, Lot G, et al. Spinal melanotic schwannoma: a tumour with poor prognosis. *Histopathology.*1999;35(6):558–566.
36. Zhang HY, Yang GH, Chen HJ, et al. Clinicopathological, immunohistochemical, and ultrastructural study of 13 cases of melanotic schwannoma. *Chin Med J (Engl).* 2005; 118(17):1451–1461.
37. Ducatman BS, Scheithauer BW, Piepgras DG, et al. Malignant peripheral nerve sheath tumors. A clinicopathologic study of 120 cases. *Cancer.* 1986;57(10):2006–2021.
38. Hruban RH, Shiu MH, Senie RT, et al. Malignant peripheral nerve sheath tumors of the buttock and lower extremity. A study of 43 cases. *Cancer.* 1990;66(6):1253–1265.
39. Ducatman BS, Scheithauer BW, Piepgras DG, et al. Malignant peripheral nerve sheath tumors in childhood. *J Neuro Oncol.* 1984;2(3):241–248.
40. Wanebo JE, Malik JM, VandenBerg SR, et al. Malignant peripheral nerve sheath tumors. A clinicopathologic study of 28 cases. *Cancer.* 1993;71(4):1247–1253.
41. Evans DG, Baser ME, McGaughran J, et al. Malignant peripheral nerve sheath tumours in neurofibromatosis 1. *J Med Genet.* 2002;39(5):311–314.
42. Sorensen SA, Mulvihill JJ, Nielsen A. Long-term follow-up of von Recklinghausen neurofibromatosis. Survival and malignant neoplasms. *N Engl J Medicine.* 1986;314(16):1010–1015.
43. Ducatman BS, Scheithauer BW. Postirradiation neurofibrosarcoma. *Cancer.* 1983;51(6): 1028–1033.
44. Foley KM, Woodruff JM, Ellis FT, et al. Radiation-induced malignant and atypical peripheral nerve sheath tumors. *Ann Neurol.* 1980;7(4):311–318.
45. Friedrich RE, Kluwe L, Funsterer C, et al. Malignant peripheral nerve sheath tumors (MPNST) in neurofibromatosis type 1 (NF1): diagnostic findings on magnetic resonance images and mutation analysis of the NF1 gene. *Anticancer Res.* 2005;25(3A):1699–1702.

46. Mautner VF, Friedrich RE, von Deimling A, et al. Malignant peripheral nerve sheath tumours in neurofibromatosis type 1: MRI supports the diagnosis of malignant plexiform-neurofibroma. *Neuroradiology*. 2003;45(9):618–625.
47. Hagel C, Zils U, Peiper M, et al. Histopathology and clinical outcome of NF1-associated vs. sporadic malignant peripheral nerve sheath tumors. *J Neurooncol*. 2007;82(2):187–192.
48. Wong WW, Hirose T, Scheithauer BW, et al. Malignant peripheral nerve sheath tumor: analysis of treatment outcome. *Int J Radiat Oncol Biol Phys*. 1998;42(2):351–360.
49. Woodruff JM, Chernik NL, Smith MC, et al. Peripheral nerve tumors with rhabdomyosarcomatous differentiation (malignant "Triton" tumors). *Cancer*. 1973;32(2):426–439.
50. Wick MR, Swanson PE, Scheithauer BW, et al. Malignant peripheral nerve sheath tumor. An immunohistochemical study of 62 cases. *Am J Clin Pathol*. 1987;87(4):425–433.
51. Halling KC, Scheithauer BW, Halling AC, et al. p53 expression in neurofibroma and malignant peripheral nerve sheath tumor. An immunohistochemical study of sporadic and NF1-associated tumors. *Am J Clin Pathol*. 1996;106(3):282–288.
52. Brekke HR, Kolberg M, Skotheim RI, et al. Identification of p53 as a strong predictor of survival for patients with malignant peripheral nerve sheath tumors. *Neuro Oncol*. 2009;11(5):514–528.
53. Cleven AH, Sannaa GA, Briaire-de BruijnI, et al. Loss of H3K27 tri-methylation is a diagnostic marker for malignant peripheral nerve sheath tumors and an indicator for an inferior survival. *Mod Pathol*. 2016;29(6):582–590.
54. Schaefer IM, Fletcher CD, Hornick JL. Loss of H3K27 trimethylation distinguishes malignant peripheral nerve sheath tumors from histologic mimics. *Mod Pathol*. 2016; 29(1):4–13.
55. Christoforidis M, Buhl R, Paulus W, et al. Intraneuralperineurioma of the VIIIth cranial nerve: case report. *Neurosurgery*. 2007;61(3):E652; discussion E652.
56. Rickert CH, Schwering EM, Siebers J, et al. Chromosomal imbalances and NF2 mutational analysis in a series of 10 spinal nerve sheath myxomas. *Histopathology*. 2007;50(2): 252–257.

14

VASCULAR MALFORMATIONS AND OTHER SELECT VASCULAR LESIONS

ARTERIOVENOUS MALFORMATION

Clinical Context

Arteriovenous malformations (AVMs) are congenital vascular abnormalities that typically present between the ages of 20 and 40 years with spontaneous hemorrhage or, less commonly, seizure (1,2). A slight male predominance may be present among AVM patients, but not more than 3:2 (1,2). AVMs have been reported throughout the central nervous system (CNS), but they are most common in the cerebral hemispheres. Rare cases of AVM occur in familial clusters, sometimes as part of the Wyburn-Mason syndrome (3,4). Imaging of AVMs includes angiography by traditional methods as well as magnetic resonance (MR) and computed tomography (CT). In the classical setting, AVMs appear as superficial intraparenchymal tangles of large and small blood vessels with a *nidus*, or focal dense collection of vessels, present centrally (5). In a longitudinal study, the risk of hemorrhage in an AVM patient following diagnosis was approximately 4% per year, with a 1% annual risk of mortality (2).

Treatment for AVM comprises three approaches that may be used in combination with the goal of reducing risk of future hemorrhage. The therapeutic approach in any individual case is determined by the risk of surgical resection, as defined by the Spetzler-Martin grading scale, which awards risk for lesion size, location in an eloquent site, and the presence of deep venous drainage (6). Stereotactic radiosurgery is the least invasive modality and is effective for low-risk lesions, whereas endovascular catheter embolization is the initial treatment for high-risk cases. Surgery may be used as an initial approach in low-risk lesions but often follows reduction by one of the other modalities in high-risk cases.

Histopathology

The microscopic appearance of AVMs reflects their gross configuration, with disorganized arrays of individual vessels penetrating through the

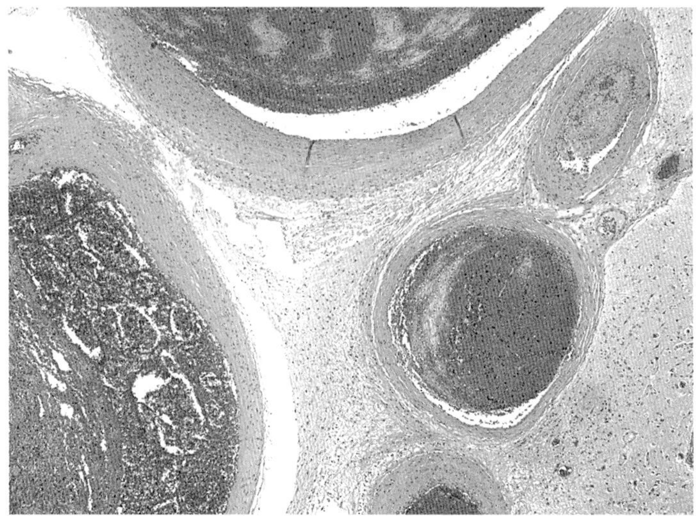

FIGURE 14-1 Arteriovenous malformations are composed of thick- and thin-walled vessels with intervening brain tissue.

brain parenchyma, each separated from each other by gliotic brain tissue (Figure 14-1). The component vessels vary in caliber and wall thickness, some with muscular arterial sides and internal elastic lamina (Figure 14-2) and others with thinner venous walls lacking smooth muscle or elastic lamina. Intermediate forms may also be seen. Variable amounts of inflammation, gliosis, and hemosiderin-laden macrophages are common in the

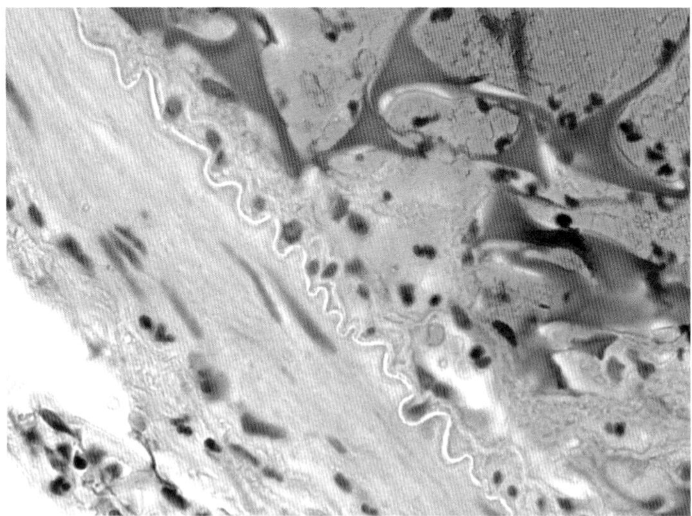

FIGURE 14-2 By definition, arteriovenous malformations must contain arteries, unequivocally identified here by the presence of a prominent elastic lamina.

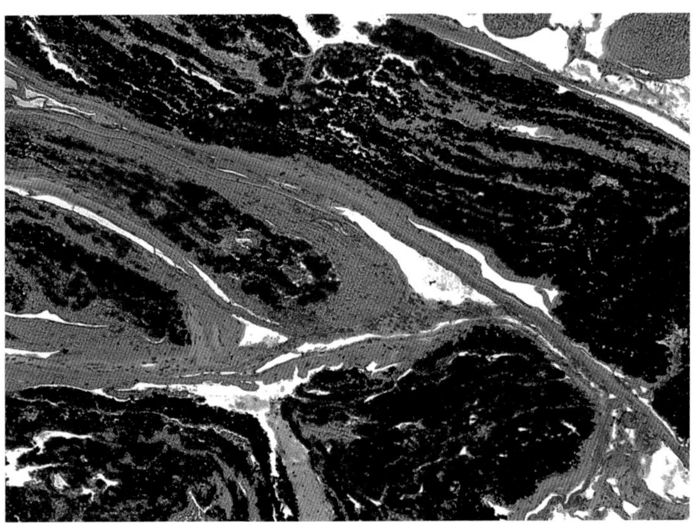

FIGURE 14-3 Some areas within arteriovenous malformations may contain back-to-back thin-walled vessels, imitating a cavernous malformation. Note intraluminal therapeutic embolic material (Onyx).

intervening brain tissue. Previously embolized resections contain intravascular foreign material.

Because the histologic appearance of AVM can overlap significantly with cavernous malformations (Figure 14-3), and clinical diagnoses incorporate in vivo observations (A-V shunting) that are not evident histologically, a more generic diagnosis of "vascular malformation" may be appropriate when the histology is unclear.

CAVERNOUS MALFORMATION (CAVERNOUS ANGIOMA, CAVERNOUS HEMANGIOMA)

Clinical Context

The age and anatomic distributions of cavernous malformations are similar to those of AVM, being most commonly diagnosed in the third through fifth decades (mean, ~35 years) in the cerebral hemispheres (6,7). No significant sex predilections exist. Most cavernous malformation patients present with seizures, focal deficits, or headaches, but only 10% or fewer present with hemorrhage, compared with 30% to 70% for AVMs (7,8). As with AVMs, some families show a predisposition toward cavernous malformations (9). The classic appearance of cavernous malformation on magnetic resonance imaging (MRI) is of a discreet, well-circumscribed nodular mass with no significant edema and little mass effect. T2-weighted images show a mixed intensity "core" and a characteristic hypointense penumbra of hemosiderin deposition (10).

Most cavernous malformations occur sporadically and are widely considered congenital. A much smaller subset develops *de novo* years after cranial irradiation for a neoplastic process (10). Ironically, radiosurgery is also a common method for reducing or involuting symptomatic cavernous malformations (11).

In contrast to AVMs, cavernous malformations contain no arteriovenous shunt; thus, they are less likely to have thin-walled vessels exposed to arterial pressures and less likely to hemorrhage. The annual risk of hemorrhage in a cavernous malformation is less than 1%, a fact underscoring the importance of distinguishing them from AVMs. Only when cavernous malformations produce significant symptoms, are they resected or undergo radiosurgery. Occasional resections are performed to rule out a radiologic suspicion for a hemorrhagic neoplasm.

Histopathology

A cohesive, solid mass of back-to-back, thin-walled blood vessels is cordoned from the surrounding brain within a discreet perimeter, beyond which gliosis, inflammation, and hemosiderin impregnate the parenchyma (Figure 14-4). The lumina may contain calcifications and remote thromboses. Although collagen may occupy space between vessels, brain is generally absent (Figure 14-5). Some cases deviate from the classical description and have features of AVM, with less defined borders and a small amount of intervascular brain, but should not contain any vessels with muscular walls or elastic lamina. As with AVMs, occasional cases with inconclusive or ambiguous histologic features should be generically labeled as "vascular malformations."

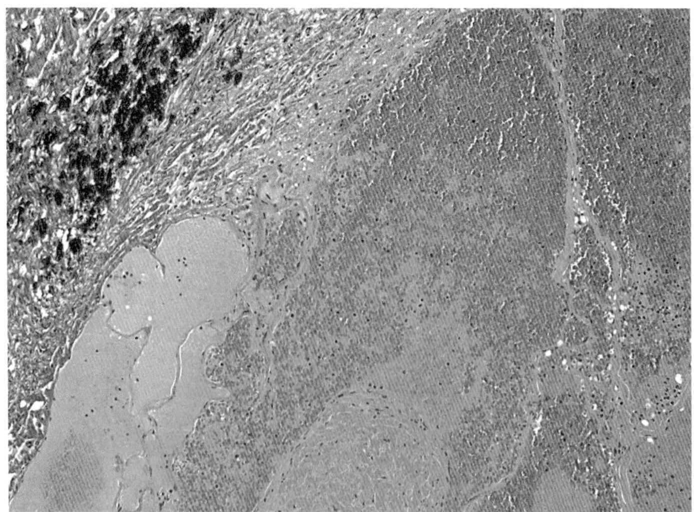

FIGURE 14-4 Cavernous malformations are well circumscribed and comprise back-to-back thin-walled vessels. The surrounding brain tissue is typically inflamed and has dense hemosiderin deposits (upper left).

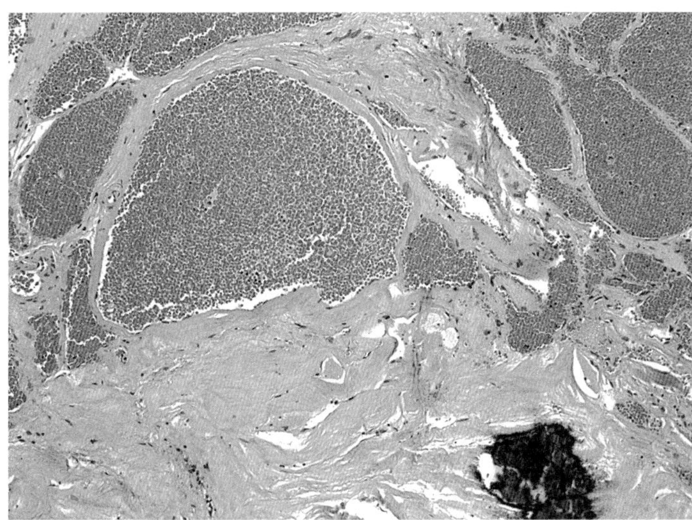

FIGURE 14-5 Dense collagen may surround a cavernous malformation and separate the vessels, but little or no brain is seen within.

CAPILLARY TELANGIECTASIA

This static vascular lesion is frequently identified on neuroimaging, but it is very rarely biopsied because its features are so characteristic. MRI reveals a patch of mild contrast enhancement within otherwise unremarkable surroundings, typically in the brainstem. Tissue sections show normal parenchyma perforated by scattered dilated capillaries.

CEREBRAL AMYLOID ANGIOPATHY

Clinical Context

Elderly patients, particularly those suffering from Alzheimer disease, tend to develop spontaneous intracranial hemorrhages in distributions that are unusual for hypertensive or aneurysmal bleeds. The resulting areas of hemorrhage may be mistaken clinically for hemorrhagic tumor masses and biopsied. Although cerebral amyloid angiopathy (CAA) is tightly linked with the development of Alzheimer-type dementia, patients occasionally present due to hemorrhages before their dementia comes to clinical attention. Some patients develop destructive granulomatous vasculitis in the setting of amyloid angiopathy, frequently referred to as amyloid β-related angiitis, or ABRA (see below).

Histopathology

CAA is most evident in superficial arteries of the leptomeninges and cortex but is not uniformly distributed. In the earliest stages, affected vessels retain a rigid, inflated contour with subtle thickening of the media by amyloid. In

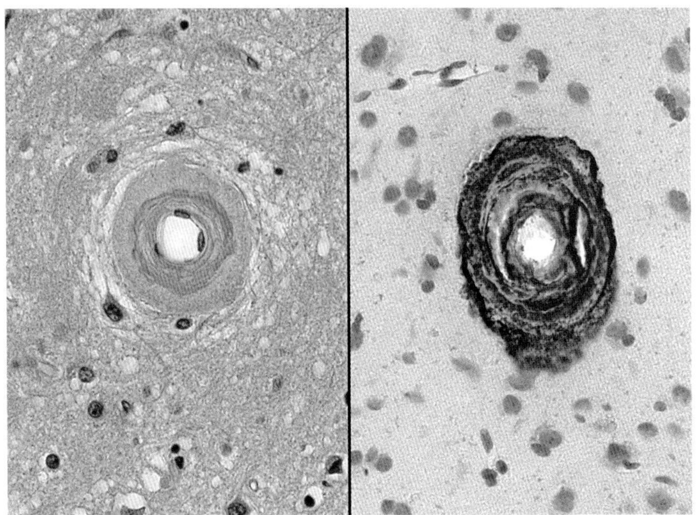

FIGURE 14-6 Amyloid angiopathy nearly replaces vessels with amorphous protein when severe (H&E, left). Affected vessels can be readily identified by Aβ amyloid immunohistochemistry (right).

severely compromised vessels, amyloid completely replaces the vessel wall and creates a thickened and brittle pipe-like channel (Figure 14-6). Some cases may have nondestructive perivascular lymphocytic inflammation that does not cause additional symptoms beyond those of CAA. Anti-Aβ antibodies have been detected in the cerebrospinal fluid (CSF) of one such patient, possibly suggesting that it is an early stage of ABRA (12). Immunohistochemistry for Aβ amyloid highlights the presence of amyloid (Figure 14-6), as do Congo red, crystal violet, and thioflavin B histochemical stains. This is the same type of amyloid found in the plaques of Alzheimer disease.

GIANT CELL ARTERITIS (TEMPORAL ARTERITIS, CRANIAL ARTERITIS)

This entity is also frequently called cranial arteritis to more accurately reflect its anatomic distribution, or giant cell arteritis to reflect its histologic appearance, although giant cells are also present in Takayasu arteritis.

Clinical Context

Temporal arteritis occurs almost exclusively after the age of 50 years and usually in the setting of the generalized inflammatory condition *Polymyalgia rheumatica.* Caucasians, particularly those of Scandinavian descent, account for the vast majority of cases (13). Women are affected almost two times as often as men. Patients present with persistent throbbing headaches and jaw claudication. In the setting of polymyalgia rheumatica, patients also have fatigue, muscle pain and tenderness, joint pain, and elevated erythrocyte

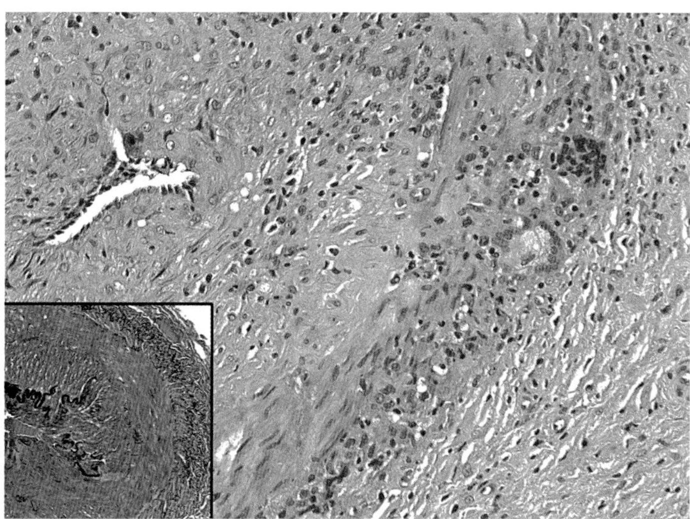

FIGURE 14-7 Temporal (giant cell) arteritis showing a thickened intima, infiltration of the elastica and adventitia by lymphohistiocytic inflammation, with destruction of the elastic layer (inset, Verhoeff elastic stain).

sedimentation rate (14). Although temporal arteritis responds well to steroids, vascular occlusion can cause permanent blindness if treatment is delayed. Biopsy of the temporal artery is the gold standard for diagnosing temporal arteritis. However, the characteristic pathologic findings may not be noted, even in patients with classic clinical disease because the changes are segmental. Complete submission of the specimen is required.

Histopathology

The histologic features of temporal arteritis vary somewhat depending on the severity of disease and whether corticosteroids have been given. The classic constellation of findings includes a T-lymphocytic infiltrate in the adventitia, multinucleate giant cells and epithelioid histiocytes around the intima-media junction, fragmentation and calcification of elastic fibers, and fibrosis and thickening of the intima (Figure 14-7). As more of these features are identified, the certainty of the histologic diagnosis increases. Giant cells are not necessary for the diagnosis and are absent in many, if not most, cases. Neutrophils should not be seen, while occasional eosinophils are allowable (15). Corticosteroids are frequently administered prior to biopsy, but most of the above features are present for at least a week after the first dose (16,17).

PRIMARY CNS VASCULITIS (PRIMARY ANGIITIS OF THE CNS)

Clinical Context

Patients with primary CNS vasculitis (PCNSV) can be sorted into two general clinicopathologic groups—amyloid β-related and idiopathic. ABRA occurs in older patients, median age around 66 years, who have a somewhat higher rate of cognitive disturbance and seizures than idiopathic PCNSV, but are otherwise similar. The idiopathic PCNSV patients have a median age around 47 years and tend to have higher rates of hemiparesis and visual disturbance (18). Other clinical subdivisions are sometimes made based on whether it was detected by angiogram, presented with hemorrhage, involved the spinal cord, or was rapidly progressive (19).

Angiography, which is confirmatory in over two-thirds of cases, shows focal and segmental areas of dilation, stenosis, and occlusion of cerebral arteries and multiple small infarcts of different ages. MRI may reveal stenosis or hemorrhage in some cases of PCNSV, yet does not show any consistent specific finding (20). Most cases abate following treatment with prednisone or cyclophosphamide with low rates of relapse, and a small number die or are left with persistent neurologic deficit (21,22).

Histopathology

PCNSV displays one of three histologic patterns—granulomatous, necrotizing, and lymphocytic. The *granulomatous pattern* consists of transmural vascular monocytic inflammation with scattered granulomas and giant cells (Figure 14-8). Almost half of granulomatous cases show deposition of Aβ-amyloid within the media, qualifying them for a diagnosis of ABRA (Figure 14-9). The amyloid in these cases is thought to be target of the immune response rather than the vessel itself, anti-β amyloid antibodies having been identified in the CSF (23). Granulomatous cases of PCNSV without amyloid remain idiopathic. The *lymphocytic pattern* comprises distorted

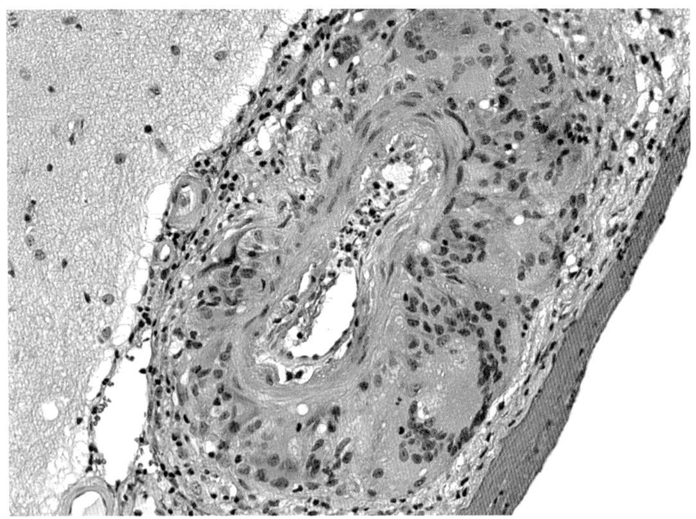

FIGURE 14-8 Granulomatous primary central nervous system vasculitis shows florid destruction of cerebral artery walls by histiocytes intermittently forming giant cells and granulomas.

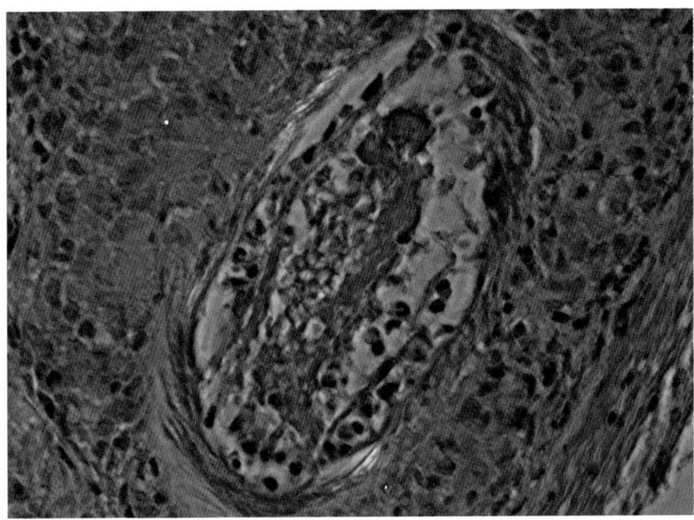

FIGURE 14-9 Amyloid β-related angiitis accounts for almost half of granulomatous central nervous system vasculitis, seen here as "apple-green" birefringence after Congo red staining.

and damaged vessels with transmural infiltrates of lymphocytes and occasional plasma cells. Transmural fibrinoid necrosis of small muscular arteries constitutes the *necrotizing pattern*. Nondiagnostic biopsies in PCNSV patients may show acute/subacute infarct and/or mild perivascular mononuclear infiltrates (24). In any case of vasculitis, an elastin stain is helpful to highlight the destruction of the arterial elastic layer.

OTHER VASCULITIDES

Several systemic autoimmune diseases can manifest as vasculitis in the CNS, including rheumatoid arthritis, lupus, Behcet disease, polyarteritis-nodosa, and others. No specific histopathologic findings characterize any one of these lesions, and the diagnosis for each depends heavily on clinical and laboratory data. Biopsies from this group of diseases are rare.

REFERENCES

1. da Costa L, Wallace MC, TerBrugge KG, et al. The natural history and predictive features of hemorrhage from brain arteriovenous malformations. *Stroke*. 2009;40(1):100–105.
2. Ondra SL, Troupp H, George ED, et al. The natural history of symptomatic arteriovenous malformations of the brain: a 24-year follow-up assessment. *J Neurosurg*. 1990;73(3):387–391.
3. Oikawa M, Kuniba H, Kondoh T, et al. Familial brain arteriovenous malformation maps to 5p13-q14, 15q11-q13 or 18p11: linkage analysis with clipped fingernail DNA on high-density SNP array. *Eur J Med Genet*. 2010;53(5):244–249.
4. Wyburn-Mason R. Arteriovenous aneurysm of midbrain and retina, facial naevi and mental changes. *Brain*. 1943;66(3):163–203.

5. Wallace RC, Flom RA, Khayata MH, et al. The safety and effectiveness of brain arteriovenous malformation embolization using acrylic and particles: the experiences of a single institution. *Neurosurgery*. 1995;37(4):606–615; discussion 615–608.
6. Spetzler RF, Martin NA. A proposed grading system for arteriovenous malformations. *J Neurosurg*. 1986;65(4):476–483.
7. Kondziolka D, Lunsford LD, Kestle JR. The natural history of cerebral cavernous malformations. *J Neurosurg*. 1995;83(5):820–824.
8. Robinson JR, Awad IA, Little JR. Natural history of the cavernous angioma. *J Neurosurg*. 1991;75(5):709–714.
9. Siegel AM, Andermann E, Badhwar A, et al. Anticipation in familial cavernous angioma: a study of 52 families from International Familial Cavernous Angioma Study. IFCAS Group. *Lancet*. 1998;352(9141):1676–1677.
10. Rigamonti D, Drayer BP, Johnson PC, et al. The MRI appearance of cavernous malformations (angiomas). *J Neurosurg*. 1987;67(4):518–524.
11. Lunsford LD, Khan AA, Niranjan A, et al. Stereotactic radiosurgery for symptomatic solitary cerebral cavernous malformations considered high risk for resection. *J Neurosurg*.2010;113(1):23–29.
12. DiFrancesco JC, Brioschi M, Brighina L, et al. Anti-Aβ autoantibodies in the CSF of a patient with CAA-related inflammation: a case report. *Neurology*. 2011;76(9):842–844.
13. Hoffman GS. Giant cell arteritis. *Ann Intern Med*. 2016;165(9):ITC65–ITC80.
14. Mertens JC, Willemsen G, Van Saase JL, et al. Polymyalgia rheumatica and temporal arteritis: a retrospective study of 111 patients. *Clin Rheumatol*. 1995;14(6):650–655.
15. Nordborg E, Nordborg C. Giant cell arteritis. In: KalimoH, ed. Cerebrovascular Diseases. Basel, Switzerland: International Society of Neuropathology; 2005:134–139.
16. Achkar AA, Lie JT, Hunder GG, et al. How does previous corticosteroid treatment affect the biopsy findings in giant cell (temporal) arteritis? *Ann Intern Med*. 1994;120(12):987–992.
17. Font RL, Prabhakaran VC. Histological parameters helpful in recognising steroid-treated temporal arteritis: an analysis of 35 cases. *Br J Ophthalmol*. 2007;91(2):204–209.
18. SalvaraniC, HunderGG, MorrisJM, et al. Aβ-related angiitis: comparison with CAA without inflammation and primary CNS vasculitis. *Neurology*. 2013;81(18):1596–1603.
19. Giannini C, Salvarani C, Hunder G, et al. Primary central nervous system vasculitis: pathology and mechanisms. *Acta Neuropathol*. 2012;123(6):759–772.
20. Boulouis G, de Boysson H, Zuber M, et al. Primary angiitis of the central nervous system: magnetic resonance imaging spectrum of parenchymal, meningeal, and vascular lesions at baseline. *Stroke*. 2017;48(5):1248–1255.
21. Salvarani C, Brown RD, Jr., Calamia KT, et al. Primary central nervous system vasculitis: comparison of patients with and without cerebral amyloid angiopathy. *Rheumatology (Oxford)*. 2008;47(11):1671–1677.
22. Salvarani C, Brown RD, Jr., Calamia KT, et al. Primary central nervous system vasculitis: analysis of 101 patients. *Ann Neurol*. 2007;62(5):442–451.
23. Piazza F, Greenberg SM, Savoiardo M, et al. Anti-amyloid β autoantibodies in cerebral amyloid angiopathy-related inflammation: implications for amyloid-modifying therapies. *Ann Neurol*. 2013;73(4):449–458.
24. Miller DV, Salvarani C, Hunder GG, et al. Biopsy findings in primary angiitis of the central nervous system. *Am J Surg Pathol*. 2009;33(1):35–43.

15

GERM CELL TUMORS

CLINICAL CONTEXT

Extragonadal germ cell neoplasms are uncommon in the central nervous system (CNS), accounting for less than 1% of all primary CNS tumors in the United States (1) and around 4% of primary CNS tumors in children (2). They recapitulate many of the features of extragonadal germ cell tumors at other sites, being midline, mostly in adolescent or young adult males and mostly seminoma/germinoma histology. CNS germ cell tumors include germinoma, immature and mature teratoma, choriocarcinoma, yolk sac (endodermal sinus) tumor, and embryonal carcinoma, with many lesions exhibiting a combination of histologies (*mixed malignant germ cell tumor*). Clinically, CNS germ cell tumors are grouped broadly into pure germinomatous and nongerminomatous types, based on prognosis and response to therapy.

CNS germ cell tumors most commonly affect males (~3:1 male: female) and have an increased incidence among people of Asian descent, accounting for up to 15% of all primary brain tumors in Taiwan (3). The incidence for CNS germ cell tumors peaks in the second decade when most cases occur, with a median age around 17 years regardless of sex or race (4,5). Although very rare, CNS germ cell tumors also occur in older adults, reported up to 86 years of age (5).

Although germ cell tumors can occur at any level of the neuraxis, the vast majority occur in the midline, with only rare cases found laterally. The most common sites for germ cell tumors within the CNS are the pineal gland and suprasellar region, with the anatomic distribution varying by sex. In males, pineal cases outnumber all other CNS sites, whereas females tend to develop suprasellar lesions (4). When considering only lesions of the pineal gland, the germ cell tumor patient population skews even further toward males, giving a ratio of 15:1 (5). Multifocal disease, usually pineal and suprasellar, is present in a minority of cases, around 15% (6,7).

Neuroimaging of germ cell tumors yields varying results, with no reliable features for distinguishing any one of them. Signal characteristics are variable and heterogeneous on both T1- and T2-weighted series, with occasional intratumoral cysts and calcification that may suggest teratoma, although both can be seen in other lesions (6). Germinomas occasionally extend along the ventricular walls in a plaque-like fashion, radiologically simulating the periventricular distribution of some primary CNS lymphomas.

The clinical workup for CNS germ cell tumors includes examination of cerebrospinal fluid (CSF) and blood for markers of differentiation, specifically β-hCG and α-fetoprotein (AFP). In cases where surgery is contraindicated, they may form the diagnostic basis for aggressive treatment (8). β-hCG in the CSF is presumptive evidence that the tumor contains choriocarcinoma elements, and AFP indicates yolk sac or immature teratoma elements. The prognostic impact of these tumor markers in the CSF is incompletely understood, but they may be associated with a small decrease in survival in patients with nongerminomatous lesions (9). One series showed frequent production of β-hCG by histologically pure germinomas that was associated with higher rates of recurrence (10).

Treatment for germ cell tumors in the CNS depends on tumor type. Pure germinomas, which are exquisitely radiosensitive, typically receive radiotherapy that is targeted to include the third ventricle, whole brain, or the entire craniospinal axis to treat potential microscopic dissemination (11). Because of greater side effects in children from cerebral irradiation, some dose-sparing approaches utilizing pre-radiation chemotherapy have been developed and show promise in reducing radiation exposure in that population (12,13). Given their rarity and heterogeneous compositions, other malignant germ cell tumors do not receive any standard regimen, except that most cases are treated with some form of radiation therapy. Pure mature teratomas are the only CNS germ cell tumor that can be approached successfully with resection alone (14).

The outcomes for pure germinomas and mature teratomas are favorable, with greater than 90% survival for both in one large series. Immature teratomas and other malignant germ cell tumors, however, had survival rates of 70% or less at 3 years (7). The presence of choriocarcinoma, yolk sac tumor, or embryonal carcinoma was associated with 38% 5-year survival in another series (15).

GERMINOMA

Primary CNS germinomas resemble those at other extragonadal sites, with large round cells containing moderate amounts of clear or partially clear cytoplasm around large nuclei with vesicular chromatin and prominent eosinophilic nucleoli (Figure 15-1). The cells vary in distribution from solid sheets with few other cell types to individually scattered almost imperceptibly among inflammatory cells and native tissue, traversed by delicate collagenous septa. Germinomas are among the few nonneuroepithelial CNS neoplasms that can infiltrate over limited distances as single cells into the surrounding tissue.

Germinoma is particularly susceptible to crush artifact and the lesion's overall histology can be obscured by it. Careful handling can minimize this effect. Immunostaining crushed areas can demonstrate distorted

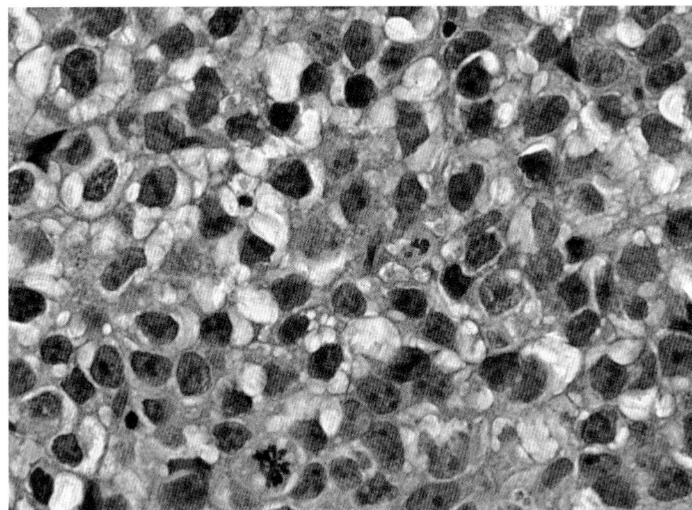

FIGURE 15-1 The cells of germinoma are large with clear cytoplasm, open chromatin, and prominent nucleoli.

positivity for germinoma markers (Figure 15-2), but diagnosing based on such findings is risky, especially with CD117, which is also expressed by mast cells.

An inflammatory infiltrate almost always accompanies the neoplastic element of germinomas, usually in the form of T-lymphocytes with or without granulomas (Figure 15-3). The lymphocytes are a mixture of CD4+ and

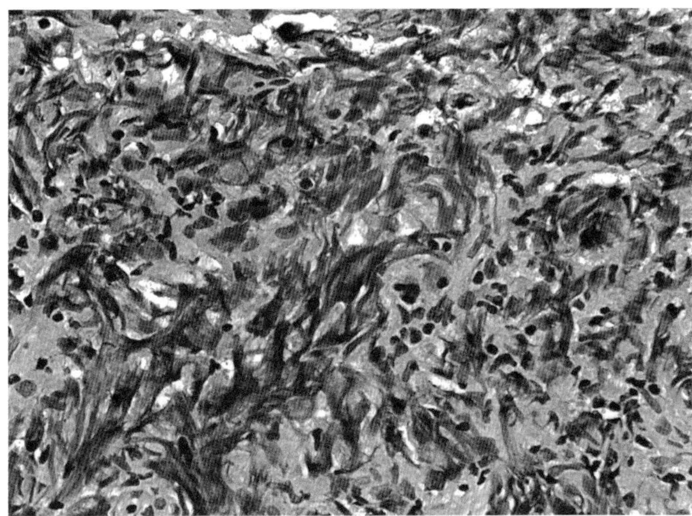

FIGURE 15-2 Crush artifact obscures many germinomas and is especially problematic for intraoperative consultation, although some immunoreactivity can still be demonstrated on permanent sections.

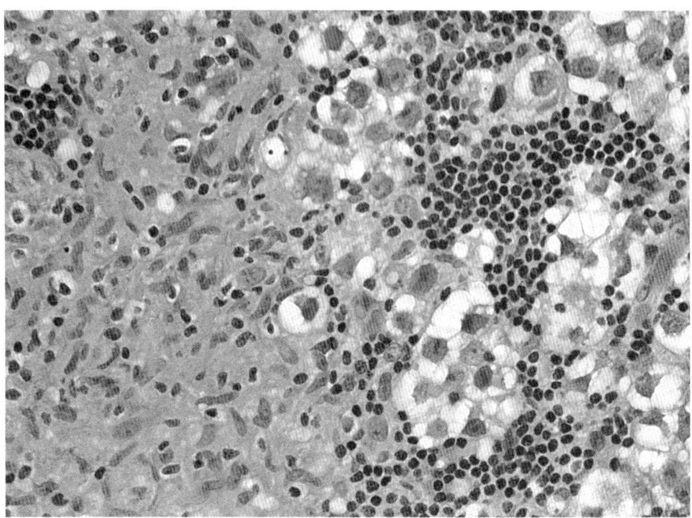

FIGURE 15-3 Granulomas and lymphocytic infiltrates are common in germinomas.

CD8+ cells that are thought to be reactive to antigens expressed by the tumor, inducing oligoclonal expansions of T-cells, a hypothetical pitfall if receptor rearrangement studies are ordered to evaluate for lymphoma (16). Small epithelioid granulomas are common and can cause confusion of germinoma with neurosarcoidosis or other granulomatous processes (17). Granulomas in a biopsy from the pineal region or suprasellar area should prompt a close examination for the presence of germinoma, which can be present as only a few scattered cells.

A fraction of otherwise pure germinoma cases contain scattered multinucleate syncytiotrophoblastic cells that are immunoreactive for β-hCG and secrete it into the CSF. Although only a small number of cases are reported in the literature with follow-up data, they appear to be more likely to recur than pure germinomas, especially when the CSF β-hCG levels are elevated (18,19). The presence of any other germ cell tumor types warrants classification as a mixed malignant germ cell tumor.

Most germinomas are immunoreactive for placenta-like alkaline phosphatase (PLAP) and CD117 (c-kit) (20). A more specific marker for germinoma is the transcriptional regulator OCT4, which shows a strong nuclear pattern in the vast majority of germinomas, and is negative in other entities in the differential diagnosis (21,22). OCT4, or the anti-OCT3/4 antibody mixture, is also positive in most cases of embryonal carcinoma, but germinoma fails to express cytokeratin and CD30, making the distinction between these two straightforward. Periodic acid-Schiff (PAS) staining often highlights diastase-labile glycogen granules within germinoma cell cytoplasm.

The differential diagnosis for germinoma includes large cell lymphoma, metastatic carcinoma/melanoma, and, in granulomatous cases, neurosarcoidosis. Immunohistochemistry is very helpful when needed because germinoma is negative for CD20, CD45, keratin, S100, and melan-A. Neurosarcoidosis should not contain any cells with OCT4 positivity.

IMMATURE TERATOMA, MATURE TERATOMA

The *sine qua non* of teratoma is the presence of structures derived from each of the three embryologic germ layers—ectoderm, mesoderm, and endoderm. Most teratomas in the CNS are immature, with poorly differentiated, mitotically active, primordial cells accompanying more identifiable tissues, and the remaining minority contain only differentiated elements (Figure 15-4). Other germ cell tumors also frequently lurk among the teratomatous elements. Any tissue type at any stage of development can be seen in teratomas, with skin, brain, cartilage, intestine, muscle, and fat being common. The diagnostic distinction between mature and immature teratoma is paramount because of the increased incidence of recurrence among the latter (23,24). Immature elements include neuroepithelial/neuroblastic, mesenchymal, or primitive glandular tissues and typically have high mitotic rates.

The individual tissue types within a teratoma may give rise to secondary malignancies specific to that tissue type, for example, medulloblastoma arising from neural tissue or adenocarcinoma arising from an epithelium (25,26). In such cases, the diagnostic term *teratoma with malignant transformation* can be used.

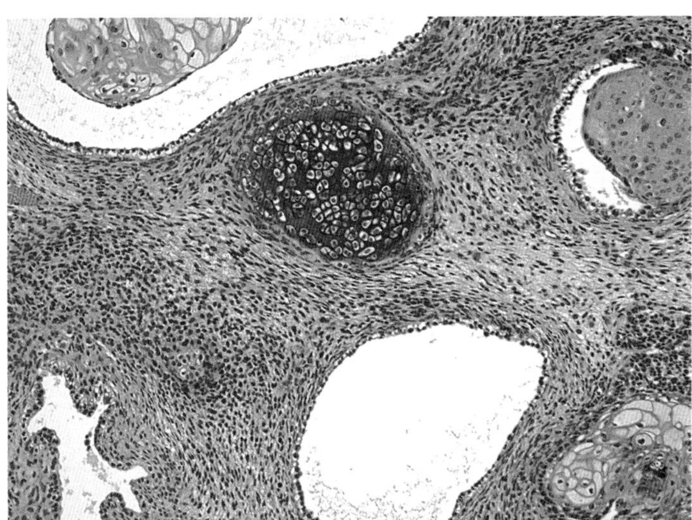

FIGURE 15-4 Immatureteratomas contain poorly differentiated embryonal elements and scattered tissues from multiple germ layers.

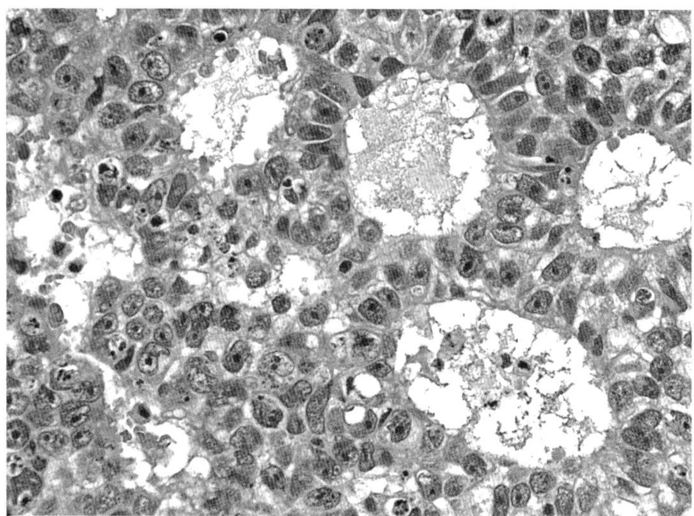

FIGURE 15-5 Embryonal carcinoma has nuclear features similar to germinoma, but it is cohesive and attempts to form epithelial structures.

The diagnosis of dermoid cyst around the pineal gland or sella should be issued with caution for limited specimens, given the likelihood that the tissue represents part of a teratoma potentially with malignant elements in the unresected portions.

EMBRYONAL CARCINOMA

Cohesive large epithelial cells with high nucleocytoplasmic ratio, open chromatin, and prominent nucleoli grow in sheets and/or attempt to form occasional glandular and tubular structures (Figure 15-5), with the effect of a highly anaplastic and poorly differentiated adenocarcinoma. The nuclear features of this tumor can closely mimic those of seminoma. As mentioned above, embryonal carcinoma expresses OCT3/4 like germinoma and additionally expresses CD30 and cytokeratin.

YOLK SAC TUMOR

Also known as endodermal sinus tumor, yolk sac tumor assumes a multiplicity of histologic patterns, often with several in a single lesion, yet with several key features seen in the vast majority of cases. Ribbons of tumor cells "festooned" around fibrovascular cores and blood vessels with intervening irregular channels create the archetypical endodermal sinus pattern. Areas of vacuolated microcystic cells and solid sheets of polygonal cells are common (Figure 15-6). The tumor cells are generally intermediate to large epithelioid cells with large vesicular nuclei and prominent nuclei,

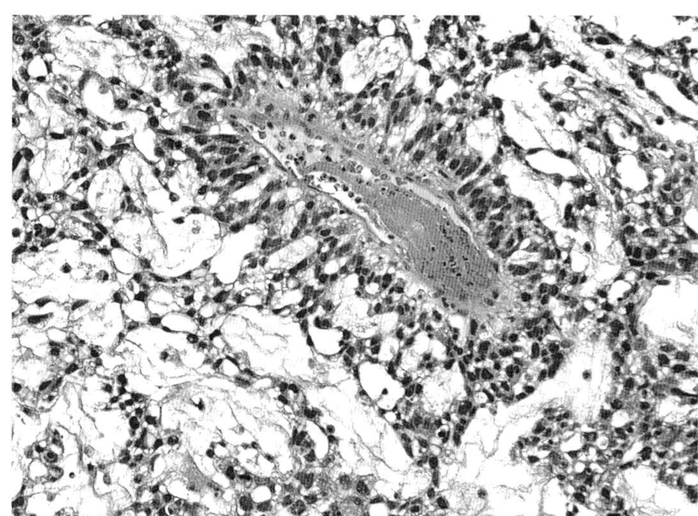

FIGURE 15-6 Yolk sac tumor frequently has a myxoidmicrocystic appearance with perivascular tumor cell arrays.

not unlike those of embryonal carcinoma and germinoma. Scattered among the cells are spherical, eosinophilic, hyaline globules that are roughly the size of the tumor nuclei. PAS staining highlights these diastase-resistant structures and aids in differentiating solid areas from embryonal carcinoma and germinoma.

Immunohistochemistry demonstrates an adenocarcinoma-like profile of reactivity, with positivity for cytokeratin and carcinoembryonic antigen (CEA), although it does not stain with EMA. AFP staining is usually positive but can be patchy or even negative. Glypican-3 is a sensitive marker for yolk sac tumor, although it can also be seen in some choriocarcinomas(27). SALL4 is another marker that has been used to identify yolk sac elements among germ cell tumors (28).

CHORIOCARCINOMA

A high degree of cellular pleomorphism and a biphenotypic cell population characterize the appearance of choriocarcinoma. The syncytiotrophoblast cells are large with amphophilic cytoplasm and multiple large irregular nuclei, sometimes with "smudgy" chromatin. The cytotrophoblasts are, in contrast, mononucleate with multiple clear intracytoplasmic vacuoles. Although the presence of syncytiotrophoblast cells should be reported, they are insufficient by themselves to change the diagnosis of a lesion and can be seen in germinoma and embryonal carcinoma. Choriocarcinomas are positive for β-hCG and cytokeratin by immunohistochemistry.

REFERENCES

1. Ostrom QT, Gittleman H, Xu J, et al. CBTRUS statistical report: primary brain and other central nervous system tumors diagnosed in the United States in 2009–2013. *Neuro Oncol.* 2016;18(suppl 5):v1–v75.
2. Ostrom QT, de Blank PM, Kruchko C, et al. Alex's Lemonade stand foundation infant and childhood primary brain and central nervous system tumors diagnosed in the United States in 2007–2011. *Neuro Oncol.* 2015;16(suppl 10):x1–x36.
3. Wong TT, Ho DM, Chang KP, et al. Primary pediatric brain tumors: statistics of Taipei VGH, Taiwan (1975–2004). *Cancer.* 2005;104(10):2156–2167.
4. Goodwin TL, Sainani K, Fisher PG. Incidence patterns of central nervous system germ cell tumors: a SEER Study. *J Pediatr Hematol Oncol.* 2009;31(8):541–544.
5. Villano JL, Propp JM, Porter KR, et al. Malignant pineal germ-cell tumors: an analysis of cases from three tumor registries. *Neuro Oncol.* 2008;10(2):121–130.
6. Liang L, Korogi Y, Sugahara T, et al. MRI of intracranial germ-cell tumours. *Neuroradiology.* 2002;44(5):382–388.
7. Matsutani M, Sano K, Takakura K, et al. Primary intracranial germ cell tumors: a clinical analysis of 153 histologically verified cases. *J Neurosurg.* 1997;86(3):446–455.
8. Qaddoumi I, Sane M, Li S, et al. Diagnostic utility and correlation of tumor markers in the serum and cerebrospinal fluid of children with intracranial germ cell tumors. *Childs Nerv Syst.* 2012;28(7):1017–1024.
9. Kim A, Ji L, Balmaceda C, et al. The prognostic value of tumor markers in newly diagnosed patients with primary central nervous system germ cell tumors. *Pediatr Blood Cancer.* 2008;51(6):768–773.
10. Fukuoka K, Yanagisawa T, Suzuki T, et al. Human chorionic gonadotropin detection in cerebrospinal fluid of patients with a germinoma and its prognostic significance: assessment by using a highly sensitive enzyme immunoassay. *J Neurosurg Pediatr.* 2016;18(5): 573–577.
11. Aoyama H, Shirato H, Kakuto Y, et al. Pathologically-proven intracranial germinoma treated with radiation therapy. *Radiother Oncol.* 1998;47(2):201–205.
12. Cheng S, Kilday JP, Laperriere N, et al. Outcomes of children with central nervous system germinoma treated with multi-agent chemotherapy followed by reduced radiation. *J Neurooncol.* 2016;127(1):173–180.
13. Calaminus G, Kortmann R, Worch J, et al. SIOP CNS GCT 96: final report of outcome of a prospective, multinational nonrandomized trial for children and adults with intracranial germinoma, comparing craniospinal irradiation alone with chemotherapy followed by focal primary site irradiation for patients with localized disease. *Neuro Oncol.* 2013; 15(6):788–796.
14. Phi JH, Kim SK, Park SH, et al. Immature teratomas of the central nervous system: is adjuvant therapy mandatory? *J Neurosurg.* 2005;103(suppl 6):524–530.
15. Sawamura Y, Ikeda J, Shirato H, et al. Germ cell tumours of the central nervous system: treatment consideration based on 111 cases and their long-term clinical outcomes. *Eur J Cancer.*1998;34(1):104–110.
16. Hadrup SR, Braendstrup O, Jacobsen GK, et al. Tumor infiltrating lymphocytes in seminoma lesions comprise clonally expanded cytotoxic T cells. *Int J Cancer.* 2006;119(4):831–838.
17. Mueller W, Schneider GH, Hoffmann KT, et al. Granulomatous tissue response in germinoma, a diagnostic pitfall in endoscopic biopsy. *Neuropathol.* 2007;27(2):127–132.
18. Uematsu Y, Tsuura Y, Miyamoto K, et al. The recurrence of primary intracranial germinomas. Special reference to germinoma with STGC (syncytiotrophoblastic giant cell). *J Neuro Oncol.* 1992;13(3):247–256.

19. Utsuki S, Kawano N, Oka H, et al. Cerebral germinoma with syncytiotrophoblastic giant cells: feasibility of predicting prognosis using the serum hCG level. *Acta Neurochir.* 1999;141(9):975–977; discussion 977–978.
20. Nakamura H, Takeshima H, Makino K, et al. C-kit expression in germinoma: an immunohistochemistry-based study. *J Neurooncol.* 2005;75(2):163–167.
21. Biermann K, Klingmuller D, Koch A, et al. Diagnostic value of markers M2A, OCT3/4, AP-2gamma, PLAP and c-KIT in the detection of extragonadal seminomas. *Histopathology.* 2006;49(3):290–297.
22. Hattab EM, Tu PH, Wilson JD, et al. OCT4 immunohistochemistry is superior to placental alkaline phosphatase (PLAP) in the diagnosis of central nervous system germinoma. *Am J Surg Pathol.* 2005;29(3):368–371.
23. Lee YH, Park EK, Park YS, et al. Treatment and outcomes of primary intracranial teratoma. *Childs Nerv Syst.* 2009;25(12):1581–1587.
24. Sawamura Y, Kato T, Ikeda J, et al. Teratomas of the central nervous system: treatment considerations based on 34 cases. *J Neurosurg.* 1998;89(5):728–737.
25. Das S, Muro K, Goldman S, et al. Medulloblastoma arising from an immature teratoma of the posterior fossa. Case report. *J Neurosurg.* 2007;106(suppl 1):61–64.
26. Freilich RJ, Thompson SJ, Walker RW, et al. Adenocarcinomatous transformation of intracranial germ cell tumors. *Am J Surg Pathol.* 1995;19(5):537–544.
27. Zynger DL, McCallum JC, Luan C, et al. Glypican 3 has a higher sensitivity than alphafetoprotein for testicular and ovarian yolk sac tumour: immunohistochemical investigation with analysis of histological growth patterns. *Histopathology.* 2010;56(6):750–757.
28. Mei K, Liu A, Allan RW, et al. Diagnostic utility of SALL4 in primary germ cell tumors of the central nervous system: a study of 77 cases. *Mod Pathol.* 2009;22(12):1628–1636.

16

HEMATOLYMPHOID NEOPLASMS

PRIMARY CNS LYMPHOMA

Although primary central nervous system lymphoma (PCNSL) technically includes any lymphocytic neoplasms restricted to the central nervous system (CNS), the term is usually understood to refer to diffuse large B-cell lymphoma (DLBCL), which accounts for around 95% of PCNSL. Low-grade B-cell lymphomas are much less common in the CNS than their higher-grade counterparts, only accounting for about 3% of PCNSL in one large European series (1). The incidence of T-cell PCNSL is low in the West, only around 2%, but makes up to 17% of PCNSL cases in some Asian countries (2). Except when otherwise stated below, PCNSL here is synonymous with DLBCL of the CNS.

PCNSL accounts for approximately 2% of primary brain tumors, 6% of malignant primary brain tumors (3), and less than 1% of non-Hodgkin lymphoma diagnoses. The incidence of PCNSL has been increasing in recent years among the elderly people in some series, although no cause for it has been determined (4–6).

Clinical Context

The population of patients with PCNSL consists of two main groups, the immunocompromised and immunocompetent, who differ in many epidemiologic and clinical variables as well as the fundamental pathophysiology of their disease (7).

Among immunocompromised patients, PCNSL is most clearly associated with HIV/AIDS and is less common in transplant recipients and others on chronic immunosuppressive therapy, or with congenital immune defects (8–10). Patients in this group are generally young adults and male, roughly reflecting the population characteristics of the HIV-infected in the West (11). Rates of immunodeficiency-related PCNSL have been decreasing along with increased use of highly active antiretroviral therapy (HAART) in HIV infection.

In contrast, immunocompetent hosts of PCNSL are older (mean age, 61 years) and are evenly split between males and females (12). Pediatric cases of PCNSL are rare, though can occur in either immunocompetent or immunocompromised hosts, with overall better outcomes than adult patients (13).

Epstein–Barr virus (EBV) is important in the pathogenesis of PCNSL in the immunocompromised, one series showing a consistent presence of EBV in immunodeficient PCNSL, but not in sporadic cases (14). In AIDS patients, the term ***AIDS-related diffuse large B-cell lymphoma*** is used, whereas other EBV-related PCNSLs, typically in elderly patients, are termed ***EBV-positive, diffuse large B-cell lymphoma, NOS***.

A small number of PCNSL are low-grade B-cell lymphomas, which differ from those that are higher grade in both prognosis and anatomic distribution. In general, low-grade lymphomas tend to arise from the dura and have an indolent course, while those of higher grade are intra-axial and aggressive. Dural lymphomas are often the marginal zone variety but can also be any other B-cell type.

The radiologic appearance of PCNSL also differs depending on whether the patient is immunocompromised. Although almost all of PCNSLs show contrast enhancement, lesions with central necrosis are much more likely in immunocompromised patients, whereas those in immunocompetent hosts are solidly contrast enhancing (15,16). In both patient groups, the lesions are located in the deep cerebral hemispheres, basal ganglia, or corpus callosum in most cases, almost always in contact with a ventricular wall and without substantial mass effect. Multiple lesions are present in fewer than half of cases (15,16). T-cell PCNSLs show similar findings, but may be more subcortical than periventricular and have a higher rate of necrosis and peripheral enhancement, even in immunocompetent hosts (17). Intraparenchymal small B-cell lesions have more variable radiologic appearance without any specific characteristic findings, while dura-based lesions have a radiologic picture similar to meningioma.

As with lymphomas elsewhere in the body, surgical intervention has no role in therapy beyond securing a tissue diagnosis, usually by stereotactic biopsy. Debulking excisions are sometimes performed on an emergent basis before the diagnosis is known, but partial resection has been associated with poorer survival (12).

Chemotherapy and radiation are the principle treatment modalities for PCNSL, yet because the CNS is impervious to many of the chemotherapeutic agents used for systemic lymphomas, many of them have limited or no effect in PCNSL. Methotrexate, when given rapidly in high doses, crosses the blood–brain barrier to provide an effective treatment, as do anthracycline agents. Radiation is also effective in treating PCNSL, often with rapid and striking reductions in tumor following treatment; however, recurrence is highly likely. Radiation monotherapy resulted in 18% 5-year survival in one series (18).

Corticosteroids also have a remarkable effect on PCNSL, sometimes causing complete radiologic remission and emptying lesional tissue of neoplastic cells. Unfortunately, the effect is temporary. Because of the dramatic effects of corticosteroid on the histologic picture of PCNSL, its use is avoided until after biopsy in suspected cases.

Survival of patients with PCNSL varies greatly depending on the patient's immune status. A meta-analysis covering 792 cases showed median survival for immunocompromised/AIDS patients to be 2.6 months, whereas median survival for sporadic cases was 18.9 months (7). A more recent series showed a significant survival gain for PCNSL-AIDS patients treated with HAART, although median survival for the HAART-treated patients was still only 8 months (19). Age younger than 60 years is also associated with improved survival (12).

Histopathology and Immunohistochemistry

LARGE B-CELL LYMPHOMA. Intraparenchymal brain lymphomas are distributed angiocentrically, collecting in the perivascular space before infiltrating the surrounding tissue (Figure 16-1). Lymphomas, at least over short distances, may invade the brain as individual cells, creating a gradient of cellularity similar to that of infiltrating gliomas. In some cases, these perivascular gradients collide, coalescing to form a sheetlike pattern that superficially mimics other "small blue cell" malignancies. Vascular destruction is a prominent feature of CNS lymphomas, with ranks of cells invading and dissecting the vessel walls, dividing them into thin concentric strands, an effect exaggerated by reticulin staining (Figure 16-2). Necrosis is common.

The cells of PCNSL are morphologically indistinguishable from those of other DLBCLs, with scant cytoplasm, vesicular chromatin, and prominent nucleoli. Even when closely packed, there is space between individual cells and the plasma membranes are clearly separate, lacking the intercellular cohesion of carcinomas. Numerous scattered apoptotic nuclei may be present, a helpful diagnostic feature because such amounts of karyorrhectic debris are rare in other lesions.

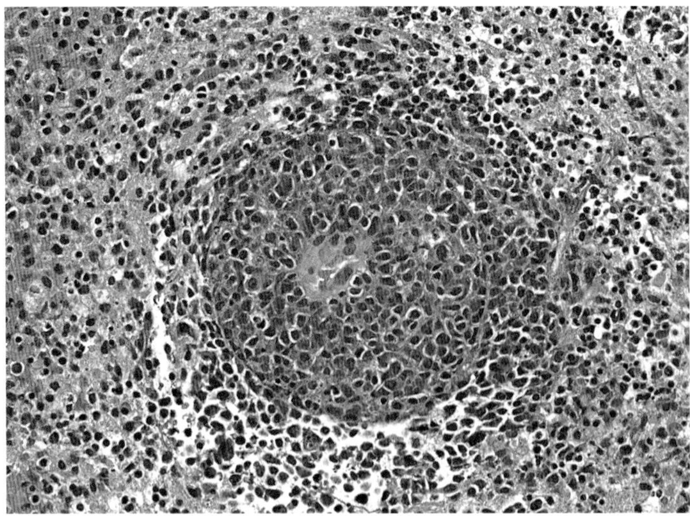

FIGURE 16-1 Typical primary CNS large B-cell lymphoma destroying the vessel wall, filling the perivascular space and infiltrating the parenchyma.

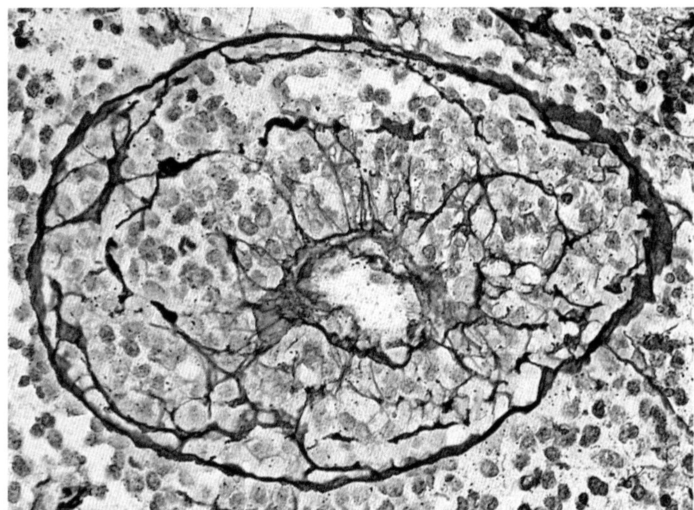

FIGURE 16-2 Reticulin staining highlights the dissection of the vascular wall by malignant cells.

A smaller component of nonneoplastic, mature T-lymphocytes and histiocytes usually accompanies the tumor cells in PCNSL, but only rarely is this constituent prominent enough to qualify a lesion as ***T-cell/histiocyte-rich large B-cell lymphoma***, which requires them to form the majority of the lesion, with only dispersed individual malignant B-cells (Figure 16-3) (20). This lymphoma is uncommon as a CNS primary.

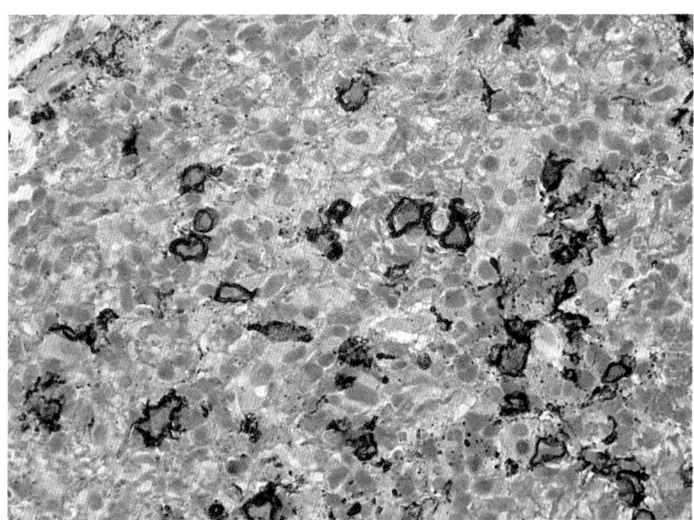

FIGURE 16-3 CD20 immunostaining unmasks the malignant B-cells among nonneoplastic T-cells in this T-cell–rich large B-cell lymphoma.

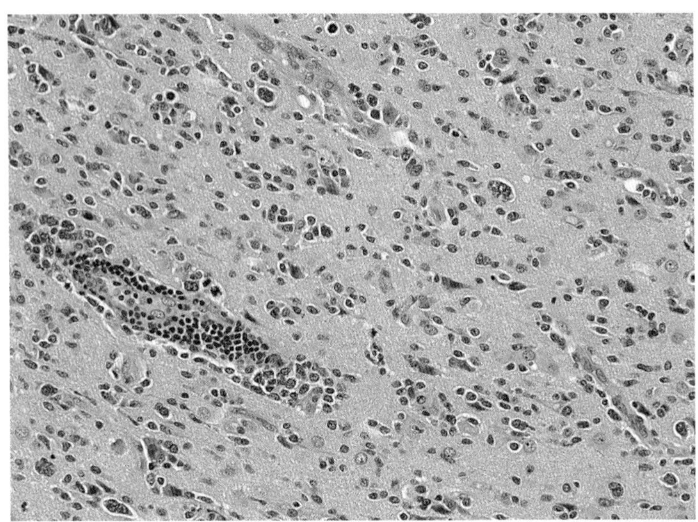

FIGURE 16-4 Primary CNS T-cell lymphomas are often less cellular, more infiltrative, and more mature appearing than B-cell primary CNS lymphoma.

The typical PCNSL shows a B-cell immunophenotype, expressing Pax5, CD19, CD20, CD22, CD45, and CD79a. Further subcategorization by immunohistochemistry into stages of B-cell development is possible with antibodies against MUM1, BCL6, and CD10, although the role of this classification in PCNSL is unclear (20–22).

T-CELL LYMPHOMAS. Angiocentric infiltrates are also characteristic of T-cell PCNSL, although with generally less cellular density and more infiltration than the large B-cell types (Figure 16-4) (2). The tumor cells are more often small and mature appearing in T-cell lesions, although cases of large T-cell PCNSL also occur (23). The lymphoma T-cells are immunoreactive for CD3 and may show any combination of CD4, CD5, CD7, and CD8 staining.

LOW-GRADE B-CELL LYMPHOMAS. In the CNS, low-grade B-cell lymphomas are usually dura-based (Figure 16-5) and are marginal zone ("MALT-derived") types, which comprise small B-cells that express CD20, but lack CD5, CD10, and CD23. Other types also rarely develop. Very rare intraparenchymal small B-cell lymphomas can also be of any of the many small B-cell subtypes, but are most often lymphoplasmacytic lymphoma (1), with monotonous populations of lymphocytes and plasmacytoidlymphocytes, often with scattered intranuclear immunoglobulin aggregates (Dutcher bodies), mast cells, and hemosiderin granules. As with other PCNSL, these cells are angiocentrically arranged and modestly infiltrate the surrounding brain tissue (Figure 16-6).

PLASMACYTOMA. Most neurosurgical specimens containing plasmacytoma are taken from bony or dural lesions in the context of multiple myeloma, which is systemic in nature. Only rarely are plasmacytomas

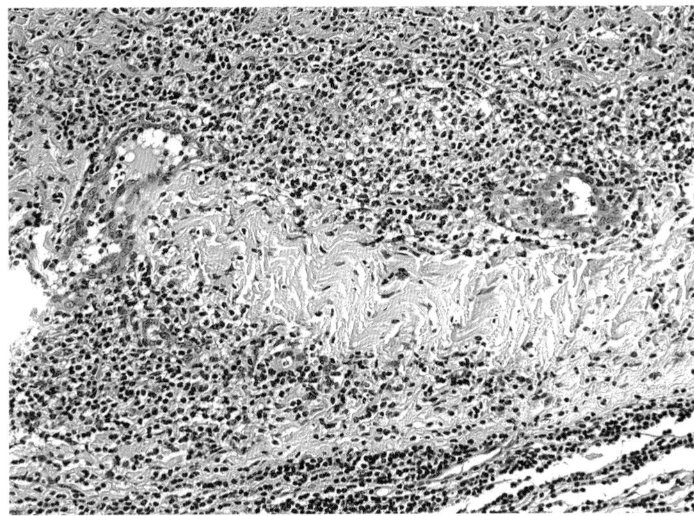

FIGURE 16-5 Marginal zone lymphomas usually occur on the dura and infiltrate the involved structures.

found in the CNS without bone marrow disease, usually as dura-based lesions (24,25). Most cases have the classic histology of small monotonous cells with eccentric round nuclei, perinuclear *hof*, and coarsely clumped chromatin.

Ancillary Testing

Testing beyond histology and immunohistochemistry is not necessary in the vast majority of brain lymphomas but may be necessary to establish the

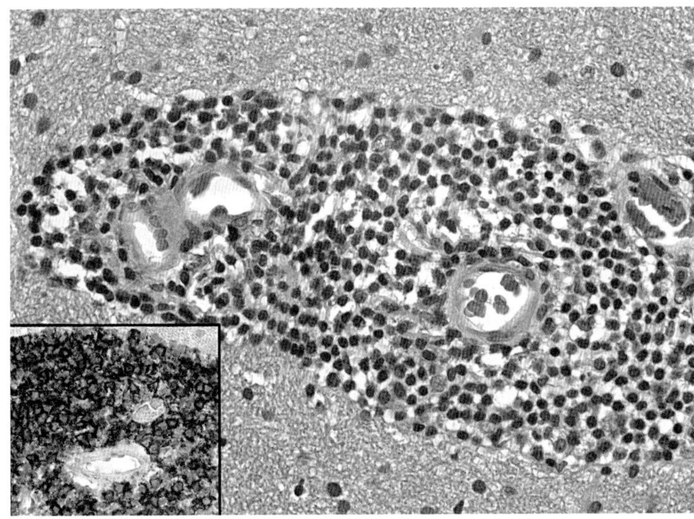

FIGURE 16-6 Parenchymal primary CNS marginal zone lymphoma is exceedingly rare and can appear like an inflammatory lesion, except for its preponderance of CD20+ B-cells (inset).

diagnosis in unusual cases. Because many hematolymphoid neoplasms contain chromosomal translocations, testing by FISH, PCR, or other DNA-based assay may help to make a specific diagnosis in such cases.

Nonneoplastic B- and T-cells undergo "somatic hypermutation" of their immunoglobulin heavy chain (IgH) and T-cell receptor genes, respectively, giving each cell a different gene length, resulting in a Gaussian distribution of gene sizes to nonneoplastic infiltrates. In contrast, lymphomas are clonal and contain only a single IgH or T-cell receptor gene size, which can be differentiated from polyclonal mixtures by PCR. This testing, when available, is a powerful tool for ruling in or out neoplastic lymphocytic infiltrates, but only in the context of a histologic picture that would be consistent with lymphoma.

Flow cytometry may be difficult in many cases of PCNSL because of specimen size, yet it can provide a rapid and sensitive classification and should be attempted when possible.

Differential Diagnosis

PCNSL, by definition, only includes processes that are limited to the confines of the CNS, so its diagnosis rests on clinical information that is not always available to the pathologist. To avoid confusion in cases where a peripheral lymphoma has extended into the CNS, the diagnostic line of the surgical pathology report should avoid the term "primary CNS lymphoma," in favor of the specific lymphoma subtype, for instance DLBCL or marginal zone lymphoma.

Most cases of PCNSL conform to the classical pattern of high-grade B-cell lymphoma with a striking perivascular distribution, but occasionally other CNS malignancies can mimic this appearance. Glioblastomas and oligodendrogliomas can show striking angiocentricity although lack the vascular destruction of lymphoma. The infiltrative frontiers of lymphomas starkly contrast to those of most metastatic lesions, but small cell neuroendocrine carcinomas can both track down perivascular spaces and invade modestly as single cells, rarely creating a superficial resemblance to lymphoma. Medulloblastoma also may extend down perivascular spaces and appear similar to lymphoma.

Following corticosteroid treatment, PCNSL lesions involute and the tumor cells become scarce, or even undetectable on tissue sections, although the collateral nonneoplastic lymphocytes and macrophages often persist and create a picture of a reactive process, such as a demyelinating lesion. Apoptotic debris from recently departed lymphoma cells may pepper the tissue.

Some of the less common lymphomas present a more significant challenge because they either lack the obvious cytologic malignancy of usual PCNSL or are obscured by an entourage of nonneoplastic inflammatory cells. T-cell lymphomas are the most prone to attracting diverse mixtures of inflammatory cells, closely simulating a reactive infiltrate such as what one might see in a vasculitis or encephalitis. Some such lymphomas are extremely difficult to diagnose with certainty, even with molecular genetic tools. Rare T-cell/histiocyte-rich large B-cell lymphomas will display the same phenomenon but have at least scattered large malignant cells as clues.

Mature T-cell lymphomas can also be diffusely infiltrative and less cellular, giving the impression of an infiltrating glioma, although subtle angiocentricity can betray the lymphoid nature of such lesions. A clinical history of marked response to steroids is a helpful clue that any lesion is not a diffuse glioma.

AMYLOIDOMA

The brains of middle-aged and elderly adults will rarely shelter a mass of aggregated immunoglobulin lambda-light chain comprising crystallized beta-pleated sheets, or amyloidoma. These lesions present with nonspecific mass lesion symptoms and afflict men and women at similar rates (26–28). Neuroimaging shows an enhancing mass in the cerebral white matter that is often ring-shaped or multifocal (28). Extra-axial examples favor the trigeminal nerve ganglion (29). Systemic amyloidoses are not associated with cerebral amyloidomas, and although the lesions contain monoclonal cells, the process is focal and indolent.

The microscopic appearance is that of amorphous, amphophilic protein in large parenchymal or perivascular fragments, around which scant lymphoplasmacytic infiltrates occur (Figure 16-7). Congo red stains the amyloid a cheerful rose color and produces the famous apple-green

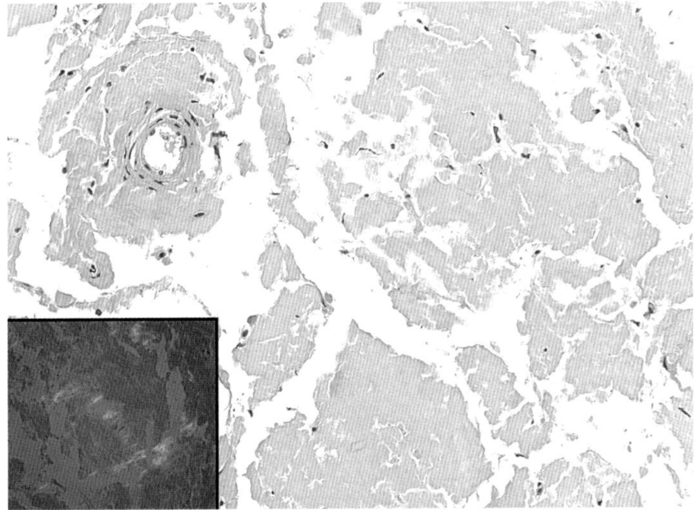

FIGURE 16-7 Amyloidomas are paucicellular and composed of masses and fragments of glassy hyaline material with apple-green birefringence after Congo red staining (inset), deposited by a scant clonal B-cell population.

birefringence in polarized light. The lambda-light chains that form the bulk of the amyloid originate from mature monoclonal B-cells that show monoclonal immunoglobulin heavy chain rearrangement, suggesting these lesions may be fundamentally neoplastic (27).

INTRAVASCULAR LYMPHOMA (ANGIOTROPIC LARGE CELL LYMPHOMA)

Clinical Context

Intravascular large B-cell lymphoma is a rare systemic hematolymphoid malignancy that most commonly affects the skin and brain in the elderly people (30). Although disease may only be symptomatic in the brain and not be radiologically detectable elsewhere, the process is thought to be widespread and systemic, hence not a PCNSL (32). Patients with CNS involvement generally present with recent onset of rapidly progressive cognitive decline or multifocal motor and/or sensory symptoms. Skin involvement manifests as an indurated red rash. Imaging shows multiple small cortical areas of T2/FLAIR hyperintensity that suggest areas of infarction without any identifiable mass lesions (31).

Intravascular lymphomas are highly aggressive, especially when involving the CNS. Not including cases diagnosed at autopsy, one series showed overall survival of 32% at 3 years, although not all of those patients had CNS involvement (30). Methotrexate has been used with some success (32).

Histopathology and Immunohistochemistry

The intravascular lymphoma is, except in extraordinary cases, a large B-cell malignancy, but it is distributed primarily within the lumens of cerebral blood vessels and occasionally percolates into the perivascular spaces. The plainly malignant tumor cells are large with open chromatin and prominent nucleoli, frequently obliterating the affected channel (Figure 16-8) and causing infarct of nearby tissue. Although blood flow is disrupted, the vessels remain intact, with little destruction of the vessel wall. The microscopic foci of intravascular lymphoma can be scattered and missed by small biopsies, or present as only a few cells in a single microscopic vessel profile. In one series, premortem tissue diagnosis could only be made in three of seven patients with intravascular lymphoma, the remainder being discovered at autopsy (32).

LANGERHANS CELL HISTIOCYTOSIS (EOSINOPHILIC GRANULOMA)

This tumor type was formerly considered a nonneoplastic, reactive process but has been shown more recently to be clonal and neoplastic, around half of cases having the *BRAF* V600E point mutation (33,34). It occurs most

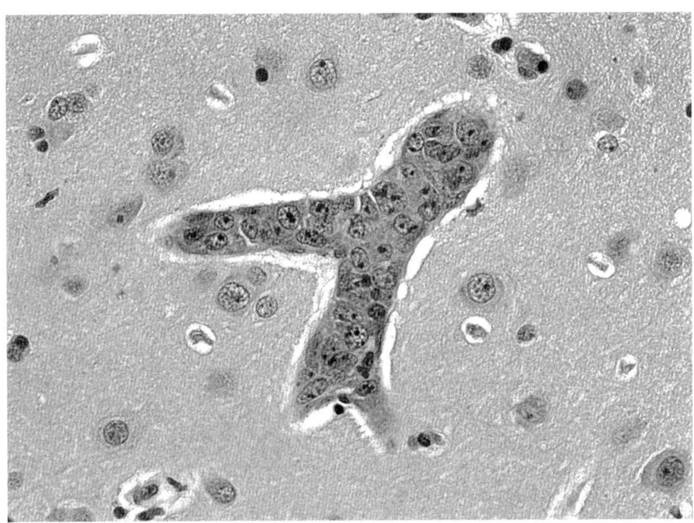

FIGURE 16-8 Intravascular lymphomas occlude small vessels with large malignant cells.

often in children younger than 15 years, only occasionally affecting adults, and ranges in extent from a single lesion to widespread systemic involvement, generally increasing in severity with decreasing patient age. The skull is one of the most common sites of disease, and the CNS is usually affected by lesions that intrude from the skull base and disrupt functions of the hypothalamic-pituitary axis, often leading to diabetes insipidus or anterior pituitary hormone deficiency (35). Other CNS lesions of Langerhans cell histiocytosis (LCH) include intracranial extra-axial mass lesions either of the dura or the circumventricular organs, and symmetrical degenerative lesions of the cerebellum and brainstem (35). Rare examples have been reported arising within the brain parenchyma (36,37). White matter changes are present in many cases of LCH that represent neurodegenerative changes (see below), although the mechanism by which these changes occur is unknown at this time.

Focal disease can be excised and treated with local radiotherapy with an excellent prognosis. More extensive disease is treated with chemotherapeutics and corticosteroids, which are variably effective (38). One series of 314 patients showed a 10-year survival rate of more than 90% (39). Because many cases have *BRAF* V600E mutations, the additional option of the small molecule inhibitor, vemurafenib, is available for refractory cases or even as first-line therapy (40).

Histopathology and Immunohistochemistry

The microscopic appearance of mass lesions in CNS LCH mirrors that of lesions in other systems. The core neoplastic element in this lesion comprises Langerhans cells, which are tissue histiocytes that are oval, intermediate in size, and monotonous. The moderately abundant cytoplasm is

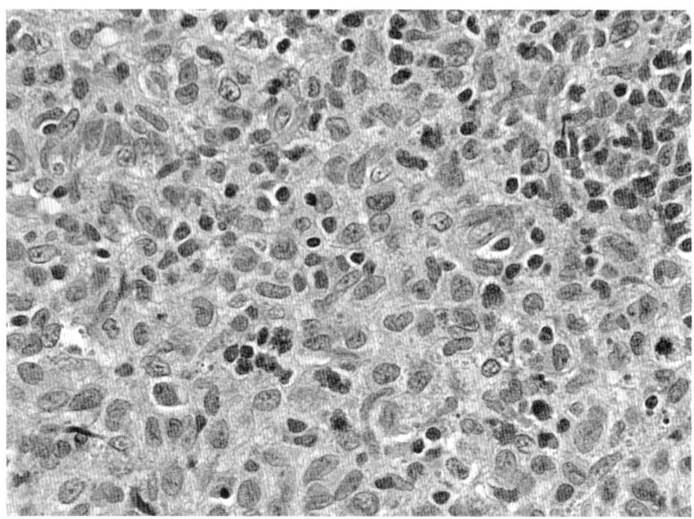

FIGURE 16-9 Langerhans cell histiocytosis is characterized by monotonous cells with irregular folded nuclei and scattered eosinophils.

slightly eosinophilic, containing irregularly shaped nuclei characterized by folds, indentations, and grooves that inspire comparisons with kidneys, horseshoes, and coffee beans (Figure 16-9). Fine chromatin surrounds apparent, but not prominent, nucleoli. Mitotic figures may be seen but should not be atypical. Among the tumor cells are a mixed population of several other inflammatory cells lineages, including eosinophils, neutrophils, lymphocytes, and other histiocytes, which can form multinucleate giant cells. Eosinophils are a consistent feature, reflected in the obsolete term for these tumors, *eosinophilic granuloma*. Plasma cells are usually a minor component. Necrosis is present sometimes and not indicative of increased aggressiveness.

The Langerhans cells are immunoreactive for generic histiocytic antigens such as CD68 and HAM56 and uniquely coexpress S100 protein and CD1a, a profile specific for Langerhans cells. Immunostaining for the cell specific protein langerin (CD207) is highly sensitive and specific for LCH (41). MIB1 nuclear staining is typically present in scattered cells, with rates occasionally exceeding 50% (42). BRAF V600E immunostaining (VE1) generally shows high levels of expression in LCH cases harboring the mutation.

Although rarely sampled *intra vitam*, neurodegenerative lesions in some cases of LCH may potentially arrive in biopsy form. Microscopically, they are devoid of Langerhans cells, instead containing cytotoxic CD8+ T-cells in perivascular cuffs and permeating the tissue. Occasional B-cells loiter in the perivascular space, and other reactive cells are present in variable numbers, including microglia and reactive astrocytes. Granulomas are not seen. In white matter, demyelination and loss of axons are present, with concomitant loss of neurons and atrophy in associated areas of cortex (43).

The differential diagnosis of LCH includes other hematopoietic lesions that typically contain eosinophils. The most common of these is probably extramedullary myeloid tumor, which can be distinguished immunohistochemically by the absence of CD1a and S100 protein reactive histiocytes and histologically by its various immature myeloid precursor cells. T-cell lymphomas and Hodgkin lymphoma also frequently contain eosinophils but are negative for S100 and CD1a.

ERDHEIM–CHESTER DISEASE

Conceptually similar to LCH, Erdheim–Chester disease (ECD) is a histiocytic neoplasm that may occur in any location and involve multiple organs. In contrast to LCH, most ECD cases are diagnosed in adulthood, from the third to seventh decades, where they present with a wide array of possible symptoms and signs, depending on the areas involved. Both LCH and ECD may occasionally be present in the same patient (44).

Virtually all patients have sclerotic lesions in the appendicular skeleton, and a few may have axial lesions. The vast majority of patients will also have neurologic effects, typically cognitive impairment, brainstem symptoms, cerebellar ataxia, and/or peripheral neuropathy. Almost half of patients have pituitary involvement that leads to diabetes insipidus and/or other endocrine defects. Cardiovascular and renal effects are common (44,45). Treatment for ECD usually includes an immune modifier like interferon or anakinra, or conventional chemotherapy like methotrexate or cladribine. Cases with *BRAF* V600E mutations may be treated with vemurafenib.

Histologically, most cases of ECD consist of foamy histiocytes, fibrosis, and Touton giant cells with a sprinkling of other inflammatory components (Figure 16-10). The histiocytes are immunoreactive for CD68, CD163, and factor XVIIIa, and negative for S100, CD1a, and CD207 (langerin) (44). Around half of ECD examples have a *BRAF* V600E mutation (46).

JUVENILE XANTHOGRANULOMA

Intracranial incursion of juvenile xanthogranuloma (JXG) is rare and essentially limited to the first few years of life. CNS JXG lesions are usually part of a multifocal process with lesions in the skin and at other peripheral sites. Surgical resection is curative in most cases, although systemic disease may be treated with chemotherapy (47). *BRAF* V600E mutations are present in a subset of JXG, providing an opportunity for targeted therapy (48).

Histologically, JXG is a cellular mixture spindled and epithelioid cells with multinucleate giant cells of the Touton or foreign body type. This mixture can give the mistaken impression of anaplasia. Immunostaining reveals expression of CD68 and factor XIIIa, but not CD1a or S100.

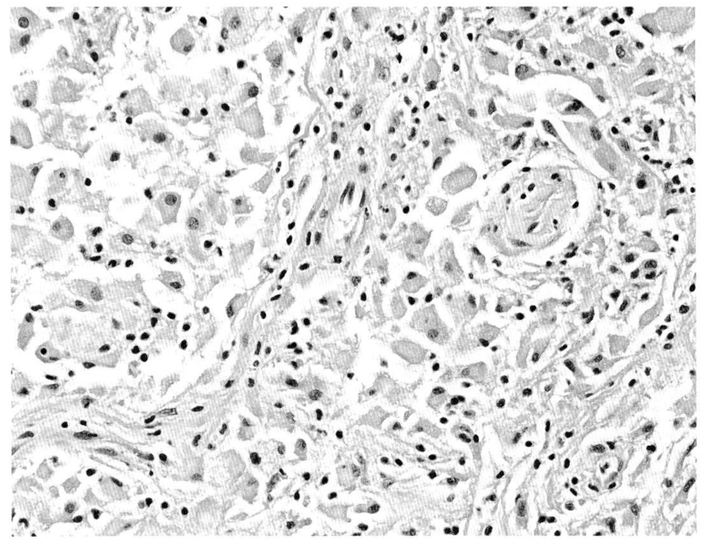

FIGURE 16-10 Erdheim–Chester disease with foamy histiocytes and fibrosis. Touton giant cells (not shown) are also typically present (image courtesy of Jose Velazquez-Vega, MD).

HISTIOCYTIC SARCOMA

Histiocytic sarcoma is a rare, malignant, hematolymphoid tumor that can arise anywhere and rarely involves the CNS. Histologically, they consist of sheets of polygonal to spindled cells with moderate to ample eosinophilic cytoplasm and pale, irregular nuclei with coarsely clumped chromatin and visible nucleoli. By immunohistochemistry, they express CD45, CD68, CD163, and lysozyme (49).

LEUKEMIAS

Any of the major categories of acute and chronic leukemia can involve the CNS, with acute lymphoblastic leukemia being the most common. Acute myeloid and chronic lymphocytic leukemias affect the CNS less often and chronic myelogenous leukemia does only rarely (50). The tumors usually form meningeal infiltrates or solid tumor masses but can also cause intraparenchymal lesions where leukemia cells infarct tissue by "sludging" or leukostasis, causing hemorrhages and even expanding to solid tumor foci. Acute myeloid leukemia can produce solid extramedullary myeloid tumors, which were formerly known as *chloromas* and *granulocytic sarcomas*.

HODGKIN LYMPHOMA

CNS involvement is very rare in Hodgkin lymphoma, much less than 1% of Hodgkin patients. About half of CNS cases have involvement at presentation, and the other half develop it during disease relapse. The majority of cases will involve the brain parenchyma, with a large minority affecting the dura. The histologic picture of CNS Hodgkin lymphoma reflects that of peripheral disease, most commonly being of the classic nodular sclerosis type. A few cases have shown CNS-restricted disease (51–53).

REFERENCES

1. Jahnke K, Thiel E, Schilling A, et al. Low-grade primary central nervous system lymphoma in immunocompetent patients. *Br J Haematol.* 2005;128(5):616–624.
2. Choi JS, Nam DH, Ko YH, et al. Primary central nervous system lymphoma in Korea: comparison of B- and T-cell lymphomas. *Am J Surg Pathol.* 2003;27(7):919–928.
3. Ostrom QT, Gittleman H, Xu J, et al. CBTRUS statistical report: primary brain and other central nervous system tumors diagnosed in the United States in 2009–2013. *Neuro Oncol.* 2016;18(suppl 5):v1–v75.
4. Olson JE, Janney CA, Rao RD, et al. The continuing increase in the incidence of primary central nervous system non-Hodgkin lymphoma: a surveillance, epidemiology, and end results analysis. *Cancer.* 2002;95(7):1504–1510.
5. Shiels MS, Pfeiffer RM, Besson C, et al. Trends in primary central nervous system lymphoma incidence and survival in the U.S. *Br J Haematol.* 2016;174(3):417–424.
6. Villano JL, Koshy M, Shaikh H, et al. Age, gender, and racial differences in incidence and survival in primary CNS lymphoma. *Br J Cancer.* 2011;105(9):1414–1418.
7. Fine HA, Mayer RJ. Primary central nervous system lymphoma. *Ann Intern Med.* 1993; 119(11):1093–1104.
8. Penn I, Porat G. Central nervous system lymphomas in organ allograft recipients. *Transplantation.*1995;59(2):240–244.
9. Phan TG, O'Neill BP, Kurtin PJ. Posttransplant primary CNS lymphoma. *Neuro Oncol.* 2000;2(4):229–238.
10. Tsang HH, Trendell-Smith NJ, Wu AK, et al. Diffuse large B-cell lymphoma of the central nervous system in mycophenolatemofetil-treated patients with systemic lupus erythematosus. *Lupus.* 2010;19(3):330–333.
11. Cote TR, Manns A, Hardy CR, et al. Epidemiology of brain lymphoma among people with or without acquired immunodeficiency syndrome. AIDS/Cancer Study Group. *J Natl Cancer Inst.* 1996;88(10):675–679.
12. Bataille B, Delwail V, Menet E, et al. Primary intracerebral malignant lymphoma: report of 248 cases. *J Neurosurg.* 2000;92(2):261–266.
13. Abla O, Sandlund JT, Sung L, et al. A case series of pediatric primary central nervous system lymphoma: favorable outcome without cranial irradiation. *Pediatr Blood Cancer.* 2006;47(7):880–885.
14. Nakhleh RE, Manivel JC, Copenhaver CM, et al. In situ hybridization for the detection of Epstein-Barr virus in central nervous system lymphomas. *Cancer.*1991;67(2):444–448.
15. Kuker W, Nagele T, Korfel A, et al. Primary central nervous system lymphomas (PCNSL): MRI features at presentation in 100 patients. *J Neurooncol.* 2005;72(2):169-177.
16. Lanfermann H, Heindel W, Schaper J, et al. CT and MR imaging in primary cerebral non-Hodgkin's lymphoma. *Acta Radiol.* 1997;38(2):259–267.
17. Kim EY, Kim SS. Magnetic resonance findings of primary central nervous system T-cell lymphoma in immunocompetent patients. *Acta Radiol.* 2005;46(2):187–192.
18. Shibamoto Y, Ogino H, Hasegawa M, et al. Results of radiation monotherapy for primary central nervous system lymphoma in the 1990s. *Int J Radiat Oncol Biol Phys.* 2005; 62(3):809–813.

19. Diamond C, Taylor TH, Im T, et al. Highly active antiretroviral therapy is associated with improved survival among patients with AIDS-related primary central nervous system non-Hodgkin's lymphoma. *Curr HIV Res.* 2006;4(3):375–378.
20. Kinoshita M, Hashimoto N, Izumoto S, et al. Immunohistological profiling by B-cell differentiation status of primary central nervous system lymphoma treated by high-dose methotrexate chemotherapy. *J Neurooncol.* 2010;99(1):95–101.
21. Larocca LM, Capello D, Rinelli A, et al. The molecular and phenotypic profile of primary central nervous system lymphoma identifies distinct categories of the disease and is consistent with histogenetic derivation from germinal center-related B cells. *Blood.* 1998; 92(3):1011–1019.
22. Momota H, Narita Y, Maeshima AM, et al. Prognostic value of immunohistochemical profile and response to high-dose methotrexate therapy in primary CNS lymphoma. *J Neurooncol.* 2010;98(3):341–348.
23. Shenkier TN, Blay JY, O'Neill BP, et al. Primary CNS lymphoma of T-cell origin: a descriptive analysis from the international primary CNS lymphoma collaborative group. *J Clin Oncol.* 2005;23(10):2233–2239.
24. Krumholz A, Weiss HD, Jiji VH, et al. Solitary intracranial plasmacytoma: two patients with extended follow-up. *Ann Neurol.* 1982;11(5):529–532.
25. Liebross RH, Ha CS, Cox JD, et al. Clinical course of solitary extramedullaryplasmacytoma. *Radiother Oncol.* 1999;52(3):245–249.
26. Gallucci M, Caulo M, Splendiani A, et al. Neuroradiological findings in two cases of isolated amyloidoma of the central nervous system. *Neuroradiology.* 2002;44(4):333–337.
27. Laeng RH, Altermatt HJ, Scheithauer BW, et al. Amyloidomas of the nervous system: a monoclonal B-cell disorder with monotypic amyloid light chain lambda amyloid production. *Cancer.* 1998;82(2):362–374.
28. Rodriguez FJ, Gamez JD, Vrana JA, et al. Immunoglobulin derived depositions in the nervous system: novel mass spectrometry application for protein characterization in formalin-fixed tissues. *Lab Invest.* 2008;88(10):1024–1037.
29. Gottfried ON, Chin S, Davidson HC, et al. Trigeminal amyloidoma: case report and review of the literature. *Skull Base.* 2007;17(5):317–324.
30. Ferreri AJ, Campo E, Seymour JF, et al. Intravascular lymphoma: clinical presentation, natural history, management and prognostic factors in a series of 38 cases, with special emphasis on the 'cutaneous variant'. *Br J Haematol.* 2004;127(2):173–183.
31. Baehring JM, Henchcliffe C, Ledezma CJ, et al. Intravascular lymphoma: magnetic resonance imaging correlates of disease dynamics within the central nervous system. *J Neurology Neurosurg Psychiatry.* 2005;76(4):540–544.
32. Baehring JM, Longtine J, Hochberg FH. A new approach to the diagnosis and treatment of intravascular lymphoma.*J Neurooncol.* 2003;61(3):237–248.
33. Willman CL, Busque L, Griffith BB, et al. Langerhans'-cell histiocytosis (histiocytosis X)—a clonal proliferative disease. *N Engl J Med.* 1994;331(3):154–160.
34. Badalian-Very G, Vergilio JA, Degar BA, et al. Recurrent BRAF mutations in Langerhans cell histiocytosis. *Blood.* 2010;116(11):1919–1923.
35. D'Ambrosio N, Soohoo S, Warshall C, et al. Craniofacial and intracranial manifestations of langerhans cell histiocytosis: report of findings in 100 patients. *AJR Am J Roentgenol.* 2008;191(2):589–597.
36. Bergmann M, Yuan Y, Bruck W, et al. Solitary langerhans cell histiocytosis lesion of the parieto-occipital lobe: a case report and review of the literature. *Clin Neurol Neurosurg.* 1997;99(1):50–55.
37. Montine TJ, Hollensead SC, Ellis WG, et al. Solitary eosinophilic granuloma of the temporal lobe: a case report and long-term follow-up of previously reported cases. *Clin Neuropathol.* 1994;13(4):225–228.

38. Weitzman S, Braier J, Donadieu J, et al. 2'-Chlorodeoxyadenosine (2-CdA) as salvage therapy for Langerhans cell histiocytosis (LCH). Results of the LCH-S-98 protocol of the Histiocyte Society. *Pediatr Blood Cancer*. 2009;53(7):1271–1276.
39. Howarth DM, Gilchrist GS, Mullan BP, et al. Langerhans cell histiocytosis: diagnosis, natural history, management, and outcome. *Cancer*. 1999;85(10):2278–2290.
40. Haroche J, Cohen-Aubart F, Emile JF, et al. Vemurafenib as first line therapy in BRAF-mutated Langerhans cell histiocytosis. *J Am Acad Dermatol*. 2015;73(1):e29–e30.
41. Lau SK, Chu PG, Weiss LM. Immunohistochemical expression of Langerin in Langerhans cell histiocytosis and non-Langerhans cell histiocytic disorders.*Am J Surg Pathol*. 2008;32(4):615–619.
42. Schouten B, Egeler RM, Leenen PJ, et al. Expression of cell cycle-related gene products in Langerhans cell histiocytosis. *J Pediatr Hematol Oncol*. 2002;24(9):727–732.
43. Grois N, Prayer D, Prosch H, et al. Group CLC-o. Neuropathology of CNS disease in Langerhans cell histiocytosis. *Brain*. 2005;128(Pt 4):829–838.
44. Estrada-Veras JI, O'Brien KJ, Boyd LC, et al. The clinical spectrum of Erdheim-Chester disease: an observational cohort study. *Blood Adv*. 2017;1(6):357–366.
45. Lachenal F, Cotton F, Desmurs-Clavel H, et al. Neurological manifestations and neuroradiological presentation of Erdheim-Chester disease: report of 6 cases and systematic review of the literature.*J Neurol*. 2006;253(10):1267–1277.
46. Haroche J, Charlotte F, Arnaud L, et al. High prevalence of BRAF V600E mutations in Erdheim-Chester disease but not in other non-Langerhans cell histiocytoses. *Blood*. 2012;120(13):2700–2703.
47. Deisch JK, Patel R, Koral K, et al. Juvenile xanthogranulomas of the nervous system: a report of two cases and review of the literature. *Neuropathology*. 2013;33(1):39–46.
48. Techavichit P, Sosothikul D, Chaichana T, et al. BRAF V600E mutation in pediatric intracranial and cranial juvenile Xanthogranuloma. *Hum Pathol*. 2017. pii: S0046-8177(17)30156-9. doi: 10.1016/j.humpath.2017.04.026.
49. Vos JA, Abbondanzo SL, Barekman CL, et al. Histiocytic sarcoma: a study of five cases including the histiocyte marker CD163. *Mod Pathol*. 2005;18(5):693–704.
50. Bojsen-Moller M, Nielsen JL. CNS involvement in leukaemia. An autopsy study of 100 consecutive patients. *Acta Pathol Microbiol Immunol Scand A*. 1983;91(4):209–216.
51. Cuttner J, Meyer R, Huang YP. Intracerebral involvement in Hodgkin's disease: a report of 6 cases and review of the literature. *Cancer*. 1979;43(4):1497–1506.
52. Gerstner ER, Abrey LE, Schiff D, et al. CNS Hodgkin lymphoma. *Blood*. 2008;112(5): 1658–1661.
53. Sapozink MD, Kaplan HS. Intracranial Hodgkin's disease. A report of 12 cases and review of the literature. *Cancer*. 1983;52(7):1301–1307.

17

SELECT TUMORS OF INDETERMINATE OR MESENCHYMAL DIFFERENTIATION

HEMANGIOBLASTOMA (WHO GRADE I)

Clinical Context

Hemangioblastomas are among the small group of central nervous system (CNS) tumors that often occur in the setting of an inherited tumor predisposition syndrome, with approximately 40% of patients expressing features of the von Hipple–Lindau syndrome (VHL; see below) (1,2). This tumor has a slight predilection for males and may present at any age, but most occur after the age of 21 years (1,3). Common presenting signs and symptoms include headache, nausea/vomiting, and ataxia. Only rare cases hemorrhage (4). The variable secretion of erythropoietin by hemangioblastomas induces an erythrocytosis in a subset of patients (5). Most hemangioblastomas (~90%) occur in the posterior fossa, but have been described in other sites throughout the CNS. Those in the spinal cord, the second most common site, are more common in patients with VHL and almost always (>95%) noted on the dorsal aspect (2,6). Retinal hemangioblastomas may be seen in VHL patients. Compared with sporadic cases, those in VHL present at a younger age, are more likely multifocal, and more likely to recur.

Neuroimaging reveals two major configurations of hemangioblastoma, "cyst with mural nodule" and solid, although a small number either lack an identifiable solid component or contain internal cystic spaces (7,8). Cystic lesions are more common and can develop over time from solid ones, eliciting symptoms through cyst expansion rather than tumor growth (6,9). Larger vascular channels in the solid portion appear as dark "flow voids" on magnetic resonance imaging (MRI), most notable on T2/FLAIR images against a backdrop of hyperintense tumor (7).

Hemangioblastomas are low-grade neoplasms that are curable by complete excision. The risk of recurrence increases with younger age, VHL diagnosis, and multicentric disease (10). For both recurrent and initial hemangioblastomas, stereotactic radiosurgery is effective at controlling most lesions (11).

Genetics

VHL syndrome is an autosomal dominant tumor predisposition that results from loss of function mutations in the gene *VHL*, encoded at locus 3p25. The normal gene product, the protein VHL, is a ubiquitin ligase involved in targeting hypoxia-inducible factor-1α (HIF) for destruction in the proteosome. Loss-of-function mutations in VHL cause a buildup of HIF within cells, triggering a cascade of signals that normally promote the cell's response to hypoxia, including the excess production of vascular endothelial growth factor (VEGF), accounting for the tumor's high vascularity and erythropoietin production. Syndromic patients have a heterozygous germline mutation in every cell and develop VHL-associated tumors where a second somatic mutation or deletion of *VHL* removes the remaining inhibition of HIF. Other tumors in VHL include renal clear cell carcinoma, pheochromocytoma, and papillary endolymphatic sac tumors. Because of its association with VHL, a diagnosis of hemangioblastoma should precipitate genetic testing because VHL patients require lifelong surveillance for malignancy.

Histopathology

Hemangioblastomas comprise two major cellular elements—endothelial cells that form the rich vasculature and stromal cells that occupy the intervascular areas. The endothelial cells are nonneoplastic and form a rich vasculature that grows at least partially in response to VEGF signals from the neoplastic stromal cells. The stromal cells are polygonal with small hyperchromatic nuclei and ample cytoplasm that varies from vacuolated with clear spherical lipid droplets (Figure 17-1) to faintly eosinophilic and

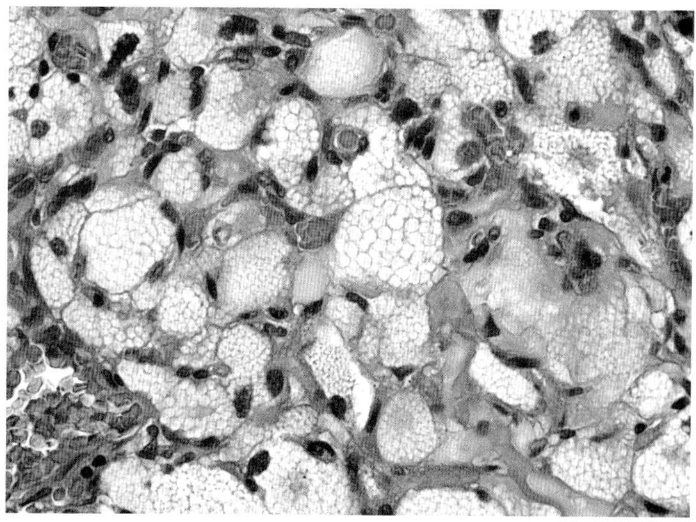

FIGURE 17-1 Hemangioblastoma stromal cells are frequently loaded with clear spherical cytoplasmic vacuoles that contain lipid material.

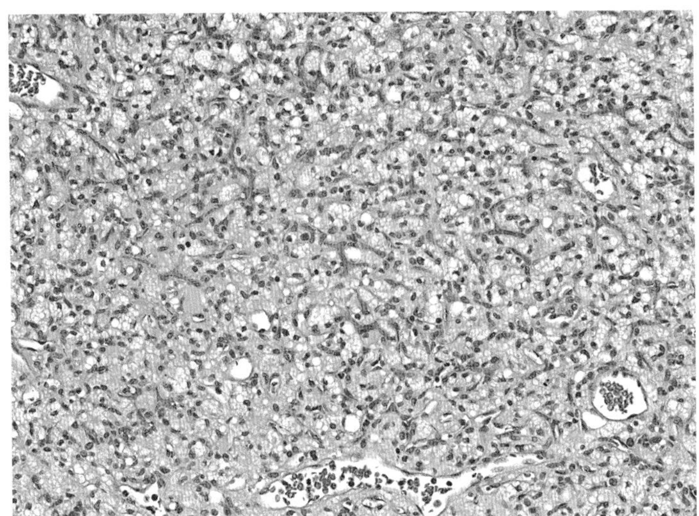

FIGURE 17-2 Reticular pattern of hemangioblastoma has a dense capillary meshwork and finely interspersed, vacuolated stromal cells.

finely granular. These components combine in two major architectural patterns—reticular and cellular. The more common reticular pattern is characterized by a dense network of capillaries with homogenously interspersed stromal cells that are more likely to be vacuolated and lipidized (Figure 17-2). In contrast, the cellular variant has large irregular vascular channels that encircle organoid nests of stromal cells that have a tendency toward smaller amounts of finely granular cytoplasm (Figure 17-3).

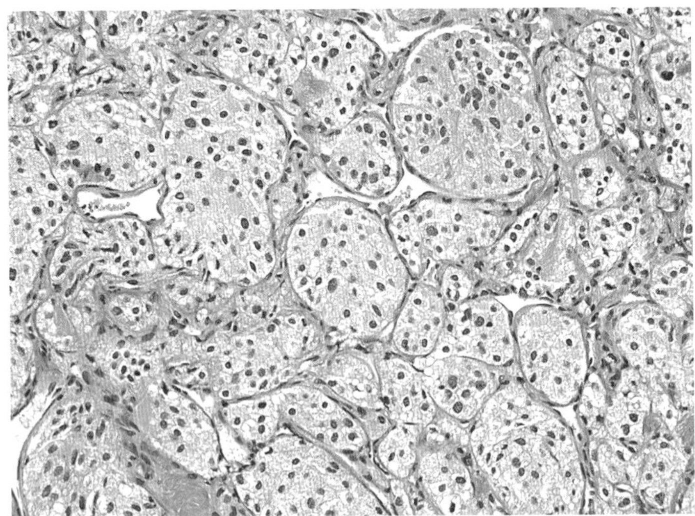

FIGURE 17-3 Cellular pattern of hemangioblastoma has nests of granular stromal cells between irregular vascular channels.

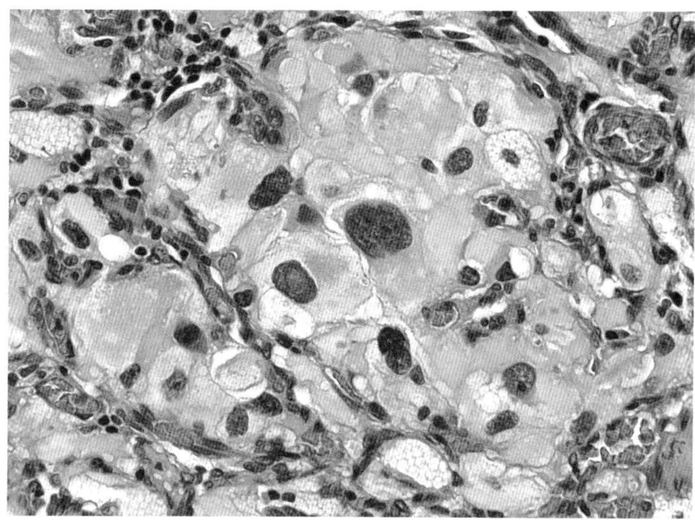

FIGURE 17-4 Nuclear atypia is normal in hemangioblastomas and reflects degenerative changes.

Although both are World Health Organization (WHO) grade I, the cellular pattern has features that overlap significantly with some metastatic carcinomas and is more likely to recur than the reticular pattern (10,12).

Mitosis and necrosis are rare in hemangioblastoma, but degenerative nuclear atypia is commonplace (Figure 17-4). Collagen occasionally deposits to form sclerotic tumors. A sparse infiltrate of mast cells is usually present.

Immunohistochemical stains for inhibin and neuron-specific enolase are usually positive, but few other markers react reliably. Glial fibrillary acidic protein (GFAP) is occasionally present within stromal cells and reactive immigrant astrocytes, both more often in the cellular pattern (12). Cytoplasmic staining for the notochordal marker brachyury has been described in hemangioblastoma and suggested as a specific marker (13). Brachyury immunostaining is typically observed in the nuclei of chordomas. Apparent ependymal differentiation has also been described (14,15).

Differential Diagnosis

Because of their histologic overlap and tendency to arise in VHL patients, renal clear cell carcinoma and hemangioblastoma are always considered together. At intraoperative consultation, distinguishing these can be very challenging and definitive diagnosis may necessarily await permanent sections and immunohistochemistry. Cytology, architecture, vascular pattern, and mast cell infiltrates are all comparable, but hemangioblastomas are inhibin immunoreactive and epithelial membrane antigen (EMA) negative, whereas renal cell carcinomas show the opposite pattern (16). Pax-8 and Pax-2 are transcription factors expressed in most renal clear cell carcinomas

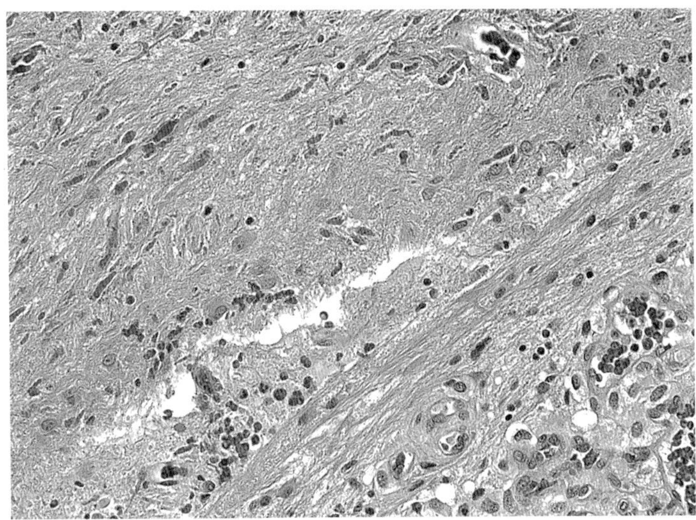

FIGURE 17-5 Rosenthal fibers are typical of the slowly compressed tissue surrounding hemangioblastomas, potentially mimicking pilocytic astrocytoma in small, nonrepresentative samples.

and not in hemangioblastomas (17,18). Rarely, renal cell carcinoma metastasizes to hemangioblastoma (19).

In young patients, a cerebellar cyst with mural nodule is most often a pilocytic astrocytoma; however, hemangioblastoma may present identically. Inclusion of perilesional tissue can yield piloid gliosis (Figure 17-5) with Rosenthal fibers that may provoke a mistaken intraoperative diagnosis of pilocytic astrocytoma. Simple awareness of this situation and recognition of the histology of hemangioblastoma should mitigate risk of this error.

The cellularity and pleomorphism of hemangioblastoma can cause concern for high-grade glioma intraoperatively, especially with noncystic cases outside of the cerebellum. Tight cohesion on smear preparation, paucity of fibrillar processes, and the presence of lipid droplets and mast cells all strongly favor hemangioblastoma in such a case. Retention of aqueous oil red-O and toluidine blue stains in the frozen section lab facilitates recognition of the latter two (Figure 17-6).

CHORDOMA

Clinical Context

Patients of all ages may present with a chordoma but most are in the third through fifth decades of life. The vast majority of cases occur in the sacrum, clivus, or cervical vertebrae (20), where notochordal cells are seeded during embryogenesis and presumably germinate into chordomas. Clival

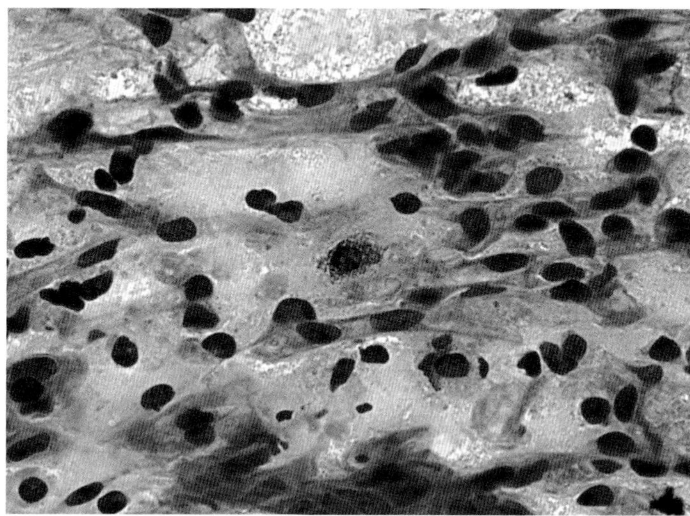

FIGURE 17-6 Aqueous toluidine blue offers a rapid intraoperative method for identifying scarlet metachromatic mast cells and lipid vacuoles (not pictured) simultaneously.

cases tend to present with cranial nerve palsies, especially of cranial nerve VI (21). In all locations, the tumor is midline, extradural, and involving bone; the pretest probability of a lesion being chordoma without the three features is low and other tumor types should be expected. Of course, rare chordomas violating these characteristics occur. The radiologic features of chordoma and chondrosarcoma, other than midline location favoring chordoma, are not helpful diagnostically (22).

Complete surgical resection is attempted in cervical and clival chordomas, although half of initial operations fall short of gross total resection (23). Proton- or photon-based radiation therapy has become standard of care following excision; however, it has not been prospectively demonstrated to significantly alter the course of disease. A recent comprehensive review of the literature concludes that age younger than 21 years and radiation therapy are clinical variables associated with lower rates of recurrence (24). One series shows a significantly higher rate of survival among patients younger than 40 years (25). Overall, survival for skull-base chordoma patients is between 40% and 60% at 5 years and 30% and 40% at 10 years (21,23,25,26).

Histopathology

Chordomas resemble notochordal tissue, with scattered clusters and cords of vacuolated cells in a basophilic chondromyxoid background. The cells have monotonous hyperchromatic nuclei and abundant cytoplasm that varies from smooth and pink (Figure 17-7) without vacuoles to completely vacuolated (Figure 17-8). Those with many vacuoles carry the descriptive label "physaliphorous," from the Greek roots for bubble and bearer. In

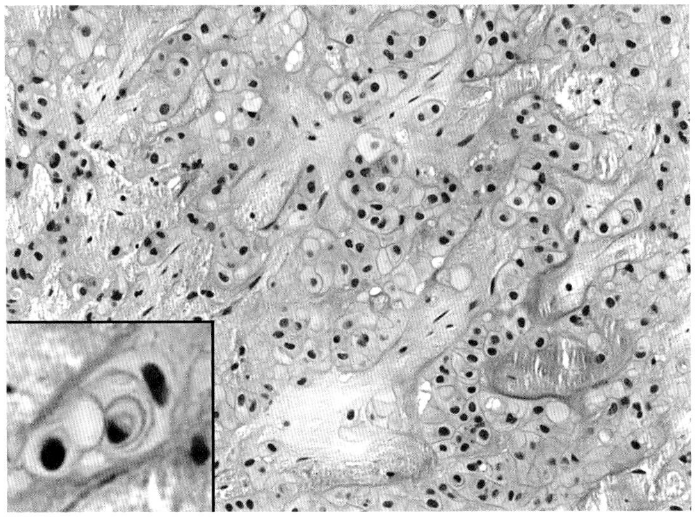

FIGURE 17-7 Chordomas may contain cords and nest of polygonal pink cells that show focal cell–cell wrapping (inset).

either case, the cells are mostly clustered and in close apposition to one another with easily apparent cell–cell borders. Cell–cell wrapping or "cannibalism" is seen frequently in chordomas and is another feature that distinguishes it from chondrosarcoma (Figure 17-7) (27). Necrosis (>10%) is the only histologic parameter associated with a significant decrease in survival, whereas nuclear pleomorphism, rare mitosis, vascular invasion, and nucleoli are not (28). Pediatric chordomas may be more cellular and less

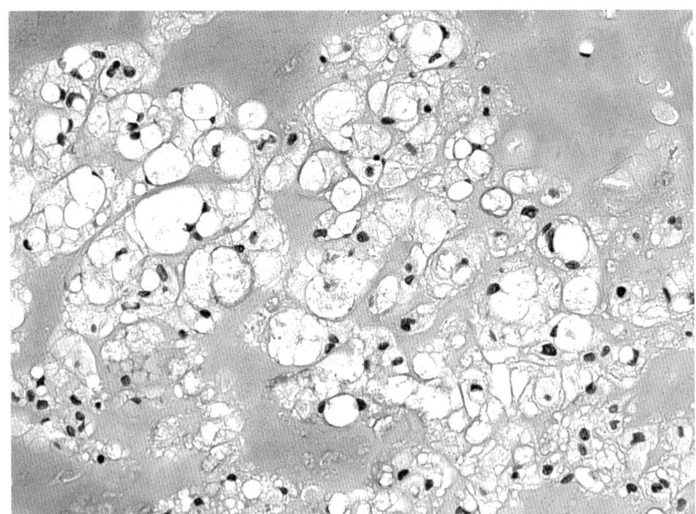

FIGURE 17-8 Chordomas also contain vacuolated "physaliphorous cells," also in cords and nests.

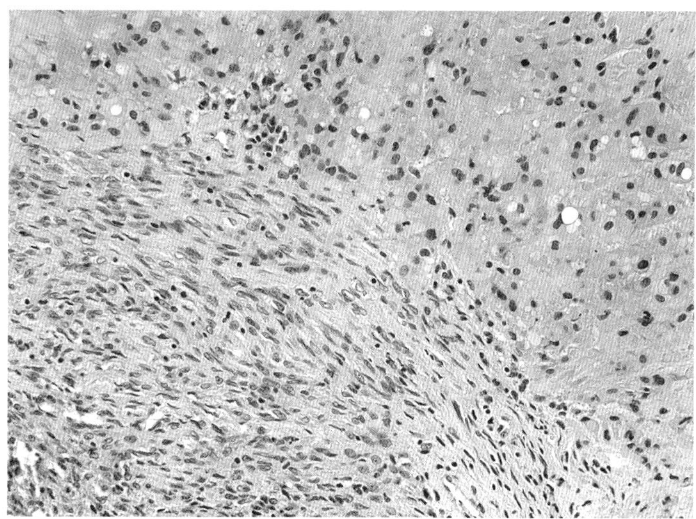

FIGURE 17-9 Chordomas rarely "dedifferentiate" into high-grade sarcomas.

overtly chordoid than adult cases. Such examples are called poorly differentiated chordoma and have a high rate of SMARCB1/INI1 loss by immunohistochemistry and aggressive clinical course (29). Poorly differentiated chordomas with SMARCB1 loss may be a novel tumor entity from either atypical teratoid/rhabdoid tumor or chordoma (30).

Rarely, chordomas develop overtly malignant sarcomatous elements (Figure 17-9) that drive the clinical course, which is typically short. The sarcomatous element varies; pleomorphic undifferentiated sarcoma, rhabdomyosarcoma, fibrosarcoma, and osteosarcoma have been described (31–34).

There may be areas within a chordoma that show chondroid differentiation, with individually dispersed cells in lacunae. In the context of foci of unequivocal chordoma, this finding is grounds for diagnosing *chondroidchordoma*, which has been associated in several series with improved survival over conventional chordoma, although this effect diminishes after sorting by patient age (25,26).

Chordomas show immunoreactivity for cytokeratins, EMA, and S100, with keratins being the most widely expressed (26). The transcription factor brachyury is expressed in fetal notochord cells and is a sensitive and specific immunohistochemical marker for chordoma (34,35). Nuclear reactivity is reliably present in chordomas and has not yet been described in other tumors in the differential diagnosis.

Differential Diagnosis

Ecchordosis physaliphora is the nonneoplastic, nonproliferative equivalent of chordoma, usually found intradurally as a small translucent nodule anterior to the brainstem. Distinction between ecchordosis and chordomas is discussed in Chapter 1 among developmental lesions and benign cysts.

Chordoid meningiomas are in the histologic differential diagnosis with chordoma, but are rarely confused clinically or radiologically since they are usually intradural, off the midline, and do not destroy adjacent bone. If a rare case were to fulfill these criteria, lack of cytokeratin and brachyury immunoreactivity and expression of somatostatin receptor 2A would distinguish it from chordoma.

Extraskeletal myxoid chondrosarcoma histologically consists of loose cords and strands of monomorphic cells and round pseudoacinar spaces in a myxoid background. Eosinophilic cytoplasm and occasional vacuolated cells are common. The cytoplasm is usually stretched into narrow strands between cells, giving a fibroblastic outline, but can be polygonal and epithelioid. In the former case, confusion with chordoma is unlikely, but epithelioid cases may appear more similar. Reactivity for brachyury and/or cytokeratin rules out extraskeletal myxoid chondrosarcoma in this instance.

CHONDROSARCOMA

Clinical Context

All primary intracranial sarcomas, only a small fraction of which are chondrosarcoma, collectively account for less than 1% of intracranial neoplasms. Of intracranial chondrosarcomas, the majority are conventional, and less than 15% of reported cases exhibit mesenchymal histology. Although rare, low-grade chondrosarcoma can appear similar to chordoma, a more common and much more aggressive neoplasm, necessitating their distinction. In the largest published series, the mean age of intracranial conventional chondrosarcoma patients was 39 years and ranged from 10 to 79 years (27). Most arise around the junctions of the occipital and temporal skull bones in the lateral base of the skull. Importantly, almost a third form in or around the clivus. Rare dural chondrosarcomas have been reported (36). Neuroimaging reveals a well-circumscribed lobulated mass that is T2-hyperintense and enhances after gadolinium contrast administration. Many cases contain calcifications on computed tomography (CT) imaging. Treatment is based on surgical resection followed by radiation therapy, achieving 99% 10-year disease-specific survival in a series of 200 patients with conventional chondrosarcoma(27). Mesenchymal chondrosarcomas are substantially more aggressive, showing 54% 5-year mortality in a large review (37).

Histopathology

Conventional chondrosarcoma has two major patterns—hyaline and myxoid. Hyaline cases resemble nonneoplastic cartilage, with glassy chondroidstroma

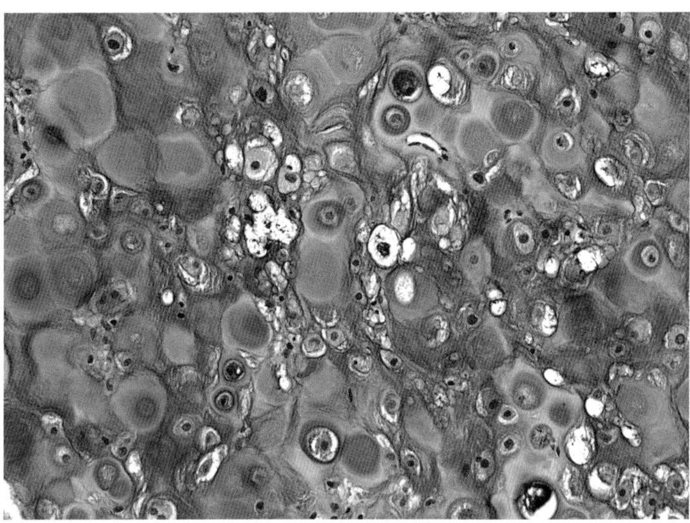

FIGURE 17-10 Chondrosarcomas maintain separation between tumor cells, even when clustered together.

dotted with individually dispersed chondrocytes within lacunae. Although the lacunae may contain two or three chondrocytes and loosely cluster in lobules, cells with cohesive borders in cords and nests are absent (Figure 17-10). This separation of cells is a key histologic feature distinguishing low-grade chondrosarcoma from chordoma. Some chondrosarcomas also contain vacuolated cells similar to physaliphorous cells in chordoma (Figure 17-11). Examination of conventional chondrosarcoma for chordoma elements is

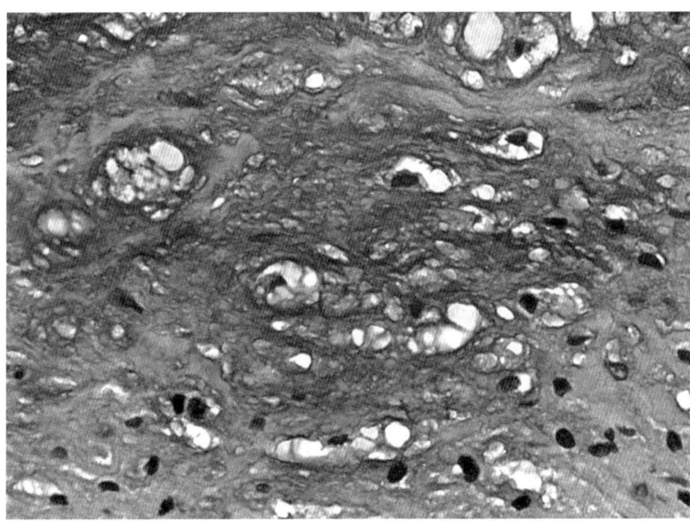

FIGURE 17-11 Chondrosarcomas may contain vacuolated cells that resemble those of chordoma.

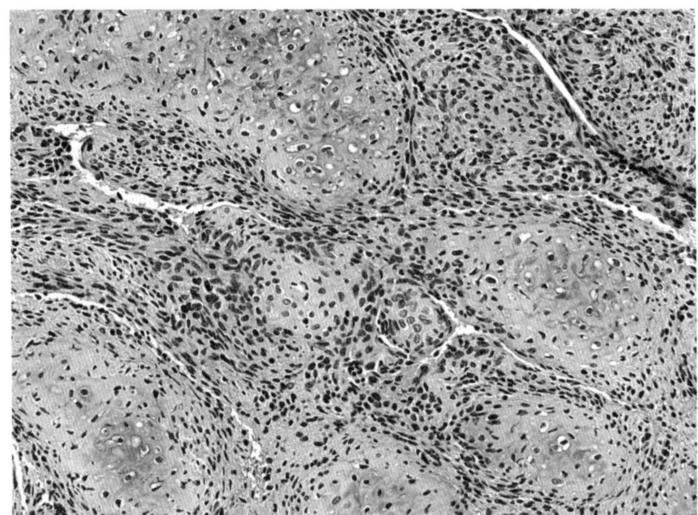

FIGURE 17-12 Mesenchymal chondrosarcomas are biphasic, with nodules of conventional chondrosarcoma in a background of embryonal mesenchyme.

imperative because areas of cartilaginous differentiation are seen in *chondroidchordomas*, which are more aggressive than chondrosarcoma (26,27). Chondrosarcomas express nuclear S100 and lack cytokeratin and brachyury expression.

Mesenchymal chondrosarcomas are biphasic tumors composed of poorly differentiated embryonal mesenchyme studded with islands of conventional chondrosarcoma (Figure 17-12). The mesenchymal component is fascicular and hypercellular, often with jagged hemangiopericytoma-like vascular channels. Immunohistochemistry for CD99 is positive (38).

CALCIFYING PSEUDONEOPLASM OF THE NEURAXIS (FIBRO-OSSEOUS LESION OF THE CNS)

Clinical Context

This curious entity was first described in 1978 and is still occasionally referred to as a fibro-osseous lesion (39). Calcifying pseudoneoplasms are uncommon, with only fewer than 50 cases reported in the literature (40). The range of patients' ages extends from 12 to 83 years with 2:1 ratio of males to females. A subset is found incidentally at autopsy, but the remainder present with a variety of signs and symptoms (40). The lesions are round, circumscribed, and usually measure 1 to 3 cm in diameter, although sizes up to 10 cm have been reported (41). Location is highly variable, ranging from extra-axial to intraventricular and from frontal lobe to lumbar spinal cord (40). CT shows prominent calcification, and MRI reveals a markedly hypointense mass on both T1- and T2-weighted sequences with internal linear and peripheral rim enhancement (40). These lesions are

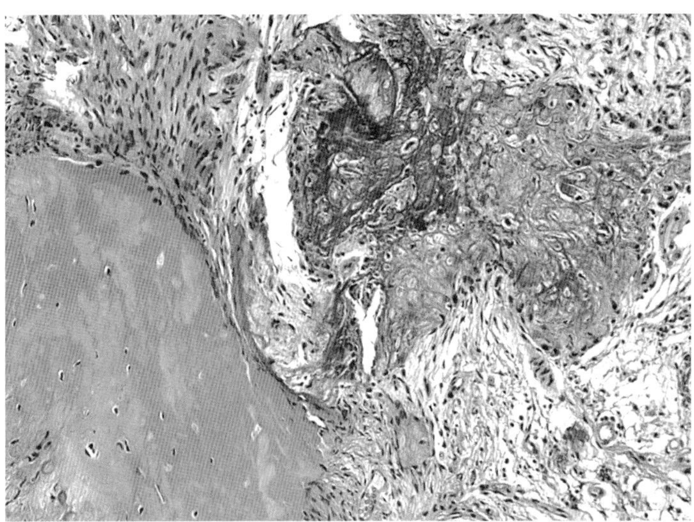

FIGURE 17-13 Calcifying pseudoneoplasm of the neuraxis with lobules and focal ossification.

benign and generally cured by complete resection without recurrence or further treatment.

Histopathology

There are several consistent microscopic features of calcifying pseudoneoplasm, including lobular organization, calcifying chondromyxoid material, and a thin rim of epithelioid and spindle cells around the lobules. Many cases also show at least focal ossification (Figure 17-13). The stromal

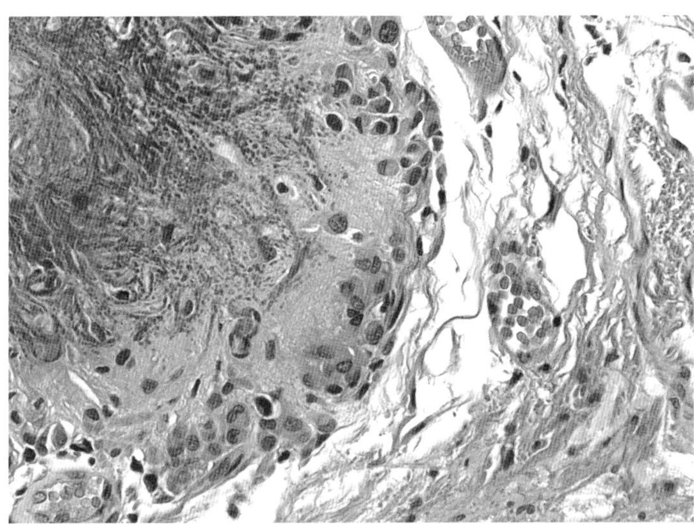

FIGURE 17-14 Strands and fragments of matrix trail behind the outwardly migrating epithelial and osteoblastoid cells, the rim calcifying pseudoneoplasm of the neuraxis.

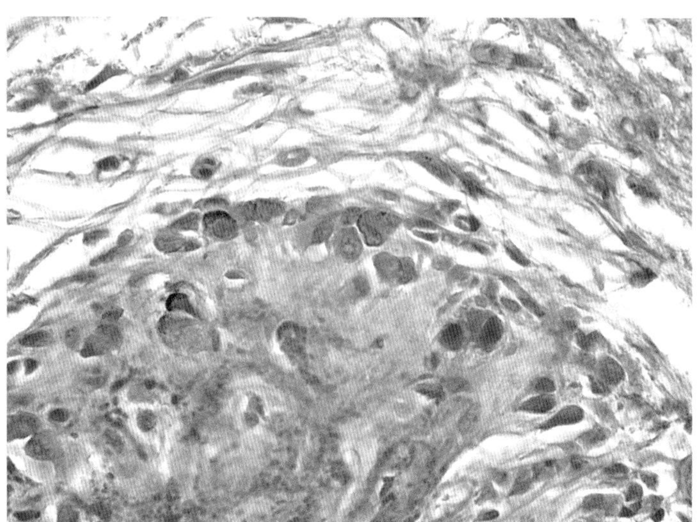

FIGURE 17-15 EMA immunostaining variably marks the peripheral cells in calcifying pseudoneoplasm of the neuraxis.

material is composed of granules and strands of basophilic and amphophilic calcified chondroid-like material that is vaguely radially oriented (Figure 17-14). A scalloped rim of epithelioid osteoblast-like cells rings the lobules, as if traveling outward on a slow wave of matrix deposition that enlarges the lesion. A thin concentric rim of spindle-shaped cells lies just beyond the lobule edges. The epithelioid cells often show focal EMA reactivity (Figure 17-15).

REFERENCES

1. Boughey AM, Fletcher NA, Harding AE. Central nervous system haemangioblastoma: a clinical and genetic study of 52 cases. *J Neurol Neurosurg Psychiatry*. 1990;53(8):644–648.
2. Conway JE, Chou D, Clatterbuck RE, et al. Hemangioblastomas of the central nervous system in von Hippel-Lindau syndrome and sporadic disease. *Neurosurgery*. 2001; 48(1):55–62; discussion 62–53.
3. Silver ML, Hennigar G. Cerebellar hemangioma (hemangioblastoma): a clinicopathological review of 40 cases. *J Neurosurg*. 1952;9(5):484–494.
4. Berlis A, Schumacher M, Spreer J, et al. Subarachnoid haemorrhage due to cervical spinal cord haemangioblastomas in a patient with von Hippel-Lindau disease. *Acta Neurochir*. 2003;145(11):1009–1013; discussion 1013.
5. So CC, Ho LC. Polycythemia secondary to cerebellar hemangioblastoma. *Am J Hematol*. 2002;71(4):346–347.
6. Wanebo JE, Lonser RR, Glenn GM, et al. The natural history of hemangioblastomas of the central nervous system in patients with von Hippel-Lindau disease. *J Neurosurg*. 2003;98(1):82–94.
7. Elster AD, Arthur DW. Intracranial hemangioblastomas: CT and MR findings. *J Comput Assist Tomogr*. 1988;12(5):736–739.

8. Lee SR, Sanches J, Mark AS, et al. Posterior fossa hemangioblastomas: MR imaging. *Radiology*. 1989;171(2):463–468.
9. Slater A, Moore NR, Huson SM. The natural history of cerebellar hemangioblastomas in von Hippel-Lindau disease. *AJNR Am J Neuroradiol*. 2003;24(8):1570–1574.
10. de la Monte SM, Horowitz SA. Hemangioblastomas: clinical and histopathological factors correlated with recurrence. *Neurosurgery*. 1989;25(5):695–698.
11. Patrice SJ, Sneed PK, Flickinger JC, et al. Radiosurgery for hemangioblastoma: results of a multiinstitutional experience. *Int J Radiat Oncol Biol Phys*. 1996;35(3):493–499.
12. Hasselblatt M, Jeibmann A, Gerss J, et al. Cellular and reticular variants of haemangioblastoma revisited: a clinicopathologic study of 88 cases. *Neuropathol Appl Neurobiol*. 2005;31(6):618–622.
13. Barresi V, Vitarelli E, Branca G, et al. Expression of brachyury in hemangioblastoma: potential use in differential diagnosis. *Am J Surg Pathol*. 2012;36(7):1052–1057.
14. Yang QX, Li Y, Tian XY, et al. Bilateral cerebellar epithelioid hemangioblastoma with possible ependymal differentiation in a patient with von Hippel-Lindau disease. *Neuropathology*. 2012;32(6):662–667.
15. Wang J, Lin XY, Qiu XS, et al. Cerebellar hemangioblastoma with perivascular pseudorosette formation and glial differentiation: a case report. *Neuropathology*. 2017;37(2):105–109.
16. Hoang MP, Amirkhan RH. Inhibin alpha distinguishes hemangioblastoma from clear cell renal cell carcinoma. *Am J Surg Pathol*. 2003;27(8):1152–1156.
17. Barr ML, Jilaveanu LB, Camp RL, et al. PAX-8 expression in renal tumours and distant sites: a useful marker of primary and metastatic renal cell carcinoma? *J Clin Pathol*. 2015;68(1):12–17.
18. Ozcan A, Zhai Q, Javed R, et al. PAX-2 is a helpful marker for diagnosing metastatic renal cell carcinoma: comparison with the renal cell carcinoma marker antigen and kidney-specific cadherin. *Arch Pathol Lab Med*. 2010;134(8):1121–1129.
19. Jarrell ST, Vortmeyer AO, Linehan WM, et al. Metastases to hemangioblastomas in von Hippel-Lindau disease. *J Neurosurg*. 2006;105(2):256–263.
20. Eriksson B, Gunterberg B, Kindblom LG. Chordoma. A clinicopathologic and prognostic study of a Swedish national series. *Acta Orthop Scand*. 1981;52(1):49–58.
21. Samii A, Gerganov VM, Herold C, et al. Chordomas of the skull base: surgical management and outcome. *J Neurosurg*. 2007;107(2):319–324.
22. Sze G, Uichanco LS, 3rd, Brant-Zawadzki MN, et al. Chordomas: MR imaging. *Radiology*. 1988;166(1 Pt 1):187–191.
23. Choi D, Melcher R, Harms J, et al. Outcome of 132 operations in 97 patients with chordomas of the craniocervical junction and upper cervical spine. *Neurosurgery*. 2010; 66(1):59–65; discussion 65.
24. Jian BJ, Bloch OG, Yang I, et al. Adjuvant radiation therapy and chondroidchordoma subtype are associated with a lower tumor recurrence rate of cranial chordoma. *J Neurooncol*. 2010;98(1):101–108.
25. Mitchell A, Scheithauer BW, Unni KK, et al. Chordoma and chondroid neoplasms of the spheno-occiput. An immunohistochemical study of 41 cases with prognostic and nosologic implications. *Cancer*. 1993;72(10):2943–2949.
26. Forsyth PA, Cascino TL, Shaw EG, et al. Intracranial chordomas: a clinicopathological and prognostic study of 51 cases. *J Neurosurg*. 1993;78(5):741–747.
27. Rosenberg AE, Nielsen GP, Keel SB, et al. Chondrosarcoma of the base of the skull: a clinicopathologic study of 200 cases with emphasis on its distinction from chordoma. *Am J Surg Pathol*. 1999;23(11):1370–1378.
28. O'Connell JX, Renard LG, Liebsch NJ, et al. Base of skull chordoma. A correlative study of histologic and clinical features of 62 cases. *Cancer*. 1994;74(8):2261–2267.

29. Mobley BC, McKenney JK, Bangs CD, et al. Loss of SMARCB1/INI1 expression in poorly differentiated chordomas. *Acta Neuropathol.* 2010;120(6):745–753.
30. Hasselblatt M, Thomas C, Hovestadt V, et al. Poorly differentiated chordoma with SMARCB1/INI1 loss: a distinct molecular entity with dismal prognosis. *Acta Neuropathol.* 2016;132(1):149–151.
31. Bisceglia M, D'Angelo VA, Guglielmi G, et al. Dedifferentiated chordoma of the thoracic spine with rhabdomyosarcomatous differentiation. Report of a case and review of the literature. *Ann Diagn Pathol.* 2007;11(4):262–273.
32. Hanna SA, Tirabosco R, Amin A, et al. Dedifferentiated chordoma: a report of four cases arising 'de novo'. *J Bone Joint Surg Br.* 2008;90(5):652–656.
33. Meis JM, Raymond AK, Evans HL, et al. "Dedifferentiated" chordoma. A clinicopathologic and immunohistochemical study of three cases. *Am J Surg Pathol.* 1987;11(7):516–525.
34. Sangoi AR, Dulai MS, Beck AH, et al. Distinguishing chordoidmeningiomas from their histologic mimics: an immunohistochemical evaluation. *Am J Surg Pathol.* 2009;33(5):669–681.
35. Vujovic S, Henderson S, Presneau N, et al. Brachyury, a crucial regulator of notochordal development, is a novel biomarker for chordomas. *J Pathol.* 2006;209(2):157–165.
36. Lee YY, Van Tassel P, Raymond AK. Intracranial duralchondrosarcoma. *AJNR Am J Neuroradiol.* 1988;9(6):1189–1193.
37. Bloch OG, Jian BJ, Yang I, et al. A systematic review of intracranial chondrosarcoma and survival. *J Clin Neurosci.* 2009;16(12):1547–1551.
38. Granter SR, Renshaw AA, Fletcher CD, et al. CD99 reactivity in mesenchymalchondrosarcoma. *Hum Pathol.* 1996;27(12):1273–1276.
39. Rhodes RH, Davis RL. An unusual fibro-osseous component in intracranial lesions. *Hum Pathol.* 1978;9(3):309–319.
40. Aiken AH, Akgun H, Tihan T, et al. Calcifying pseudoneoplasms of the neuraxis: CT, MR imaging, and histologic features. *AJNR Am J Neuroradiol.* 2009;30(6):1256–1260.
41. Bertoni F, Unni KK, Dahlin DC, et al. Calcifying pseudoneoplasms of the neural axis. *J Neurosurg.* 1990;72(1):42–48.

18

METASTASES

CLINICAL CONTEXT

Metastases are the most common tumors in the central nervous system (CNS), accounting for more lesions than all primary tumors combined (1), and affecting just over half of the total number of brain tumor patients. Even these estimates are most likely low due to ascertainment bias among the terminally ill patients with cancer (2). The age distribution of patients with CNS metastases parallels the primary incidence of the most common metastasizing malignancies, increasing throughout adulthood. Although the presentation of metastatic disease in the CNS varies greatly, most patients present with sudden onset of mental status changes or seizures. Whereas many cancers are detected clinically when they interfere with function of the respective primary organ, a significant number of brain metastases are discovered before a primary diagnosis, adding to the importance of accurately classifying them (3,4).

Essentially all metastases reach the CNS by hematogenous spread, usually first establishing tumor in the lungs where malignant cells likely gain access to the systemic arterial circulation (2). Most often, the metastatic cells then lodge within the capillaries at the gray-white matter junction of the cerebral cortex, although metastatic lesions have been documented in every location in the CNS. Radiologically, suspicion for metastasis rises when there are multiple lesions (especially at the gray-white junction) or when the patient has a history of prior malignancy. Most metastases are approximately spherical with well-circumscribed, pushing borders and prominent adjacent edema, which appears on magnetic resonance imaging as T2-signal hyperintensity. Areas of necrosis and hemorrhage are common. Because of the paramagnetic qualities of melanin, intrinsic, bright T1 signal is characteristic of pigmented metastatic melanomas.

Only a few histologic types of cancer account for >90% of CNS metastases observed in practice, the majority of which are carcinomas, with melanomas making up most of the remainder. Lymphomas are considered systemic diseases, therefore not metastatic when involving the brain. The frequencies of metastases from particular organs do not reflect the rates of primary lesions in those sites. Pulmonary and mammary carcinomas account for roughly 60% of all brain metastases (5,6) but only

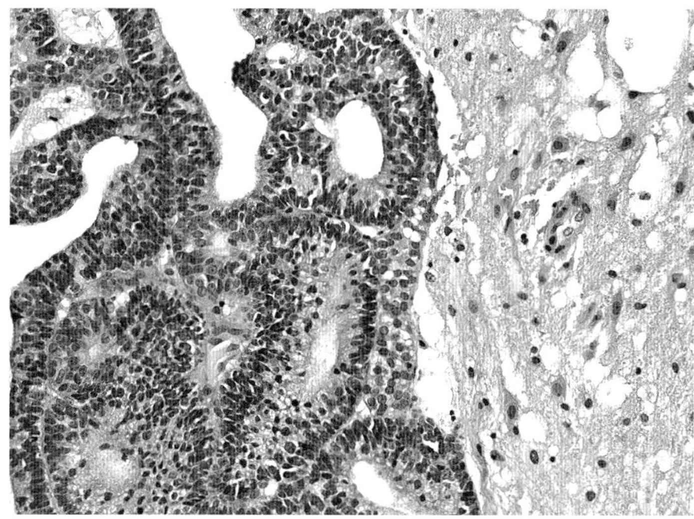

FIGURE 18-1 Pulmonary adenocarcinoma is the most common metastasis to the central nervous system, where it and other metastases form discreet sharply circumscribed lesions.

around 30% of all primary solid malignancies (6,7). In contrast, carcinomas of bladder, thyroid, and prostate are common as primaries but account for only a few percentage of all CNS metastases (2,5). Of bronchopulmonary carcinomas, adenocarcinoma is the most common (Figure 18-1), followed by neuroendocrine carcinoma, with only occasional metastases from squamous cell cancers. Renal cell and colorectal carcinomas also metastasize to the CNS but represent a small minority. Melanomas follow carcinomas in incidence among cerebral metastases, accounting for about 8% of all cases (5,8).

Only a few small series examine CNS metastases from sarcomas, emphasizing their relative rarity (9–12). Although still rare in pediatric populations, sarcomas account for a larger proportion of CNS metastases in those patients, from a third to half in two single-institution series (13,14). The most common histologic subtypes include osteosarcoma, pleomorphic undifferentiated sarcoma (malignant fibrous histiosarcoma), Ewing sarcoma, and leiomyosarcoma (9,11,12). Notable for its tendency to metastasize to the CNS is alveolar soft part sarcoma (Figure 18-2), which is represented among CNS-metastatic sarcomas far out of proportion to its primary incidence (9–12). It is rare for sarcomas to present with brain metastases, yet alveolar soft part sarcoma and synovial sarcoma have a greater propensity to do so.

Diffuse Leptomeningeal Metastasis (Meningeal Carcinomatosis, Carcinomatous Meningitis)

Some malignancies diffusely infiltrate the leptomeningeal space, spreading through the cerebrospinal fluid (CSF) and forming a sheet of malignant

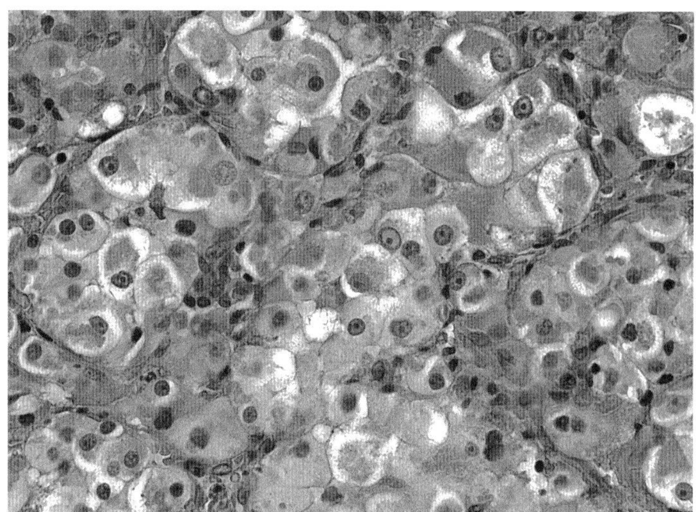

FIGURE 18-2 Alveolar soft part sarcoma, composed of large cells with abundant granular eosinophilic cytoplasm and prominent nucleoli arranged in nests, is uncommon but shows a high rate of cerebral metastasis.

cells over the pial surface. Although frequently referred to as "carcinomatous meningitis" because it usually originates from carcinoma and presents with symptoms similar to meningitis, melanomas and occasional sarcomas also diffusely involve the CSF space (15). Even with intrathecal chemotherapy and radiation treatment, the outlook for patients with diffuse leptomeningeal metastasis is grim, with a median survival of <6 months after diagnosis in one series (16). Malignant cells fill the subarachnoid space and often extend into the brain along the perivascular spaces (Figure 18-3).

CNS Metastases in Children

Metastases are distinctly uncommon in the pediatric population, representing only about 2% of all pediatric brain tumors (13,14,17). Overall survival in children with CNS metastases is poor, with median survivals around a year or less (13,14). Some metastases in children may mimic primary CNS malignancies, including neuroblastoma, blastema-predominant Wilms tumor, alveolar rhabdomyosarcoma, and undifferentiated midline carcinoma (NUT1-related carcinoma).

Sellar/Parasellar Metastases

Only a very small fraction of intracerebral metastases occur in the pituitary gland, and even fewer are symptomatic (18–20). The metastases mostly originate from primaries in the breast for women and lung for men. Unlike pituitary adenomas, which present with abnormalities in anterior lobe hormones, metastases often present with acute onset of diabetes insipidus because of their tendency to occur in the posterior lobe (20).

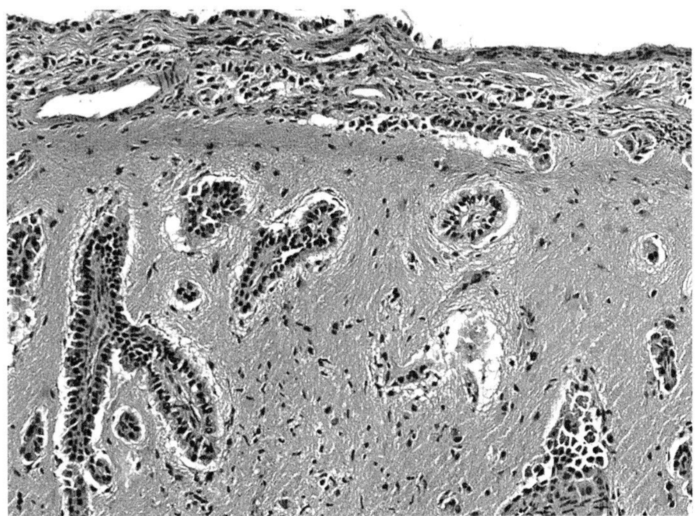

FIGURE 18-3 Diffuse leptomeningeal metastases fill the subarachnoid space and frequently invade along perivascular spaces.

Spinal Cord Metastases

Most metastatic involvement of the spinal cord results from compression by epidural masses from the vertebral bones or paravertebral soft tissue. Intramedullary lesions also occur, though at a much lower rate (21).

HISTOPATHOLOGY

The specific features of CNS metastases vary greatly depending on the primary lesion and the pattern of involvement, yet several features are fairly consistent among all cases. With few exceptions, metastatic malignancies grow as well-delineated round masses that do not entrap indigenous cells as they expand (see Figure 18-1). Diffuse leptomeningeal metastases, some small cell neuroendocrine carcinomas, and melanomas are exceptions, with the latter two occasionally invading along blood vessels (Figure 18-4) or in a "pseudogliomatous" pattern (Figure 18-5). This modestly infiltrative pattern of growth is an issue in very small tissue samples at a lesion's edge because it typically extends <0.3 cm into the surrounding brain (22).

Necrosis often forms the vast majority of the specimen, especially if the lesion has been previously irradiated. Residual tumor cells are most often found around the periphery of the lesion, consistent with a radiologic appearance of ring enhancement. Residual tumor cells around blood vessels create a pseudopapillary, or peritheliomatous, architecture with intervening debris. Many metastases also form thick and collagenous perivascular connective tissue, which is generally not seen in primary neoplasms.

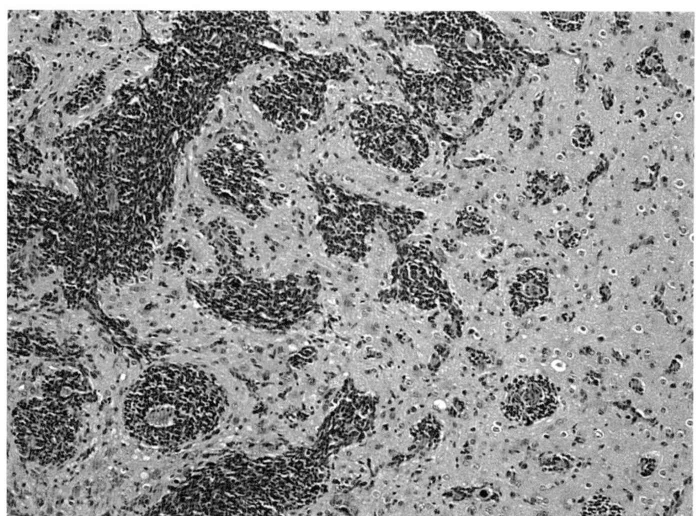

FIGURE 18-4 Small cell neuroendocrine carcinoma spreading along perivascular spaces, a pattern also seen in some metastatic melanomas.

The tissue around a metastasis usually shows reactive changes, with prominent reactive astrocytes and scattered lymphocytes.

During intraoperative consultation, cytologic preparations may be the most helpful tools with which to differentiate metastases from primary brain tumors. The cells of carcinoma are round or polygonal, form cohesive clusters, and have sharply defined cytoplasm without fibrillar cytoplasmic extensions (Figure 18-6). Melanomas are less cohesive and often

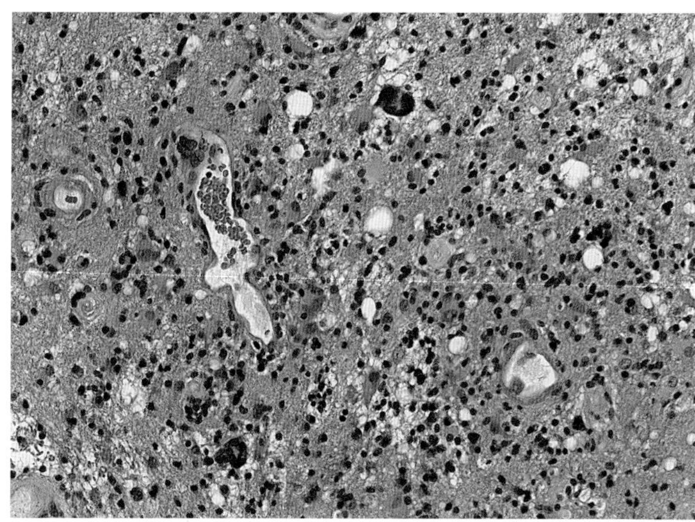

FIGURE 18-5 "Pseudogliomatous" invasion of individual neuroendocrine carcinoma cells can be seen within a few millimeters of the primary lesion.

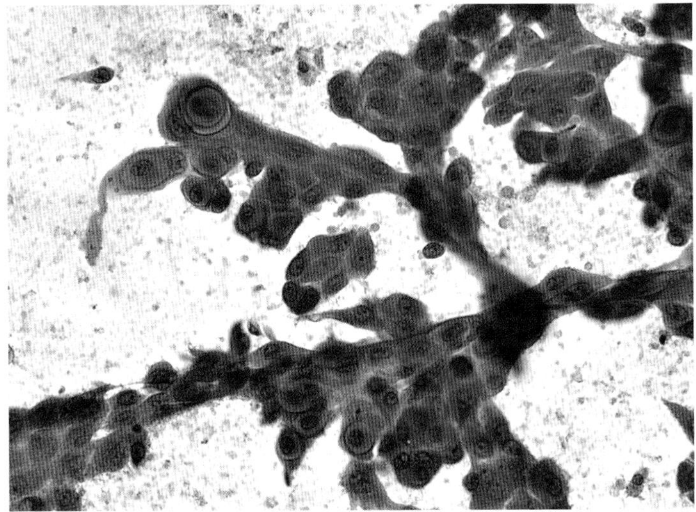

FIGURE 18-6 Cohesive clusters of polygonal cells with prominent borders typify carcinomas but are not seen in glial neoplasms.

have prominent nucleoli, nuclear pseudoinclusions, and background lymphocytes (Figure 18-7).

IMMUNOHISTOCHEMISTRY

Most cases require fewer immunostains because a history of cancer will guide the selection of confirmatory markers; however, a significant subset

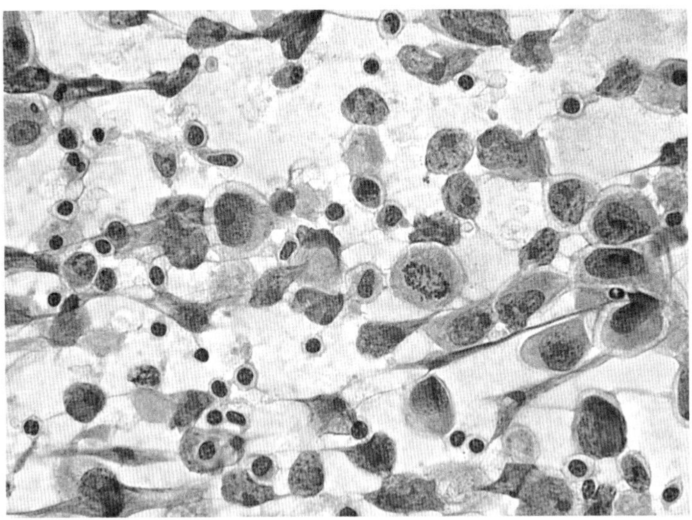

FIGURE 18-7 Classic smear preparation of melanoma shows poorly cohesive cells with prominent nucleoli and background lymphocytes.

TABLE 18-1 Most Common Metastases to the CNS

Tumor Type	Supportive Positive Immunomarkers
Pulmonary adenocarcinoma	Napsin A, TTF-1, CK7(CK20-)
Pulmonary small cell carcinoma	Synaptophysin, TTF-1, CD56
Melanoma	SOX10, HMB-45, Melan A/MART-1, MITF, S100
Breast carcinoma	GATA-3, mammaglobin, GCDFP-15, ER, PR, CK7(CK20-)
Colorectal carcinoma	SATB2, CDX2, CK20(CK7-)
Gastroesophageal carcinoma	CDX2, CK7, & CK20
Renal cell carcinoma	PAX8, PAX2, RCC, carbonic anhydrase IX, vimentin
Squamous cell carcinoma	CK5/6, p63

of brain metastases are the first presentation of a malignancy and may require immunohistochemistry to suggest a primary source (3). In such cases, the workup for tumor origin parallels that for metastases in any other location, a complete discussion of which is beyond the scope of this text. The immunophenotypes of the most common metastases (Table 18-1) are discussed below.

Pulmonary adenocarcinomas express cytokeratin 7 (CK7) and generally lack cytokeratin 20 (CK20) reactivity. Because breast carcinomas also show similar CK7 staining and are common CNS metastases, other markers are required to suggest pulmonary origin. Thyroid transcription factor-1 (TTF-1) is a nuclear protein expressed in about 75% of pulmonary adenocarcinomas and rarely in those from other organs (23,24). However, neuroendocrine carcinomas of both pulmonary and nonpulmonary origin may also express TTF-1, so concurrent neuroendocrine antibodies may be advised if morphologically ambiguous. Napsin A shows higher specificity for pulmonary adenocarcinoma and may be used in conjunction with TTF-1 (23,25). Napsin A immunoreactivity has been demonstrated in some renal tumors (26) and ovarian or endometrial clear cell carcinoma (27).

Neuroendocrine carcinomas, the vast majority of which are of lung origin, express synaptophysin, chromogranin, and CD56 in addition to cytokeratins. Almost all pulmonary neuroendocrine carcinomas also express TTF-1, but nuclear reactivity also decorates some extrapulmonary cases. Cytokeratin 20 should be performed when Merkel cell carcinoma is suspected because it creates a perinuclear dot-like pattern of reactivity that is unique among neuroendocrine carcinomas.

Metastatic mammary carcinoma will express nuclear GATA3 in nearly all cases; however, as with other markers, morphology and other markers need to be ordered in parallel due to expression by other carcinoma types, in the case of GATA3 from skin, cervix, and bladder. Estrogen receptor, progesterone receptor, mammaglobin, and gross cystic disease fluid protein 15 (GCDFP-15) are all only intermittently present in breast carcinoma metastases (28). Cytokeratin 7 reactivity is reliably present but does not help distinguish breast from lung origin. Mammary origin can sometimes only be suggested by the patient's history.

Adenocarcinomas of any of the digestive organs may express the nuclear protein CDX2, although CDX2 reactivity is also common in adenocarcinoma from ovary and bladder (29). CDX2 reactivity is useful, however, because nuclear reactivity supports a nonbreast, nonlung origin. Another nuclear transcription factor, SATB2, is sensitive and relatively specific for colorectal carcinoma, though also with the caveat that müllerian carcinomas may also show expression (30,31). Cytokeratin staining can further suggest whether the primary lesion is colonic, if the metastasis expresses CK20 and not CK7, but other gastrointestinal carcinomas have variable patterns of reactivity for these markers and cannot be localized based on CK7 and 20 immunostaining (32).

Renal clear cell carcinoma usually requires no confirmatory immunohistochemistry, but it must be distinguished from cellular hemangioblastoma, particularly in patients with von Hipple–Lindau syndrome who are predisposed to developing both. Renal cell carcinoma (RCC) immunohistochemically expresses CD10, RCC antigen, EMA, cytokeratin (AE1/3), PAX2, and PAX8 (33–35). Aquaporin 1, inhibin-alpha, and neuron-specific enolase immunostains are negative in RCCs and positive in many hemangioblastomas, making them useful in combination to support the diagnosis of hemangioblastoma (34).

Squamous carcinomas are uncommon CNS metastases and can be identified by expression of cytokeratin 5/6 and nuclear reactivity for p63.

Many gliomas express two of the major immunomarkers of melanoma, S100 protein and SOX10, yet the morphologic differences ensure that there are fewer circumstances where this would result in misdiagnosis. Furthermore, it is highly unusual for gliomas to have immunoreactivity for other melanocytic markers, such as HMB-45 or Melan A/MART-1. A more challenging distinction to make is between CNS melanocytic tumors and metastatic ones. CNS melanocytic tumors express all of the same immunohistochemical markers as extra-CNS melanomas, yet they are more similar to melanocytic tumors of the uvea, harboring *GNAQ* and *GNA11* activating mutations rather than mutations in *BRAF, HRAS,* and *NRAS.*

Differential Diagnosis

The primary CNS neoplasm most often in the differential diagnosis with metastases is glioblastoma. Most of the time, any resemblance is superficial, but some features may raise doubt as to a glioblastoma's identity. Rare cases have foci of polygonal epithelioid cells with well-defined cell–cell borders similar to carcinoma or melanoma. In the majority of such cases, epithelioid cells generally lack the extent of cohesion seen in carcinoma.

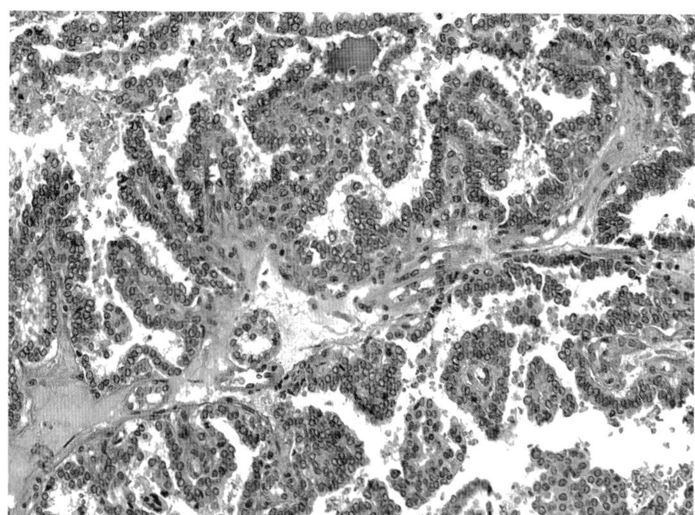

FIGURE 18-8 Although uncommon, metastatic papillary thyroid carcinomas can closely resemble choroid plexus neoplasms.

More infiltrative areas should also be seen in glioblastoma and not metastasis. Palisading necrosis, entrapped neurons, glomeruloid vascular proliferation, and minimal perivascular collagen, all favor glioblastoma. Strong, diffuse glial fibrillary acidic protein (GFAP) reactivity essentially rules out any metastatic neoplasm, as does the demonstration of entrapped axons by neurofilament staining. This distinction is discussed further in the section on glioblastoma.

Gliosarcomas may appear similar to metastatic sarcoma when the glial element is largely overrun. Support for the diagnosis of gliosarcoma comes from GFAP immunostaining that should show at least scattered pockets of glial tumor cells. It is also highly unusual for a metastatic sarcoma to present without a previous history or radiologically obvious extracranial primary.

One of the most difficult diagnostic decisions can be between anaplastic meningioma and metastatic carcinoma. Only rarely does a meningioma lose all identifying histologic features, usually retaining at least vague whorls and bland nuclear features. Somatostatin receptor 2A immunostaining is also retained in most high-grade meningiomas only expressed in a few types of metastatic carcinoma. This differential diagnosis is discussed in more detail in the section on anaplastic meningioma.

Infrequently, papillary thyroid carcinoma metastasizes to the brain, impersonating a choroid plexus neoplasm when it displays the classic papillary architecture (Figure 18-8). Morphologic differentiation can be difficult, but immunoreactivity for thyroglobulin and TTF-1 rules out a primary process. Choroid plexus neoplasms also lack the pale chromatin and nuclear grooves and pseudoinclusions of papillary thyroid carcinoma.

REFERENCES

1. Walker AE, Robins M, Weinfeld FD. Epidemiology of brain tumors: the national survey of intracranial neoplasms. *Neurology*. 1985;35(2):219–226.
2. Gavrilovic IT, Posner JB. Brain metastases: epidemiology and pathophysiology. *J Neurooncol*. 2005;75(1):5–14.
3. Giordana MT, Cordera S, Boghi A. Cerebral metastases as first symptom of cancer: a clinico-pathologic study. *J Neurooncol*. 2000;50(3):265–273.
4. Merchut MP. Brain metastases from undiagnosed systemic neoplasms. *Arch Intern Med*. 1989;149(5):1076–1080.
5. Berghoff AS, Schur S, Fureder LM, et al. Descriptive statistical analysis of a real life cohort of 2419 patients with brain metastases of solid cancers. *ESMO Open*. 2016;1(2): e000024.
6. Preusser M, Capper D, Ilhan-Mutlu A, et al. Brain metastases: pathobiology and emerging targeted therapies. *Acta Neuropathol*. 2012;123(2):205–222.
7. American Cancer Society. Cancer Facts and Figures 2017. Atlanta: American Cancer Society; 2017.
8. Schouten LJ, Rutten J, Huveneers HA, et al. Incidence of brain metastases in a cohort of patients with carcinoma of the breast, colon, kidney, and lung and melanoma. *Cancer*. 2002;94(10):2698–2705.
9. Bindal RK, Sawaya RE, Leavens ME, et al. Sarcoma metastatic to the brain: results of surgical treatment. *Neurosurgery*. 1994;35(2):185–190; discussion 190–181.
10. Gercovich FG, Luna MA, Gottlieb JA. Increased incidence of cerebral metastases in sarcoma patients with prolonged survival from chemotherapy. Report of cases of leiomysarcoma and chondrosarcoma. *Cancer*. 1975;36(5):1843–1851.
11. Salvati M, D'Elia A, Frati A, et al. Sarcoma metastatic to the brain: a series of 35 cases and considerations from 27 years of experience. *J Neurooncol*. 2010;98(3):373–377.
12. Yoshida S, Morii K, Watanabe M, et al. Brain metastasis in patients with sarcoma: an analysis of histological subtypes, clinical characteristics, and outcomes. *Surg Neurol*. 2000;54(2):160–164.
13. Suki D, Khoury Abdulla R, Ding M, et al. Brain metastases in patients diagnosed with a solid primary cancer during childhood: experience from a single referral cancer center. *J Neurosurg Pediatr*. 2014;14(4):372–385.
14. Wiens AL, Hattab EM. The pathological spectrum of solid CNS metastases in the pediatric population. *J Neurosurg Pediatr*. 2014;14(2):129–135.
15. Taillibert S, Laigle-Donadey F, Chodkiewicz C, et al. Leptomeningeal metastases from solid malignancy: a review. *J Neurooncol*. 2005;75(1):85–99.
16. Wasserstrom WR, Glass JP, Posner JB. Diagnosis and treatment of leptomeningeal metastases from solid tumors: experience with 90 patients. *Cancer*. 1982;49(4):759–772.
17. Kebudi R, Ayan I, Gorgun O, et al. Brain metastasis in pediatric extracranial solid tumors: survey and literature review. *J Neurooncol*. 2005;71(1):43–48.
18. Abrams HL, Spiro R, Goldstein N. Metastases in carcinoma; analysis of 1000 autopsied cases. *Cancer*. 1950;3(1):74–85.
19. Max MB, Deck MD, Rottenberg DA. Pituitary metastasis: incidence in cancer patients and clinical differentiation from pituitary adenoma. *Neurology*.1981;31(8):998–1002.
20. Teears RJ, Silverman EM. Clinicopathologic review of 88 cases of carcinoma metastatic to the putuitary gland. *Cancer*. 1975;36(1):216–220.
21. Grem JL, Burgess J, Trump DL. Clinical features and natural history of intramedullary spinal cord metastasis. *Cancer*. 1985;56(9):2305–2314.
22. Neves S, Mazal PR, Wanschitz J, et al. Pseudogliomatous growth pattern of anaplastic small cell carcinomas metastatic to the brain. *Clin Neuropathol*. 2001;20(1):38–42.

23. Bishop JA, Sharma R, Illei PB. Napsin A and thyroid transcription factor-1 expression in carcinomas of the lung, breast, pancreas, colon, kidney, thyroid, and malignant mesothelioma. *Hum Pathol.* 2010;41(1):20–25.
24. Kaufmann O, Dietel M. Thyroid transcription factor-1 is the superior immunohistochemical marker for pulmonary adenocarcinomas and large cell carcinomas compared to surfactant proteins A and B. *Histopathology.* 2000;36(1):8–16.
25. Stoll LM, Johnson MW, Gabrielson E, et al. The utility of napsin-A in the identification of primary and metastatic lung adenocarcinoma among cytologically poorly differentiated carcinomas. *Cancer Cytopathol.* 2010;118(6):441–449.
26. Zhu B, Rohan SM, Lin X. Immunoexpression of napsin A in renal neoplasms. *Diagn Pathol.* 2015;10:4.
27. Iwamoto M, Nakatani Y, Fugo K, et al. Napsin A is frequently expressed in clear cell carcinoma of the ovary and endometrium. *Hum Pathol.* 2015;46(7):957–962.
28. Bhargava R, Dabbs DJ. Use of immunohistochemistry in diagnosis of breast epithelial lesions. *Adv Anat Pathol.* 2007;14(2):93–107.
29. Werling RW, Yaziji H, Bacchi CE, et al. CDX2, a highly sensitive and specific marker of adenocarcinomas of intestinal origin: an immunohistochemical survey of 476 primary and metastatic carcinomas. *Am J Surg Pathol.* 2003;27(3):303–310.
30. Dragomir A, de Wit M, Johansson C, et al. The role of SATB2 as a diagnostic marker for tumors of colorectal origin: results of a pathology-based clinical prospective study. *Am J Clin Pathol.* 2014;141(5):630–638.
31. Magnusson K, de Wit M, Brennan DJ, et al. SATB2 in combination with cytokeratin 20 identifies over 95% of all colorectal carcinomas. *Am J Surg Pathol.* 2011;35(7):937–948.
32. Chu P, Wu E, Weiss LM. Cytokeratin 7 and cytokeratin 20 expression in epithelial neoplasms: a survey of 435 cases. *Mod Pathol.* 2000;13(9):962–972.
33. Rivera AL, Takei H, Zhai J, et al. Useful immunohistochemical markers in differentiating hemangioblastoma versus metastatic renal cell carcinoma. *Neuropathology.* 2010;30(6): 580–585.
34. Weinbreck N, Marie B, Bressenot A, et al. Immunohistochemical markers to distinguish between hemangioblastoma and metastatic clear-cell renal cell carcinoma in the brain: utility of aquaporin1 combined with cytokeratin AE1/AE3 immunostaining. *Am J Surg Pathol.* 2008;32(7):1051–1059.
35. Ozcan A, de la Roza G, Ro JY, et al. PAX2 and PAX8 expression in primary and metastatic renal tumors: a comprehensive comparison. *Arch Pathol Lab Med.* 2012;136(12): 1541–1551.

19

INTRAOPERATIVE CONSULTATION

Intraoperative neuropathology consultation can be a significant source of anxiety to the general surgical pathologist who covers only an occasional neurosurgical specimen, particularly early in one's career. It seems anecdotally commonplace that one's first after-hours frozen section case at a new job is courtesy of a neurosurgeon. It is for such pathologists that this chapter is written, with a focus in mind to cover the absolute essentials of neuropathology intraoperative consultation (IC) necessary to provide the surgeon adequate guidance and service. The intent of this chapter is not to extensively review frozen section pathology, nor review all of the possible situations and diagnoses, rather to provide a starting place and framework for successful IC that covers the most common specimen types (Table 19-1). Several reviews of this subject are available in the literature (1–4).

PREPARATION

Preparation for an IC begins with a careful review of the patient's clinical history. Based on the age, clinical history, lesion location, and other neuroimaging findings, one can establish a preoperative list of potential diagnoses (see Chapter 20). This list of diagnoses allows for assessment of whether the observed histology is representative of the targeted lesion and can frame the degree of certainty one should place in the interpretation of that histology. For instance, a stereotactic biopsy in a 65-year-old of a ring-enhancing hemispheric lesion that reveals mildly hypercellular brain tissue with scattered atypical glial cells and no mitosis or other findings was probably taken in the vicinity of a glioblastoma and not sufficient for that diagnosis. In such cases, more tissue should be requested.

Neuroimaging is a crucial component of surgical neuropathology, serving as a sort of gross examination of the entire lesion in the context of the adjacent structures. Although it's not practical to know neuroradiology in detail, the pathologist should know what helpful features to look for in the imaging report, if not the images themselves. Some important questions include: What is the location? Is it intrinsic or extra-axial? Is it circumscribed and discrete, or ill-defined? Is it cystic? Is it multifocal? Does it have associated edema (T2/FLAIR signal)? Does it expand involved structures or have other mass effect? Is it contrast-enhancing? Does it demonstrate restricted diffusion? At a minimum, one should be familiar

TABLE 19-1 **General Tips for Successful Neuropathology Intraoperative Consultation**
Review the patient's clinical history and neuroimaging findings prior to the procedure.
Communicate directly with the surgeon.
Have a preoperative differential diagnosis.
Reserve some of the IC specimen for routine processing, even when told more is coming.
Perform smear preparations or touch imprints.
If tissue is limited, use only a cytologic preparation and submit the rest for routine processing.
For better histologic detail, freeze tissue as rapidly as possible.
Ask for more tissue if there is any uncertainty about adequacy.

with the findings of the neuroimaging report and the radiologist's opinion as to what the findings represent.

Although not always feasible, direct communication with the surgeon prior to the procedure can be helpful to fill in potential gaps in the patient's history that may not be fully communicated in the medical record. In emergent cases, direct communication may be the only source of patient history. The pathologist should also inquire as to whether there are any special considerations for allotment of tissue, such as for research, culturing, clinical trials, or molecular testing. In cases where lymphoma is suspected, it is crucial to know whether the patient received corticosteroids because it can drastically alter and obscure the usual histopathology.

One should be vigilant when reviewing clinical histories of prospective IC patients for potential cases of Creutzfeldt-Jakob disease (CJD). Such patients are typically at least 60 years of age and have rapidly progressive dementia, visual impairment, and myoclonus. When a brain biopsy is undertaken in a potential case of CJD, the tissue should not be examined intraoperatively, rather it should be processed separately from all other tissue using a special protocol for potential prion disease specimens. Contamination of the frozen section laboratory with prion protein from such specimens could potentially halt IC operations while decontamination is performed. A protocol for handling potential prion disease specimens is publicly available on the Internet from the United States National Prion Disease Pathology Surveillance Center at Case Western Reserve University.

TISSUE HANDLING

There are three types of specimens that account for most neurosurgical ICs; from largest to smallest they are: open biopsy/resection, stereotactic needle biopsy, and endoscopic biopsy. Open biopsies or resections are typically large, and there is no question as to whether the lesion has been sampled, rather the purpose of ordering an IC is to identify the general tumor type, which may impact how aggressively the lesion is excised, or, in the case of metastasis or infectious lesion, what other testing or imaging may be needed. Needle core biopsies, on the other hand, are performed by stereotactic coordinates without direct visual guidance, introducing a number of factors that may result in unsatisfactory or nonrepresentative tissue cores. For these specimens, the IC is primarily for ensuring tissue adequacy for diagnosis and ancillary testing. Endoscopic biopsies are under direct visual guidance, but are only able to collect minute fragments of tissue that may not be representative.

Regardless of the type of IC specimen, a few principles should guide the triage and apportionment of tissue. The most important is to always reserve some of the tissue sent for IC for routine paraffin embedding. Most of the time, a separate specimen will be sent for routine processing, but conditions may prevent the surgeon from collecting additional tissue, or the additional tissue may be unsatisfactory. Not only does frozen tissue have degraded histomorphology, freezing can alter the immunoreactivity of the tissue for some antibodies, making it less suitable for establishing the final diagnosis. In the event that all of the tissue must be used for IC, that should be communicated to the surgeon so that more can be collected if possible. In IC cases with limited tissue, cytologic preparation alone without frozen section is better to preserve tissue for processing.

Beyond retaining some of the tissue for paraffin embedding and depending on the IC diagnosis, additional tissue may need to be submitted for other testing, such as flow cytometry for lymphoma, culturing for infectious process, or frozen tissue for clinical trial eligibility or molecular testing. Communication with the surgeon about who is responsible for submitting what testing is crucial to avoiding duplicate efforts or lost opportunities.

GROSS EXAMINATION

Although most neuropathology IC specimens are small, many of the common diagnostic entities have typical gross appearances that can further inform histopathologic observations (Table 19-2). With experience, one can anticipate the histologic diagnosis in many cases by gross examination, as can some experienced neurosurgeons.

CYTOLOGIC PREPARATIONS

An important and time-honored component of neuropathology IC is the smear or squash preparation, in which a small amount (1 to 2 mm^3) of fresh tissue is placed on a glass slide and smeared across the surface by another slide (Figure 19-1), spreading out the cellular elements and allowing for examination of the cytologic details without the distortion caused

TABLE 19-2 Typical Gross Findings of Common Intraoperative Consult Specimens

Gross Features	Diagnosis/Diagnoses
Mildly/moderately firm, solid red throughout, obvious widespread cautery	Solitary fibrous tumor, hemangioblastoma
Clear mucoid/semi-liquid with small vessels and whitish areas	Dysembryoplastic neuroepithelial tumor, pilocytic astrocytoma, rosette-forming glioneuronal tumor
Firm, tan, nodular, cohesive, homogeneous cut surface	Meningioma, some metastases
Soft, semi-solid, red and tan perhaps with areas of whitish necrosis, congested and/or dark (thrombotic) blood vessels	Glioblastoma, lymphoma, some metastases
Firm, friable, ragged surfaces, hemorrhagic or prominent small blood vessels, pale areas of necrosis	Metastatic carcinoma, other metastases
Red-tan, opaque, slimy texture, leaves thick deposits on touch imprints	Pituitary adenoma
Firm, tan-red, leaves mostly blood and few pituitary cells on touch imprints	Adenohypophysis/anterior pituitary
Rubbery membranous tissue with flaky, white, friable material that washes off of smear slides during staining	Dermoid/epidermoid cysts, teratoma

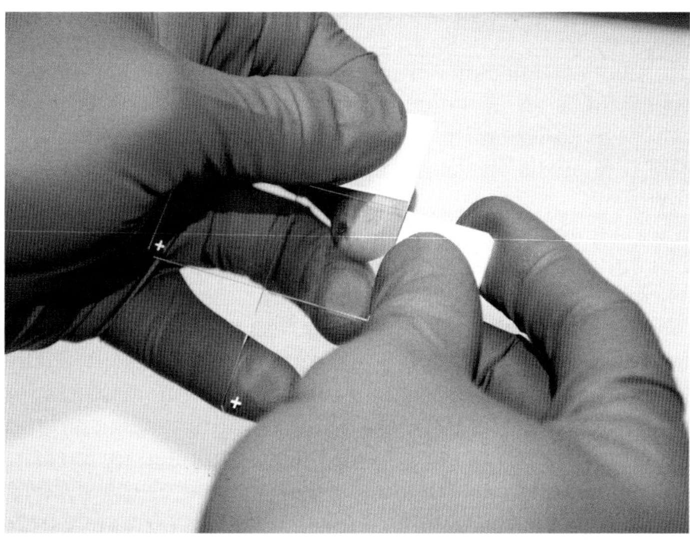

FIGURE 19-1 Smear preparations are made by spreading a small fragment of tissue across the surface of a slide with another slide. The pressure applied should be enough to distribute the cells thinly without destroying them.

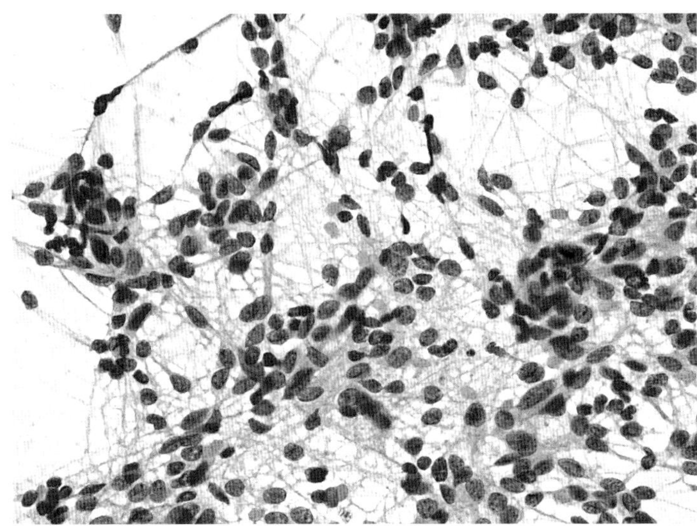

FIGURE 19-2 A major advantage of smear preparations is that they demonstrate the fibrillar cytoplasmic process of glial cells, seen here in a smear from an ependymoma.

by the freezing process. Smear preparations are alone sufficient in many cases to identify lesional tissue and are used for IC without concurrent frozen section in some institutions, allowing for more tissue to remain unfrozen for routine processing. Indeed, if tissue is limited, frozen section should be omitted and only cytologic examination should be performed, preserving the maximal amount of specimen for paraffin embedding.

Smear preparations have an advantage over frozen section in demonstrating fibrillar cytoplasmic processes (Figure 19-2), cellular cohesion, and nuclear details, all of which provide important clues to the diagnosis in most cases. Even when the tissue fails to smear, it contributes information for the diagnosis by suggesting the presence of collagen or other resilient matrix.

Several elements of technique are important to producing optimal smear preparations. The amount of tissue should be no more than 1 to 2 mm^3 per slide, otherwise the resulting thickness and large spread can hinder microscopic examination. The pieces should be nicked from larger fragments with a scalpel blade or put on the slide directly if already the correct size, in either case taking care not to crush the tissue before it gets to the slide. Each area of the tissue with a different gross appearance should be sampled. Sufficient pressure must be applied to smear the tissue thinly, but not so much that the tissue is destroyed or the slide is broken. To provide strong and even support, grasp the end of the slide between the thumb and forefinger and place the tips of the third through fifth fingers along the bottom of the slide. After the tissue is smeared, the slide should be placed in fixative as quickly as possible to avoid air-drying artifact.

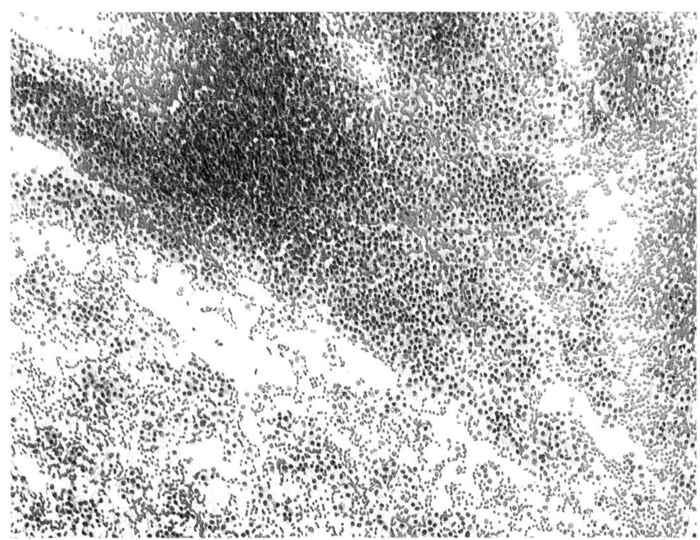

FIGURE 19-3 Gentle blotting of a pituitary adenoma on a glass slide leaves numerous cells on the surface, a helpful finding not seen with normal anterior pituitary tissue.

Although generally less effective than smears, there are at least two IC situations in which touch imprints are preferable. The most common is that of a sellar mass suspected to be pituitary adenoma. Mere gentle dabbing of an adenoma leaves piles of intact individual cells on a slide surface (Figure 19-3), in contrast to adenohypophysis, which is more firm and stingily releases only occasional small clusters and individual cells for examination. Abundant shedding of neuroendocrine cells on touch imprint is essentially diagnostic in itself for pituitary adenoma; other patterns should be followed with frozen sections.

Touch imprints are also helpful when germinoma is a potential diagnosis, typically in a younger person with either a pineal or midline sella region mass. The large and delicate cells of germinoma rarely survive even gentle smearing, but will remain more intact when gently touched. The gentlest handling should be used at all times with such specimens. Some hematopoietic lesions are also somewhat better preserved on touch preparations.

FROZEN SECTIONS

Freezing necessarily disrupts the fine structures of tissue and results in suboptimal histology. This is caused primarily by the formation of ice crystals that displace the surrounding milieu, stretching and distorting the cells and leaving angular empty spaces on the finished slide (Figure 19-4). The degree of ice crystal artifact is directly related to the amount of time that it takes the tissue to freeze; the slower the freeze, the worse the histology.

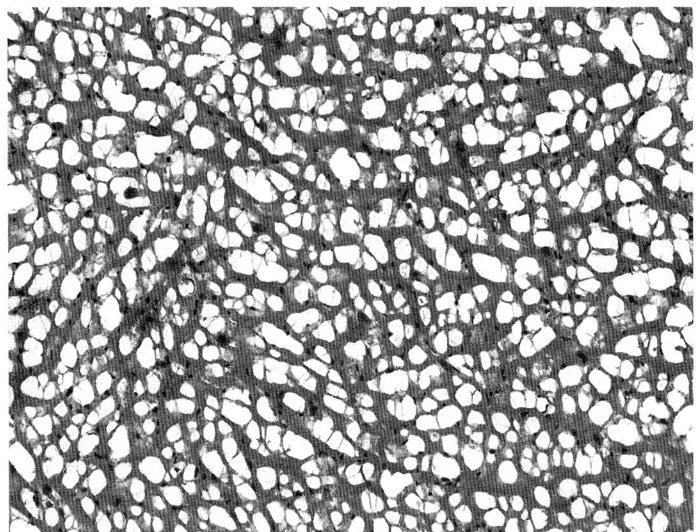

FIGURE 19-4 Slow freezing caused marked ice crystal artifact in this edematous brain tissue, evident in the numerous small spaces in the section and poor histologic detail.

Isopentane cooled in liquid nitrogen can produce tissue sections that rival paraffin sections in quality (Figure 19-5), whereas tissue just placed in the cryostat and frozen passively may be uninterpretable. This effect is particularly pronounced in tissues with richly myxoid backgrounds.

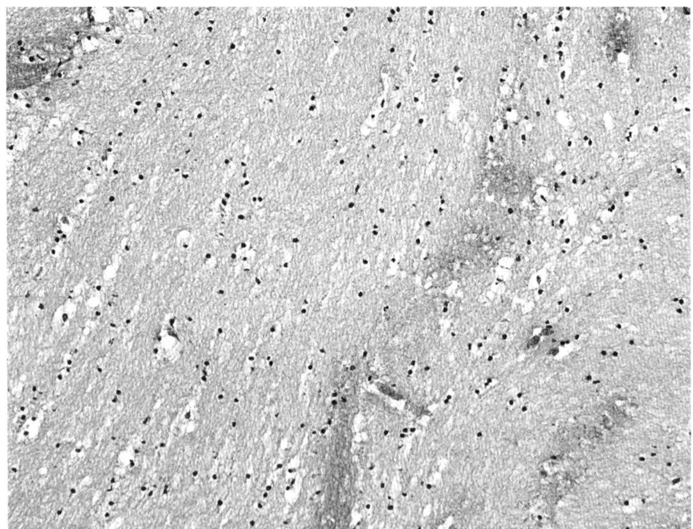

FIGURE 19-5 Tissue from the same specimen as Figure 19-3, but snap-frozen with refrigerant spray and resulting in less freezing artifact.

Frozen sections have the advantages over cytologic preparations of demonstrating the architecture of a lesion and representing a larger sampling of the tissue. Although not always informative, architectural features add another layer of potentially helpful information in difficult cases. In larger pieces of tissue, a frozen section can more easily sample a larger area and detect potentially important focal findings, such as an area of higher proliferation or necrosis.

DIAGNOSTIC INTERPRETATION

The IC diagnosis is mostly for the purpose of tissue adequacy in the case of stereotactic biopsies and to categorize the lesion in open excisions to the degree that it may impact the extent of resection. Beyond these two aims, the scope of the IC diagnosis should be limited to only what is unequivocal. To do that while still providing helpful information, one may use less specific diagnoses that cover two or more potential specific diagnoses (Table 19-3). Such less specific diagnoses are useful to avoid discrepancies and wholly appropriate as long as they satisfy the surgeon's needs.

Intraoperative diagnosis follows the same algorithm as regular surgical neuropathology, starting with determination of whether the tissue is normal or not. Familiarization with normal histology of different areas of brain and spinal cord in unremarkable autopsy tissue is helpful in establishing a feeling for this. One may even want to keep autopsy brain slides in the frozen section laboratory for comparison of cellularity during IC. If the tissue is normal, it is helpful to the surgeon to provide feedback on the likely location of the said tissue. Is it gray matter? Is it white matter? Is there ependymal lining? Is it cerebellum?

If the tissue is not normal, the next determination is if it's reactive or neoplastic. One should run through a list of reactive, infectious or inflammatory conditions that could explain the histology. Descriptive diagnoses often suffice for this category. Among the most challenging ICs is the distinction between gliosis and lower-grade infiltrating glioma (see Chapter 3 and below). If neoplastic, then the usual examination of tissue architecture and cellular features proceeds with the determination of whether it is metastatic or primary and ultimately what specific tumor type.

Grading is not necessary in most neuropathology IC cases. Because the IC tissue is only a portion of the total tissue to be examined, it may not be representative. This is more of a problem when the IC material indicates a lower grade, because additional findings that constitute high grade may be revealed in the paraffin tissue. In such cases, the phrase "no evidence of high-grade features" may be used, particularly if imaging suggests aggressive findings that are not observed in the IC. On the other hand, if high-grade features are unambiguously present in the IC material, it should be stated because they will not go away with additional sampling. In the case of a histologically classic glioblastoma, one may give that as the IC diagnosis because the grade can go neither up nor down.

TABLE 19-3 Example Generic Intraoperative Consult Diagnoses

Intraoperative Diagnosis	Potential Final Diagnoses
Lesional/pathologic tissue present	Minimum feedback for CNS biopsy, implies that the tissue is representative and sufficient for diagnosis (must be correlated with surgeon's expectations and neuroimaging findings)
Low-grade neuroepithelial neoplasm	Pilocytic astrocytoma, ganglioglioma, dysembryoplastic neuroepithelial tumor, pleomorphic xanthoastrocytoma, (most WHO grade I–II intrinsic brain/spinal cord tumors)
High-grade neuroepithelial neoplasm	Glioblastoma, anaplastic oligodendroglioma, anaplastic ependymoma, medulloblastoma, other embryonal tumors (most WHO grade III–IV intrinsic brain/spinal cord tumors)
Infiltrating glioma	Diffuse astrocytoma, anaplastic astrocytoma, glioblastoma, oligodendroglioma
Astrocytoma	Pilocytic vs. diffuse astrocytoma
Malignant embryonal neoplasm	Medulloblastoma, AT/RT, embryonal tumor with multilayered rosettes, CNS neuroblastoma
Metastatic malignant neoplasm	Metastatic carcinoma, melanoma, sarcoma
Macrophage-rich lesion	Demyelinating lesion (including progressive multifocal leukoencephalopathy), infarct, treated lymphoma
Hypercellular neuroglial tissue	Abnormal; gliosis vs. infiltrating glioma
Granulomatous lesion	Neurosarcoidosis, fungal or *M. tuberculosis* infection, germinoma, amebiasis, granulomatous vasculitis (incl. Aβ-related)
Low-grade spindle cell neoplasm	Schwannoma, fibrous meningioma, most low-grade mesenchymal tumors
High-grade spindle cell neoplasm	High-grade sarcomas, gliosarcoma, sarcomatoid renal cell carcinoma

COMMON PITFALLS

Oligodendrogliomas and infiltrating astrocytomas are common sources of discrepancies between IC diagnosis and final diagnosis. This is due to the distortion of oligodendroglioma nuclei on frozen section to appear hyperchromatic and irregular, thus more like those of an astrocytoma, all in a setting of overlapping clinical and radiologic features. In cases of infiltrating gliomas, one should not assert astrocytic or oligodendroglial differentiation, especially now that those terms are largely based on genetic findings that supersede histomorphology. "Infiltrating glioma" will usually suffice, possibly modified with "high-grade" or "no evidence of high-grade features" as appropriate to the situation.

Infiltrating gliomas may be difficult to distinguish from **reactive gliosis** even for experienced neuropathologists. There are several morphologic features that can be helpful in making this distinction intraoperatively. In smear preparations, reactive astrocytes have large, eccentric cytoplasm with abundant fibrillar cytoplasmic extensions that are fairly uniform in size and dispersion and nuclei that contain generally smooth chromatin and subtle, enlarged nucleoli. In contrast, neoplastic astrocytes have fewer cytoplasmic processes that are more irregularly spaced. On tissue section, reactive astrocytesare evenly spaced from one another and extend processes in all directions, whereas neoplastic astrocytes usually appear as naked nuclei on a fibrillary background. Gemistocytic astrocytoma cells have eccentric prominent cytoplasm, but more disorganized processes and atypical nuclei. Oligodendrogliomas are more subtle and may appear as mildly increased cellularity with no apparent atypia. Unless it is unambiguous, the IC diagnosis for lesions that could be reactive or infiltrative tumor should be termed "hypercellularneuroglial tissue" and further worked up on paraffin-embedded tissue. Again, the IC diagnosis should be consistent with the imaging findings.

Piloid gliosis, in which reactive astrocytes produce Rosenthal fibers in response to slowly increasing pressure, can be mistaken for **pilocytic astrocytoma**. This finding can be seen around any slowly expanding, circumscribed mass and is most commonly seen in the tissue around craniopharyngiomas, hemangioblastomas, and spinal cord syrinx. The potential risk to the patient is probably the highest in the latter case, where a biopsy is performed to assess for infiltrating glioma around a syrinx. A mistaken IC diagnosis of pilocytic astrocytoma could potentially lead to unnecessary resection of non-tumoral tissue. Pilocytic astrocytomas are generally more cellular and myxoid than piloid gliosis and usually have a biphasic pattern. In ambiguous cases, the term "piloid astroglial tissue" can be used as the IC diagnosis.

Pituitary adenomas are among the most common neurosurgical specimens and have a significant potential for IC misdiagnosis. The most common difficulty is determining adenoma from adenohypophysis. Adenohypophysis has multiple cell types, which should not be seen in adenomas, yet compressed gland around adenomas usually loses cytoplasmic detail and becomes monomorphic. Such tissue generally still has a nested architecture but can still be difficult to tell from adenoma. The gross examination and touch preparation are very helpful in identifying adenoma; compared to anterior pituitary, adenomas are much softer and the vast majority of them leave abundant cells on touch imprints.

The morphology of pituitary adenomas is variable to the degree that they can potentially overlap with a number of malignant tumors that occasionally occur in or metastasize to the sella. The most common of these are plasmacytoma, lymphoma, metastatic melanoma, and metastatic carcinoma. The vast majority of these other entities will not present a challenge; however, rare cases can defy confident IC diagnosis. Descriptive terms such as "epithelioid neoplasm" or "plasmacytoid neoplasm" may be appropriate in those circumstances.

Spindle cell neoplasms are commonly misdiagnosed on IC. Schwannoma and fibrous meningioma can have similar presentations and histologic features and probably account for most IC discrepancies in this category. Meningiomas usually have an attachment to the dura that is lacking in schwannomas; review of neuroimaging findings can assist determining that. The nuclear features of fibrous meningiomas are also more monotonous. If ultimately unclear on IC examination, a diagnosis of "low-grade spindle cell tumor" can be issued.

Lymphomas can be tricky IC specimens, especially when the patient has received corticosteroid treatment. Such therapy causes rapid death among the tumor cells and triggers infiltrates of macrophages, leading to histologic resemblance to **demyelinating lesions**. Demyelinating lesions have macrophage-rich infiltrates and less-prominent lymphocytic infiltrates, but do not have widespread apoptosis or necrosis.

In the acute phase, **demyelinating lesions** can have a deceptive appearance of infiltrating glioma before the cytoplasm of the macrophages is fully developed and enlarged. Smear preparations are excellent in this situation for demonstrating the macrophages' subtle foamy cytoplasm and lack of fibrillar processes.

The densely cellular **cerebellar granule layer** has occasionally been interpreted as a malignant neoplasm on IC. The small and numerous granule neurons can give the impression of a "small, round, blue cell tumor," particularly medulloblastoma because both have small, fibrillar rosette structures. The keys to recognizing cerebellar granule layer are to notice the high degree of monotony of granule neurons and utter lack of mitotic figures and apoptotic nuclei. Large Purkinje neurons lie just superficial to the granule layer and are usually included in any tissue from that area.

REFERENCES

1. Lee HS, Tihan T. The basics of intraoperative diagnosis in neuropathology. *Surg Pathol Clin*. 2015;8(1):27–47.
2. Powell SZ. Intraoperative consultation, cytologic preparations, and frozen section in the central nervous system. *Arch Pathol Lab Med*. 2005;129(12):1635–1652.
3. Yachnis AT. Intraoperative consultation for nervous system lesions. *Semin Diagn Pathol*. 2002;19(4):192–206.
4. Somerset HL, Kleinschmidt-DeMasters BK. Approach to the intraoperative consultation for neurosurgical specimens. *Adv Anat Pathol*. 2011;18(6):446–449.

20

GENERAL APPROACH AND DIFFERENTIAL DIAGNOSIS

CLINICAL AND NEUROIMAGING VARIABLES

The interpretation of routine H&E-stained sections and immunohistochemistry from CNS lesions can be difficult and risky when performed outside of the context of clinical and neuroimaging data. Indeed, many difficulties may arise from attempts to establish a diagnosis based on morphology alone. As detailed in the preceding chapters, the differential diagnosis for surgical neuropathology specimens varies widely depending on the lesion location, imaging characteristics, and patient age. Together, these variables should guide the establishment of pretest probabilities of diagnoses and streamline the interpretation of histologic findings, winnowing numerous distinct entities to a manageable few. Outside of the context of these clues, some CNS lesions with vastly divergent outcomes may differ only very subtly from one another histologically. Simply put, surgical neuropathology cannot be practiced in a vacuum, and the most appropriate diagnosis will only be reached consistently with a disciplined approach that includes input from as much clinical and neuroimaging information as is available.

The following series of tables lists differential diagnoses based on clinical/imaging information (Tables 20-1 to 20-8) and covers most surgical neuropathology specimens but is not intended to be exhaustive.

APPROACH TO HISTOLOGIC DIAGNOSIS

After establishing a differential diagnosis based on age and neuroimaging, microscopic examination in surgical neuropathology progresses in an algorithmic fashion, starting with a determination of whether the tissue is normal. This can be a daunting task in some cases where the histologic findings are minimal, as in some lower-grade infiltrating gliomas. Abnormal tissue can then be categorized into one of several general pathophysiologic processes, such as reactive/inflammatory, infectious, or neoplastic, from which more specific diagnoses are developed. Another approach is to separate lesions by overall low-magnification pattern, such as circumscribed, infiltrative, perivascular, and leptomeningeal, which to some

TABLE 20-1 Tumors of the Posterior Fossa

Pediatric
Pilocytic astrocytoma
Medulloblastoma
Ependymoma
Infiltrating astrocytoma (brainstem)
Atypical teratoid/rhabdoid tumor
Dermoid cyst
Hemangioblastoma
Embryonal tumor with multilayered rosettes
Rosette-forming glioneuronal tumor
Ganglioglioma
Adult
Metastasis
Meningioma
Hemangioblastoma
Subependymoma
Infiltrating astrocytoma
Dysplastic cerebellar gangliocytoma (Lhermitte–Duclos disease) (rare)
Rosette-forming glioneuronal tumor (rare)
Cerebellopontine angle
Schwannoma
Meningioma
Epidermoid cyst
Choroid plexus papilloma
Endolymphatic sac tumor

extent recapitulates neuroimaging data. Regardless of approach, systematic histologic evaluation for all entities consistent with a particular lesion's clinical/imaging features is encouraged and will help to prevent inadvertent omission of the correct diagnosis from consideration.

TABLE 20-2 Lesions of the Spine

Intramedullary spinal cord
Poorly-circumscribed
Infiltrating astrocytoma
Sarcoidosis or other inflammatory process
Reactive changes around syrinx or kyphosis
Well-circumscribed
Ependymoma
Hemangioblastoma (typically dorsal)
Pilocytic astrocytoma (often cystic)
Metastasis
Demyelinating lesion
Abscess
Germinoma (rare, can also be infiltrative)

TABLE 20-2 Lesions of the Spine (continued)
Intradural, extramedullary
Meningioma
Schwannoma
Neurofibroma
Malignant peripheral nerve sheath tumor
Solitary fibrous tumor/hemangiopericytoma
Calcifying pseudoneoplasm of the neuraxis
Ependymoma (rare)
Melanocytoma (rare)
Epidural
Metastasis
Herniated intervertebral disc
Plasmacytoma
Abscess
Calcifying pseudoneoplasm of the neuraxis
Bone and soft tissue tumors
Cauda equina, filum terminale
Myxopapillary ependymoma
Schwannoma
Neurofibroma
Meningioma (sometimes clear cell)
Malignant peripheral nerve sheath tumor
Paraganglioma of the filum terminale
Metastasis

TABLE 20-3 Dura-Based Lesions
Meningioma
Metastasis
Solitary fibrous tumor/hemangiopericytoma
Primary meningeal melanocytic neoplasm
Sarcoidosis
Sarcoma
Rosai–Dorfman disease/extranodal histiocytosis
Low-grade lymphoma
Idiopathic pachymeningitis
Granulomatous polyangiitis

TABLE 20-4 Tumors of the Ventricles

- Lateral ventricles
  - Meningioma (posterior/trigone)
  - Central neurocytoma
  - Ependymoma (children)
  - Subependymoma (adults)
  - Subependymal giant cell astrocytoma
  - Choroid plexus xanthoma
  - Choroid plexus tumor (children > adults)
  - Dysembryoplastic neuroepithelial tumor (septum pellucidum)
- Third ventricle
  - Pilocytic astrocytoma (children, anterior)
  - Endodermal/colloid cyst
  - Chordoid glioma (anterior)
  - Germinoma or other germ cell tumor
  - Pineal parenchymal tumors (posterior)
  - Papillary tumor of the pineal region (posterior)
- Fourth ventricle
  - Ependymoma
  - Medulloblastoma
  - Pilocytic astrocytoma
  - Subependymoma
  - Choroid plexus neoplasms (adult, papilloma > child, carcinoma)
  - Rosette-forming glioneuronal tumor of the fourth ventricle

TABLE 20-5 Sellar and Parasellar Mass Lesions

- Pituitary adenoma
- Rathke cleft cyst
- Craniopharyngioma
- Meningioma
- Pilocytic astrocytoma
- Metastasis
- Lymphoma
- Xanthogranuloma
- Germinoma or other germ cell tumor
- Chordoma
- Granular cell tumor
- Pituicytoma
- Spindle cell oncocytoma of the adenohypophysis
- Hypophysitis, primary or secondary

TABLE 20-6 Mass Lesions Associated With Epilepsy (>2-Year Duration)
Ganglioglioma
Dysembryoplastic neuroepithelial tumor
Angiocentric glioma
Meningioangiomatosis
Cortical tuber
Cortical heterotopia
Cavernous malformation
Hypothalamic hamartoma (often gelastic, or laughing, seizures)
Focal cortical dysplasia (rarely mass-like)

TABLE 20-7 Distinctive Neuroimaging Findings
Multifocal
Metastases
Lymphoma, especially intravascular
Disseminated infection/abscesses
Vasculitis
Multiple sclerosis
Progressive multifocal leukoencephalopathy
Glioblastoma (less common)
Parasitic cysts
Ring/rim-enhancing
Glioblastoma
Metastases
Abscess
Demyelinating lesion (gap at superficial aspect)
Radiation necrosis
Intraparenchymal hemorrhage
Lymphoma
Low-grade tumors (occasional; pilocytic astrocytoma, DNT)
Cyst with mural nodule
Ganglioglioma (supratentorial)
Pleomorphic xanthoastrocytoma (supratentorial)
Hemangioblastoma (infratentorial/posterior fossa)
Pilocytic astrocytoma (infratentorial/posterior fossa)
Papillary glioneuronal tumor

(*continued*)

TABLE 20-7 Distinctive Neuroimaging Findings (continued)

Internally cystic
- Craniopharyngioma
- Pilocytic astrocytoma
- Desmoplastic infantile ganglioglioma/astrocytoma
- Ependymoma
- Astroblastoma
- Papillary glioneuronal tumor
- Teratoma
- Developmental cyst
- Parasitic cyst
- Pineal cyst

Calcifications
- Oligodendroglioma
- Central neurocytoma
- Ependymoma
- Craniopharyngioma
- Cortical tuber
- Calcifying pseudoneoplasm of the neuraxis
- Subependymal giant cell astrocytoma
- Vascular malformation
- Teratoma

Corticotropic
- Oligodendroglioma
- Dysembryoplastic neuroepithelial tumor
- Cortical dysplasia
- Dysplastic cerebellar gangliocytoma (cerebellar cortex)

Intrinsically T1-hyperintense on MRI (lipid, protein, hemosiderin, melanin)
- Lipoma
- Melanoma or melanocytoma
- Craniopharyngioma
- Endodermal cyst
- Teratoma
- Xanthogranuloma
- Hematoma
- Vascular malformations, especially cavernous malformation
- Meningioma (uncommon)
- Cerebellar liponeurocytoma (rare)

Restricted diffusion on diffusion-weighted MRI
- Abscess
- Infarct
- Epidermoid cyst
- Metastasis with central necrosis
- Glioblastoma
- Acute demyelination
- Densely cellular neoplasms (e.g., embryonal tumors)

TABLE 20-8 Tumors Associated With Familial Tumor Predispositions, Approximate Frequency of Syndrome, Given Presence of Specified Tumor

Tumor	Syndrome: frequency
Optic pathway pilocytic astrocytoma	NF1: 60%, lower at ages <1 year
Malignant peripheral nerve sheath tumor	NF1: 50%
Vestibular schwannoma	
Unilateral, age <20 years	NF2: 20%
Unilateral, age >20 years	NF2: <1%
Bilateral	NF2: ~100%
Meningioangiomatosis	NF2: 20%
Subependymal giant cell astrocytoma	Tuberous sclerosis: ~100%
Atypical teratoid/rhabdoid tumor	Rhabdoid tumor syndrome: 20%–30%
Hemangioblastoma	
Cerebellar	von Hipple–Lindau: 20%–40%
Spinal/brainstem	von Hipple–Lindau: 60%–80%
Dysplastic cerebellar gangliocytoma (Lhermitte–Duclos disease)	Cowden syndrome: ~100%
Nodular-desmoplastic medulloblastoma (SHH molecular group)	Gorlin syndrome: unknown, thought to be high among patients <2 years old
Choroid plexus carcinoma	Li–Fraumeni syndrome: unknown

INDEX

Note: Page locators followed by f and t indicates figure and table respectively.

N

R